Contents

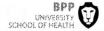

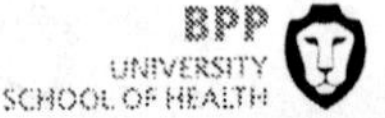

BPP
UNIVERSITY
SCHOOL OF HEALTH

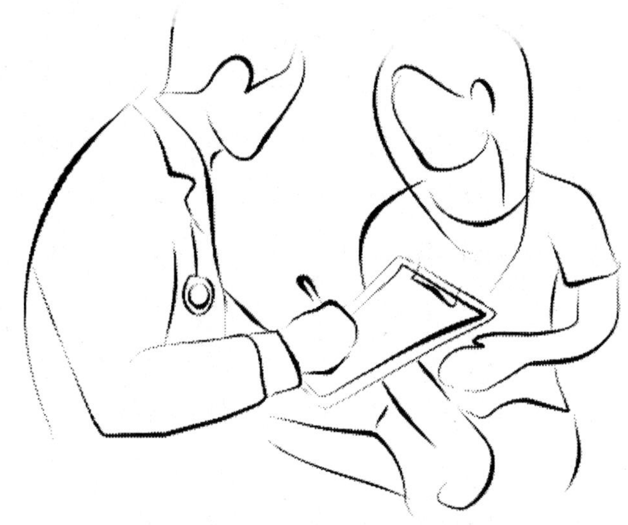

The Essential Clinical Handbook for the Foundation Programme

A comprehensive guide for Foundation doctors

Third Edition

Edited by
Emma Ladds and Rameen Shakur

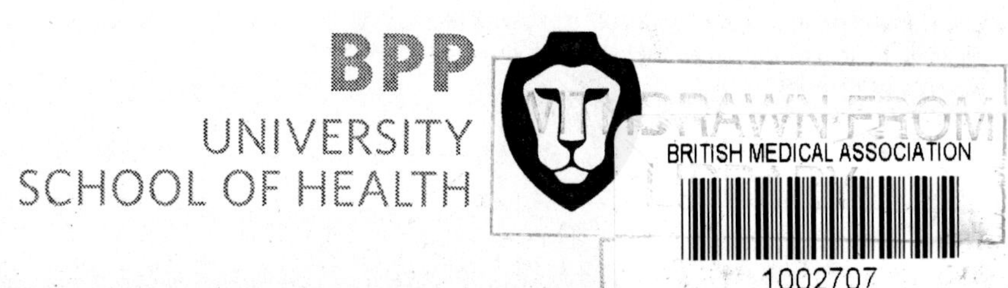

First edition November 2010
Third edition January 2017

ISBN 9781 5097 0235 0
Previous ISBN 9781 4453 8163 3
e-ISBN 9781 5097 0240 4
e-ISBN 9781 5097 0238 1

British Library Cataloguing-in-Publication Data
A catalogue record for this book is available from the British Library

Published by
BPP Learning Media Ltd
BPP House, Aldine Place
London W12 8AA

www.bpp.com/health

Printed in the United Kingdom by

RICOH UK Limited
Unit 2
Wells Place
Merstham
RH1 3LG

Your learning materials, published by BPP Learning Media Ltd, are printed on paper sourced from sustainable, managed forests.

The views expressed in this book are those of BPP Learning Media and not those of any medical schools, the NHS or NICE. BPP Learning Media are in no way associated with or endorsed by any medical schools, the NHS or NICE.

The contents of this book are intended as a guide and not professional advice. Although every effort has been made to ensure that the contents of this book are correct at the time of going to press, BPP Learning Media, the Editor and the Author make no warranty that the information in this book is accurate or complete and accept no liability for any loss or damage suffered by any tperson acting or refraining from acting as a result of the material in this book.

Every effort has been made to contact the copyright holders of any material reproduced within this publication. If any have been inadvertently overlooked, BPP Learning Media will be pleased to make the appropriate credits in any subsequent reprints or editions.

A note about copyright

Dear Customer

What does the little © mean and why does it matter?

Your market-leading BPP books, course materials and e-learning materials do not write and update themselves. People write them on their own behalf or as employees of an organisation that invests in this activity. Copyright law protects their livelihoods. It does so by creating rights over the use of the content.

Breach of copyright is a form of theft – as well as being a criminal offence in some jurisdictions, it is potentially a serious beach of professional ethics.

With current technology, things might seem a bit hazy but, basically, without the express permission of BPP Learning Media:

- Photocopying our materials is a breach of copyright
- Scanning, ripcasting or conversion of our digital materials into different file formats, uploading them to facebook or e-mailing them to your friends is a breach of copyright

You can, of course, sell your books, in the form in which you have bought them – once you have finished with them. (Is this fair to your fellow students? We update for a reason.) But the e-products are sold on a single user license basis: we do not supply 'unlock' codes to people who have bought them secondhand.

And what about outside the UK? BPP Learning Media strives to make our materials available at prices students can afford by local printing arrangements, pricing policies and partnerships which are clearly listed on our website. A tiny minority ignore this and indulge in criminal activity by illegally photocopying our material or supporting organisations that do. If they act illegally and unethically in one area, can you really trust them?

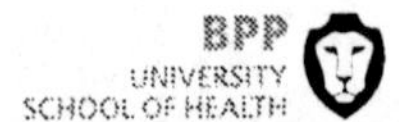

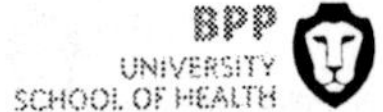
BPP
UNIVERSITY
SCHOOL OF HEALTH

About the Publisher

The UK's only university solely dedicated to business and the professions.

We are dedicated to preparing you for a professional career. We offer a strong commercial approach, within a business culture designed to help you stand out in the workplace after you graduate. Our programmes are designed in partnership with employers and respected professionals in the fields of law, business, finance and health.

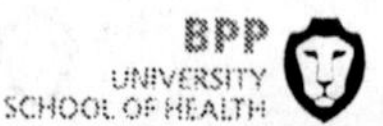

About the Contributors

Editor

Miss Emma Ladds is a GP trainee currently working in paediatrics at the Oxford University Hospitals NHS Foundation Trust. She completed her MA(Oxon) MBBCh at Somerville and Magdalen Colleges in Oxford and subsequently undertook her foundation placements in Bristol, which included a rotation in Academic Public Health. After a year as a plastic surgery core surgical trainee, she was offered an NIHR-funded academic clinical fellowship in General Practice and subsequently gained a place to study for a Master's in Public Health at Harvard University from 2017-2018. She enjoys the stories in medicine and the challenge of trying to answer research questions that are relevant for the problems of patients' daily lives. She also holds a lectureship at Magdalen College, Oxford, providing tutorials for undergraduates and clinical medical students and hopes to continue to combine academic research and teaching alongside her clinical work as a GP. She has a particular interest in interventions to improve health promotion and also enjoys escaping the hospital to cycle, sail or dig on her allotment.

Major contributors

Chapter 3

Dr Christian Brown graduated from the University of Oxford and is now a core psychiatry CT2 at the South West London and St George's Mental Health NHS Trust. He has a particular interest in forensic psychiatry and the application of philosophy to medicine.

Dr Aaron Dehghan graduated with a BSc (Hons) in Anatomical Sciences from The University of Manchester and subsequently graduated from Imperial College School of Medicine as a doctor. He is currently working as an academic Foundation Year doctor at Oxford University Hospitals.

Dr Stephanie Lawrie is currently an FY2 doctor working in the Thames Valley region. She completed medical school in Scotland and her FY1 jobs at Buckinghamshire healthcare NHS Trust. She plans to pursue a medical career path.

Chapter 4

Dr Natalie Redgrave graduated from the University of Oxford Medical School. She is currently an FY2 doctor in the Oxford Deanery, working in the department of General Surgery at Milton Keynes University Hospital.

Chapter 7

Dr Anna Francis is a CT2 in Brighton. She completed foundation training in Gloucester, following a slightly unconventional route into clinical medicine that included an MSc in Neurosciences after her third year and a spell of research in Cambridge. She has a particular interest in Neurology.

Chapter 8

Dr Oliver Manley trained at Manchester Medical School where he completed a Master's in Tissue Engineering for Regenerative Medicine. He completed the academic foundation programme in Oxford where he is currently a core surgical trainee.

Miss Emma Ladds contributed to all chapters

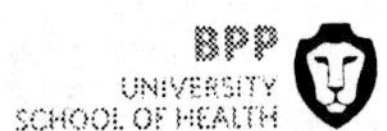

Contributors from previous edition

Editor

Dr Rameen Shakur

Major chapter section contributors

Dr Sandeep Panikker

Mrs Ruth Green

Dr Simon Green

Dr Prita Rughani

Mr Ravivarma Balasubramaniam

Dr Mandeep Kaler

Dr Vimal Raj

Dr Tabitha Turner-Stokes

Dr John Apps

Dr Abhishek Joshi

Dr Geraldine McElligott

Dr Rashmi Patel

Professor David Scott

Acknowledgements (figures)

Illustrations in previous and current edition provided by:

Dr John Apps
Dr Tabitha Turner-Stokes
Mr Ravivarma Balasubramaniam
Dr Mandeep Kaler
Dr Sandeep Panniker
Dr Rashmi Patel
Dr Vimal Raj
Mr Santron Sathasivam
Professor David Scott
Mr Christopher Yu

Thank you to the National Institute for Health and Clinical Excellence (NICE); The Resuscitation Council UK; The United Kingdom Foundation Programme Office; The British Thoracic Society; Professor PA Routledge at the Cardiff University Therapeutics and Toxicology Centre; and Andrew Goldberg and Gerard Stansby for kind permission to include illustrations from their publications, which are acknowledged in full where they appear.

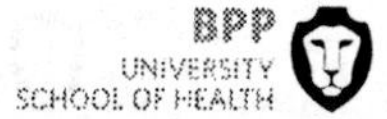

Abbreviations

5HIAA	5-hydroxyindoleacetic acid
5HT	5-hydroxytryptamine
A&E	Accident & Emergency
AAA	Abdominal aortic aneurysm
ABC	Airway, breathing, circulation
ABCDE	Airway, breathing, circulation, disability, exposure
ABG	Arterial blood gas
ABPI	Ankle brachial pressure index
ABX	Abdominal X-ray
AC	Adenocarcinoma
ACE	Angiotensin converting enzyme
ACS	Acute coronary syndrome
ACTH	Adrenocorticotrophic hormone
ADAM 33	ADAM metallopeptidase domain 33
ADH	Anti-diuretic hormone
ADLs	Activities of daily living
AEDs	Anti-epileptic drugs
AF	Atrial fibrillation
AFB	Acid fast bacillus
AFFIRM	Atrial fibrilation followup investigation of rhythm management
AFP	Serum a-feloprotein
AIDS	Acquired immunodeficiency syndrome
AL	Amyloid light chain
ALP	Alkaline phosphatase
ALS	Advanced Life Support
ALT	Alanine aminotransferase
AMA	Anti-mitochondrial antibodies
AMTS	Abbreviated mental test score
ANA	Antinuclear antibodies
ANCA	Antineutrophil cytoplasmic antibodies
Anti-LKM antibodies	Anti-liver/kidney/microsomal antibodies
Anti-SLA	Anti-soluble liver antigen
AP	Anterio-posterior
APTT	Activated partial thromboplastin time
APUD cells	Amine precursor uptake and decarboxylation cells
ARVC	Arrhythm ogenic right ventricular cardiomyopathy
ASIS	Anterior superior iliac spine
ASO	Anti-streptolysin-O
AST	Aspartate aminotransferase
A-V	Arterio-venous
AVNRT	Atrioventricular nodal re-entrant tachycardia
AVRT	Atrioventricular re-entrant tachycardia
AXR	Abdominal X-ray
BCC	Basal cell carcinoma
BCG	Bacille Calmette-Guérin
BD	*Bis die* (twice a day)
BE	Base excess
BIPAP	Biphasic positive airway pressure
BMI	Body mass index
BNF	British National Formulary
BNP	Brain-type natriuretic peptide
BOOP	Bronchiolitis obliterans organising pneumonia
BP	Blood pressure
BPAGl	Bullous pemphigoid antigens 1
BPH	Benign prostatic hyperplasia
Bpm	Beats per minute
BRCA	Breast cancer gene
BTS	British Thoracic Society
BXO	Balanitis xerotica obliterans
CA 19-9	Carbohydrate antigen 19-9
CABG	Coronary artery bypass graft
CAGE	Cutting, annoyed, guilty, eye-opener
CARD	Caspase Recruitment Domain
CbDs	Case-based Discussions
CBG	Capillary blood glucose
CCF	Congestive cardiac failure
CD	Crohn's disease
CEA	Carcinoembyronic antigen
Ch	French gauge
CHART	Continuous hyperfractionated accelerated radiotherapy
CHF	Congestive heart failure
CK	Creatinine kinase

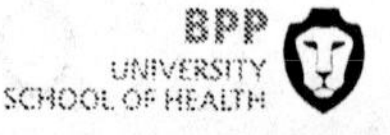

CK-MB	Creatinine kinase muscle/brain type
CLL	Chronic lymphocytic leukaemia
CLO	Campylobacter-like organism
CML	Chronic myeloid leukaemia
CMV	Cytomegalovirus
CNS	Central nervous system
COPD	Chronic obstructive pulmonary disease
COX	Cyclo-oxygenase
CPAP	Continuous positive airway pressure
CPPD	Calcium pyrophosphate dehydrate
CPR	Cardiopulmonary resuscitation
CRH	Corticotrophin releasing hormone
CRP	C-reactive protein
CSF	Cerebrospinal fluid
CT	Computer tomography
CTPA	Computer tomography pulmonary angiogram
CVP	Central venous pressure
Cx	Circumflex artery
CXR	Chest X-ray
DC	Direct Current cardioversion
DCIS	Ductal carcinoma *in situ*
DCM	Dilated cardiomyopathy
DEXA	Dual energy X-ray absorptiometry
DIC	Disseminated intravascular coagulation
DMARDs	Disease modifying anti-rheumatic drugs
DMSA	Dimercaptosuccinic acid
DNA	Deoxyribonucleic acid
DNAR	Decision not to attempt resuscitation
DOB	Date of birth
DOPS	Direct observation of procedural skills
DOT	Directly observed therapy
DSH	Deliberate self-harm
DTs	Delirium tremens
DVLA	Driver and Vehicle Licensing Agency
DVT	Deep vein thrombosis
EADs	Early after depolarisations
EAU	Emergency Assessment Unit
EBV	Epstein-Barr virus
ECG	Electrocardiogram
ED	Emergency Department
EEG	Electroencephalography
EF	Ejection fraction
ELISA	Enzyme-linked immunosorbent assay
EMF	Endomyocardial fibrosis
ENT	Ears, Nose, and Throat
ERCP	Endoscopic retrograde cholangio-pancreatography
ERDS	End-stage renal failure
ESR	Erythrocyte sedimentation rate
ESWL	Extracorporeal shock wave lithotripsy
ET	Endotracheal
EVAR	Endovascular aneurysm repair
EVLA	Endovenous laser ablation
FAP	Familial adenomatous polyposis
FBC	Full blood count
FER	Forced expiratory ratio
FEV1	Forced expiratory volume in one second
FFP	Fresh frozen plasma
FNA	Fine needle aspiration
FVC	Forced vital capacity
FY	Foundation Year
G6PD	Glucose-6-phosphate dehydrogenase
GABA	Gamma-aminobutyric acid
GALS	Gait, arms, legs, and spine
GCS	Glasgow coma scale
GGT	Gamma-glutamyl transferase
GHB	Gamma-hydroxybutyrate
GI	Gastrointestinal
GMC	General Medical Council
GOR	Gastro-oesophageal reflux
GORD	Gastro-oesophageal reflux disease
GP	General practitioner
GTN	Glyceryl trinitrate
GUM	Genitourinary medicine
HAV	Hepatitis A virus
Hb	Haemoglobin
HBcAg	Core antigen
HBeAg	Pre-core antigen
HBsAg	Surface antigen

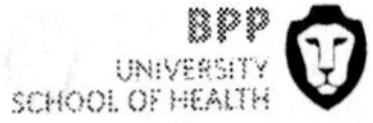

HBV	Hepatitis B virus
HCG	Human chorionic gonadotropin
HCM	Hypertrophic cardiomyopathy
HCV	Hepatitis C virus
HDU	High dependency unit
HDV	Hepatitis D virus
HER2	Human epidermal growth factor receptor 2
HIV	Human immunodeficiency virus
HLA	Human leukocyte antigen
HNPCC	Hereditary non-polyposis colon cancer
HO	House Officer
HPV	Human papilloma virus
HRT	Hormone replacement therapy
HSV	Herpes simplex virus
IBD	Inflammatory bowel disease
IBS	Irritable bowel syndrome
ICP	Intracranial pressure
ICU	Intensive care unit
Ig	Immunoglobulin
IHD	Ischaemic heart disease
ILS	Immediate life support
IM	Intramuscular
INR	International normalised ratio
ISDN	Isosorbide dinitrate
IUCD	Intrauterine coil device
IV	Intravenous
IVP	Intravenous pyelogram
IVU	Intravenous urogram
JVP	Jugular venous pressure
KUB	Kidneys-ureters-bladder
LA	Local anaesthetic
LAD	Left anterior descending artery
LBBB	Left bundle branch block
LCIS	Lobular carcinoma in situ
LDH	Lactate dehydrogenase
LFTs	Liver function tests
LHRH	Luteinising-hormone releasing hormone
LMWH	Low molecular weight heparin
LOS	Lower oesophageal sphincter
LP	Lumbar puncture
LQTS	Long QT syndrome
LSD	Lysergic acid diethylamide
LV	Left ventricle
LVP	Large-volume paracentesis
MAO	Monoamine oxidase
MC+S	Microscopy, culture and sensitivity
MCP	Metacarpophalangeal
MCV	Mean cell volume
MDCT	Multi-detector computer tomography
MDMA	3,4-methylenedioxymetham-phetamine ectasy
MDRTB	Multi-drug resistant TB
MDT	Multidisciplinary team
MEN	Multiple endocrine neoplasia
MEWS	Modified early warning score
MHC	Major histocompatibility complex
MI	Myocardial infarction
Mini-CEX	Mini clinical evaluation exercise
Mini-PAT	Mini peer assessment tool
MMSE	Mini mental state examination
MRCP	Magnetic resonance cholangiopancreatography
MRI	Magnetic resonance imaging
IvIRSA	Methicillin-resistant *Staphylococclis aureus*
MS	Multiple sclerosis
MST	Morphine sulphate tablets
MSU	Mid-stream urine
NAC	N-acetylcysteine
NAFLD	Non-alcoholic fatty liver disease
NAPQI	N-acetyl-p-benzoquinoneimine
NBM	Nil by mouth
Nd:YAO	Neodymium-doped yttrium aluminium garnet
NO	Nasogastric
NHS	National Health Service
NICE	National Institute for Health and Clinical Excellence
NTV	Non-invasive ventilation
NOD	Nucleotide-binding oligomerization domain
NSAID	Non-steroidal anti-inflammatory drug
NSCLC	Non-small-cell lung cancer
NSOCT	Non-seminomatous germ cell tumours
NSTEMI	Non-ST elevation myocardial infarction
NYHA	New York Heart Association
OCP	Oral contraceptive pill
OD	*Omin die* (once daily)

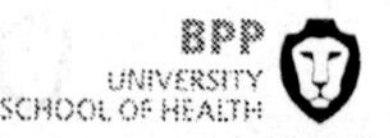

OGD	Oesophagogastroduodenoscopy
OGTT	Oral glucose tolerance test
OSCE	Objective structured clinical examination
OTC	Over the counter
PA	Postero-anterior
PALS	Patient Advice and Liaison Services
PBC	Primary biliary cirrhosis
PCR	Percutaneous coronary intervention
PCNL	Percutaneous nephrolithotomy
PCP	*Pneumocystitis carinii*
PCR	Polymerase chain reaction
PE	Pulmonary embolism
PEA	Pulseless electrical activity
PEF	Peak expiratory flow
PEFR	Peak expiratory flow rale
PET	Positron emission tomography
PIP	Proximal inter-phalangeal
pND	Paroxysmal nocturnal dyspnoea
pNS	Peripheral nervous system
PO	Per oral
PPI	Proton pump inhibitor
PR	Per rectum
lORN	Pro re nata (as needed)
PSA	Prostate specific antigen
PI'	Prothrombin time
PTFE	Polytetrafluroethylene
PTH	Parathyroid hormone
PUO	Pyrexia of unknown origin
PUVA	Psoralens and ultraviolet A phototherapy
RA	Rheumatoid arthritis
RBBB	Right bundle branch block
RBC	Red blood cell
RCA	Right coronary artery
RCM	Restrictive cardiomyopathy
RCR	Royal College of Radiologists
RTF	Right iliac fossa
RNA	Ribonucleic acid
ROSC	Return of spontaneous circulation
RTA	Road traffic accident
SA	Sino-atrial node
SAAG	Serum-ascitic albumin gradient
SAH	Subarachnoid haemorrhage
SANAD	Study of Standard and New Anti-Epileptic Drugs
SCC	Squamous cell carcinoma
SCLC	Small-cell lung cancer
SDH	Subdural haemorrhage
SHO	Senior House Officer
SIADH	Syndrome of inappropriate antidiuretic hormone secretion
SIRS	Systemic inflammatory response syndrome
SLE	Systemic lupus erythematosus
SMA	Smooth muscle antibodies
SMR	Standard mortality ratio
SOB	Shortness of breath
SOL	Space occupying lesion
SpR	Specialist Registrar
SSRI	Selective serotonin re-uptake inhibitors
ST	Specialist Trainee
STEMI	ST elevation myocardial infarction
SUDEP	Sudden unexplained death in epilepsy
SVT	Supra-ventricular tachycardia
SXR	Skull X-ray
TB	Tuberculosis
TCA	Tricyclic antidepressants
TDS	Ter die sumendus (three times a day)
TENS	Transcutaneous electrical nerve stimulator
TFT	Thyroid function tests
TGF	Tumour growth factor
TIA	Transient ischaemic attack
TIPSS	Transjugular intrahepatic portasystemic stent shunt
TNF	Tumor necrosis factors
TNM	Tumour-node-metastasis
TOE	Trransoesophageal echocardiography
TP	Trombocytopenic purpura
TPA	Tissue plasminogen activator
TPN	Total parenteral nutrition
TRUS	Transrectal ultrasound scan
TSH	Thyroid stimulating hormone
tTGA	Tissue transglutaminase
TUR	Transurethral resection
TURBT	Transurethral resection of bladder tumour

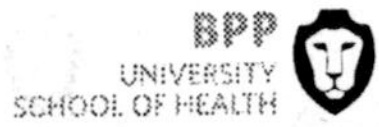

TURP	Transurethral resection of the prostate
TWOC	Trial without catheter
U&Es	Urea and electrolytes
UA	Unstable angina
UC	Ulcerative colitis
UMN	Upper motor neuron
URTI	Upper respiratory tract infcction
USS	Ultrasound scan
UTI	Urinary tract infection
V IQ scan	Ventilation perfusion
VF	Ventricular fibrillation
VT	Ventricular tachycardia
VZV	Varicella zoster virus
WBC	White blood cell
WCC	White cell count
WE	Wernicke's encephalopathy
WHO	World Health Organization
WLE	Wide local excision
WPW	Wolff-Parkinson-White
XDRTB	Extremely drug resistant TB

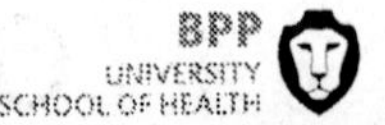

Foreword by Professor Lord Ara Darzi

The introduction of the Foundation Programme has been fundamental in helping bridge the gap for Foundation Year doctors, ensuring that high quality continuous education is provided with a rigorous curriculum.

This is a practical handbook of the Foundation Programme curriculum in medicine and surgery, incorporating current assessment tools used for postgraduate medical education as its basis, such as Direct Observation of Procedural Skills and Case-based Discussions. It provides Foundation Doctors with a valuable and practical clinical insight into their FY1 and FY2 years. It is clearly designed and laid out to aid the busy Foundation Year doctor and will enable them to successfully complete their e-portfolio to a high standard in order to achieve the best attainable scores. Key chapters include: Case Based Discussions of both core surgical and medical cases, supplemented by up-to-date guidelines from NICE; comprehensive illustrated step-by-step instructions on how to competently and safely carry out the major procedures one may experience during the Foundation training; and the Mini-Clinical Evaluation Exercise, which highlights the necessary clinical examination skills required for successful attainment of high scores in the assessments.

I have no doubt that this book will provide a valuable reference guide for medical students and junior doctors to completion of their Foundation training and their chosen postgraduate medical or surgical careers.

Professor Lord Ara Darzi

Foreword by Sir Graeme Catto

Who knows what will be expected of doctors forty years from now? The science will have changed; society's expectations will have changed – but people will not have changed. They will trust us when most burdened by ill health and worries. That need for trust and humanity in medicine is unchanging but it is conditional. It depends on our professionalism – our competence and our unfailing willingness to put the interests of our patients first.

The Foundation Programme is critically important in promoting both aspects of our professionalism. Not only does it allow the postgraduate student to integrate the knowledge, skills and behaviours acquired during the undergraduate years and provide the good quality clinical care patients expect, but it ensures a breadth of experience across a range of specialties. The well documented problems of the last few years have produced some significant benefits. Firstly they have emphasised the importance of postgraduate education in creating the well-informed, flexible medical workforce any health service will require in the years ahead. Secondly we now have a credible and creditable curriculum for the Foundation Programme in the UK.

This Handbook is not only *essential* but unique. It is the only text that covers the whole Foundation Programme curriculum, incorporating medical and surgical topics in a way that is practical and immediately relevant for the busy postgraduate student. The chapters on practical procedures and mini clinical evaluations provide detailed information and are particularly useful for doctors in training. Whatever specialty you choose to pursue, this Handbook provides the necessary basic information. Aimed at postgraduate students during the Foundation years, this text cannot but improve patient care and patient safety. Perhaps as importantly, it is an enjoyable read – for all postgraduate medical students whatever their age and stage.

Sir Graeme Catto

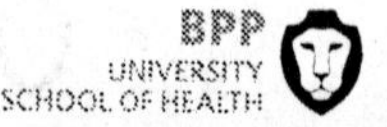

Foreword by Professor Iona Heath

Courage and Joy

As you embark on your career as a qualified doctor, I wish you both courage and joy. I want to make ten points about courage and five about joy. And, of course they are closely related and you will need the courage to realise the joy.

Courage

I wish you the courage:

1. to come close enough to each patient not only to look but to see, not only to listen but to hear. John Berger wrote almost fifty years ago in his book *A Fortunate Man*, which is an extraordinary portrait of a GP working in the Forest of Dean: '*He does not believe in maintaining his imaginative distance: he must come close enough to recognise the patient fully.*'
2. to look beyond the attenuated truth of scientific medicine and not to seek its familiar shelter too soon. Remember that doctoring is not a science but the sensitive *application* of science to the lives of unique individuals. Doctors need to be able to see and hear each successive patient in the fullness of their humanity, to minimise fear, to locate hope (however limited), to explain symptoms and diagnoses in language that make sense to each different patient, to witness courage and endurance and to accompany suffering. There is no biomedical science that I know of that helps with any of this and so you will find that while a knowledge and understanding of science is essential it is not sufficient.
3. to trust the patient's account of their experience of illness and to pay real attention to the parts of their story that do not fit with your initial diagnostic understanding.
4. to tolerate the inevitable uncertainty of applying the generalised truths of biomedical science to particular patients; to take time whenever possible; to use time as a diagnostic and a therapeutic tool and to know that you cannot get it right all the time.
5. to hold the frontier between illness and disease and to resist medicalisation. Per Fugelli, the Emeritus Professor of Social Medicine in Oslo writes: '*Modern technological medicine converts more and more of biological variation, natural stress, and the natural troubles of life into diagnoses with demands for specialized investigation and therapy. The result is a malignant combination of learned helplessness and perfectionist expectations among patients.*' You will need courage to resist this accelerating process.
6. to help patients to make their own decisions which accommodate their own values.
7. to be a partisan and an advocate. All doctors have a wider social and political responsibility to speak out on behalf of the most needy and the least heard: to speak truth to power.
8. never to assume; always to ask.
9. to be honest, not to flinch and to remain present in the face of suffering, loss and dying.
10. to know when to stop struggling to preserve life in the face of your own fears and needs, and to help the patient and their family to make it easier for each other to accept the inevitability of death.

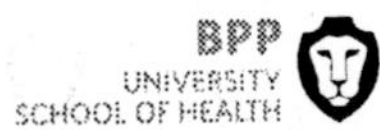

Joy

And I wish you joy in:

1. the whole of humanity. Your work will bring you into privileged contact with a quite extraordinary range of different people, life stories and contexts.
2. sharing stories. The great biographer Richard Holmes reminds us that: '*Once known in any detail and any scope, every life is something extraordinary…often containing unimagined degrees of suffering or heroism, and invariably touching extreme moments of triumph and despair, though frequently unexpressed.*'
3. the intensity and breadth of your work. John Berger writes: '*Happiness occurs when people can give the whole of themselves to the moment being lived.*'
4. making a difference through science, skill, witnessing, and advocacy.
5. the amazing opportunities that medicine gives you to find colleagues and to make friends around the world.

So I wish you luck and joy and courage in equal measure!

Professor Iona Heath

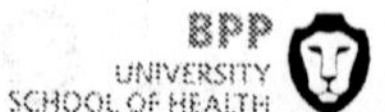

Acknowledgements

Kindness is the language which the deaf can hear and the blind can see.

Mark Twain

When somebody asks you to start a project, and promises it won't be much work, never believe them! Editing the latest edition of this book has been quite an undertaking and I am indebted to many people for their support and advice. First of all, I would like to thank Dr Helen Ashdown, who suggested I take it on, and the contributors and editors to the previous edition who worked so hard to put the original book together.

I am very grateful to my colleagues who have contributed to this edition, both in terms of chapter contributions, personal case studies and useful tips for newly qualified doctors. Your help has been hugely appreciated. Professor Iona Heath's foreword is both thought-provoking and inspiring and, in a time when medicine is suffering from depressed morale and great difficulties recruiting and retaining staff, such words are deeply encouraging – thank you.

Finally, I would like to thank the patients I have already seen in my career and the stories and emotions they have shared. Although there are days when going to work is the last thing you want to do, working in medicine has already been a huge privilege, and for all its challenges, I cannot think of anything else I would rather do.

Miss Emma Ladds

Dedication

To all those I love, and who love me. You are my world.

How to use this book

Every effort has been made to ensure the accuracy of the material contained within this guide. However it must be noted that medical treatments, drug dosages/formulations, equipment, procedures and best practice are currently evolving within the field of medicine.

Readers are therefore advised always to check the most up-to-date information relating to:

- The applicable drug manufacturer's product information and data sheets relating to recommended dose/formulation, administration and contraindications.
- The latest applicable local and national guidelines.
- The latest applicable local and national codes of conduct and safety protocols.

It is the responsibility of the practitioner, based on their own knowledge and expertise, to diagnose, treat and ensure the safety and best interests of the patient are maintained.

This book, written by doctors, is intended for Foundation Year doctors, medical students and educational and clinical supervisors. The book has been designed to cover the Foundation Programme curriculum. The top 20 symptoms/presentations mentioned in the curriculum are covered in the medical and surgical chapters of this book. A differential diagnosis table for each symptom/presentation exists at the beginning of each subchapter. **The differentials in bold are covered in the subchapter. Please note that the differentials not in bold may be covered in other subchapters of the book and thus you may need to refer to the Index.** The 'Top Tips' boxes are comprised of clinical and practical hints from current junior doctors, including the key pieces of information they wish they had known when starting their foundation years.

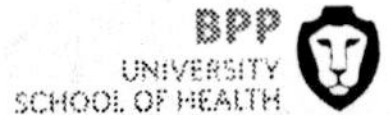

Chapter 1

So you have finally made it: Doctor

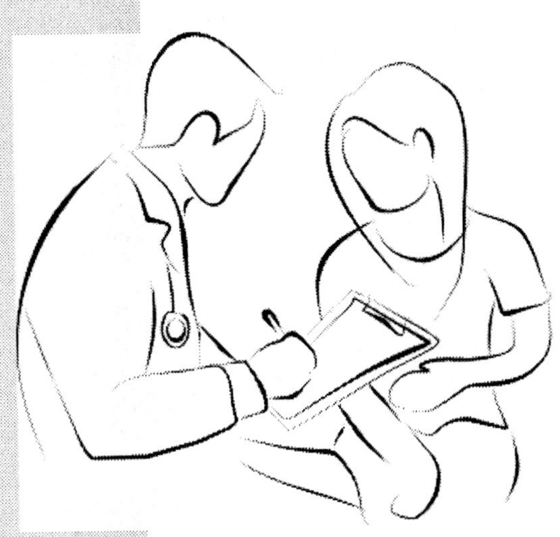

So you have finally made it: Doctor

Doctors are men who prescribe medicines of which they know little, to cure diseases of which they know less, in human beings of whom they know nothing.
François-Marie Arouet ('Voltaire' 1694–1778)

Despite William Harvey's discovery of the circulatory system, van Leeuwenhoek's identification of micro-organisms and Jenner's development of vaccines, medicine and surgery in the 1700s remained crude, brutal and mostly ineffective. Chance played as great a role in patient recovery as any medical skill and Voltaire's satirical quip about doctors was well justified. Many might argue that little has changed. Although great advances have been and continue to be made, it is tempting as doctors to imagine we know all the answers to the problems of the human body. The truth is that we do not.

Our patients are not just bodies. They are people, full of hopes and dreams, worries and fears, plans for the future and memories of the past. The art of medicine lies in acknowledging this individuality and learning how to develop and apply our knowledge meaningfully so that the the logical scientist combines with the humanitarian. The best teachers along this path are the people we meet as patients. If we listen carefully, we can at least become doctors who *'prescribe medicines in human beings of which we know a little'*.

The doctor

The medical profession is currently going through a period of change and adjustment. Many clinical roles are evolving from those of specialised generalists to highly specialised individuals within

Case Study: A patient, friend and meaningful moments...

I had last seen Mrs A as the porters wheeled her to theatre on the morning of her operation. We met the evening before, when she was admitted. Her CT scan revealed a large tumour and brought a continuous stream of neurosurgeons to her room that evening. They held long discussions with Mrs A, which she neither understood nor remembered, and left her none-the-wiser about their plans.

We sat that evening, after the torrent of surgeons had diminished, and watched as a beautiful rainbow emerged from the gloomy day. We talked through what the neurosurgeons were planning – as far as I understood, anyway! Although overwhelmed, Mrs A was also positive. 'But I've had such a good life,' she kept repeating, such a good life and she recounted slurred tales of her days in Malaysia and Singapore. As she was wheeled away, waving, on the trolley the next morning, it was impossible not to admire her spirit, and optimism. I did not think I would ever see her again and felt a pang of sadness for someone who had passed so fleetingly through my life.

Eighteen months later I was sitting in a GP consulting room, looking through the list of requested home visits. To my great surprise, I saw Mrs A listed on the screen. It must be her: palliative, hemiplegic, requesting a review of her steroids. I drove over to see her and to my great surprise she did remember me. Over the next couple of months I watched her decline. Gradually her speech became more and more incomprehensible and eventually she never left her hospital bed. It was frequently surrounded by varying combinations of relatives and carers, palliative nurses and old friends and gradually she grew weaker and weaker.

I expected her to die before I left the practice, but to my surprise she hung on and eventually I was the one who had to say goodbye. I went one lunchtime after morning surgery, a couple of days before I was moving to my next rotation. I think she understood I was leaving, but her reply was incomprehensible. However, the tears that trickled down her steroid-swollen cheeks were unmistakable. I too felt a dampness at the corner of my eyes – and then the niece began to cry and then the carer, and then we all burst out laughing.

I won't ever forget Mrs A. She died about six months after I left the GP practice – a peaceful death, I'm told. I had done little for her as a doctor but I felt she had taught me much about how to help a patient as a person. I had shared her fears before surgery and eventually her final decline, but also witnessed her enjoyment of life and the people she cared about. We had been through something together, and perhaps that is what being a doctor should be about.

a wider healthcare team. Ever-increasing technical developments, more complicated treatment pathways and rising patient demands are resulting in a complex world of healthcare, presenting diverse challenges for individual practitioners.

However, the study and practice of medicine is still one of the most interesting and rewarding professions. The pleasure felt at making a correct diagnosis or seeing the relief and gratitude of patients and families, combined with the guilt and remorse that arise when more could have been done, generate a rollercoaster of highs and lows not experienced in many other walks of life. The grip of a fearful hand evokes many powerful emotions. It is a great privilege to be part of such a world and this should not be forgotten in the stress of the many daily challenges.

The team

From the moment you start out as a foundation doctor, throughout your years as a trainee and beyond, it is important to recognise that you are part of a wider team, who share success and failure together. This may not always be easy, but working with a diverse range of highly skilled, talented and generally caring individuals will offer many opportunities for professional and personal development and should be embraced. Creating a friendly and supportive work environment is crucial for both effective clinical care and the happiness of individual team members and should not be underestimated.

You

Medics have always had a 'work-hard, play-hard' reputation. At every level medicine can be physically and emotionally demanding and it's vital to find some way of balancing these stresses in order to keep going. Despite the introduction of the European Working Time Directive, most doctors still work long, antisocial hours, often having to travel great distances from family or friends, which can lead to periods of isolation and loneliness. A profession that prides itself on caring for others all too often doesn't pay enough attention to looking after its own members. We need to remember to try and care for ourselves and colleagues as well as our patients – sometimes easier said than done.

Congratulations on making it to this point. Graduating as a doctor is a huge achievement that well deserves recognition and celebration. It is also a great responsibility. Welcome to our profession. We do hope you enjoy your work in medicine, whichever path you choose to take, and wish you the best of luck for your future progress.

This book

This book is designed to provide a clinical reference for some of the commonly encountered clinical and surgical problems during the foundation years. It is not comprehensive, nor is it a replacement for clinical experience or senior advice when you feel out of your depth. It also includes some guidance on how best to complete the training requirements of the early years as a junior doctor and some inspiration for the many possible career routes or alternatives following completion of the Foundation Programme.

We hope to provide some practical tips and advice for surviving and succeeding as a doctor and have included some of the stories and lessons we have learned from patients along the way.

Always laugh when you can. It is cheap medicine
Lord Byron (1788–1894)

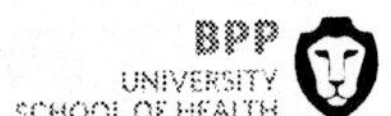

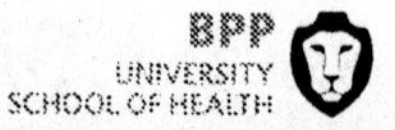

Chapter 2

An introduction to the Foundation Programme

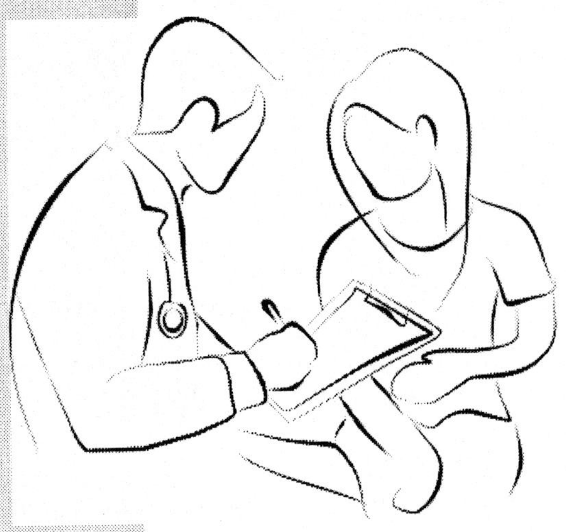

Chapter 2

An introduction to the Foundation Programme

Introduction

The life so short, the craft so long to learn
Hippocrates

The first years of practice as a doctor have always been challenging. Not only do you have to learn how to apply theoretical knowledge quickly, often in unfamiliar settings and with unfamiliar patients and medical teams, but you also have to contend with the practical demands of the job, which can seem far more daunting. Printing the patient list seems a simple task until none of the printers work and the ward clerk has not arrived, the consultant is waiting and your bleep has just gone off twice...

You will quickly pick up these skills and learn how to usefully apply your knowledge. In order to satisfy the requirements of the Foundation Programme you also need to prove that you have done so. Feedback from team members, procedural skills, practical assessments and CBDs all need to be recorded on an online e-portfolio. Being well prepared and organised, both with work and these training assessments, will make life much easier and earn you the trust of your seniors. They will then be more keen to teach, allow you greater clinical independence and offer more constructive feedback.

Despite their challenges, the Foundation years should also be enjoyable. If they are not, something is wrong and you need to tell someone. Beyond your immediate clinical team, each year you will have an assigned Educational Supervisor and a different Clinical Supervisor for each placement. They are the people to talk to if you are experiencing problems. There will also be a number of contacts within your local postgraduate department and training deanery, who should also be able to help. Never be afraid to ask for help or support at any point.

This chapter will cover some general and practical advice to try and help make the next two years enjoyable and successful.

Before you start

Shadowing

Many medical schools organise shadowing periods for medical students in their final years so they can discover what the job of a foundation doctor entails. Most hospitals also arrange a similar week for the new FY1 intake before the August handover. These can be really valuable experiences and will help give you knowledge and confidence for your first rotation. Make sure you ask the current FY1 for their top tips on doing the job effectively, especially how they manage the patient lists and handovers or any particular challenges they have found and how they have dealt with them.

Your hospital

Probably one of the greatest challenges you will face as a foundation doctor is making sure you have found all your patients. You will quickly get a rough idea of the layout of the hospital, but make sure you find the wards where you tend to have patients as soon as possible and get used to the set-up and teams there. Other useful places to be able to find will include the radiology department, your consultant's office (and perhaps more importantly his secretary's), theatres, if you have a surgical job, the postgraduate centre and above all, the doctor's mess and the nearest coffee shop.

Your job

Whether you start in a very specialist tertiary referral unit or an acute general medical ward in a District General Hospital (DGH), your job as an FY1 will be broadly similar. You will be required to know which patients are under your team's care and keep a record of them, help with the ward round and simple ward jobs, prepare discharge summaries and look after any acutely unwell patients, calling for senior back-up when needed. You will also probably be included

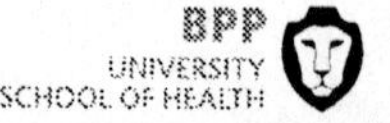

in an on-call rota to cover any urgent jobs and clerk new patients. The exact requirements of on-call roles tend to vary considerably, but you will always have senior back-up to help you.

It is helpful to learn early about your patient throughput ie where/how do patients arrive, stay and leave your care and what is your specific input at each of these different stages. The senior nurse on the ward, ward manager or ward clerk can help with this and you will soon pick it up. It is also useful to know where different members of your team will be on different days – your consultant's secretary is a good person to ask if you are ever unsure.

Your team

There will be different members of the team depending on the job. Don't worry if you can't immediately remember everybody's name – that will quickly come and bleep numbers may be more important. It's useful to make a note of these on your phone on day 1 or write them at the top of your patient list, so you always have someone you can call for advice or help.

The team members will normally include:

The consultant

The most senior, fully trained doctor who holds ultimate responsibility for the care of their patients and therefore your actions. They are responsible for organising your induction to the team when you arrive and overseeing your training during your placement. They will also probably be your Clinical Supervisor for the duration of that post.

Different consultants have different likes and dislikes and you will quickly work this out! It is worth asking the outgoing FY1/2 if they have any specific tips for keeping the boss happy, and the registrar is always a good person to ask if you have any queries about this.

One of the worst mistakes you can make is to be frightened of your consultant and fail to ask them questions. The majority are very approachable and it is better to ask if you are ever in doubt – most doctors would rather head off any problems early with their patients, rather than have to deal with them later. They are also people who generally like meeting trainees and getting to know you.

It is also vital to have a good relationship with your consultant's secretary, who will often be a gold mine of useful information and can help you get forms signed etc.

Specialist Trainee (ST) doctors

These are junior doctors beyond FY2, and are in a training scheme to become a consultant in a particular speciality. They are referred to by the number of years' training they have had – ST1 onwards. They will be involved in outpatient clinics, theatre or procedure lists, working on the wards and doing on-calls. They tend to make most of the day-to-day management decisions and lead the ward rounds. When things get frightening, they are the people to call.

ST1 and ST2 doctors will often be on the ward and may have a similar job to you. They are particularly useful people to help complete assessments. Along with FY2 doctors they make up the old 'Senior House Officer' grade.

The House Officer (FY1 doctor)

The most junior, but very important, member of the team, who is crucial to help the daily ward round and general ward work smoothly.

The wider team

Nurses

Nurses are without doubt some of the most important people to you and can make the difference between things going smoothly and completely falling apart. You need to have them on your side.

Find out who is in charge of the ward (Senior Sister/Charge Nurse) and make a special effort to introduce yourself. This person will be incredibly useful to you both practically and educationally. They can solve problems that you might be having trouble with. Remember: you work on their ward, and they will know the systems and the other staff better than you do.

Ensure you know who the other nurses and healthcare assistants are, and what skills they have. This may take some time, but it means you can ask the right favour from the right person. Knowing the people you work with on a day-to-day basis will also make for a much easier start to your job.

You may also work with a number of specialist nurses, who are highly trained in a single field. They are often very experienced and knowledgeable and can be a great resource, as well as providing practical help if you need it.

Pharmacists

The ward pharmacist will be able to give any advice you need about prescribing medications, or which drugs are on the hospital formulary. They help ensure that no medication errors arise by checking the drug charts and also are responsible for getting drugs up to the ward – they can be particularly useful if you need something urgently or to try and facilitate a prompt discharge.

Physiotherapists (PTs)

PTs use physical therapies such as breathing exercises, muscular training and motivational strategies to improve your patient's stability, strength, stamina and confidence. They often use frames and walking aids to get patients moving, especially after operations. They work in rehabilitation, and are an essential part of your discharge planning, but will also help in acute illnesses such as pneumonia or other respiratory conditions.

Occupational therapists (OTs)

If your patient has any persisting difficulties after they have been treated for their illness, the OT will try and help them to find solutions. These will often include modifications to a patient's home environment that aim to maximise independence. Again they are an essential part of your discharge team and should be involved in patient care from an early stage.

Social workers

If your patient needs support when leaving hospital, the social worker will help to co-ordinate and find funding for it. They are invaluable when aiming to discharge elderly patients, who may need carers at home or funding for nursing home placements. Along with the ward discharge co-ordinator, they are essential to help maximise patient throughput – which sadly is becoming increasingly pressurised and challenging for many teams.

Case Study: The sadness of a delayed discharge

Mr and Mrs Jones had lived in a little village in South Wales all of their married life. For their ruby wedding anniversary, they decided to go on holiday to France. Unfortunately, on the way home, Mrs Jones tripped over a curb and sustained an open tibia/fibula ankle fracture. She was taken to the nearest trauma centre, where they fixed the fracture and covered the defect with a free gracilis flap.

The team referred Mrs Jones to the local hospital in South Wales so that she could continue her rehabilitation closer to home. They were happy to accept her but there was no bed. Mr and Mrs Jones had never been apart before and he completed a 6-hour round journey to visit his wife every other day throughout her stay. Occasionally his son drove him, but most of the time the 76-year-old came on his own.

Initially Mrs Jones recovered well and she eagerly anticipated going home. However, over time complications developed. Much of the skin graft over the flap failed and further reconstructive procedures had to be performed, necessitating a longer stay in hospital. Mrs Jones sank into a deep depression and became unwell, suffering a chest and then urinary infection, which necessitated a stay on the High Dependency Unit. Mr Jones was distraught. Gradually she improved, the Welsh hospital found a bed and Mr and Mrs Jones were delightedly reunited.

Although Mrs Jones suffered a nasty injury and a series of medical complications, it is difficult not to speculate about how different her story might have been, had she been closer to home, without the stress of separation from friends and family.

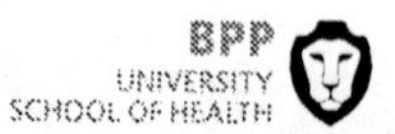

How to be a good Foundation Year doctor

You have three things to achieve as an FY doctor.

1. To learn and develop
2. To prove you have learned and developed
3. To ensure the smooth running of your clinical team and take good care of your patients

If you concentrate on the last point the others will follow. Try and be organised, friendly and approachable, know your limits and when to ask for help and you will be safe and an enjoyable member of the team.

The ward round

The ward round usually happens in the morning and sets the tone for your day. The aim is for a review of all the patients under your team's care in order to move their management forwards. Your job as an FY doctor is to ensure the ward round moves smoothly, that decisions and plans are documented, and that the jobs that are generated are done quickly and effectively.

There are various different ward rounds:

Consultant ward rounds

The consultant sees all their patients and makes decisions about their progress. They will often only have a limited amount of time, so you should be well prepared with notes, investigation results etc.

Post-take ward rounds

All new admissions are seen by the consultant. If you have clerked the patient you will be required to present them to the team, which can be nerve-wracking, but again just try and be organised and practice will help. Your most important job is to make sure all the patients are added to the list.

Business round

The most senior doctor, usually a Registrar, leads a ward round to ensure that the management of patients is progressing. These are often a bit more laid-back and may be a better time to ask any non-urgent questions you have regarding the patients.

During the ward round you will need to guide the team from patient to patient, finding the notes en route. It is often helpful if there's more than one of you to do this. You will also need the observation and drug charts by the time you arrive at the bedside.

It can be helpful for the team if you give a brief presentation of each patient and any recent changes. As the team discuss the case, you need to note and record the observations, the consultation that takes place and the plan that is reached.

There may be a ward round proforma, but if not, it is important to note down:

- Date, time and the person leading the round
- Diagnosis +/- procedure or any current issues
- How the patient is feeling that morning – any new complaints
- Observations
- Any examination findings
- The impression and plan

If you are unsure at any point or miss something, ask. Everybody understands that ward rounds are busy, especially for FY1 and 2 doctors, and it is much better for patient and team to take a few moments now than implement the wrong management plan.

Top tips for the ward round

- ☑ A well-organised list
- ☑ The exact location of all your patients
- ☑ Blank request forms
- ☑ Continuation sheets for the notes
- ☑ The latest investigation results
- ☑ Easy access to the medical notes
- ☑ Easy access to the observation charts
- ☑ Easy access to the drug chart
- ☑ A nurse, to tell you of any recent changes and to inform of management plans
- ☑ Two or three pens – you will definitely lose one!

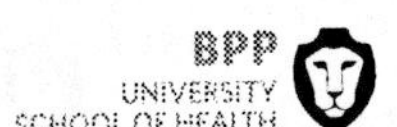

The list

Every patient list varies, but it is essential that it includes the following information:

- Patient's name
- Date of birth
- Hospital number
- Location in the hospital
- Presenting complaint and diagnosis
- Jobs that they need doing

Make enough copies of the list for all the members of your team, and circulate these at the beginning of the ward round. Keeping a good list is probably the most important thing an FY doctor can do. If you can't find a patient, you can't look after them.

Jobs

During the ward round, more difficult jobs may be taken up by the consultant or more senior trainees. After the ward wound it is a good idea if all remaining junior doctors sit down and make sure you have written down all the jobs. Prioritise and divide them between you – it may be more appropriate for FY1 doctors to do the bloods and discharge summaries etc and the FY2s to make referrals.

Getting the jobs done can be more complicated than it sounds. Make sure you prioritise and are organised to minimise your workload eg if you need to talk to the radiologists about some investigations, collect them all together so you only have to make one trip, or sit down and order all the laboratory investigations in one go.

The jobs normally fall into the following categories:

- Jobs that need to be done immediately
- Radiological investigations
- Laboratory investigations
- Referrals
- Discharges
- Other jobs

Prioritise

Working out which jobs to do first can be difficult. The following tips may help, but you need to be flexible and work as a team – you never know when you may be bleeped in an emergency:

- Who are the sickest patients? Do their jobs first.
- If you need an investigation by the end of the day, focus on it early.
- If you need to involve someone who works regular office hours, do these jobs before 5pm.
- Do clinical jobs before clerical jobs.

Immediate jobs

If you discover a sick patient on the ward round, or something that needs to be done immediately, it has to be prioritised. If the team is big enough, it may be possible to peel off the ward round and do the job then before catching the team up later on.

Radiological investigations

Find out on day 1 exactly how your hospital processes requests for radiological intervention. Most now use a computer based system, but some use handwritten forms. You will need to know the quickest and most effective ways of doing this. It is also important to know how to actually make an investigation happen – different to making the request – often involving a trip to the radiology department to chat to the on-call radiologist and radiographers. Your seniors will be able to offer you advice on this.

Radiologists are legally responsible for the radiation dose they expose patients to, which means every investigation must be justified. Moreover, computer tomography (CT) and magnetic resonance imaging (MRI) machines are coming under increasing pressure to deliver more and more investigations, so it can sometimes be very challenging to get an urgent scan. It is important to know when to escalate this to your seniors and when to accept the limitations of the system – if in doubt, ask.

Top tips for getting an urgent scan

- ☑ Talk to the consultant radiologist in person
- ☑ Ensure you have the patient's details including hospital number
- ☑ **Briefly** summarise the patient concluding with, 'I would like the scan to answer [this clinical question] because it will alter their management in this way....'
- ☑ Do not discuss non-urgent requests otherwise you may not be able to get an urgent scan when you truly need it
- ☑ If you get stuck, escalate early to a more senior member of the team

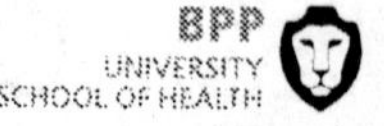

Beware...

Every doctor has a list of radiological images that stick in the mind. There is the chest radiograph with a tension pneumothorax where, instead of treating the clinical signs with an urgent needle thoracocentesis, time was wasted ordering an investigation and the patient died.

There is another showing bilateral chest drains because the radiograph was mistakenly uploaded as a mirror image and the initial drain inserted on the side with clinically no haemothorax, necessitating a second invasive procedure. There is the aspiration pneumonia with a nasogastric tube in the right main bronchus, or the tortuous subclavian line sitting in the left ventricle – the list goes on...

Investigations complement clinical history and examinations. It is essential to know when to, and when not to, perform such tests and how to interpret and act on the information they provide. Know and respect your limitations and ask for help! Radiologists sometimes seem scary, but they are an excellent source of advice – use them.

Laboratory investigations

Like radiological investigations, it is crucial you know how to request laboratory tests for biochemistry, haematology and microbiology specimens. Some more specialist tests may have to be sent away for processing. Find out how to contact these labs directly, in and out of office hours, as sometimes you need a result quickly, or advice about how to do a specific test.

Learn which colour blood bottles are required for each test. This varies slightly from hospital to hospital. All samples sent to any laboratory should be labelled with:

- The patient's name
- Date of birth
- Unique identifying number
- Date and time

They should be accompanied by a request form with as much clinical detail as you can, and the exact nature of the test required. In many hospitals this is now done through an electronic requesting system. When making group and hold or cross-match requests, it is essential to send two temporally distinct samples with separate request forms. It is often a good idea to confirm with the transfusion service exactly what is required for each patient before you take any blood.

If the result of a laboratory test is needed urgently, then you will have to either collect the blood yourself or ask another team member – many nurses and HCAs can take blood and are a valuable resource. If the test can wait until the next day, then you can ask the phlebotomists to do it – if you are lucky enough to have them! You will need to know your local policy for making such requests – and double check the blood is taken the next day.

In an emergency you can get urgent results by running some venous blood through a blood gas analyser. These often provide a haemoglobin count, basic electrolytes, glucose and lactate levels and a guide to the metabolic state of the patient. The machines are found in Accident and Emergency departments and intensive care, respiratory and renal wards and sometimes acute medical admission units. You should find out where your nearest one is, how they work and any code you might need to access it. If in doubt, there is often a friendly nurse or doctor around who can help you run the sample.

Referrals

Referrals to other consultants are the way your team can get other specialists' opinions on your patient's condition and management. They are an important part of the patient's care, because they ensure optimal management in all aspects, and are often made when you reach the extent of your team's expertise. It is important to try and make these requests as early in the day as possible, as this allows the other team time to organise their own work and increases the likelihood of a timely review for your patient.

Most inpatient referrals are organised by phone conversations between junior members of the two teams. However, some may be done through online forms eg referrals to multidisciplinary teams, and some will be done via letter – this is often more common in an outpatient setting.

When making any kind of referral, make sure you:

- Contact the appropriate member of the other team – requests for urgent clinical reviews should go straight to the registrar, whereas more routine requests could go via more junior levels

- Use a standardised communication style to avoid waffling such as Situation, Background, Assessment, Response Required (SBAR)
- Make sure the priority of the referral is clear; for example, it is helpful to know that this is not urgent clinically, but may facilitate a speedy discharge
- Ensure you get the name of the person to whom you made the referral and leave several suitable contacts for your team
- Clearly document all aspects of the conversation, especially the other team's response

Discharges

When a patient leaves hospital, it is essential there is an effective handover to the primary care team and that they leave with appropriate medications. The discharge summary provides this means of communication, summarising the hospital stay, any significant management steps and, most importantly, what needs to be done in primary care when the patient returns home.

Discharges are **crucial** to allow a patient to leave on time ie to tie in with transport, carer packages, medications, district nurse visits etc, therefore it is essential you make sure they are ready on time. Try to anticipate discharges and begin the letters well in advance, preferably from when the patient is admitted.

How to write a discharge summary

Many hospitals now have electronic discharge templates, which require you to fill in specific information. Essentially, the GP needs to know when, why and under whose care the patient went into hospital; what happened to them and what was done; and anything further they need to do to look after them. It is good practice to make sure all of the following are communicated:

- Patient identifying details
- Presenting complaint
- Physical findings
- Results of investigations
- Diagnosis
- Management
- Medications on discharge, including any changes to long-term medication and why
- Any follow-up planned by the hospital
- Any follow-up suggestions to the GP
- Your name and contact details

Other jobs

These can include a whole range of non-clinical, often menial, chores ranging from important conversations with family members to fetching the coffee! Use your initiative and try not to think about how long you spent at medical school to be able to carry a request form to the relevant department!

Being efficient

Foundation doctors have always had to work very hard. This is not going to change. If you are not strategic and intelligent about the way in which you go about the job you will quickly be snowed under by more and more work. This is depressing and stressful, and will prevent you from learning. There are a number of ways you can try and improve how efficiently you work.

Invest in your reputation

This is not as superficial as it seems. A reputation for being polite, kind, caring and considerate of the people around you, patients and professionals, will be your most useful asset for your foundation years and beyond. If you obviously care for your patients and their relatives, then it is much more likely that the professionals around you will want to help you. This will help you with requesting services from other specialties, and will encourage other staff around you to support you.

Delegate

When all the jobs are delegated to you, it may often seem like there is no one left on the team who can help. However, nurses, HCAs and other professionals often share many of your practical skills and, whilst busy, may be able to help. This is often particularly true when you are on-call. Don't be afraid to ask (politely); they can always say no. Utilising other resources available to you such as the phlebotomy team will also ensure that you are free to do the tasks that only a doctor can do, such as referrals.

Again, make sure you have a good relationship with the phlebotomists, so you can always ask for an extra favour if needed. Be polite, grateful and strategic in your requests; phlebotomists work to time, not to workload, so if you give them too many bloods to take, you may well end up having to do them yourself. You should really only ever request investigations (including bloods) when they are clinically indicated.

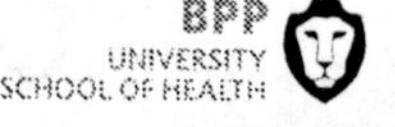

Shortcuts

There are always shortcuts – physical or to negotiate systems and tasks – that you will learn for each job. Try and find them early, as they really will save you time, but be careful never to take any that might compromise patient care.

Being effective

Getting your jobs done quickly is very different to getting them done well. Most of the work of a junior doctor will involve getting the most appropriate investigation or review for your patient, and there are some strategies that may be used to help you do this:

Know your patient

Whenever you approach a senior about something, always try and know everything you can about the patient. Take a few minutes to read through the notes from the current admission and previous discharge letters and correspondence may also be helpful.

Have a focused question

Explain exactly what the clinical (or other) question is that you are facing and what you need from the other person or team. Listen to any alternatives and try and justify why the team has taken this management strategy.

Confirm the plan

After the discussion, make sure you confirm the steps agreed. Repeat back what you are expecting to happen or what you need to do, to avoid any misunderstanding. Ambiguity in communication is very often the cause of mistakes or the reason for delays in patient management. Always remember to document the discussion and the agreed plan.

Asking for help

If you are ever stuck or need technical assistance, your immediate seniors are the people to ask, escalating up the ladder as needed. If you are worried about an acutely unwell patient, never be afraid to call for help from any grade of doctor. If you cannot get hold of the registrar, most consultants would want to know immediately that you were concerned and struggling and will find you another source of help if they cannot come themselves.

There are also a number of more specialist teams available to provide assistance if needed. For example, there may be an IV team who can help you with IV access, or there may be a urology specialist nurse to help with catheterisations. Other team members or nurses may know what is available in your hospital.

Going home

Going home on time is one of the most important things you can do, for you, your family and the team. Of course there will be times when this is not possible, but try not to become sucked into the vortex of work. It is vital you have time to recover between shifts and the importance of a meaningful work-life balance cannot be overstated.

Before leaving each day the following needs to have been accomplished:

- Any changes documented in the notes, with a plan for treatment
- All jobs from the ward round done
- All investigation results reviewed and actioned
- Any sick patients stabilised, or handed over to the on-call team
- All fluids prescribed for the night
- All monitored drugs prescribed eg warfarin, monitored antibiotics such as gentamicin
- Any drug charts rewritten if needed

Once you are satisfied that you have done all these things, leave.

Professionalism

In a very unsatisfying way, it is difficult to define professionalism. We all know it when it is there and recognise the lack when it is not. A sense of integrity combined with the following elements all contribute to developing professionalism:

- Punctuality
- Honesty
- Politeness
- Knowing your limits
- Being willing to admit to mistakes
- Being willing to improve

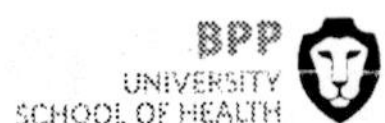

Whistle-blowing

The term whistle-blowing tends to invoke unsavoury connotations. However, if one of your colleagues or seniors is not up to scratch, not coping with the job, or is lying or covering up mistakes, it is your professional duty to your patients to do something about it. Each trust has its own whistle-blowing procedures; however, as a foundation doctor, you should speak to your consultant and follow their guidance on what to do next. Other options can include your clinical or educational supervisors.

If you are worried no one is taking your concern seriously, put it in writing to your Foundation Supervisor. This will give you a record of the communication, and will encourage action on the part of your seniors.

'Professional' is not a label you give yourself – it is a description you hope others may apply to you.

David Maister

(*True Professionalism*, Free Press, 1997)

On-call shifts

On-call shifts add variety to your daily work, provide excellent learning opportunities and often allow you greater autonomy and independence. However, they are also often busy, stressful and tiring.

As an FY1 doctor on-calls will consist of:

- Clerking new patients
- Emergency jobs for acutely unwell patients
- Maintenance jobs for stable patients

Whilst the breakdown of these components will vary, the unpredictability of an on-call remains the greatest challenge in all rotations.

Unpredictability and uncertainty

As the FY1 on-call, you are the first port of call for any simple jobs that need to be done and for any acutely ill patients that need assessing. The nature of the job means that you can never fully predict what will happen, and when. You will have to deal with an unpredictable workload and uncertain diagnoses in unwell patients. Somehow you have to work with that uncertainty.

One of the greatest challenges is ordering this workload in some kind of organised manner. Prioritise your jobs. If they are emergencies or urgent, do them as soon as you can; if they are routine, try and do them geographically. Write down the details of every phone call and all the patient details so you remember everything you have been asked to do.

Handover processes and the way you structure your on-call shift may help you minimise the uncertainty you are facing.

Handover

At the beginning of your shift it is vital to have a good handover about any sick patients and jobs that need doing. Many hospitals organise formal team handovers and this can be a useful opportunity to discuss how you will manage these patients throughout the shift and any senior support that may be required.

If you receive verbal handovers from separate teams, make sure you take a note of all the patient details and what the plan is for them. If you are asked to follow up investigations, make sure you ask the team how they were planning to alter management depending on the results.

Structuring your shift

When you arrive, the first thing you should do is find out who your seniors are for that shift and how to contact them. It is often worth touching base with them before you start so that they know that they are working with you.

At the beginning of the shift, it is a good idea to proactively visit the wards for which you're responsible and ask the nurses if they have any jobs that you can get out of the way. These normally include:

- Prescribing fluids
- Prescribing warfarin
- Prescribing simple analgesia
- Rewriting drug charts
- Taking drug levels for monitoring eg gentamicin

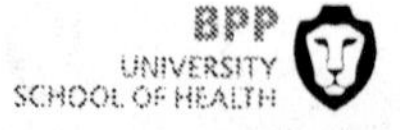

If it is safe to do so, prescribe enough fluids and warfarin to last until the end of your on-call period eg the whole weekend. Find out if the nurses on the ward are able to help you with levels or routine bloods etc. The more of this routine work you can do early, or delegate, the less pressured you will feel when you are called to deal with urgent reviews.

Clerking new patients

You might have to clerk new patients whilst on-call, which is time consuming. As soon as you are bleeped, ask the nurse calling you what the basic presenting complaint is, what the observations are and whether the patient looks well or not. Also ask if anyone can take bloods from the patient.

You can review the patient briefly and assess how unwell they are. If they are stable, then you can do any more urgent jobs and return later, but if they are acutely unwell, then you may have to break off and work on them now.

Dealing with the sick patient

Inevitably during your on-call, a nurse will bleep you and tell you about a patient they are worried about, that they would like you to see. It is almost impossible to judge how sick a patient is on the other end of a telephone, so never try to do it. Nevertheless, try to get as much information as you can on the first call – what are the symptoms and the observations and why in particular is the nurse worried **now**?

It might be tempting to dismiss a bleep as somebody being overcautious, or having little substance, but many nurses have a lot of experience and can recognise when someone is ill, whether the observations indicate it or not. Ask the nurse to do a fresh set of observations and electrocardiogram (ECG) and put the patient on high flow oxygen while you are on your way. If the blood pressure is low, ask them to get a bag of fluids ready for when you arrive.

On the way, run through some of the possible differentials in your head. Stay calm. When you arrive, make a quick airway, breathing, circulation, disability, exposure (ABCDE) assessment and put out an immediate arrest call if any of these are compromised (see Chapter 5). If you are happy the patient does not warrant an arrest call, briefly look at the notes and ask the patient and nurses what the latest problem seems to be. Examine the patient, observation chart and ECG and perform some basic investigations – commonly venous or arterial blood gases, blood and urine cultures and appropriate radiological tests. Ensure the patient has intravenous access.

Often it will not be immediately clear what the underlying diagnosis is. Treat the symptoms and signs as you progress through your ABCDE assessment to stabilise the patient. If there is any suspicion of sepsis (see Chapter 3), ensure the Sepsis 6 bundle has been enacted:

- High flow oxygen
- IV fluids
- Empirical antibiotics
- Blood cultures
- Lactate
- Monitoring urine output – possibly with a catheter

When you have performed these steps, notify your senior and let them know the status of the patient and what your management plan currently is.

Two sick patients

If you have two patients that are sick, you are not going to be able to do everything for both of them. Call for help from your seniors and take their advice. They will help you prioritise and develop a strategy for dealing with both patients safely. Never be afraid to ask for an early senior review – most people would prefer to know of any concerning patients early, to help head off any trouble.

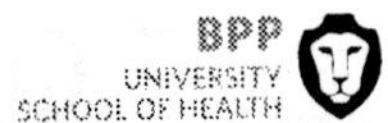

A day in the life of an on-call Trauma and Orthopaedic FY1 doctor

Saturday morning and I long for a lie-in. Instead I leave the house at 6:30, to organise the lists before the trauma meeting at 8:00. I doze gratefully as the registrar and SHO present the X-rays for the day's operating lists, post-operative patients and referrals.

Then the ward round, as busy as ever. The SHO and I scrabble to make sure the consultant has seen all the patients before they head off to theatre. A brief respite for coffee – essential – and then we return to the ward. There are three cannulas awaiting us, several drug charts and an anxious nurse requesting a discharge summary for a patient who has suddenly been offered a nursing home bed – worth its weight in gold. I start the discharge summary and the SHO does a round of cannulas.

She is soon bleeped from A&E to admit a new patient and disappears. Mrs Jones has a low blood pressure, which magically returns to normal when we repeat it. Then a bleep from a distant ward – Mr Hughes has low saturations. Has he been out for another cigarette? I wonder, but go to review him anyway. This is lucky as he is tachycardic and quite unwell. The SHO runs up briefly from A&E to review him and asks me to send off some bloods and cultures and request an X-ray, she starts some fluids and antibiotics and disappears again. I finish the jobs and return to the ward – two more cannulas and another urgent discharge summary are waiting.

Luckily the phlebotomists have been round, so it is soon time to do the warfarin prescriptions and order the bloods for tomorrow. I chase some results and discover Mr Prewitt's abdominal ultrasound has shown moderate ascites – secondary to his liver metastases, poor man. A phone call to the medical registrar earns him an ascitic tap and it's time for a (very brief) late lunch. The afternoon is similar – checking bloods, giving fluids, a few cannulas, drug charts and so on until finally, exhausted, I hand over to the night team, desperate to get home for some food and sleep before beginning all over again tomorrow!

Dealing with death

People in hospital are sick and some of them will die. Death is never far away and you will need to get used to this. When a patient dies, you should quickly confirm their death, otherwise the rest of the hospital cannot get on with dealing with the death. You may also be required to write a death certificate and a cremation form.

Confirming death

As an FY doctor, it will be your job to confirm their death:

1. Ask the nurses to ensure that any relatives have left the bedside
2. Check that the patient does not respond to verbal and pain stimuli
3. Feel for a central pulse for three minutes, whilst listening for heart sounds
4. Feel for respiratory effort for three minutes, whilst listening for breath sounds
5. Inspect the pupils and confirm that they are fixed and dilated

When you are satisfied the patient is dead, check if there is a pacemaker by feeling over the chest. Note the time of death with your findings in the notes, writing out the patient's full name, date of birth and hospital number yourself. You also need to document those present at the time of death, anybody you spoke to and mention if you spoke to anyone present about the death and document whether or not they had any concerns, and make it clear whether or not there was a pacemaker present.

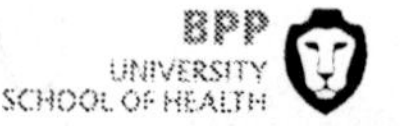

The death certificate

Once your patient is confirmed dead, they need to have a certificate written so that their death can be registered and their funeral planned. Death certificates may be issued by any doctor, confident about the cause of death, who provided care during the last illness and who saw the deceased within 14 days of death. Often this will be the doctor who verifies the death. You will often have to write this.

The information that must be included on the death certificate includes:

- The patient's name
- The place of death
- The last time you saw the patient alive
- The causes of death:
  - Ia the immediate cause
  - Ib the condition causing Ia
  - Ic the condition causing Ib
  - II conditions contributing to the death, but not directly causing it
- Your name and signature
- Your qualifications
- The consultant responsible for the patient's care

Part Ia

Deciding on the causes of death is often tricky. Always talk to your consultant before completing a certificate. Cause is often likely to be something like pneumonia, pulmonary embolism or ventricular tachycardia, all of which may result in a myocardial infarction (the mode of death).

Always be as specific as you can and, if there are several possible causes eg pneumonia and pulmonary oedema, use the notes and observation charts etc to try and select the most likely.

Parts Ib and Ic

These are the conditions that led directly to the immediate cause of death. For example, if your patient died of pulmonary oedema, then they most likely had left ventricular failure (Ib) which will have been caused by some form of cardiac disease, eg ischaemic heart disease or myocardial infarction (Ic). If your patient had a cerebrovascular event (Ia), then that may have been caused by AF (Ib) which may have been caused by thyrotoxicosis (Ic).

Part II

This is where you write the other conditions that your patient had, which contributed but did not directly cause death. Often, conditions such as renal failure or dementia that made treating the primary causes more difficult, are included here along with co-morbidities in the same organ system as the terminal illness.

The Coroner's Office

You have to discuss a case with the Coroner if:

- The patient was in hospital less than 24 hours
- The patient underwent an operation within the last year of life
- Death is deemed to be in any way 'unnatural', ie violent, accidental, sudden or unexplained, involving substance abuse, due to industrial disease (this includes those elderly patients who die following a neck of femur fracture)
- You cannot give a cause of death

In these cases, phone the Coroner's Office and discuss the case. They may suggest what to write, or they may suggest talking to a pathologist about the case. Sometimes they will tell you a post-mortem is required. The Coroner makes decisions about the cause of death if you cannot do so.

Cremation forms

If a patient's family have decided that their relative is to be cremated, then you will have to complete Part A of a cremation form to state that there is no reason why the body should not be cremated. Essentially, you are saying that there is no reason to suspect any foul-play in the patient's death, and so a cremation is legally acceptable. This is a big responsibility, and you should take it seriously.

The Part A section of the form consists of: more detailed information about the patient; details of their final illness and duration of your care; any individuals who were with them at the time of death; details of your inspection of the body; the reasoning behind the cause of death you have stated and whether they have any potentially dangerous implants.

Once you have completed the form, a more senior doctor checks it. They may call you and other people you have mentioned on the death certificate, so as to discuss what was written and whether anyone has any concerns about the patient's death.

Case Study: A challenging death

Mrs Smith had never wanted to live to be 100, her son explained. She had always just enjoyed life and had never experienced a day's illness until she was diagnosed with Alzheimer's Disease when she was 93. Over the next year she progressed rapidly, and her 94th birthday was spent in the residential home her family found for her when she could no longer recognise them or care for herself.

They were very pragmatic people – as indeed they reflected she had been – and had no desire to prolong her life unnecessarily. Unfortunately, one day she fell while walking with her zimmer frame and was admitted to hospital, thought to have suffered a large stroke. She became more and more unwell, developing sepsis and delirium. In her agitation she would scream and howl, throwing her arms around violently, not caring if they made contact with bed rails, people or any other parts of her own body. Her skin was bruised a deep, rich violet colour and she moaned continually.

A CT scan was performed, which was negative. She had not had a stroke. On closer examination one of her legs was shorter than the other and twisted outwards – she had a hip fracture. One night, septic and delirious, she was transferred to the orthopaedic team, who did their best to stabilise her in order to operate and fix her hip. However, she became progressively more unwell and it became evident she was dying. When she finally passed away, her pain and agitation controlled with a syringe driver and surrounded by her family, her son and daughter-in-law expressed their relief that her suffering had ended.

When it came to writing the death certificate the FY1 struggled to know what to put on the certificate. The consultant wanted 1a to be neck of femur fracture, but the FY1 knew that hadn't caused her death. She had died of sepsis, but the source was unclear – was she more likely to have had pneumonia or urosepsis or was there perhaps some other hidden cause of her infection? Did it matter? Unsure and needing to notify the Coroner of the death, she called his office and discussed the case. The Coroner agreed Mrs Smith had **not** died of her fracture and talked the FY1 through the clinical notes, finally determining that the death certificate should read Ia) urosepsis Ib) acute kidney injury II) Alzheimer's Disease and neck of femur fracture. Ultimately of course, the cause of death was far less important than the course of death, and it was sad that the attention paid to the former had not been paid earlier to the latter.

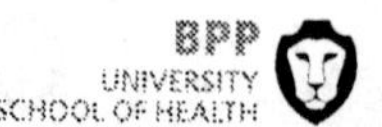

Foundation Programme summary

The job of a foundation doctor has probably not changed enormously over the last few decades. There is more paperwork, they must seek a greater number of referrals from specialist teams and there is an ever-increasing pressure caused by the rapid increase in patient throughput. However, the most important part of the FY1's role has stayed the same, and that is to ensure the smooth running of the team.

However, the introduction of the Foundation Programme, which was designed to encourage foundation doctors to take responsibility for their own learning, requires a record of a specified number of structured 'Situational Learning Events' as well as other evidence, including a demonstration of:

- Competency at core procedures
- Competency at other practical skills (using DOPS)
- Competency at assessing and managing patients (using Mini-CEXs)
- That you are developing your knowledge (using CBDs)
- That you are working well within your team (using Mini-TABs)
- That you are participating in teaching (using a Developing the Clinical Teacher SLE)
- Satisfactory reports from your Clinical and Educational Supervisor for each placement and a satisfactory end-of-year Educational Supervisor's report
- Evidence of reflective practice
- Evidence of career planning

This evidence is all recorded on the NHS e-portfolio website (https://www.nhseportfolios.org).

Up to date information regarding the Foundation Programme can be found at the following websites:

☞ www.foundationprogramme.nhs.uk
☞ www.rcplondon.ac.uk
☞ www.rcseng.ac.uk

Core procedures

In FY1, the GMC requires evidence of demonstration of competency at 15 core procedures:

- Venepuncture
- IV cannulation
- Prepare and administer IV medication, injections and fluids
- Arterial puncture in an adult
- Blood culture (peripheral)
- IV infusion including the prescription of fluids
- IV infusion of blood and blood products
- Injection of local anaesthetic to skin
- Subcutaneous injection
- Intramuscular injection
- Perform and interpret an ECG
- Perform and interpret peak flow
- Urethral catheterisation (male)
- Urethral catheterisation (female)
- Airway care including simple adjuncts

Any doctor more senior than FY1, senior nurses or allied healthcare professionals who have been trained in the procedure and assessment and feedback methodology can perform these assessments.

Mini-Clinical Evaluation Exercise

(see Chapter 10)

This is an assessment of your ability to perform a clinical evaluation of a patient; essentially taking a history, or examining them, making a diagnosis and then deciding on a management plan.

On-calls or post-take ward rounds are often good environments to complete these assessments, and it is often easier to request to send your assessor an email ticket at a later date for them to complete your report.

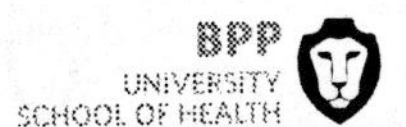

Assessments must be performed by trainees at ST1 or above. A recommended minimum of three Mini-CEX assessments is suggested for each placement in FY1 and six **must** be completed in both FY1 and FY2.

Direct Observation of Procedural Skills (DOPS)

(see Chapter 9)

DOPS are assessments of practical skills, which demonstrate your ability to perform a certain skill. They are often more specialist procedures than core procedures eg lumbar punctures or insertion of arterial line. Specialist clinics, anaesthetic rooms or theatre may be good places for these assessments.

Assessors must be competent to perform the procedure themselves and there is no minimum number that must be completed throughout the Foundation Programme; however, up to three DOPs may count towards the requirement for six Mini-CEXs.

Case-Based Discussions (CBDs)

This is an assessment of your developing clinical knowledge, to show that you are learning medical facts as well as skills. Sometimes assessors will request you to prepare in advance and sometimes they will be a more informal discussion.

A variety of assessors (ST1 and above) should be used to help you complete a minimum of two CBDs in each placement. Six must be completed in each year.

Team Assessment of Behaviour (TAB)

This is a multi-source feedback, requiring feedback from a variety of people you work with. You will receive a rating and written feedback from each person and in theory this should be done anonymously. It is an excellent way of assessing how good a team player you are and allowing any individual to raise concerns or provide particular praise about your practice.

You **must** complete one TAB per year, and it is recommended that these are started in the fourth month of the first placement of both years, so as to give you time to repeat an assessment if needed.

A minimum of ten ratings/assessors are required for each TAB, which must include at least two of:

- Doctors more senior than F2, including at least one consultant or GP principal
- Senior nurses (band 5 or above)
- Allied health professionals
- Other team members including ward clerks, secretaries and auxiliary staff

Developing the Clinical Teacher

One of these assessments must take place each year, with the aim of helping the doctor develop teaching or presenting skills. Useful settings for completion might include FY1/FY2 local teaching sessions, departmental audit days or providing observed tutorials or bedside teaching sessions to medical students.

Supervisors' reports

You have one Educational Supervisor (ES) each year and one Clinical Supervisor (CS) per placement. Academic FY2 doctors also have an Academic Supervisor (AS). You must provide evidence of satisfactory end-of-placement ES and CS reports and one end-of-year ES report. Depending on the exact programme structure, AF2 doctors may need to substitute an AS for a CS report during their research block.

These reports are generated during end-of-placement meetings with the relevant supervisors and must be signed by both trainer and trainee. It is often a good idea to book these with the consultant's secretary as you start your placement in order to make sure they take place.

Reflective practice

This is an important part of medical practice and personal development in general. There will be many patients that raise challenging questions in your mind, or that you find yourself wondering what might have happened had the case been managed in an alternate way, if certain discussions had been handled differently or if particular team members had behaved otherwise.

Whilst you do not **have** to complete these assessments, demonstration of engagement with reflection provides

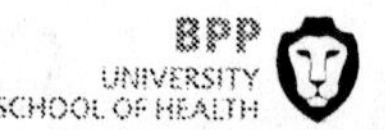

further evidence for the GMC that you are engaging with the training programme and that you are a well-rounded and thoughtful trainee.

Career development

Again, whilst you do not have to provide formal evidence about any career planning you have undertaken, recording any taster days you undertake and reflecting on what you have learned will again provide additional evidence about what sort of doctor and individual you are. It may also provide a useful stimulus for discussions with your clinical or educational supervisors, who may be able to suggest how you could explore your options further.

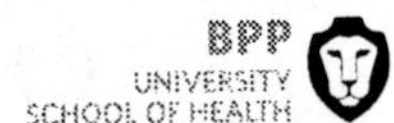

Chapter 3
Core Foundation competencies in medicine

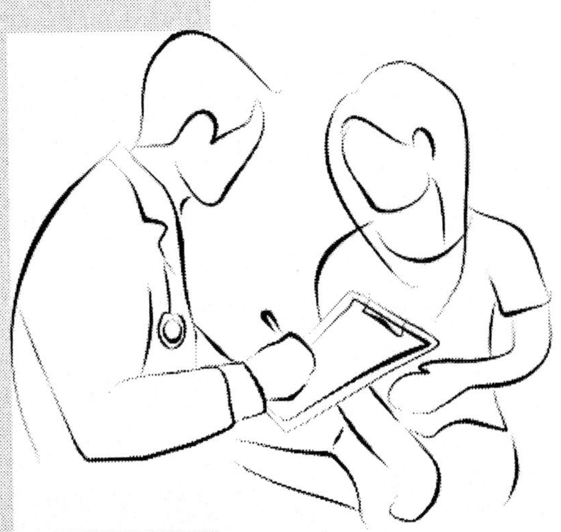

Core Foundation competencies in medicine

What we need in medical schools is not to teach empathy, as much as to preserve it – the process of learning huge volumes of information about disease, of learning a specialized language, can ironically make one lose sight of the patient one came to serve; empathy can be replaced by cynicism.

Abraham Verghese

Abdominal pain

Differential diagnosis

System/Organ	Disease
Gut	Gastritis **Gastro-oesophageal reflux disease (GORD)** **Peptic ulcer** Intestinal obstruction Diverticulitis **Inflammatory bowel disease (IBD)** **Ulcerative colitis** **Crohn's disease** Appendicitis Volvulus Gastroenteritis Strangulated hernia Constipation **Irritable bowel syndrome (IBS)**
Hepato-biliary	Cholecystitis Ascending cholangitis
Pancreatic	Acute pancreatitis Chronic pancreatitis
Splenic (referred to shoulder tip)	Infarction Rupture
Urinary tract	**Urinary tract infection (UTI)/ pyelonephritis** Acute urinary retention Polycystic kidney (eg haemorrhage into cyst) Ureteric colic
Gynaecological	Ectopic pregnancy Ovarian cyst (rupture or torsion) Endometriosis Severe dysmenorrhea
Vascular	Aortic dissection Ischaemic colitis
Peritoneum	Peritonitis
Abdominal wall	Rectus sheath haematoma
Retroperitoneal	Retroperitoneal haemorrhage
Referred	Lower lobar pneumonia Myocardial infarction (MI) Thoracic spinal disease
Other	Hypercalcaemia Diabetic ketoacidosis (DKA) Porphyria Uraemia

Table 3.1: Differential diagnosis of abdominal pain

Gastro-oesophageal reflux disease (GORD)

Epidemiology

Affects up to 30% of Western populations. There is a higher incidence in the developed countries as obesity tends to be more common in these individuals.

Aetiology

Mechanism	Precipitant
Reduced clearance from oesophagus	Poor posture, post-prandial
Reduced pressure of the lower oesophageal sphincter	Systemic sclerosis
Direct damage to the mucosa of the oesophagus	Foods with a high fat content, alcohol, caffeine, smoking, pregnancy, nitrates and channel blockers
Increased production of gastric secretions	Alcohol, hot drinks, acidic stomach contents, bile, NSAID, Zollinger-Ellison syndrome
Damage to the anti-reflux mechanism	Hiatus hernia
Delayed gastric emptying	Pyloric stenosis, gastric atony
Increased intra-abdominal pressure	Obesity, ascites, tight clothing and pregnancy

Table 3.2: Mechanism and precipitants of GORD

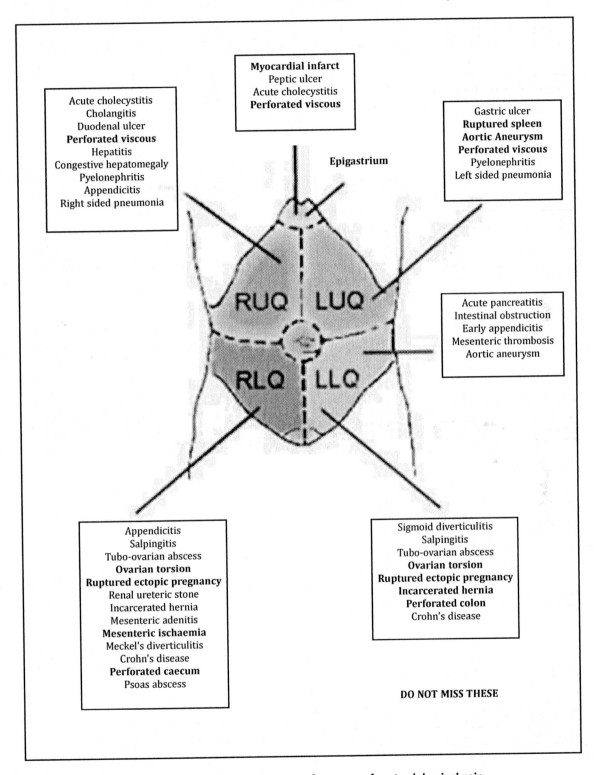

Myocardial infarct
Peptic ulcer
Acute cholecystitis
Perforated viscous

Acute cholecystitis
Cholangitis
Duodenal ulcer
Perforated viscous
Hepatitis
Congestive hepatomegaly
Pyelonephritis
Appendicitis
Right sided pneumonia

Gastric ulcer
Ruptured spleen
Aortic Aneurysm
Perforated viscous
Pyelonephritis
Left sided pneumonia

Epigastrium

RUQ
LUQ
RLQ
LLQ

Acute pancreatitis
Intestinal obstruction
Early appendicitis
Mesenteric thrombosis
Aortic aneurysm

Appendicitis
Salpingitis
Tubo-ovarian abscess
Ovarian torsion
Ruptured ectopic pregnancy
Renal ureteric stone
Incarcerated hernia
Mesenteric adenitis
Mesenteric ischaemia
Meckel's diverticulitis
Crohn's disease
Perforated caecum
Psoas abscess

Sigmoid diverticulitis
Salpingitis
Tubo-ovarian abscess
Ovarian torsion
Ruptured ectopic pregnancy
Incarcerated hernia
Perforated colon
Crohn's disease

DO NOT MISS THESE

Figure 3.1: The differential diagnoses for causes of acute abdominal pain

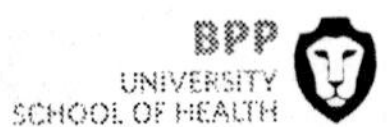

Pathophysiology

A small amount of post-prandial reflux is normal. However, GORD involves the passage of acidic gastric contents into the distal portion of the oesophagus which causes symptoms and impairs quality of life. It usually occurs where there is dysfunction of the lower oesophageal sphincter (an intrinsic muscular band around the lower 4 cm of the oesophagus and the crural diaphragm).

Oesophagitis may be evident macroscopically or microscopically but correlates poorly with symptoms. Around two-thirds of symptomatic patients have no evidence of oesophagitis on endoscopy.

Microscopically there is initial hypertrophy of the epithelial layer of the oesophagus. Subsequently, there is an infiltration of inflammatory cells resulting in macroscopic inflammation, erosions and mucosal ulceration. As healing occurs strictures may form.

With prolonged exposure to acid there is metaplasia of the normal stratified squamous epithelium and Barrett's oesophagus develops.

History/examination

- Epigastric or retrosternal burning pain – worse on lying flat, bending down or on straining
- Symptoms mostly after meals, with some symptomatic relief with the use of antacids
- Exacerbation of symptoms with large, fatty meals and tight clothing
- Waterbrash: the excessive production of saliva and bitter taste in the mouth due to acidic gastric contents refluxing into the oespohagus
- Recurrent chest infections caused by nocturnal aspiration
- Chronic cough or wheeze
- Dysphagia or odynophagia due to ulcers of the oesophageal mucosa and any resultant strictures
- Oesophageal ulceration may present with an upper GI bleed
- Nausea and vomiting
- Epigastric tenderness
- It may be difficult to distinguish between the symptoms of GORD and those of cardiac ischaemia – both may be provoked by exercise and relieved by the use of GTN spray

NICE recommendations for suspected upper GI cancer referrals:

- Dysphagia at any age
- Dyspepsia at any age + one or more of the following:
  - Weight loss
  - Proven anaemia
  - Vomiting
- Dyspepsia in a patient aged 55 years or more with at least one of the following 'high-risk' features:
  - Onset of dyspepsia <1 year previously
  - Continuous symptoms since onset
- Dyspepsia combined with at least one of the following known 'risk factors':
  - Family history of upper GI cancer in more than two first-degree relatives
  - Barrett's oesophagitis
  - Pernicious anaemia
  - Peptic ulcer surgery over 20 years previously
  - Known dysplasia, atrophic gastritis, intestinal metaplasia
  - Jaundice
  - Upper abdominal mass

In a prospective observational study, the prevalence of gastric cancer was 4% (and serious benign disease 13%) in a cohort of patients referred urgently for alarm symptoms.

Investigations

Blood tests:

- FBC and haematinics
- U&Es
- Clotting screen

Endoscopy:

- Part of urgent investigations for upper GI cancer in patients with alarm symptoms as recommended by NICE
- Not generally indicated
- Findings are normal in more than half of patients with GORD with some showing features of oesophagitis

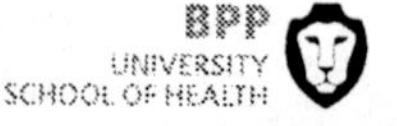

Other:

- **Barium meal:** often unhelpful as it may illustrate gastro-oesophageal reflux even in asymptomatic individuals. It can demonstrate a hiatus hernia.
- **Oesophageal pH and manometry studies:** can be performed in patients where the gastroscopy is normal despite typical features of GORD or if symptoms are unresponsive to treatment. With no erosions on endoscopy, the presence of a positive 24-hour pH study gives a diagnosis of non-erosive reflux disease (NERD) but a negative study gives a diagnosis of 'functional heartburn'.
- **Cardiac investigations** may be required for atypical pain.

Management

- **Lifestyle measures:** smoking cessation, weight loss avoidance of drugs that precipitate symptoms (NSAIDs, steroids, bisphosphonates etc), spicy foods, alcohol, large meals late at night, and hot drinks such as coffee and tea. Night-time dyspepsia may be eased by elevating the head of the bed by 15 cm.
- **Antacids** such as magnesium and aluminium hydroxide or alginates (eg gaviscon).
- **Acid suppression:** if no alarm symptoms are present and no endoscopy is planned, NICE recommends a one-month trial of a proton pump inhibitors (eg omeprazole). If symptoms persist or recur, investigation for *H. pylori* is recommended, followed by eradication therapy and treatment with the lowest dose PPI possible to control symptoms.
- **Prokinetic drugs:** can relieve nausea and vomiting, eg metoclopramide and domperidone.
- **Surgery:** patients who do not respond or are intolerant to medical therapy may require surgical management: the most common procedure is the laparoscopic Nissen fundoplication, where the fundus of the stomach is sutured around the end of the distal oesophagus. This results in a region of high pressure at the lower oesophagus reducing the volume of acid reflux.

Prognosis

Approximately 50% of patients are successfully treated with weight loss and the prescribing of simple antacids.

Dyspepsia occurs in 40% of the population annually and leads to a primary care consultation in 5% and endoscopy in 1%.

Of those who undergo endoscopy:

- **40% have functional or non-ulcer dyspepsia**
- **40% have gastro-oesophageal reflux disease (GORD)**
- **13% have ulcer disease**
- **2% have gastric cancer**
- **1% have oesophageal cancer**

Peptic ulcer disease

Epidemiology

Peptic ulceration is now decreasing in the developed world due to effective treatment of *Helicobacter pylori. H. pylori* is a Gram-negative microaerophilic flagellated bacillus, which has an incidence of 40% in the developed world and up to 80% in the developing world. It is associated with a lower socio-economic background and overcrowded living conditions.

Males are more commonly affected than females with a ratio of 4:1. Duodenal ulcers are 3–4 times more common than gastric ulcers. Duodenal ulcers are most likely between 20 and 60 years of age whereas gastric ulcers tend to present more in the elderly population.

Aetiology

The major causes are *Helicobacter pylori* infection and NSAIDs. Others include gastric cancers (adenocarcinoma and lymphoma), gastrinoma, Zollinger-Ellison Syndrome, hyperparathyroidism, radiation and severe physiological stress.

Smoking, chronic alcohol use and stress increase the likelihood of peptic ulceration.

Pathophysiology

Peptic ulcers form due to a breach in the mucosa in the stomach and duodenum. Duodenal ulcers tend to develop due to impairment in the production of gastric acid. Gastric ulcers usually result from the effects of cytotoxins produced by bacteria such as *H. pylori* and the resultant stimulation of an immune response.

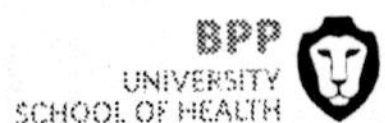

H. pylori	Chronic NSAIDs
• First described by Marshall and Warren in their Nobel-prize winning paper of 1983. • Account for 70% of gastric and 95% of duodenal ulcers. • Bacteria cause inflammation of the gastric mucosa, which is usually asymptomatic. Approximately 15% of those infected develop an ulcer. • *H.pylori* is also associated with B-cell lymphoma and Gastric Associated Lymphoid Tissue tumours.	Inhibit cyclo-oxygenase (COX 1 and 2). COX-1 is involved in the production of prostaglandins, which protect the gastric muscosa by increasing the secretion of bicarbonate, therefore COX suppression results in gastric mucosal damage.

Table 3.3: How *H. Pylori* and NSAID/Aspirin lead to peptic ulcer disease

History/examination

- Epigastric pain, related to meal times, with symptoms of nausea, heartburn, chest pain and acid reflux, bloating, haematemesis (including coffee-ground vomiting) and malaena. There may be epigastric tenderness on examination.
- Gastric ulcers classically present with epigastric pain precipitated by food. Associated symptoms of anorexia, vomiting and weight loss are common and more pronounced if there is an underlying malignant ulcer.
- Duodenal ulcers classically present with pain one to three hours after food and during the night. The pain is often relieved by milk or other neutral foods. The pain may radiate to the back in the case of a posterior ulcer.
- Symptoms respond to antacid treatment.

Complications

- Gastric outlet obstruction (pre-pyloric or duodenal ulcer) presents with projectile vomiting and a succession splash.
- Perforation (more commonly associated with duodenal ulcers) with signs of peritonitis.
- Upper GI bleeding with pallor or a more acute haemorrhage with malaena on digital rectal examination.

Investigations

Blood tests:

- FBC: to check for a drop in Hb
- U&E: an isolated raised urea is indicative of the 'protein meal' in cases of bleeding associated with the ulcer
- Clotting screen
- Cross-match
- Consider serum gastrin and calcium if clinically indicated to exclude rarer causes such as Zollinger-Ellison syndrome and hyperparathyroidism

Upper GI endoscopy:

- Peptic ulcers are most common on the gastric lesser curve and first part of the duodenum.
- Gastric carcinomas characteristically have a rolled edge, and tend to affect the greater curvature and antrum.
- A biopsy must be taken to confirm the nature of the lesion.

H. Pylori detection:

- 13C urea breath tests or stool antigen tests are the recommended way of testing for *H. pylori*, although laboratory-based serology can be used if locally validated. Stop antisecretories or bismuth two weeks before the test.

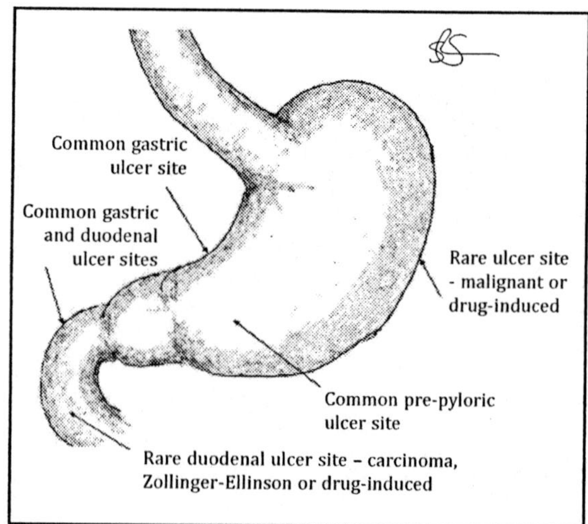

Figure 3.2: Sites of gastric ulcer disease

Management

Triple therapy for *H. pylori* eradication for 10–14 days. Either regimen is thought to be equally effective, and treatment failure with one should proceed to treatment with the other.

Regimen 1	Regimen 2
Omeprazole 20 mg or Lansoprazole 30 mg BD	
Clarithromycin 500 mg BD	
Amoxicillin 1g BD	Metronidazole 400 mg BD
> 80% of patients are cured with this combination of treatment and the relapse rate is <5%.	

Table 3.4: The common regimens of triple therapy

- **Lifestyle advice:** smoking cessation, weight loss, alcohol reduction and avoidance of NSAIDs and aspirin.
- **Proton pump inhibitors:** reduce gastric acid secretion and are effective for ulcer healing. They should be taken for at least four to eight weeks.
- **Antacids:** symptomatic relief.
- **Surgical management** if:
  - There is persistent bleeding or ulcer perforation
  - No response to maximal medical therapy
  - A malignant gastric ulcer has been diagnosed

Case Study: An unpleasant path...

Mrs Rivers had just woken up. For the past three weeks she had been unconscious – sedated, ventilated, battling for her life with the help of antibiotics and inotropes. She had barely made it. The infection that had stolen her fingers and toes and turned her legs a dusky purple had very nearly also stolen her life. Mrs Rivers lived with her husband and two young children, and her intensive care cubicle was littered with drawings and 'get well soon' cards. There was even a live photo frame, across which smiling, blond-haired little girls kept appearing.

It was all rather grim, but finally, finally she was awake and unventilated and talking. Life seemed to have turned a corner and Elizabeth was looking forward to leaving the ICU for the ward – she couldn't remember which one they were taking her to, or which group of doctors would be looking after her, but that really didn't seem to matter. At least she would be leaving the beeping, buzzing, whirring machines behind.

A few hours before she was supposed to be moved, she began to feel a bit more unwell – nauseous and with a slight aching pain in the middle of her chest. She didn't say anything; feeling unwell was part of being in intensive care. A few moments later, Elizabeth was sick. A stream of bright red blood flew onto her hospital blankets and pooled between her knees. Doctors and nurses came running towards her and merged together as her vision blurred and her head felt fuzzy and light-headed.

She was vaguely conscious of everything happening around her, but the next thing Elizabeth really remembered was the horrible, claustrophobic feel of the smooth camera tube going down her throat. She gagged and tried to pull it out, but someone held her hands and she was too weak anyway. She could feel a cold drip running through her cannula and saw two bags of blood hanging above her head. 'Ulcer,' she heard them mutter, 'just on the greater curvature. I'm not sure I've ever seen one bleeding that much before'. 'Inject it?' Another voice, this one younger. 'Yes, and zap it too I think.' Elizabeth felt a funny feeling deep inside, just beneath her rib cage and then a sharp, intense pain. She tried to cry out, but couldn't because of the tube in her throat. 'That's got it, I think,' the first voice again and she felt the tube slide quickly up her throat. She coughed and coughed as it came out and took great gasps of air.

A few hours later and she was back in intensive care with her family around her. 'It was an ulcer,' one of the young, boyish doctors was explaining, 'sometimes when people are really unwell all the stress causes them to develop and they can bleed, like yours did.' 'Can't you stop them?' John asked, squeezing Elizabeth's contracted hand. She felt too weak and sore to say anything. 'We were trying. We give you a medicine every day to try and protect the stomach, but despite that sometimes, if people have been really unwell, it's just not enough.' John and Elizabeth looked at each other. Each knew they were both thinking the same thing. She was so lucky to be here, so lucky, and the battle had really only just begun, but they would fight it, all the way, and she would get better.

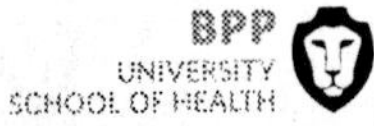

Prognosis

Patients confirmed to have a gastric ulcer require a repeat OGD in six to eight weeks to reassess the ulcer, check for healing and to repeat biopsies and cytology to exclude the diagnosis of gastric carcinoma. This is performed even if the patient is asymptomatic with initial treatment.

The annual recurrence rate is now as low as 2% since the introduction of *H. pylori* eradication therapy.

Inflammatory bowel disease (IBD)

The term IBD encompasses two chronic disease processes: ulcerative colitis (UC) and Crohn's disease (CD) which will be considered separately.

Ulcerative colitis (UC)

Epidemiology

Primarily a disease of the developed world, affecting 70 per 100,000 people are affected with an incidence of 10 per 100,000 per year. Most people present between the ages of 20 and 40 years.

Females are affected more than males and the incidence is higher in the white population, in particular Ashkenazi Jews. In Europe northern populations are affected more frequently than those in the south.

Aetiology

The aetiology remains unclear, but is thought to result from an abnormal pro-inflammatory response of the body to food products or bacteria which are present within the bowel lumen, which is determined by both genetic and environmental factors.

A family history is present in around 25–40% and an association has been demonstrated with particular HLA-DRB1 alleles, whilst other environmental factors that have been implicated include infection, abnormalities in the immune response, defective mucous production and psychosocial factors.

Interestingly cigarette smoking has a protective role but there is some mild evidence to suggest that NSAID use may increase the risk of developing, or exacerbate the severity of, IBD.

Pathophysiology

UC starts in the rectum and spreads proximally. Initially the mucosa becomes inflamed and oedematous. As the disease progresses granuloma formation, bleeding, pus production and eventually ulceration of the epithelial layer is seen. Healing is by mucosal granulation, resulting in the formation of pseudopolyps.

- **Distal disease** (left-sided colitis, proctitis or proctosigmoiditis) – 60% of patients
- **Left-sided colitis** (up to the splenic flexure) – 40% of patients
- **Extensive colitis** (up to hepatic flexure) and pancolitis – 20% of patients

Microscopic features:

- Crypt abscesses
- Mucosal oedema
- Continuous disease
- Dysplastic epithelial changes if longstanding

Macroscopic features:

- Confluent, superficial inflammation
- Pseudopolyps
- Shortened, narrowed 'hosepipe colon'

History/examination

- Bloody diarrhoea
- Colicky abdominal pain, urgency, tenesmus (procto-sigmoiditis or extensive colitis)
- Constipation and rectal bleeding (proctitis)
- Malaise, fever, weight loss
- Symptoms of extra-intestinal disease: joint, cutaneous or eye manifestations

The disease follows a chronic, relapsing-remitting course with precipitants for relapse including stress, infection, antibiotic therapy and drug use eg NSAIDs.

Investigations

Blood tests:

- FBC: anaemia and increased WBC
- Inflammatory markers: raised ESR and CRP
- Biochemistry: low albumin
- Cross-match

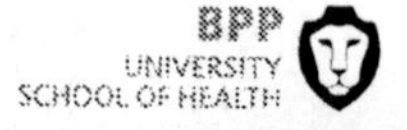

Imaging:

- Erect CXR if perforation suspected
- AXR shows dilatation of large bowel loops, toxic megacolon, mucosal oedema, and proximal faecal loading in proctitis

Sigmoidoscopy/colonoscopy:

- Inflammation of the colonic mucosa, oedema, ulceration, active bleeding and pseudopolyps.
- Colonoscopy should never be performed in acute flare-ups as there is a significant risk of perforation due to the friable nature of the mucosa. It can help to define the extent of disease and differentiate UC from Crohn's disease as well as screen for any evidence of dysplasia.

Histology:

- Biopsy confirms diagnosis and determines the extent of disease

Other:

- Stool MC&S to exclude infective diarrhoea

Management of acute flares

- A to E assessment and resuscitation
- Assess severity using Truelove and Witt's criteria
- Consider emergency surgery
- NBM with IV fluids
- Consider thromboprophylaxis
- Decompression of toxic megacolon and antibiotics if perforation

Pharmacological therapy

1. **Corticosteroids:**
   i) Topical (enema, foam or suppository) or IV
   ii) Usually orally for four weeks in mild relapse; orally for four to six weeks in moderate relapse and IV for five days then orally in severe relapse
   iii) Judicious use due to side effects (diabetes, hypertension, osteoporosis, myopathy, hypokalaemia, cataracts etc) – avoid long-term use and monitor appropriately for side effects

2. **5 - Aminosalicylates (Mesalazine or Sulphasalazine):**
   i) First-line therapy in inducing and maintaining remission in mild/moderate disease, reducing relapse from 80% to 20%
   ii) Orally/enema/suppository. Slow release preparations eg Asacol and Pentasa
   iii) Side effects: rash, headache, acid reflux, diarrhoea, blood dyscrasias

3. **Azathiprine:**
   i) Oral immunosuppressive that acts as a steroid-sparing agent
   ii) Side effects: nausea, headache, bone marrow suppression, hepatitis (monitor LFTs)

4. **Ciclosporin:**
   i) Oral immunosuppressive used in severe UC or if no response to initial treatment. Helps reduce need for urgent surgical intervention
   ii) Side effects: electrolyte disturbances, renal dysfunction, hypertension, seizures, opportunistic infection (monitor levels)

5. **Infliximab:**
   i) Monoclonal antibody against TNF
   ii) Rescue therapy for acute severe colitis or refractory disease
   iii) Only recommended in cases where ciclosporin is contraindicated

Urgent surgical intervention

- **Indications:** colonic perforation, massive haemorrhage, toxic megacolon, failure of medical therapy
- **Procedures:** total colectomy with end ileostomy; proctocolectomy with ileo-rectal anastomosis; proctocolectomy with ileao-anal pouch formation

	Mild	Moderate	Severe
Stool frequency	<4 daily	4–6 daily	>6 daily
Blood in stool	Small amounts	More blood	Visible blood
Anaemia	No	No	Yes
Heart rate	<90	<90	>90
Fever	No	No	>37.8
Inflammatory markers	normal	normal	ESR >30

Note. For severe disease, one or more features of systemic upset must be present.

Table 3.5: NICE definitions of disease severity (based on Truelove and Witt criteria)

Management of chronic disease

The aim of treatment is induction and maintenance of remission:

- Education of patient and family
- Provision of information about patient support groups eg National Association for Colitis and Crohn's disease
- Dietician referral – may need iron and nutritional supplementation
- Referral to clinical psychologist
- Long-term follow-up with gastroenterology

Pharmacological therapy:

- Topical or oral aminosalicylates
- Steroid-sparing agents if aminosalicylates not tolerated or effective

Surgical therapy:

- **Indications:** disease not controlled by maximal medical therapy; development of carcinoma (or prophylaxis); prevention of adverse effects on childhood growth
- **Procedures:** as for acute disease

Up to 30% of patients may ultimately require surgical intervention as part of the management for their UC.

Gastrointestinal complications

- **Haemorrhage:** either chronic, minimal loss, resulting in microcytic anaemia or massive haemorrhage requiring emergency intervention.
- **Toxic megacolon:** haemodynamically, rapidly deteriorating patient with AXR revealing: lack of faecal shadows, mucosal thickening, dilated loops of colon (>6 cm); urgent surgical intervention required.
- **Pouchitis:** in patients who have undergone surgery resulting in formation of an ileo-anal pouch. Infection can be managed with metronidazole and ciprofloxacin.
- **Carcinoma:** increased risk of developing colorectal carcinoma. Greater risk in patients with duration of disease, recurrent relapses and co-existing primary sclerosing cholangitis. Colonoscopic screening recommended from ten years following onset of symptoms.

Extra-intestinal manifestations/complications

- General: weight loss, lethargy, growth retardation
- Haematological: increased risk of venous and arterial thrombosis
- Eyes: episcleritis and uveitis
- Hepatobiliary: fatty changes in the liver, primary sclerosing cholangitis and cholangiocarcinoma
- Skin: erythemanodosum, pyodermagangrenosum
- Musculoskeletal: arthritis (peripheral and axial) with an identical picture to ankylosing spondylitis and sacroiliitis. Clubbing

Prognosis

The majority of patients with UC suffer from recurrent relapses; however, their overall mortality is comparable to the general population.

The main causes of morbidity and mortality are recurrent severe flare-ups of colitis which are unresponsive to therapy and the development of colon cancer in patients who have long-standing disease.

Crohn's disease (CD)

Epidemiology

Less common than UC, CD is more common in Europe and North America with a prevalence of 50 in 100,000 and an incidence of around 5 per 100,000 per year. There is a particularly increased risk in Ashkenazi Jews.

Patients present in early adulthood but there is a second peak in the seventh decade. Small bowel disease is more common in the younger population whilst older individuals tend to have more colonic features. Women are almost twice as frequently affected as men.

Aetiology

Genetic factors are thought to have a greater role than in UC. First-degree relatives of affected individuals have an increased risk (>10%) and a 40% concordance has been found in monozygotic twins. The CARD 15 gene and anti-BPI antibodies have been implicated.

Smoking increases the risk of disease four-fold and worsens progression. Other environmental factors include gut infections, diet and abnormal immune responses.

Pathophysiology

CD can affect any part of the gastrointestinal system but most commonly involves the terminal ileumand ileo-caecal regions in a discontinuous pattern.

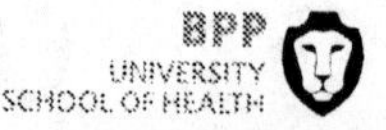

Microscopic features:

- Transmural inflammation
- Non-caseating epitheloid granuloma formation

Macroscopic features:

- Superficial discontinuous apthous ulcers that become deep fissuring ulcers (skip lesions)
- Cobblestoning
- Oedema
- Fibrosis
- Stricture, adhesion and fistula formation – may cause obstruction

History/examination

- Diarrhoea, abdominal pain, weight loss, malaise, anorexia, rectal bleeding and occasionally fever.
- Symptoms vary depending on extent and location of GI involvement.
  - Small bowel disease: steatorrhoea
  - Large bowel disease: rectal bleeding
- The patient may be thin or cachectic or have features of malabsorption: abdominal distension, pallor, oedema, bruising, and mouth ulcers.
- Perianal skin tags, fissures, fistulae and abscesses are common.
- There may be a mass in the right iliac fossa.
- Clubbing with long-standing disease.

Investigations

Blood tests:

- FBC: anaemia due to iron, vitamin B12 or folate deficiency, reactive thrombocytosis
- Inflammatory markers: increased ESR, CRP and WCC
- Biochemistry: reduced albumin, which can be a marker of malabsorption/malnutrition and reduced calcium

Microbiology:

- Stool MC&S to exclude an infective cause

Imaging:

- Ultrasound and CT scan if an intra-abdominal abscess or mass is suspected
- MRI for complicated perianal disease
- Sinogram to map an enterocutaneous fistulae tract prior to surgery

Sigmoidoscopy/colonoscopy:

- Help to determine the extent of disease and may illustrate thickened bowel wall, patchy inflammation and cobblestoning.
- Capsule endoscopy may be helpful in small bowel disease.

Histology:

- Biopsy from the rectum or large bowel is required for accurate diagnosis.

Other:

- Barium follow-through/small bowel enema will illustrate features such as strictures, fistulae, abscesses, 'rose thorn' ulcers and polyps.

Management of acute flares

See management of acute flares in UC.

Management of chronic disease

As in UC, the aim of treatment is to induce and maintain a period of remission.

- Education of patient and family
- Provision of information about patient support groups eg National Association for Colitis and Crohn's Disease
- Dietician referral and dietary modification
  - Iron and folate supplements often required
  - Elemental diets can be effective (liquid nutritionally balanced diet, without protein antigens that can trigger relapses) as steroid
  - Avoid high residue foods (sweetcorn, uncooked vegetables, nuts etc) in those with small bowel strictures, as they act as food boluses and can result in obstruction
  - Inpatients with severe relapses may need enteral or TPN
- Referral to clinical psychologist
- Long-term follow-up with gastroenterology
- Loperamide or codeine phosphate to reduce diarrhoea

Pharmacological therapy

1. **Corticosteroids:**
   i) Proven efficacy for use in the treatment of relapses
   ii) Not helpful in maintaining long-term remission

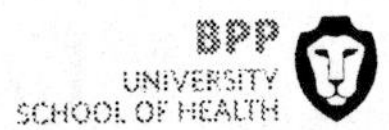

iii) Usually orally for four weeks in mild relapse with gradual reduction; IV for five days then orally in severe relapse
iv) Rectal steroids for proctitis
v) Oral budesonide in ileo-caecal involvement as the preparation releases the drug in the ileum, reducing systemic side effects
vi) Judicious use due to side effects (diabetes, hypertension, osteoporosis, myopathy, hypokalaemia, cataracts etc) – avoid long-term use and monitor appropriately for side effects

2. **5-Aminosalicylates:**
   i) Sulfasalazine is more effective in Crohn's colitis compared to small bowel disease.
   ii) Slow release preparations of mesalazine such as Pentasa are primarily active in the small bowel and is used in the treatment of active disease as well as maintenance.

3. **Azathioprine:**
   i) An immunosuppressive agent, and has a role as a steroid-sparing agent as in UC.
   ii) Indicated in refractory Crohn's.

4. **Methotrexate:**
   i) An immunosuppressive agent that can be used instead of azathioprine in patients who don't tolerate it
   ii) Indicated in refractory Crohn's
   iii) Adverse effects include bone marrow suppression, hepatic fibrosis and pneumonitis (FBC and LFT monitoring)

5. **Infliximab:**
   i) Can induce remission in patients with severe Crohn's unresponsive to maximal medical therapy.
   ii) Adverse effects include infection, infusion reaction, and rarely B cell lymphoma.

6. **Antibiotics:**
   i) Metronidazole and ciprofloxacin are usually used in active Crohn's, particularly in perianal involvement.

Surgical management

Up to 80% of Crohn's patients with long-standing relapses require surgical treatment. Due to recurrence, up to half of these patients may require a further operation within ten years.

- Strictures are managed with minimal resection or strictureplasty.
- Surgical resection depends on the location of disease. The most common procedure is excision of the caecum and terminal ileum with side-to-side anastomosis.
- Intra-abdominal abscesses are drained, often under radiological guidance and enteric fistulae are usually resected.

Gastrointestinal complications

- **Strictures:** may result in obstruction.
- **Perforation:** may result in abscess formation.
- **Abscess and fistula:** abscesses tend to form around inflamed bowel and discharge via fistulae into the colon, bladder (recurrent UTI, haematuria), skin and vagina (faeculent discharge or flatus per vagina).
- Anal fissures, abscesses and fistulae.
- Haemorrhage that is usually mild and long-standing resulting in anaemia.
- Toxic megacolon is very uncommon.
- There is a slightly higher incidence of bowel cancer in Crohn's patients compared to the general population.

Systemic features/complications

- **General:** weight loss, fever, short stature in children
- **Eyes:** episcleritis and uveitis
- **Oral:** mouth ulcers
- **Haematological:** vascular thrombosis, auto immune haemolytic anaemia
- **Renal:** uric acid calculi and/or oxalate calculi
- **Hepatobiliary:** gallstones, fatty changes, cholangiocarcinoma, sclerosing cholangitis (more common in UC)
- **Skin:** erythema nodosum, pyoder magangrenosum.
- **Musculoskeletal:** arthritis (peripheral and axial) with an identical picture to ankylosing spondylitis and sacroiliitis. Clubbing

Prognosis

Mortality is twice that of the general population but this may be decreasing with better medical management and more conservative surgical management.

There is an increased risk of both colorectal and small bowel adenocarcinoma.

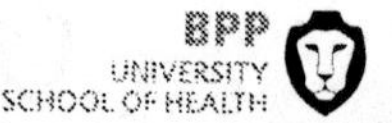

Crohn's Disease	Ulcerative Colitis
Terminal ileum, colon and anal involvement	Colon and rectum involvement
No bile duct involvement	Bile duct involvement
Patchy/skip lesions	Continuous lesions
Transmural inflammation	Shallow, mucosal
Granulomas present	Granulomas absent
Stenosis common	Stenosis rare

Table 3.6: Pathological differences between Crohn's and UC

Irritable bowel syndrome (IBS)

Epidemiology

IBS is the most common complaint in gastroenterology clinics. 1 in 10 adults have episodic symptoms with a female-to-male ratio of 3:1. Peak incidence is between the ages of 20 and 30.

Aetiology

No organic cause has been found. There is an association with abnormal intestinal motility, and may be influenced by abnormal communication between the enteric and central nervous systems.

There is also an association with affective mental disorders and food intolerance. It may result after an episode of acute infective gastroenteritis.

History/examination

The diagnosis is clinical. There is an international agreed set of diagnostic criteria known as ROME II:

- **At least three months in one year of abdominal discomfort (central/ lower) that has at least two of the following features starting with the pain:**
  - Relief on defecation
  - Change in bowel frequency
  - Change in the appearance and consistency of stool
- Other supporting symptoms:
  - Frequency of <3/week and >3/day (alternating constipation and diarrhoea)
  - Straining
  - Hard/lumpy or loose/watery stool
  - Urgency to defecate
  - Tenesmus
  - Passing mucous with stool
  - Abdominal bloating
- Other gastrointestinal features – non-diagnostic:
  - Nausea and vomiting
  - Dyspepsia and heartburn
  - Dysphagia
  - Anal pain due to levator ani spasm
- Associations:
  - Anxiety, stress, depression and obsession with bowel habit
  - History of adverse life events
  - Higher rates of reported sexual and physical abuse
  - Gynaecological symptoms such as dyspareunia, dysmenorrhoea, and bowel symptoms occurring around menstruation
  - Urinary frequency and urgency
  - Headaches, and lethargy

IBS is a diagnosis of exclusion. These ALARM symptoms require further investigation:

- Weight loss
- Rectal bleeding
- Anorexia
- Patients over 40 years
- Nocturnal abdominal pain or diarrhoea
- Mouth ulcers

- On examination the patient is generally normal.
- There may be diffuse or localised abdominal tenderness.
- Occasionally, the descending colon may be palpable and tender.

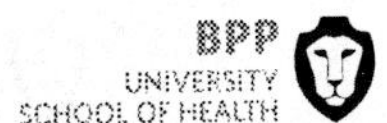

Investigations

The diagnosis is primarily clinical and investigations are primarily to exclude another cause.

Blood tests:

- FBC
- U&Es
- LFTs
- Inflammatory markers: CRP and ESR
- Thyroid function tests and anti-tissue trans-glutaminase antibodies to exclude thyrotoxicosis and coeliac disease

Sigmoidoscopy/colonoscopy:

- Rectal biopsy and barium enema can be performed if there is uncertainty regarding the diagnosis.

Other:

- Stool MC&S

Management

- Ensure an organic cause has been excluded
- Reassurance to reduce anxiety
- Relaxation classes, CBT or hypnosis to reduce anxiety

Symptom control:

- **Pain:** antispasmodics such as mebeverine or buscopan (particularly before meals), calcium channel blockers and peppermint oil, tricyclic anti-depressant and selective serotonin reuptake inhibitors
- **Diarrhoea:** loperamide or codeine
- **Constipation:** high fibre diet or bulking agents such as fybogel
- **Reducing flares:** avoidance of potential dietary triggers such as wheat, dairy or fructose

Prognosis

Most patients are symptom-free after five years.

Urinary tract infection and pyelonephritis

UTI: the presence of >10 bacteria/ml in a freshly voided sample of urine.

Pyelonephritis: an infection of the renal parenchyma, usually following ascending infection from the bladder.

Epidemiology

UTI is a very common condition worldwide, accounting for 2% of GP consultations in the UK. It is significantly more common in women, the elderly and those living in care homes.

Pyelonephritis has an incidence of approximately 10/10,000 per year in women and 2/10,000 per year in males. It is more common in younger women.

Aetiology

Infection most commonly is caused by bacteria entering the bladder via the urethra but blood borne infection is also seen.

The most common infecting organisms are part of the normal gut flora, in particular *Escherichia coli* (70–80%). Staphylococcus, Streptococcus, Pseudomonas, Klebsiella and Proteus are also common infecting organisms. Common causes of sterile pyuria include partially treated bacterial infection, tuberculosis or inflammation from a non-infective cause.

Pathophysiology

Risk factors:

- **Females:** shorter urethra allowing easier access for organisms to the bladder. During micturition, there may be backflow of urine in the shorter female urethra, which does not usually occur in the longer male urethra.
- **Sexual activity:** can predispose to infection in females especially with a change in partner. It is advised for females to empty their bladder prior to and following sexual intercourse.
- **Urinary retention and incomplete emptying of the bladder** in patients results in the static urine within the bladder increasing the likelihood of infection.
- **Chronic prostate disease** in males.
- **Urinary catheterisation:** can introduce bacteria into the urinary tract and hence a sterile technique is essential. Indwelling catheters in particular create a potential for infection, with colonisation of the biofilm within days of insertion.

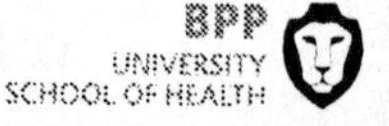

- **Immunosuppressed or diabetic** patients are at an increased risk of infection.
- **Pregnancy** increases progesterone level which causes dilatation and relaxation of the ureters. This enables reflux of urine into the ureters increasing the risk of more serious upper tract infection.

Risk factors for UTI:

- Female
- Sexual activity (particularly with change in partners)
- Urinary retention and incomplete voiding
- Previous history of UTI or pyelonephritis
- Chronic prostatic disease
- Urinary catheterisation
- Immunosuppression or diabetes
- Pregnancy

History/examination

- Presentation can vary from asymptomatic UTI to acute pyelonephritis with severe sepsis.
- UTI examination findings:
  - Possible signs of sepsis
  - Suprapubic tenderness
  - Palpable bladder if acute retention
- Pyelonephritis examination findings
  - Clearer signs of sepsis, ie fever, tachycardia, hypotension
  - Possible rigors
  - Loin/renal angle tenderness

Investigations

Urine dipstick:

- Nitrites positive, produced from bacterial conversion of urinary nitrates.
- Leucocytes positive confirms pyuria.
- A trace of protein or blood may be present.
- The dipstick does not positively diagnose or exclude an infection.

Mid-streamurine (MSU) for microscopy and culture:

- Organisms may be present and identified along with antibiotic susceptibility.
- White cells suggest infection and white cell casts indicate involvement of the upper tract as the casts are formed in the renal tubules.
- A UTI is diagnosed if there are >10 bacteria/ml of urine.
- Send a morning first-pass urine sample from the first micturition of the day for patients suspected of having mycobacterial infection.

Blood tests:

- FBC: raised white cells
- U&E: increased urea and creatinine in dehydration or if there is outflow tract obstruction
- Increased inflammatory markers
- Glucose to exclude diabetes
- Blood cultures

In children and men, patients with recurrent UTIs and all pyelonephritis further investigations are required:

- AXR to exclude calculi (see Figure 3.3)
- Ultrasound KUB
- Further tests as indicated: IVU, isotope scans such as DMSA, cystoscopy

Management

- Analgesia.
- Increased fluid intake. Pyelonephritis may require IV fluids due to more profound dehydration and associated nausea and vomiting.
- Antibiotics:
  - Empirical antibiotics according to local protocol should be commenced if symptomatic with a positive urine dip.
  - A three-day course of trimethoprim is the usual first choice for an uncomplicated UTI.
  - For pyelonephritis IV antibiotics are often required initially and should be based on local guidelines.
- An asymptomatic positive dipstick does not require treatment except in pregnant women.
- Indwelling catheters should be changed.
- In both males and females a cause should be sought in recurrent infection.

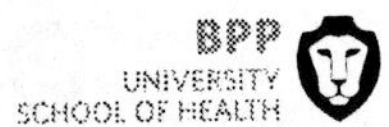

Complications of recurrent UTIs include renal scarring and chronic renal impairment.

Prevention of recurrent UTIs

- Avoid constipation as this can prevent complete bladder emptying.
- Avoid bubble baths and soapy irritants in bath water.
- Double voiding on micturition, which involves attempting to completely empty the bladder initially and then voiding again after five minutes.
- If UTI is associated with sexual intercourse, encourage micturition afterwards.
- Drinking plenty of fluid and in particular cranberry juice which has been shown to reduce the incidence of bacteruria.
- Good catheter care and early removal of unnecessary catheters.
- Prophylaxis with a low-dose of antibiotic daily but this should only be instigated on specialist advice.

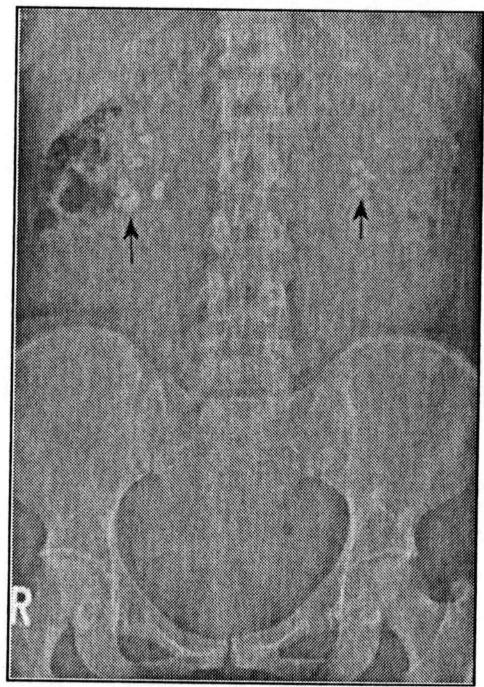

Figure 3.3: KUB X-ray showing bilateral multiple renal calculi (arrows)

Further reading and references

1. British Society of Gastroenterology. (2007) *Guidelines for osteoporosis in inflammatory bowel disease and coeliac disease.* [Online]. Available from: www.bsg.org.uk/pdf_word_docs/ost_coe_ibd.pdf [Accessed 7 November 2016].
2. British Society of Gastroenterology. (2004) *Guidelines for the management of inflammatory bowel disease in adults.* [Online]. Available from: www.bsg.org.uk/images/stories/docs/clinical/guidelines/ibd/ibd_2011.pdf [Accessed 7 November 2016].
3. Kapoor, N., Bassi, A., Sturgess, R., et al. (2005) Predictive value of alarm features in a rapid access upper gastrointestinal cancer service. *Gut* 2005; 54(1):40-5.
4. National Institute for Health and Care Excellence. (2008) *Irritable bowel syndrome* (CG061). [Online]. Available from: www.nice.org.uk/guidance/cg61/chapter/About-this-guideline [Accessed 7 November 2016].
5. National Institute for Health and Care Excellence. (2010) *Ulcerative colitis CKS.* [Online]. Available from: http://cks.nice.org.uk/ulcerative-colitis [Accessed 7 November 2016].
6. National Institute for Health and Care Excellence. (2015) *Suspected cancer: recognition and referral* (NG12). [Online] Available from: www.nice.org.uk/guidance/ng12?unlid=98748146920151291155552,5161700902016923910 [Accessed 7 November 2016].
7. Scottish Intercollegiate Guidelines Network. (2006) *Management of suspected bacterial urinary tract infection in adults.* 88. Edinburgh, Scottish Intercollegiate Guidelines Network.
8. Dent, J., Jones, R., Kahrilas, P., et al. (1996) The Montreal definition and classification of gastroesophageal reflux disease: a global evidence-based consensus. *Am J Gastroenterol* 2006; 101:1900–20.
9. Marshall, B.J. and Warren, J.R. (1986) Unidentified curved bacilli on gastric epithelium in active chronic gastritis. *Lancet* 1986; 1: 1273–5.

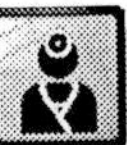

Acute back pain

Differential diagnosis

System/Organ	Disease
Mechanical back pain	**Back pain** Sciatica
Degenerative	Osteoarthritis
Traumatic	Osteoporosis (vertebral fracture)
Inflammatory	Ankylosing spondylitis
Infective	**Osteomyelitis** Tuberculosis (Pott's disease) Discitis
Tumours	Tumours of the bone (primary/metastases)

Table 3.7: Differential diagnosis for causes of acute back pain

Epidemiology

A very common complaint; around 80% of adults experience back pain at some time in their lifetime. It carries a significant level of morbidity, accounts for about 5% of GP consultations and is responsible for approximately 50 million lost working days per year in the UK.

It is mostly self-limiting, settling within two months; however, there are a number of more serious causes. The history should include the 'red and yellow flag' symptoms for chronicity. These are outlined in Table 3.7.

Mechanical back pain is most common in those aged 15–30 years. Degenerative joint disease and osteoporosis are most common in those over the age of 50 years. In middle-aged individuals (30–50 years) causes such as malignancy and a prolapsed intervertebral disc must be considered.

Aetiology

Table 3.9 outlines the various causes of back pain, relevant differentials to consider as well as ways in which to determine the cause by the clinical findings on history and examination.

Risk factors:

- Abnormal posture
- Insufficient back support
- Wearing high-heeled shoes
- Unequal leg length
- Heavy manual labour
- Heavy manual labour
- Anxiety/depression
- Pregnancy
- Ageing

Red flag symptoms	Yellow flag symptoms
• Age under 20 or over 55 • Non-mechanical pain which is worsening • Pyrexia of unknown origin • Pain in the thoracic region of the spine • Focal neurological features • Major trauma (or more minor trauma if there is a diagnosis of osteoporosis) • Cancer • Systemic features such as weight loss • Immunosuppression • Use of steroids • New structural deformity • New bladder dysfunction • New faecal incontinence • Saddle anaesthesia	• Belief that the pain is harmful and disabling • Avoidance behaviour • Reduced activity levels • Low mood/depression • Social withdrawal • Problems at work • Lack of social/family support

Table 3.8: Red and yellow flag symptoms for acute back pain

Pathophysiology

Pathophysiology is dependent on aetiology.

History/examination

- Age, sex, and occupation

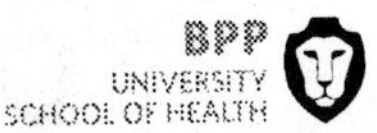

- History of trauma or injury to the back or other precipitating factors such as falls, heavy lifting or strenuous activity
- Any previous back conditions or surgery
- Onset of symptoms and duration
- Character of pain eg sharp, dull, shooting
- Radiation of pain
- Exacerbating or relieving factors
- Paraesthesia
- Weakness in leg(s)
- Bowel or bladder dysfunction
- Early morning stiffness (and duration)
- Relevant medical conditions such as rheumatoid arthritis, osteoporosis, osteoarthritis
- Any contraindications to using NSAIDs
- Any stress at work or at home

Cauda equina syndrome

- Nerve root pain in both lower limbs
- Sacral paresthesia in saddle distribution
- Flaccid paralysis of the lower limbs (may present as weakness)
- Bladder or bowel dysfunction

Acute cord compression

- Usually bilateral
- Lower motor neuron deficit at the level of cord compression with upper motor neuron features below this level – although acutely no upper motor neuron signs will be seen
- Disturbance of sphincter function

Perforated aneurysm

- Pulsatile mass in the abdomen
- Signs of peritonism
- Evidence of shock
- Radio-femoral delay

Also examine carefully for the following features:

- Scars or obvious deformity in the back, eg due to scoliosis or kyphosis.
- Observe the gait for any abnormal posture or limping.
- Palpate the spine in order to elicit any vertebral body or para-spinal tenderness.
- Check movements such as flexion, extension, lateral flexion and rotation, and also push the iliac crests together in order to elicit any restriction of movement at the sacroiliac joints.
- Look for any clubbing, muscle wasting, signs of weight loss such as cachexia, and anaemia.
- Feel for any masses in the abdomen.
- Peripheral pulses and perfusion.
- A full neurological examination.
- Straight leg raise.
- Digital rectal exam to assess anal tone.
- Perineal and perianal sensation.

Investigations

Blood tests:

- FBC: anaemia or raised WCC
- Inflammatory markers
- Bone profile: calcium, phosphate and ALP. Increased calcium and ALP may suggest bony metastases. Calcium is increased and ALP normal in myeloma and ALP increased and calcium normal in metabolic bone disease
- PSA

Microbiology:

- Blood cultures: Including AFB if spinal infection is suspected

Imaging:

- X-rays:
  - History of trauma, especially in those over the age of 55 years
  - Degenerative changes in osteoarthritis
  - Signal alignment abnormalities such as in kyphosis and scoliosis
  - Destruction of vertebral bodies by presence of infection or malignancy
  - Pathological fractures
  - Spondylolisthesis (most commonly at L5/S1 where there is forward subluxation of one vertebral body on the one below it)
- CT:
  - Imaging of the spinal canal in order to elicit any specific pathology
- MRI:
  - Indicated if any of the surgical emergencies are suspected
  - Especially useful for detecting any intervertebral disc abnormalities
  - The best investigation to demonstrate cord compression
  - Will show intra-spinal tumours, as well as any cysts or abscesses
- Bone scan:
  - 'Hot' spots will indicate infection, malignant lesions or fractures as well as degenerative disease

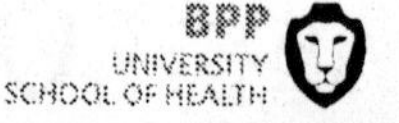

Examine for signs of medical emergencies as follows:

Causes	Differentials	Characteristics to differentiate the causes of back pain
Simple/ mechanical	• Intervertebral disc prolapse (can compress the nerve root resulting in sciatica) • Injury to facet joints, spinal ligaments or muscle • Degenerative changes including osteoarthritis • Fractures • Spondylolisthesis is when there is anterior displacement of one vertebra relative to the one below. • Spondylolysis is a stress fracture of the pars interarticularis (most commonly of L5), common in gymnasts and is a cause of Spondylolisthesis • Spinal stenosis	• Tends to be of sudden onset • Often unilateral pain affecting the leg and buttock • Pain mostly in evenings • No morning stiffness • Pain is worse on movement in particular after exercise • Relief with rest
Inflammatory/ infective	• Ankylosing spondylitis • Mycobacterium tuberculosis • Salmonella • Brucella	• More gradual onset • Often bilateral pain • Pain is constant and is at its worst in the mornings • Associated with morning stiffness • Exercise tends to relieve symptoms
Sinister cause	• Metastatic carcinoma (from carcinoma of breast, lung, kidney, thyroid, and prostate) • Myeloma • Bacterial/Tuberculosis/Osteomyelitis • Cauda equina syndrome • Cord compression	• A constant pain with no relieving factors, waking patient at night • Systemic symptoms usually present such as fever, weight loss, night sweats, anorexia • Localised bony tenderness • Neurological signs involving more than one spinal root level • Signs present in both lower limbs • Altered bowel, bladder, sexual function
Metabolic	• Osteomalacia • Osteoporosis • Wilson's disease • Haemochromatosis • Paget's disease	
Referred pain	• Pelvic disease • Vasculature for example an aortic aneurysm • Genitourinary (bladder, prostate) • Gastrointestinal disease such as pancreatitis • Retroperitoneal structures such as the uterus and kidneys	

Table 3.9: Differential diagnosis of acute back pain and differentiating features

Management

- The more sinister causes of pain must be excluded and managed accordingly before using treatments for non-specific back pain.
- Empower the patient to help manage their pain.
- Education about lower back pain and the usual course.
- Explore patient concerns and expectations.
- Encourage physical activity and avoid total bed rest. However, more strenuous activities should be moderated.
- **Pharmacological therapies** – shown in large RCTs not to be generally effective
  - Paracetamol
  - NSAIDs
  - Weak opioids
  - Muscle relaxants

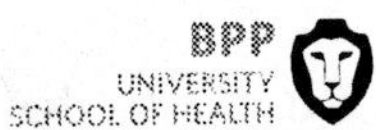

  - Low-dose antidepressants such as Amitriptylline
  - Consider strong opioids and pain clinic referral if possible

- **Non-pharmacological**
  - Physiotherapy/exercise programme: helps strengthen core muscles and improve posture
  - Manual therapy: spinal manipulation, spinal mobilisation and massage
  - Acupuncture

- **Surgical**
  - Discectomy/microdiscectomy or spinal fusion may be indicated for significant pain unresponsive to medical treatment

Prognosis

- Most patients (more than 90%) with acute back pain will be symptom-free after 6 weeks.
- A number of patients develop chronic back pain which can result in significant morbidity – as predicted by yellow flag symptoms.

Osteoarthritis

Osteoarthritis is a group of conditions affecting synovial joints characterised by loss of articular cartilage, resulting in pain, deformity and loss of function. Although previously thought of as a normal consequence of ageing associated with 'wear and tear', it is now known that it is caused by localised inflammation.

Epidemiology

Incidence and prevalence increase with age. It is the commonest cause of arthritis in the elderly, hip and knee joint replacements and GP consultations.

Aetiology

A multifactorial condition which can be primary or secondary.

Risk factors

- Increasing age
- Obesity
- Male gender <age 45; female gender >age 45
- Smoking
- Manual occupation
- Joint trauma
- Abnormal joint loading
- Genetic: polygenetic inheritance

Pathophysiology

There are three main disease mechanisms:

1. Loss of cartilage: the chondrocytes produce an increased amount of enzymes which are responsible for the degradation of cartilage.
2. Remodelling of bone: increased bone turn-over results in subchondral bone sclerosis with the formation of cysts and proliferation of new bone and osteophyte formation. The joint contour changes as a result of these.
3. Inflammation of the synovium: there is an increase in the amount of synovial fluid.

History/examination

- Joint pain:
  - Particular joints
  - Severity and nature of pain
  - Impact on activities of daily living
  - Joint stiffness: after inactivity, which is usually more problematic first thing in the morning lasting less than 30 minutes
- Hand: what daily tasks are becoming difficult
- Hip: pain in the groin, buttock or anterior thigh
- Knee: pain on kneeling, climbing stairs and getting in and out of cars
- Spine: pain on movement. The cervical and lumbar regions are more commonly affected
- On examination joint deformities lead to a reduced range of movement
  - **Hands:**
    - o Heberden's nodes (swelling at the distal interphalangeal joints)
    - o Bouchard's node (swelling at the proximal interphalangeal joints)
  - **Hip:**
    - o Pain on internal rotation is usually the first sign of osteoarthritis of the hip
    - o Mobilise and look for antalgic gait
  - **Knee:**
    - o Obvious deformity
    - o Reduced use may result in quadriceps wasting
    - o Knee pain may represent referred pain from the hip, so always examine the hip joint as well

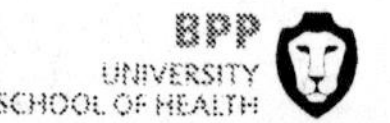

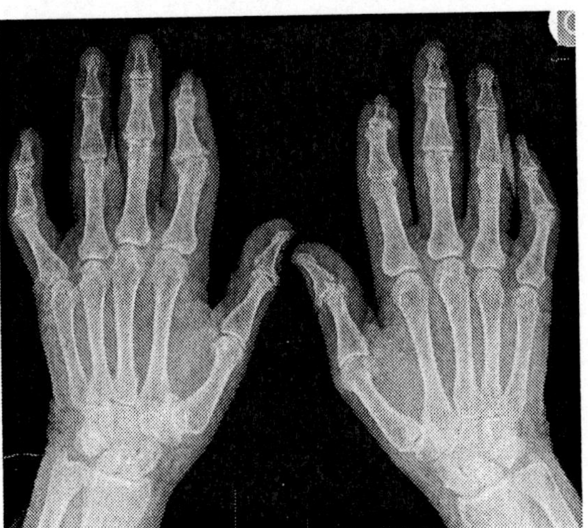

Figure 3.4: Radiograph showing osteoarthritic changes – Bouchard and Heberden's nodes, loss of joint space, subchondral sclerosis, cysts, osteophytes and joint subluxation in the hands

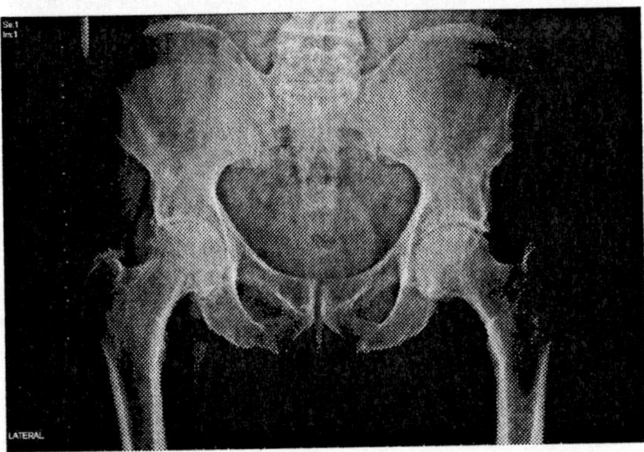

Figure 3.5: Pelvic radiograph showing arthritic changes – loss of joint space, osteophytes, subchondral cysts and sclerosis in the hip joints

- **Spine:**
    - Palpate the bony prominences of the spine for localised pain
    - Neurological examination to look for signs indicative of nerve entrapment

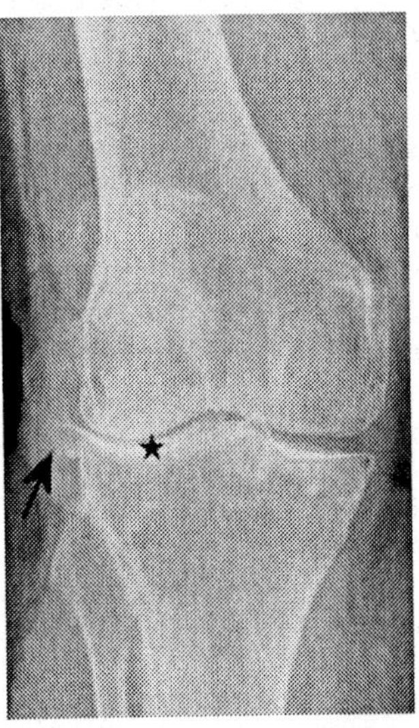

Figure 3.6: Radiograph of right knee showing decreased joint space in the lateral compartment (star) with osteophyte formation (arrow) in keeping with osteoarthritis

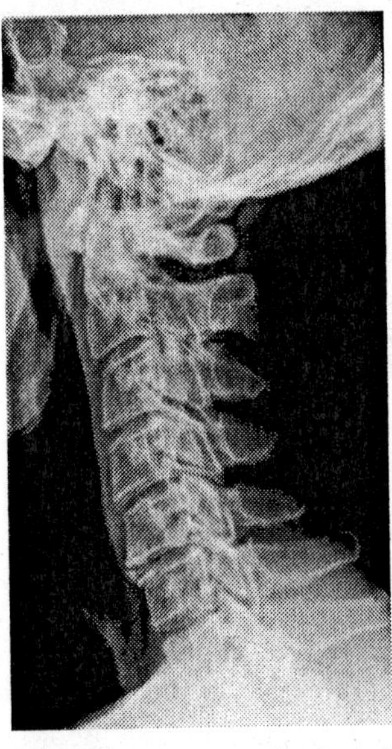

Figure 3.7: Lateral radiograph of cervical spine showing joint space narrowing and osteophytes, in keeping with osteoarthritis

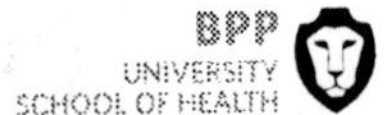

Investigations

- Mainly a clinical diagnosis confirmed by imaging.

Imaging:

- X-rays:
  - Loss of joint space
  - Osteophytes
  - Subchondral sclerosis
  - Subchondral cyst
  - Joint subluxation
  - Soft-tissue swelling
- CT/MRI scan of the spine:
  - Vertebral disc pathology
  - Spinal canal stenosis
  - Cord compression
  - Facet joint arthritis
  - Square appearance of the hand (subluxation of the base of the thumb); the wrist and MCP joints are usually not affected which can help differentiate the disease from rheumatoid arthritis

Management

This is a difficult condition to manage. Aims of treatment include: symptom relief, maintenance of function and quality of life.

Management should be patient centred and take a holistic approach (see further reading and references).

- Patient education and empowerment
- Management plan devised in conjunction with the patient, family and carers
- Weight loss and management
- Physiotherapy can aid pain reduction, increase joint mobility and strengthen supporting muscles such as the quadriceps for the knee
- Occupational therapy
- Other non-pharmacological treatments include orthotic aids, walking aids, appropriate footwear, heat/cold treatment, TENS and hydrotherapy
- **Pharmacological:**
  - Oral analgesia as per WHO analgesic ladder

Case Study: A painful journey

Mrs W had three children whom she loved dearly. The oldest two were working in London now and the youngest would be joining them next year when he finally finished university – to her great sadness, they were all so far away. While she wouldn't change her children for the world, Mrs W sometimes resented the toll that motherhood had taken on her body. She had never returned to her pre-pregnancy weight after the birth of her last child, and somehow the pounds had just piled on over the years. Housework, hours spent at a desk at work, even giving hugs, everything had worn her out and for the last few years she had felt a horrible aching pain in her knees. The left was definitely the worst, particularly in the morning or after walking and she could sometimes feel bones grinding together when she walked. She noticed that she had begun to limp and avoided stairs or uneven surfaces. She could no longer go walking with her husband and even moving around the house was beginning to be difficult. Night-time was excruciating – there just seemed no escape.

Mrs W's GP organised an X-ray of her knees, which showed degenerative osteoarthritic changes. She gave Mrs W some strengthening exercises and referred her for physiotherapy and a weight-loss programme. No painkillers seemed to help; even injections into the knee only provided only temporary relief and physiotherapy only seemed to make the pain worse. Over the years as her life shrunk around her, Mrs W became thoroughly depressed and avoided leaving the house as much as possible, frequently spending whole days just sitting sadly thinking about the past. Her GP started some antidepressants, but they didn't seem to help – nothing could take away the pain.

Eventually, Mrs W was referred to an orthopaedic surgeon who offered her a left total knee replacement. She was terrified by the prospect of an operation, even one that was planned. However, over the next few months, pre-operative assessments and education sessions helped quieten some of her anxiety and she underwent the operation smoothly. Despite only being in hospital a few days, the recovery took longer than she expected and her knee remained stiff and sore for months afterwards. However, about six months later, she walked into her follow-up outpatient appointment without a stick or a limp, a big smile on her face; 'the right one's still bad of course,' she said, when the consultant asked how things were going, 'but even with just the left one, it's like I've got a new life, not just a new knee'.

- Topical eg NSAIDs and capsacin
- Intra-articular corticosteroid injections when pain is moderate to severe

- **Surgery** (pain relief, or to increase mobility if possible):
  - Arthroscopy and debridement
  - Arthrodesis
  - Osteotomy
  - Joint replacement

Prognosis

A slowly progressive disease with significant degree of morbidity.

Osteoporosis

A systemic condition resulting from a reduction in the bone mass and quality, causing thin and fragile bones with increased susceptibility to fractures.

Epidemiology

Osteoporosis is seen most commonly in white post-menopausal women and more than 70% of osteoporotic fractures are in females. Incidence increases with age and it is more common in developed countries.

The lifetime risk of fragility fracture is 40% for a white woman and 13% for a white man. There are over 300,000 fragility fractures per year in the UK.

Hip fractures have an incidence of 4.3 per 100,000 females aged 45–64 years and 90.1 per 100,000 females aged 65–85 years per year.

Vertebral fractures occur in 1–2% of females aged 44–54, increasing to >10% in those aged over 65.

Aetiology

Risk factors:

- Female gender
- Family history of fragility fracture
- Inflammatory bowel disease and coeliac disease
- Post-menopausal
- Low BMI
- Smoking
- Caucasian
- Glucocorticoid excess
- Alcohol excess
- Age
- Hyperthyroidism
- Low dietary calcium
- Past history of fracture

Pathophysiology

Osteoporosis may result from not achieving an optimal peak bone mass in the early 20s, which is governed by both genetic and environmental factors.

The condition also results from bone loss seen with ageing. This occurs at about 1% per year except in post-menopausal women where the reduction in oestrogen causes a more rapid deterioration. There is usually an increase in bone resorption and a reduction in bone formation. Both factors contribute to thin and fragile bones which are more susceptible to fractures from low-impact trauma. Most fractures involve the hips, wrists and vertebral bodies.

History/examination

- Pain: onset, location and any deformity (especially kyphosis)
- History of trauma (including low-impact)
- Family history of osteoporosis and fragility fracture
- Menstrual history
- Corticosteroid use
- Smoking and alcohol history
- Diabetes, Cushing's syndrome, multiple myeloma
- Any reduction in height
- History of falls
- Features of steroid excess: moon facies, buffalo hump, bruising, straiae
- Gait abnormalities

Investigations

Blood tests:

- FBC
- U&Es: usually normal
- Thyroid function tests
- Calcium – high in hyperparathyroidism and low in vitamin D deficiency
- ALP – raised if recent fracture
- Further tests depend on clinical suspicion of an underlying cause, eg parathyroid hormone and vitamin D level, myeloma screen, cortisol levels

Imaging:

- **X-ray:** confirm the presence of a fracture.
- **Spinal X-rays:** vertebral body compression fractures.
- Bones may appear osteopenic on X-ray but osteoporosis cannot be diagnosed on plain X-rays.

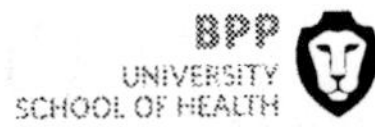

T-score	Interpretation
−1.0 or above	Normal
−2.5 to −1.0	Osteopenia
−2.5 or below	Osteoporosis

Table 3.10: Diagnostic T-score score levels set by WHO

- **Isotope bone scan:** to determine whether a vertebral body collapsed secondary to osteoporosis or if there is a more sinister cause such as malignancy.
- **Dual energy X-ray absorptiometry (DEXA) scan:**
  - Measures the bone mineral density at the proximal femur and lumbar spine (most common areas)
  - Considered the 'gold standard' diagnostic test
  - A 'T-score' is obtained which compares the tested bone mineral density to a reference population of healthy young adults, and is expressed as the number of standard deviations below this reference population, as shown in Table 3.10

When an osteoporotic fracture has occurred, the diagnosis is 'established osteoporosis'.

Management

Acute management of non-vertebral fractures will be dictated by the orthopaedic surgeons.

Acute spinal cord compression from vertebral fracture is a medical emergency (see section on weakness and paralysis).

In acute cases of vertebral fracture and collapse, the mainstay of treatment is analgesia, followed by early mobilisation and physiotherapy (employing a multidisciplinary approach).

Prevention is necessary, both primary and secondary (see further reading for current NICE guidance).

- Lifestyle changes such as more weight-bearing exercise, smoking cessation, reducing alcohol
- Calcium (1–1.5 g) and Vitamin D (400–800 units) daily
- Hormone replacement therapy
- Bisphosphonates:
  - Inhibit osteoclast activity and therefore reduce bone resorption
  - Major side effects are gastro-intestinal
  - Must be taken at least 30 minutes before food, with the patient sitting upright for that time
- Strontium ranelate, Raloxifine (a selective estrogen receptor modulator) and Teriparatide (a recombinant parathyroid hormone)
- Aim to reduce steroid therapies if possible
- Falls service referral if indicated

Prognosis

There is a high mortality in those who suffer from a hip fracture: 10% within 1 month and 30% within 1 year.

A further 30% may require institutional support following a hip fracture as it causes them to lose their independence and their level of mobility is reduced.

Osteoporotic compression fracture of the spine causes a considerable morbidity with pain and loss of independence.

Ankylosing spondylitis

Ankylosing spondylitis is a chronic inflammatory disease. It is one of the spondylarthropathies, and is characterised by sacroiliitis, peripheral arthropathy, rheumatoid factor negativity, a familial tendency and involvement of other tissues, in particular the heart, lungs, skin and eyes.

The two widely used diagnostic criteria are as shown below:

New York Criteria (1968)	European spondylarthropathy study group
• Limited movement of the lumbar spine in 3 planes • Pain in lumbar spine • Chest expansion <2.5 cm • Radiologically unilateral sacroiliitis grade III-IV or bilateral grade II	• Inflammatory spinal pain or synovitis along with at least one of: positive family history, psoriasis, IBD, buttock pain, enthesopathy, sacroiliitis

Table 3.11: Diagnostic criteria for ankylosing spondylitis

Epidemiology

Prevalence is 0.1 to 0.5% of the population, with a male preponderance (5:2). Onset is typically in the second or third decades. The disease is rare in Japanese and Black African individuals but very common in North American Pima Indians.

Aetiology

There is a combination of genetic and environmental influences.

An association with the human leukocyte antigen-B27 (HLA-B27) gene on chromosome 6 has been suggested. This is present in about 10% of the Caucasian population but in over 95% of those with the disease. In monozygotic twins with HLA-B27 positivity, concordance is over 70% but it is only about 20% for dizygotic twins.

Multiple other loci on other genes have also been identified which confer additional susceptibility. The specific role of all of these genes is unclear.

It is hypothesised that infective agents within the environment are involved in triggering ankylosing spondylitis, and these are unknown.

Pathophysiology

Affected joints become infiltrated with lymphoid and plasma cells causing bony erosions and cartilage destruction. Eventually, there is fibrosis and hence joint stiffness and immobility, which is known as ankylosis.

History/examination

- Pain, stiffness and fatigue, present for at least three months
- Stiffness that is worse in the morning and improves with exercise

Skeletal symptoms:

- Back pain, stiffness and a progressive reduction in the range of movement at the spine – worse in the morning and after prolonged periods of immobility and relieved by activity
- A 'question mark' spine due to the combination of increased thoracic kyphosis and loss of lumbar lordosis. This posture can result in reduced chest expansion and problems with mobility if severe
- Symptoms are persistent with intermittent worsening and result in deformities which develop over a period of ten or more years
- Peripheral arthropathy, especially in the lower limbs
- Enthesopthies – tenderness on the chest wall from the intercostal muscle insertions and sternocostal joints. Also plantar fasciitis and Achilles tendinitis
- Osteoporosis

Extra-articular manifestations:

- Anterior uveitis
- Apical lung fibrosis
- Cardiac involvement, ie aortic valve incompetence and AV nodal conduction defects
- Association with inflammatory bowel disease
- Amyloidosis
- On examination:
  - Ask the patient to look from side to side; they will need to turn the whole body to achieve this.
  - **The Schober test:** make two marks over the spine with the patient standing, the first at the level of the posterior superior iliac spine and the second 10 cm above that. Ask the patient to bend forward as far as possible and measure the distance between the marks. This should increase to more than 15 cm.
  - Ask the patient to stand with their heels and back flush to the wall; their occiput will not be able to touch the wall at the same time.

Investigations

Blood tests:

- FBC: a chronic anaemia is usual
- Inflammatory markers raised
- Serum IgA may be raised
- Rheumatoid factor: negative
- HLA-B27 testing – not routinely performed

Imaging:

Early disease may provide no radiological changes.

- **X-ray pelvis:** blurring of joint margins at sacroiliac joints, sclerosis and loss of joint space indicating sacroiliitis
- **X-ray spine:** with disease progression, there is squaring of the vertebral bodies, syndesmophyte

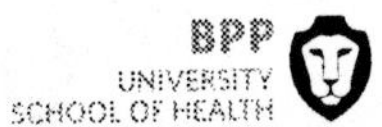

formation and bridging of the bones with fusion of the vertebrae giving the 'bamboo spine' appearance

- **CXR:** may reveal apical fibrosis

Other:

- **Pulmonary function tests:** restrictive abnormality
- **ECG:** any cardiac involvement
- **Echocardiography:** define cardiac involvement

Management

The mainstay of treatment is to relieve pain, prevent the formation of spinal deformity and to enhance mobility:

- Patient education and provision of information eg promote awareness of the National Ankylosing Spondylitis Society (www.nass.co.uk).

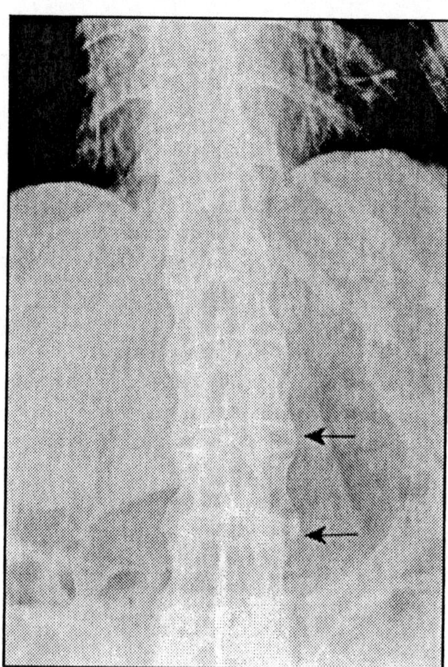

Figure 3.8: A bamboo spine: a plain frontal X-ray of the thoracolumbar spine showing flowing osteophytes in keeping with ankylosing spondylitis

- Genetic counselling may be required.
- Physiotherapy to teach exercises to maintain posture and mobility and to encourage general fitness. Swimming is especially beneficial.
- **Pharmacological**
  - Analgesia, especially NSAIDs, are effective in reducing symptoms of pain as well as morning stiffness.
  - Disease modifying agents such as Sulfasalazine and Methotrexate can help to improve any peripheral joint symptoms but have little effects on the spine.
  - Bisphosphonates.
  - Newer biological therapies such as Infliximab.
- **Surgical**
  - Intervention is rare.
  - Hip replacement for severe hip arthritis.

Prognosis

With appropriate anti-inflammatory drug therapy, disease-modifying agents, and physiotherapy there is a good chance that the patient can lead a normal life with a normal life expectancy. More than 75% of sufferers remain in full-time employment.

Tumours of the bone

Epidemiology

Primary malignant tumours affecting the bone are rare. It makes up 0.2% of all neoplasms and approximately 400 cases are diagnosed each year in the UK.

Aetiology

Tissue	Benign	Malignant
Bone	Osteoma	Osteosarcoma Ewing's sarcoma
Cartilage	Chondroma	Chondrosarcoma
Bone marrow	–	Lymphoma Myeloma
Synovium	–	Synovial sarcoma

Table 3.12: Primary tumours of the bone

Secondary malignant tumours are significantly more frequent and are most commonly from the breast, prostate, thyroid, kidney, lung and bowel (in descending order of frequency). The vertebrae are the commonest site affected by metastatic disease, but only 10% are symptomatic.

Pathophysiology

Pathophysiology is dependent on the aetiology.

History/examination

- Local pain, swelling, and signs of a pathological fracture
- Neurological symptoms from nerve root or spinal cord compression (progressive lower limb motor weakness, altered bladder and bowel function and saddle anaesthesia)
- Weight loss, lethargy and reduced appetite
- Any symptoms from a non-bone primary neoplasm

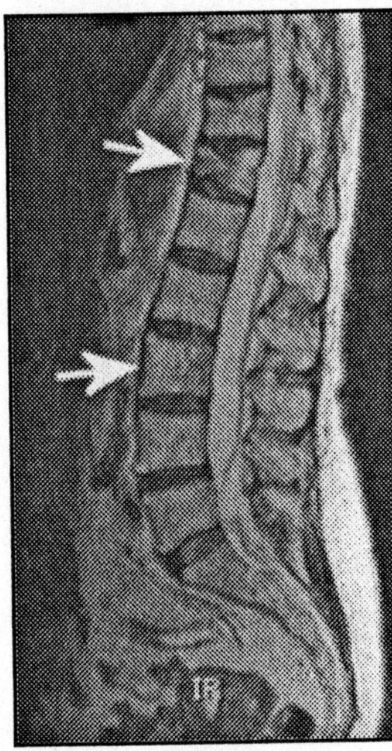

Figure 3.9: Sagittal MRI image of the lumbar spine showing multiple regions of abnormal signal intensity in keeping with bony metastases (arrows)

Blood tests:

- FBC
- U&Es
- LFT
- Bone profile
- Inflammatory markers
- Protein electrophoresis (paired serum and urine protein electrophoresis for Bence-Jones protein) and PSA

Imaging:

- X-ray spine: to check the spine for any abnormal features
- CXR: look for primary tumours in the chest
- CT/MRI:
  - Look for signs of cord compromise
  - Can also define local spread

Others:

- Bone biopsy

Management

The management of primary bone neoplasms should be dictated by a multidisciplinary team at a specialist bone unit. It will depend on tumour type and stage and may include chemotherapy, radiotherapy, and surgical resection.

The priorities when treating secondary metastatic deposits are to control pain, prevent fractures and maintain function and mobility.

- Adequate analgesia. Use the WHO analgesic ladder, but often strong opiates are required as well as adjunctive therapy for neuropathic pain.
- Bisphosphonates inhibit osteoclastic activity and can help reduce pain.
- Some types of chemotherapy/hormone.
- Therapy help eg Tamoxifen may be indicated in breast cancer.
- Radiotherapy can be useful in reducing pain and by shrinking tumours can relieve spinal cord compression.
- Surgery may be helpful in stabilising an unstable spine.

Prognosis

This varies according to the type of neoplasm and stage. Secondary metastatic deposits carry a poor prognosis.

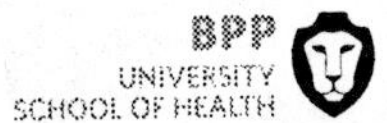

Further reading and references

1. British Orthopaedic Association. (2007) *The care of patients with fragility fracture*. [Online]. Available from: www.fractures.com/pdf/BOA-BGS-Blue-Book.pdf [Accessed 7 November 2016].
2. Day, R.O., Ferreira, M., Lin, C.C., et al. (2015) Efficacy and safety of paracetamol for spinal pain and osteoarthritis: systematic review and meta-analysis of randomised placebo controlled trials. BMJ 2015; 350:h1225.
3. National Ankylosing Spondylitis Society, www.nass.co.uk
4. National Institute for Health and Clinical Excellence. (2012) *Osteoporosis: assessing the risk of fragility fracture* (CG146). [Online]. Available from: www.nice.org.uk/guidance/cg146?unlid=7937365782016825151147 [Accessed 7 November 2016].
5. National Institute for Health and Clinical Excellence. (2009) *Low back pain in adults: early management* (CG088). [Online]. Available from: www.nice.org.uk/guidance/cg88?unlid=72906404120161251 2034 [Accessed 7 November 2016].
6. National Institute for Health and Clinical Excellence (2008). *Osteoarthritis: the care and management of osteoarthritis in adults* (CG059). [Online]. Available from: https://www.nice.org.uk/guidance/cg59 [Accessed 7 November 2016].
7. National Osteoporosis Guideline Group (2008). *Guideline for the diagnosis and management of osteoporosis in postmenopausal women and men from the age of 50 years in the UK*. [Online]. Available from: www.shef.ac.uk/NOGG/NOGG_Pocket_Guide_for_Healthcare_Professionals.pdf [Accessed 7 November 2016].

Acute confusion

Differential diagnosis

System/Organ	Disease
Central nervous system (CNS)	**Delirium (acute confusional state/toxic confusional state)**
Alcohol-related	**Alcohol withdrawal and Wernicke's encephalopathy**
Infection	**Cerebral abscess** Sepsis (UTI, chest infection, septicaemia) Encephalitis
Liver disease	**Acute hepatic failure and encephalopathy**
Drugs	Intoxication or side effects
Metabolic	Hyponatraemia Hypercalcaemia
Others	Hypoxia Post-ictal period in epileptics Intracranial bleed Stroke Post-head injury Constipation

Table 3.13: Differential diagnosis for acute confusion

Delirium

Also known as the 'Acute Confusional State', delirium is among the commonest clinical presentations a foundation doctor will encounter. It is a syndrome of impaired consciousness (poor attention, disorientation, confusion) secondary to an underlying physical condition, and is associated with significantly elevated risks of falls, dehydration, and death.

Successful management relies on timely diagnosis, and then follows two principles: treatment of the underlying condition, and management of the symptoms of delirium itself.

Epidemiology

Delirium is very common in the hospital setting, with a prevalence of up to 50% of those aged >65 in hospital. As many as 80% of people at the end of life exhibit signs of delirium, with a similar figure applying to those in ICU.

Current NICE guidance identifies four major risk factors:

- Age over 65
- Dementia

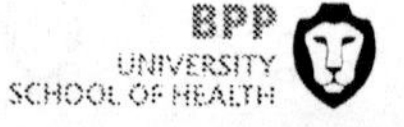

- Current hip fracture
- Severe illness

Delirium in younger patients indicates severe illness.

Aetiology

There is a great number of possible underlying causes of delirium, with presentations usually being multifactorial in their origin. It is helpful to think about predisposing and precipitating factors, eg infection (precipitating factor), on a background of dementia (predisposing factor).
Common precipitants include:

- Infection: eg urinary, respiratory, biliary, skin/soft tissue
- Metabolic disturbance: eg hypo-/hyperglycaemia, electrolyte disturbance, liver failure, renal failure, dehydration
- Hypoxia: eg secondary to pulmonary embolism or exacerbation of COPD
- Intracranial: eg space occupying lesion, encephalitis, epilepsy, stroke, subdural haematoma
- Endocrine disease: eg thyroid disease
- Cardiovascular: eg shock (eg GI bleed), MI, anaemia
- Substances: eg alcohol intoxication/withdrawal, other substance intoxication/withdrawal (eg benzodiazepines)
- Iatrogenic: eg medication, surgery, environmental change
- Severe pain
- Constipation or urinary retention

Pathophysiology

Our understanding of the pathophysiology of delirium is incomplete, but the clinical syndrome probably involves metabolic disturbances in the CNS, resulting in disordered neurotransmission.

Diagnosis

Diagnosis of delirium necessarily follows two steps: 1) identification of the clinical syndrome, and 2) diagnosis of the underlying cause.

Onset of symptoms is usually over hours to days, though there is sometimes a prodrome of mild, subclinical delirious behaviour. Symptoms and level of consciousness fluctuate markedly and are often worse at night.

Clinical features include:

- Poor attention, easily distracted, slow responses*
- Disoriented in time, place, and person
- Short-term memory loss
- Hallucinations (68% visual, 40% auditory), sometimes delusional or paranoid thinking
- Lack of co-operation*, social withdrawal*, emotional changes/lability, agitation**, or aggressive behaviour**

The asterisks indicate a distinction which is sometimes made between hyperactive** (heightened arousal, restless, agitated), hypoactive* (withdrawn, quiet, sleepy), and mixed 'motor subtypes' of delirium. Hypoactive delirium is frequently diagnosed late or missed altogether as symptoms are more subtle.

The AMTS is a quick way to quantify the degree of impairment:

AMTS
- Age (1)
- Time (to nearest hour) (1)
- Address to recall at end of test (eg 42 West Street)
- Year (1)
- Name of this place (1)
- Identification of two persons (1)
- Date of birth (1)
- Dates of World War II (1)
- Name of current prime minister (1)
- Count backwards 20-1 (do not interrupt, this is a test of attention) (1)
- Address recall (1)

The main differential diagnosis for the syndrome is that of dementia. However, an acute onset and fluctuant course are more suggestive of delirium. Insidious onset with little day-to-day variation is more suggestive of dementia.

Diagnosis of the underlying cause will be guided by a thorough and systematic approach to history and examination, with further tests and investigations as appropriate. A collateral history is almost always useful in reaching a diagnosis. Ensure that you obtain:

- Past medical history and baseline function (especially dementia, stroke, recurrent infections, malignancy)
- Drug history (especially polypharmacy, but consider anticholinergics, sedatives, analgesics)

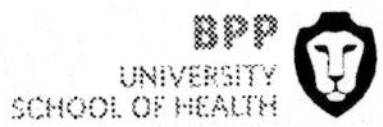

- Alcohol history (consider withdrawal syndrome)
- Drug history (acute intoxication)
- History of head injury

It would be inefficient to list all the possible tests and investigations which may be required to diagnose the underlying cause for delirium – almost any medical condition may be responsible. The following lists cover the most routine and relevant tests, but they are not comprehensive.

Blood tests should include:

- FBC, clotting screen (infection, anaemia, bleeding diathesis)
- U+Es, magnesium, calcium, phosphate
- LFTs, TSH, B12, Folate
- Blood glucose
- Blood cultures (if history suggestive of infection, **even if apyrexial**)

Common further tests, depending on the presentation, include:

- CXR (infection/mass)
- Urine dip/culture (infection)
- ECG (MI or arrhythmia)

Depending on the history, the following may also be necessary:

- CT brain (stroke, bleed, hydrocephalus, space-occupying lesion)
- ABG (acid-base, oxygenation status)
- EEG (diffuse slowing in delirium, useful to differentiate from dementia if there is diagnostic uncertainty)
- CSF sample (encephalitis/meningitis/SAH)

Management

The most important aspect of the management of delirium involves timely identification and treatment of the underlying cause, and optimisation of co-morbid medical conditions. The identification of delirium should prompt a thorough history, examination, and a battery of appropriate tests to identify the cause. **The essential message is that if a patient develops delirium, there is an underlying physical cause,** which must be identified and treated.

Non-pharmacological management is an essential component of the approach:

- Keep the patient safe (eg cot-sides on bed to prevent falls, removal of unsafe objects from near the patient, one-to-one nursing or being near to the nursing station)
- Orientation aids: visible clock, calendar, natural light, reassuring patient verbally
- Communication aids: glasses, hearing aids, staff introducing themselves
- Verbal de-escalation of agitation/aggression

Note that both excessive and insufficient sensory stimulation can exacerbate delirium.

Though there is a role for medication (usually antipsychotics) in extreme agitation/distress, these should be considered last-line, and ought to be prescribed only after senior review or following discussion with the liaison psychiatrist. Consideration should be made of the risk currently posed by the patient to themselves and to others, and the success/failure of verbal, behavioural, or environmental de-escalation techniques.

Older adults tend to be much more susceptible to the adverse effects of medication, so prescribing should be cautious, usually aiming for half the working-age adult dose. An adage to keep in mind regarding dosing in the elderly is 'start low, go slow'.

Haloperidol is the most commonly used antipsychotic in this context, but bear in mind its QTc-prolonging effects (always obtain a pre-treatment ECG), and the risk of Extra-Pyramidal Side Effects (EPSEs), stroke, and death. Antipsychotics are contraindicated in Parkinson's disease and dementia with Lewy bodies. Benzodiazepines are not recommended for non-alcohol-related delirium.

Further reading and references

1. National Institute for Health and Clinical Excellence. (2010) *Delirium: prevention, diagnosis and management* (CG103). [Online]. Available from: www.nice.org.uk/guidance/cg103?unlid=63448807120161011215839 [Accessed 7 November 2016].
2. Lloyd, G.G. and Guthrie, E. (eds.) (2007) *Handbook of Liaison Psychiatry*. Cambridge, Cambridge University Press.
3. Burns, A., Byrne, J., and Gallagley, A. (2003) Delirium (review). *J Neurol Neurosurg Psychiatry* 2003; 75:(3) 362-367.

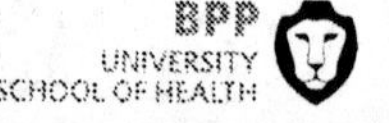

Alcohol withdrawal and Wernicke-Korsakoff Syndromes

The cessation of alcohol consumption in an alcohol-dependent individual, for example on admission to hospital, can precipitate a withdrawal syndrome, ranging from mild to life-threatening. Detection of alcohol dependence on admission allows for prophylactic treatment, avoiding potentially serious consequences.

Definitions

A pattern of alcohol consumption which carries a risk of physical or psychological harm is known as **hazardous drinking**. The most severe kind of hazardous drinking, in which harm is **likely**, is termed **harmful drinking**.

In this section, the term **alcohol dependence** will be used to refer to a biological dependence on alcohol, which may be associated with a morning tremor or anxiety relieved by further alcohol consumption.

The 'CAGE questionnaire' (see below) is useful in detecting very hazardous drinking, but the ten-question 'AUDIT' tool is preferred in primary care.

The CAGE questionnaire

Have you:

- Tried to Cut back on your drinking? (1)
- Been Annoyed because of criticism of your drinking? (1)
- Felt Guilty about your drinking? (1)
- Used alcohol as an Eye-opener? (1)

Score ≥ 2 indicates probable alcohol dependence

Delirium tremens is the name given to the syndrome of severe, as opposed to **mild** or **moderate**, alcohol withdrawal.

Wernicke's syndrome/encephalopathy are synonymous terms which describe an acute syndrome consisting of the classic triad of opthalmoplegia, altered mental state, and ataxia. **Korsakoff's syndrome/psychosis** describes a chronic syndrome of anterograde and retrograde amnesia, confabulation, poor insight, and apathy. The syndromes are often described together as **Wernicke-Korsakoff Syndrome (WKS)**. Both relate to low vitamin B levels, usually dietary in cause. Heavy alcohol consumption is a significant risk factor, but WKS also occurs in other contexts (eg extreme malnutrition in anorexia).

Epidemiology

- Hazardous drinking: 33% of all men, 16% of all women.
- Harmful drinking: 6% of all men, 2% of all women.
- Dependence: 9% of all men (highest between ages 25–34), and 3% of all women (highest between ages 16–24), most of which is mild, with only 0.4% and 0.1% of all adults reporting moderate and severe dependence respectively.

Around 5% of patients admitted with alcohol withdrawal will develop delirium tremens which, untreated, has a mortality of 20%.

Aetiology

Harmful drinking often has a complex aetiology which must account for biological, psychological, and social factors in the patient's background. Low mood and anxiety may play a part. Alcohol dependence occurs due to a regular (usually large) consumption of alcohol, and withdrawal is due to the abrupt reduction in intake in a dependent individual.

Pathophysiology

In alcohol dependence, tolerance occurs as a result of an upregulation in NMDA receptors and a downregulation in GABA(A) receptors. Following cessation of alcohol intake, the resultant imbalance of inhibitory and excitatory neurotransmission causes the withdrawal syndrome.

Heavy alcohol consumption causes gastrointestinal malabsorption of nutrients and vitamins, commonly resulting in severe deficiencies of B vitamins. Thiamine is an essential cofactor in CNS glucose metabolism, and deficiency can cause atrophy / infarction in certain areas of the brain – underlying WKS.

History/examination

Always ask about alcohol consumption when clerking a patient. It is important to ascertain:

- The quantity of alcohol being consumed (Do you drink alcohol? What do you drink? How much? How often?). Calculate the number of units consumed daily.

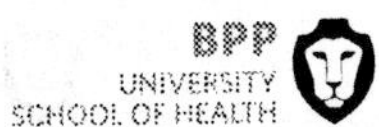

- Whether they ever abstain for more than 24–48 hours, and whether they experience any withdrawal effects, including:
  - Tremor, nausea, vomiting, anxiety
  - Whether they have ever had withdrawal seizures

Units of alcohol

1 unit is equivalent to:

- ½ pint of ordinary beer
- 1 glass of wine
- 1 measure of 40% spirits

Mild withdrawal presents with anxiety or irritability, tachycardia, and sweating.

Moderate withdrawal may additionally include hypertension, confusion, and increased agitation.

Severe withdrawal, or *delirium tremens*, will include hallucinations (visual, tactile), seizures, arrhythmias, or shock.

Onset is usually between 24 and 72 hours from the last drink, but can occur earlier.

Standardised tools such as the Clinical Institute Withdrawal Assessment for Alcohol (revised), or CIWA-Ar, are useful for monitoring withdrawal symptoms and titrating PRN benzodiazepines.

Wernicke-Korsakoff Syndrome is suggested when a heavy drinker presents with any of: memory disturbances, confusion, confabulation, nystagmus, diplopia (or other opthalmoplegia), or low GCS.

Investigations

There are no specific tests for alcohol withdrawal – 'normal' blood test results do not rule out the syndrome:

- MCV is raised in only 30% of heavy drinkers.
- GGT is raised acutely in 60% of heavy drinkers.
- Abnormal clotting may result from decreased hepatic synthetic function.
- Blood glucose may be low.
- Thiamine, folate, B12, may be low.

Always consider CT/MRI brain if WKS is suspected.

Do not fall foul of 'diagnostic overshadowing' in which alternative aetiologies are missed because a patient's symptoms are ascribed to a significant alcohol history without adequately investigating alternative causes.

Management

Management should address the following:

- Treatment of the withdrawal syndrome (reducing regimen of benzodiazepines)
- Prevention/treatment of WKS, nutritional support (B-vitamin, multivitamin supplements)
- Treatment of psychosis in *delirium tremens*

Withdrawal should be anticipated by obtaining an **accurate alcohol history.** Depending on the risks of withdrawal and WKS, an appropriate dose of benzodiazepine and parenteral B vitamins should be started prophylactically. This is usually in the form of a reducing regimen of benzodiazepine.

Your hospital should have a **local guideline** depending on which benzodiazepine (usually chlordiazepoxide [Librium], or diazepam [Valium]) and B vitamin preparation (usually Pabrinex) are available. Prescription is usually risk-stratified by daily alcohol consumption, and will include a reducing regimen of benzodiazepine, plus PRN benzodiazepine (as titrated according to the CIWA-Ar).

NICE guidance recommends parenteral B vitamin administration in the context of A&E attendance and acute illness/injury. Diagnostic suspicion for WKS should be high, due to the risk of irreversible brain damage. Pabrinex is usually given IV or IM for three to five days, after which a B vitamin preparation (eg thiamine + Vitamin B Co-Strong) may be administered orally.

Haloperidol may be used for management of psychosis in *delirium tremens*. Be aware of the risks of prolonged QTc (obtain an ECG prior to treatment), and EPSEs. Senior review is warranted in this situation.

Seizures should be managed acutely as any other seizure, following an ABC approach, with short-acting benzodiazepines usually being the definitive treatment.

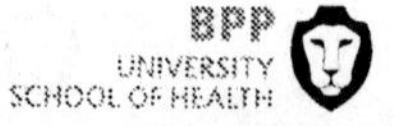

Further reading and references

1. Delanty, N., Frye, M.A., and McKeon, A. (2008) The Alcohol Withdrawal Syndrome. *J Neurol Neurosurg Psychiatry* 2008; doi: 10.1136/jnnp.2007.128322.
2. Health & Social Care Information Centre. (2015) *Statistics on Alcohol.* [Online]. Available from: http://content.digital.nhs.uk/catalogue/pub17712/alc-eng-2015-rep.pdf [Accessed 7 November 2016].
3. Lloyd, G.G. and Guthrie, E. (eds.) (2007). *Handbook of Liaison Psychiatry*. Cambridge, Cambridge University Press.
4. Sadock, B. and Sadock, V.A. (2007) *Kaplan and Sadock's Synopsis of Psychiatry*, 10th edition. Philadelphia, Lippincott Williams and Wilkins.
5. National Institute of Clinical Excellence. (2011) *Alcohol-use disorders: diagnosis, assessment and management of harmful drinking and alcohol dependence* (CG115). [Online]. Available from: www.nice.org.uk/guidance/cg115?unlid=1275530362015121015426 [Accessed 7 November 2016].
6. National Institute of Clinical Excellence. (2010) *Alcohol-use disorders: diagnosis and management of physical complications* (CG100). [Online]. Available from: www.nice.org.uk/guidance/cg100 [Accessed 7 November 2016].

Dementia

Dementia is the chronic or progressive disturbance of higher cortical functions, such as memory, language, visuospatial processing, or emotional cognition, due to an underlying disease of the brain, and without clouding of consciousness (*cf.* delirium).

There are multiple underlying diseases which cause dementia (demanding different approaches to management), as well as there being numerous non-dementia illnesses which present similarly (and may be fully treatable). Therefore, the diagnostic process should first exclude these non-dementia illnesses, and only then should one attempt to classify the underlying dementia subtype.

This section will first describe a general approach to the diagnosis of dementia, and subsequently provide a brief overview of the specific features of the commonest subtypes.

Epidemiology

Dementia is becoming increasingly common in the UK's ageing population. Prevalence increases with age:

- 1.5% in people aged 65–69 years
- 20% in people aged 85–89 years

Screening for dementia is recommended in those with Down's syndrome, post-stroke, and Parkinson's disease, but not in the general population.

Diagnosis

Common conditions which present similarly to dementia are:

- Delirium (usually more rapid in onset and with a fluctuating course and impairment of consciousness).
- Depression (usually more rapid in onset, with low mood, and good insight into memory difficulties).
- Mild Cognitive Impairment (MCI). MCI is a poorly defined entity which progresses to dementia (usually of Alzheimer's type) in around 50% of patients. By definition, MCI does not cause a functional impairment.

The commonest dementias are:

- Alzheimer's Disease (AD, 50%)
- Vascular dementia (25%)
- Dementia with Lewy Bodies (DLB, 15%)
- Frontotemporal dementias (FTD, <5%)

Other causes include: Parkinson's disease, multiple head traumas, prion diseases, Huntington's disease, normal pressure hydrocephalus, space occupying lesions, infections (syphilis, HIV), excess alcohol intake, and endocrine/metabolic disturbances (eg hypothyroidism/hyponatremia/vitamin B deficiencies).

Except in special cases, dementia is a clinical diagnosis, relying on the exclusion of other causes, and a history consistent with the condition. Many cases of dementia have a mixed aetiology.

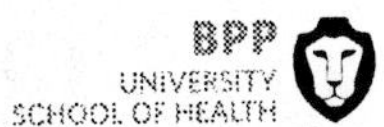

History/examination

Obtain a reliable collateral history with permission. If recent and sudden onset confusion, first rule out delirium.

History:

- Memory loss, particularly short-term. Word finding difficulties, repetitiveness, disorientation. Timing of onset (sudden/gradual), duration (<6 months is less suggestive of dementia), course (gradual, stepwise, fluctuant). Degree of insight.
- Functional deficits: effect of memory loss on activities of daily living, current care needs/care package.
- Change in personality (disinhibition suggestive of frontotemporal or vascular cause, apathy is less specific).
- Symptoms of depression: low mood, disturbed sleep, anhedonia, poor appetite, anxiety or agitation, feelings of hopelessness, suicidal ideation.
- Hallucinations (DLB).
- Agitation, or aggression. Carer stress/support.
- Positive family history.
- Always consider medication as a cause, and obtain a medication history (common culprits are benzodiazepines, analgesia, anticholinergics, steroids).
- Alcohol history.

Examination:

- 'Head turn sign', turning to carer first when asked a question.
- Vascular risk: Arcus senilis, focal weakness/ evidence of stroke, peripheral vascular disease.
- Tremor, rigidity, bradykinesia (Parkinsonian triad), shuffling gait, mask-like facies. Dementia in Parkinson's disease, or Dementia with Lewy Bodies.

Cognitive testing:

- The Montreal Cognitive Assessment (MoCA) is a free, brief cognitive screening tool, which is reportedly more useful than the MMSE in the early stages of dementia.
- The sMMSE, GPCOG, and 6-CIT are all also recommended for the brief assessment of cognition in dementia.
- The Addenbrooke Cognitive Examination (ACE-III) is a more extensive tool which may be used in secondary care.
- Domain-specific neuropsychological testing may be carried out by a specialist psychologist.

Investigations

NICE recommends the following routine tests: FBC, U+Es, Ca, glucose, LFTs, TFTs, B12 and Folate levels.

Depending on the clinical situation, NICE suggests that the following may be appropriate: midstream urine culture, XR chest, syphilis or HIV serology, ECG, brain imaging.

Management

Management of the cognitive symptoms of dementia depends on the underlying diagnosis. An overview of the management of the three commonest dementia subtypes is presented below.

General principles:

Patient and carer education is important following diagnosis. The Alzheimer's Society is a good starting point for individuals and families to find local support, though there are many other resources available. Development of coping strategies (eg keeping a diary, writing down a daily routine) is practical, intuitive, and effective.

Currently, NICE requires that drug therapy for AD and DLB (eg acetylcholinesterase inhibitors) is started by a specialist.

There are no specific pharmacological treatments for vascular dementia, though vascular risk factors may be appropriately managed with medication, in addition to lifestyle alterations.

Managing aggression and agitation:

A new onset of behavioural disturbance in persons with dementia should prompt a thorough review of physical health, in order to exclude delirium. Also consider a new onset of:

- Depression;
- Pain;
- Medication side effects; and
- Environmental factors (such as a change in location).

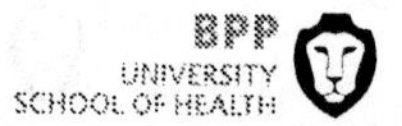

Non-pharmacological approaches should be tried first. NICE recommends consideration of: aromatherapy, therapeutic use of music or dancing, animal-assisted therapy, and massage.

Pharmacological therapy is appropriate only if the patient is severely distressed, or there is immediate risk to the patient or others. Antipsychotics (eg risperidone) may be used, though they are contraindicated in DLB/Parkinson's disease, and incur a significant risk of stroke and death.

Acute and severe agitation or aggression, which is refractory to de-escalation techniques (listening, redirection), may be treated cautiously using benzodiazepines, or haloperidol.

Courses of sedatives and antipsychotics should be regularly reviewed such that the minimum effective dose is used, and for the shortest duration possible. Use the oral route of medication administration if possible, and for parenteral administration, IM is preferred to IV.

Frequent monitoring of vital signs (eg every 15 minutes for the first hour) should follow administration of sedatives, due to the risk of respiratory depression and death, particularly if the patient falls asleep/ unconscious.

Most trusts will have local guidance with regards to the pharmacological management of acute behavioural disturbance. Consider referral to secondary mental healthcare or liaison psychiatry.

Risk assessment:

Particular risks to be aware of in dementia are self-neglect, falls, accidents (leaving the stove on, fires), medication risk (accidental overdose), driving (the DVLA must be informed of a diagnosis of dementia), and risk to carers (aggression/burnout). If you are concerned about any of these, a referral to occupational therapy will facilitate safe discharge.

Capacity:

Valid consent to investigation and treatment should be sought if possible. If you are concerned about a person with dementia's capacity, refer to the Mental Capacity Act.

Further reading and references

1. National Institute of Clinical Excellence. (2006) Dementia: *supporting people with dementia and their carers in health and social care* (CG42). [Online]. Available from: www.nice.org.uk/guidance/cg42 [Accessed 7 November 2016].

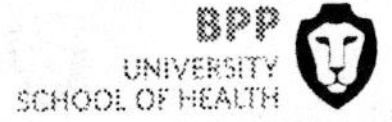

Type	Pathophysiology	Risk factors	Clinical findings	Treatment	Prognosis
Alzheimer's Dementia (AD)	Primary neurodegenerative condition characterised by microscopic findings of β-amyloid plaques and neurofibrillary tangles.	Increasing age, family history. Genetic: ApoE variants confer variable risk, trisomy 21 (Down's syndrome) carries significant risk. Environmental: low educational attainment, depression.	Gradual onset and progression of impairment: first of short-term memory, then language (word-finding), and ultimately all aspects of cognitive function. Insight into memory loss tends to be poor.	Acetylcholinesterase inhibitors are safe and effective in mild-moderate AD. Glutamate-blockers (memantine) are neuroprotective, and useful in moderate-severe AD.	Gradual decline, average survival 5–7 years from diagnosis. Rapid decline associated with shorter survival. Early-onset AD is an aggressive disease with a poorer prognosis.
Dementia with Lewy Bodies (DLB)	Primary neurodegenerative condition characterised by presence of Lewy Bodies (α-synuclein-predominant cytoplasmic inclusion bodies) in cerebral cortex and Substantia Nigra (hence Parkinsonian symptoms).	Increasing age, family history. Otherwise as yet poorly understood.	Simultaneous onset of dementia with Parkinsonian motor-symptoms. Fluctuating level of consciousness (may make differentiation from delirium difficult). Vivid visual hallucinations.	Limited evidence but solid theoretical basis suggesting efficacy of anticholinesterase inhibitors in DLB. Antipsychotic medication must be avoided.	Average survival 5–7 years.
Vascular Dementia (VD)	Dementia due to multiple cerebral infarcts/ cerebrovascular disease.	Increasing age, male sex. Vascular risk factors including hypertension, high cholesterol, diabetes, smoking. Previous stroke.	Rapid/subacute onset, with stepwise deterioration in cognitive function. History of stroke is supportive of diagnosis. Highly variable symptom profile, memory may be preserved in early stages. Insight into memory difficulties often retained.	Control vascular risk factors (treat hypertension, high cholesterol, diabetes; stop smoking, encourage physical activity). Treatment is otherwise supportive and symptom-directed.	Stepwise deterioration. Highly variable survival from time of diagnosis.

Table 3.14: Pathophysiology, risk factors, clinical findings, treatment, and prognosis, for three of the commonest causes of dementia

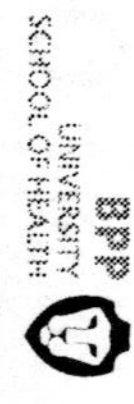

Medical ethics and the law

It is essential to have an understanding of the legal frameworks within which we treat patients.

Confidentiality

Caldicott Principles, and justification for information sharing, eg with police.

Consent

For consent to be **valid**, it must be informed and voluntary, and the patient must have **capacity** regarding the specific decision.

Voluntariness is the degree to which a patient has made a decision of their own volition, rather than having been forced or coerced into it by someone else – be it a family member, or perhaps their doctor.

To be **informed** means to be made aware of two categories of information: firstly, the nature of the procedure, or therapy being offered, eg practically what an operation entails. Secondly, the patient should be told (in intelligible terms) what the intended **benefits**, **risks**, and **alternatives**, are to the intervention. The standard of information expected to be communicated to patients has risen in recent years following the 'Montgomery' case in 2015 – to quote from the Supreme Court ruling:

> *The test of materiality [with regards to risk] is whether, in the circumstances of the particular case, a reasonable person in the patient's position would be likely to attach significance to the risk, or the doctor is or should reasonably be aware that the particular patient would be likely to attach significance to it.*

Consent cannot be general (eg 'you can do whatever you like to me'); it must relate to specific interventions. It may be explicit (eg verbal or written), or implicit (eg giving arm to doctor for blood to be taken). Significant interventions like surgery usually involve written consent, and you should make yourself aware of any local specific procedures or forms relevant to your speciality.

Capacity

A person has capacity with regards to a specific decision if they are able to:

- **Understand** the relevant facts
- **Retain** the facts for the duration required to make the decision
- **Weigh up** the facts with the relevant values
- **Communicate** their decision

This is sometimes referred to as the 'four-stage' test of capacity. If there are concerns that an individual may be lacking in capacity, referral should be made to the principles of the Mental Capacity Act (MCA, 2005):

- Assume that the patient has capacity until incapacity is established.
- All practicable steps to help the patient make the decision must be taken prior to treatment (eg hearing aids, reading glasses, interpreter).
- Patients are allowed to make **unwise** decisions without being deemed incapacitated.
- Decisions made for or on behalf of the patient must be in their **best interests**, and
- Follow an approach which is **least restrictive** to the person's rights and freedoms.

The MCA should only be used if there is:

- A **specific** decision to be made **now; and**
- The inability to make the decision is due to an impairment of or disturbance in the functioning of the mind or brain.

If the answers to both of the above are yes, then the four-stage test of capacity should be employed with regards to each specific decision, and a judgement made on the **balance of probability** (ie with >50% certainty).

The person who should perform the capacity test should be whoever is best informed about the specific decision – for example, a social worker if it relates to financing a nursing-home placement, or a surgeon if it relates to an operation.

'Best interests decisions' should take into consideration the prior wishes of the patient, and will often be informed by discussion with the patient's friends/ relatives.

Deprivation of Liberty Safeguards (DoLS)

The DoLS were introduced in order to provide a framework (not dissimilar in principle to the Mental Health Act) to protect individuals who lack capacity, and whose liberty may be restricted as a result of care or treatment. It only applies to the hospital and care home settings.

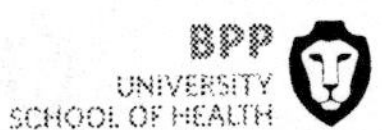

If an incapacitated individual is felt to be subject to a deprivation of liberty (eg sedation, constant supervision, inability to leave premises), the **managing authority** (eg care-home manager) must apply to the **supervisory body** (eg local authority) for authorisation of the deprivation of liberty. This consists of a six-part assessment made by a Best Interests Assessor and a doctor. Authorisation can last for up to a year.

The Mental Health Act (MHA)

The MHA provides a legal framework for the detention and treatment, without consent, of people:

- Who have a mental disorder of a nature or degree which warrants admission to hospital; and
- For whom admission is in the interests of the patient's health or safety, or the protection of others.

If a patient lacks the capacity to consent to admission/treatment for an acute mental disorder, they should also be detained under the MHA.

The MHA provides safeguards against arbitrary detention, including: tribunal, with legal representation of patients, the right for patients to appeal their section, and limited time periods for detention. An incapacitated patient admitted 'informally' would not have these rights and could be detained indefinitely without review – hence the requirement for the MHA in this instance, or DoLS if appropriate.

For the purposes of foundation training (outside of psychiatric placements), it is important to be familiar with Section 5 of the MHA, and useful to be aware of Sections 2 and 3.

Section 5 relates to patients already admitted to hospital (ie in a ward, not A&E or an outpatient clinic). It is a 'holding power', providing a legal basis for preventing a patient from leaving the hospital, in order that they have a full MHA assessment and consideration of Section 2 or 3. It does not allow involuntary treatment, therefore whilst held under Section 5, treatment must either be voluntary or, in an emergency, in line with the Common Law 'doctrine of necessity in his/her best interests' or the Mental Capacity Act.

Section 5(2) is invoked by the 'approved clinician in charge of the patient's treatment' (eg the responsible medical consultant on a medical ward), or an appointed deputy, and lasts for 72 hours. If a doctor is not available, Section 5(4) may be invoked by a member of nursing staff, and lasts for 6 hours. Sections 5(2) and 5(4) cannot be renewed.

Practically speaking, invoking Section 5(2) involves filling out a brief form, which is passed on to the 'authorised officer' (who will set about arranging the MHA assessment). If you do not know where 5(2) forms are kept in your ward/hospital, call your liaison psychiatry team for advice as to where to find them, how to fill them out, and who to give them to.

Section 2 of the MHA lasts up to 28 days and is for **assessment** of a patient. It should be used when there is diagnostic uncertainty about the patient's presentation. If a patient has an established diagnosis, and there is appropriate treatment available, then Section 3 may be used. Section 3 lasts up to 6 months in the first instance, and can be renewed.

Further reading and references

1. Mental Health Act. (1983) [Online]. Available from: www.legislation.gov.uk/ukpga/1983/20/contents [Accessed 7 November 2016].
2. Mental Capacity Act. (2005) [Online]. Available from: www.legislation.gov.uk/ukpga/2005/9/contents [Accessed 7 November 2016].
3. *Montgomery (Appellant) v Lanarkshire Health Board (Respondent) (Scotland) (2015)* UKSC 11.

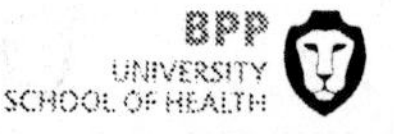

Breathlessness

Differential diagnosis

System/Organ	Disease
Respiratory	**Pneumothorax** **Pulmonary embolism** Pneumonia **Asthma** **Chronic obstructive pulmonary disease (COPD)** Pleural effusion Interstitial lung disease Lung cancer
Cardiac	**Pulmonary oedema** Acute myocardial infarction Arrhythmia Valvular heart disease
Other	Anaemia Anaphylaxis Airway obstruction Anxiety Metabolic acidosis Neuromuscular disorders Pain

Table 3.15: Differential diagnosis of breathlessness

Pneumothorax

Epidemiology

The incidence is roughly 18–28 in 100,000 for males and 1.2–6 in 100,000 for females. It tends to affect either young adults or older individuals with underlying lung disease.

Aetiology

Primary spontaneous pneumothorax: occurs where there is no underlying lung condition. It typically affects tall, young, thin males and is thought to be due to rupture of small sub-pleural blebs and bullae at the lung apex. The risk is increased by:

- Smoking
- Marfan syndrome
- Homocystinuria
- Family history

Secondary spontaneous pneumothorax occurs as a complication of underlying respiratory disease, for example:

- Bullous emphysema
- Infections (eg tuberculosis or *pneumocystic jerovici* pneumonia)
- Malignancy
- Idiopathic pulmonary fibrosis

Trauma can also lead to a pneumothorax. This can be as a result of either a penetrating or blunt chest wall injury. Traumatic pneumothorax can be iatrogenic (for example, as a consequence of pleural aspiration or subclavian central line insertion).

Tension pneumothorax can occur with any of these types. It is a rare but life-threatening condition that requires immediate management.

Pathophysiology

Pneumothorax refers to a collection of air in the pleural cavity, resulting in ipsilateral lung collapse. A break in the integrity of the alveoli, pleura or chest wall leads to the movement of air from the higher pressure alveoli to the lower pressure intrapleural space. The air flow will continue until the pressure gradient is equalised or the break in integrity has been sealed.

Tension pneumothorax occurs when a one-way valve develops that allows accumulation of air during inspiration with no release during expiration. The volume of air and pressure within the pleural space increases, resulting in breathlessness, mediastinal shift, hypoxia and shock (due to reduced venous return to the heart).

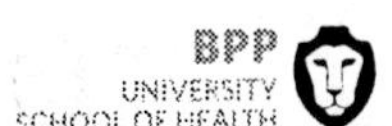

History/examination

History	• Sudden onset • Pleuritic chest pain • Shortness of breath • Past medical history of respiratory disease, previous pneumothorax or Marfan's syndrome • History of trauma • Family history of pneumothorax • Smoking
Exam	• Respiratory distress • Hypoxia • Tachycardia • Hypotension (late) • Tracheal deviation • Ipsilteral reduced chest wall expansion • Ipsilateral hyper-resonant percussion • Ipsilateral reduced/absent breath sounds • Distended neck veins (late)

Table 3.16: History/examination findings in the breathless patient

A patient with severe symptoms, clinical features of pneumothorax and haemodynamic compromise should raise suspicion for tension pneumothorax.

Investigations

Tension pneumothorax is a clinical diagnosis and no initial investigations are required.

Blood tests:

- ABG: hyperventilation and respiratory alkalosis, type 1 respiratory failure

Imaging:

- Chest X-ray: standard erect inspiratory film
- CT chest: may be required in uncertain or complex cases

Management

All patients should be referred to the respiratory team within 24 hours of diagnosis. The respective management pathways are shown in Figure 3.10.

Primary spontaneous pneumothorax:

For more information on pleural aspiration and chest drain insertion, see Chapter 8.

Secondary spontaneous pneumothorax (SSP):

Any patient aged over 50 years old, with a significant smoking history and/or evidence of underlying respiratory disease, should be treated as an SSP.

Traumatic pneumothorax:

The management is similar to SSP (see above). Surgical thoracotomy may be required if the patient continues to deteriorate.

Tension pneumothorax:

Tension pneumothorax requires immediate decompression by inserting a 14 or 16G cannula into the second intercostal space, mid-clavicular line followed by chest drain insertion.

- Patients should be advised not to fly until resolution confirmed and not to dive.
- Every patient should have respiratory follow-up until full resolution of the pneumothorax.

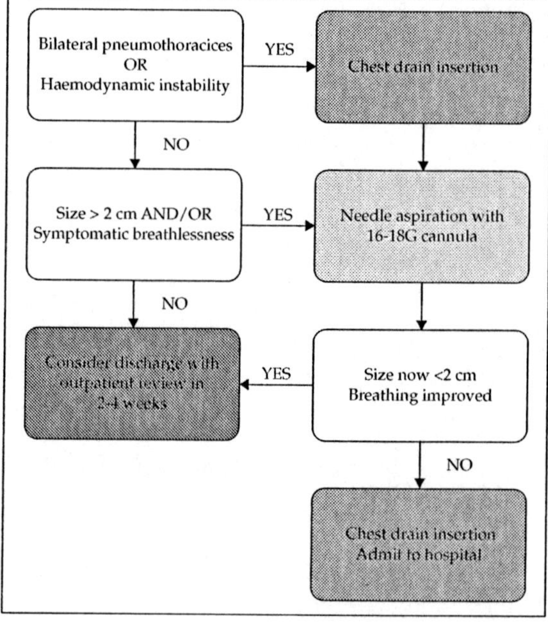

Figure 3.10: Management of primary spontaneous pneumothorax

Prognosis

- 1 in 5 patients with PSP will have recurrence on the same side. This risk increases with each subsequent pneumothorax.
- Patients with SSP are at greater risk of recurrence.
- Recurrent pneumothoraces can be treated with pleurodesis or by surgery.

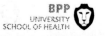

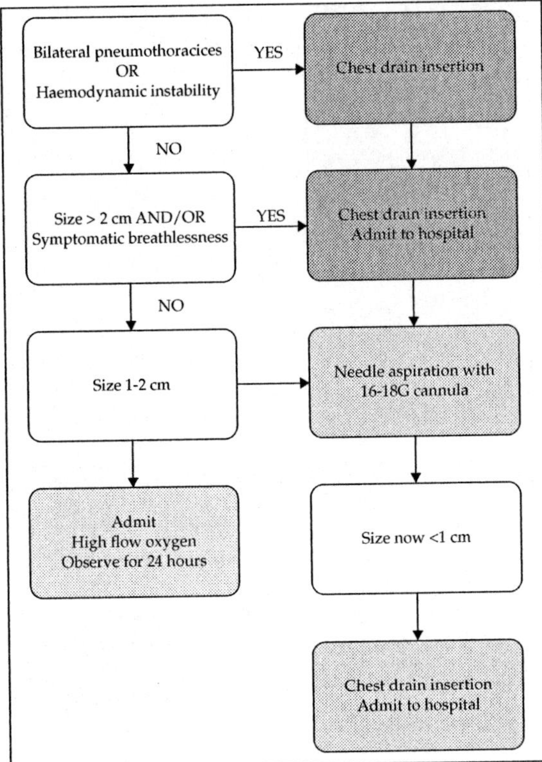

Figure 3.11: Management of bilateral pneumothoraces or in a haemodynamically unstable patient

Pulmonary oedema

Epidemiology

Pulmonary oedema is common, affecting over 1% of individuals over the age of 65.

Aetiology

Cardiac	• Ischaemic heart disease • Valvular heart disease • Mechanical complications of acute coronary syndromes • Hypertensive crisis • Acute arrhythmia • Acute myocarditis • Cardiac tamponade • Aortic dissection • Cardiomyopathies
Renal	• Acute and chronic renal failure • Renal artery stenosis

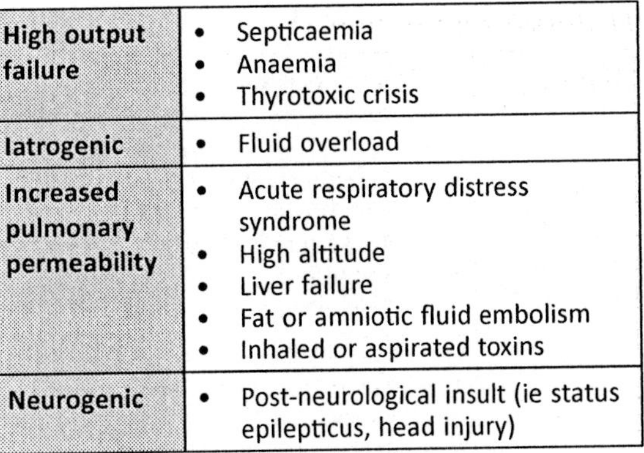

High output failure	• Septicaemia • Anaemia • Thyrotoxic crisis
Iatrogenic	• Fluid overload
Increased pulmonary permeability	• Acute respiratory distress syndrome • High altitude • Liver failure • Fat or amniotic fluid embolism • Inhaled or aspirated toxins
Neurogenic	• Post-neurological insult (ie status epilepticus, head injury)

Table 3.17: Aetiology of pulmonary oedema

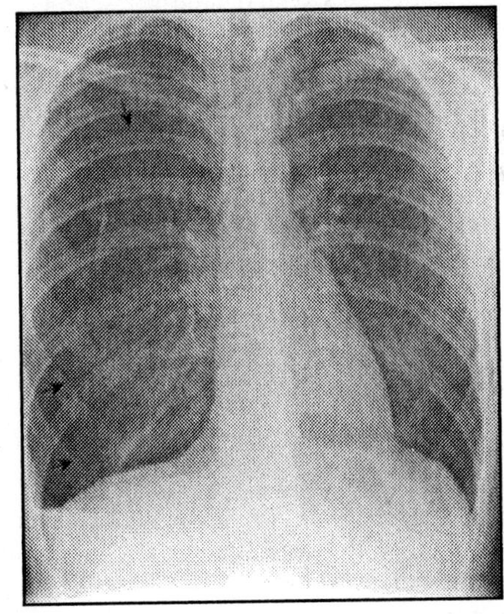

Figure 3.12: Chest X-ray showing a large right pneumothorax. Note the absence of lung markers in the periphery and the edge of the collapsed lung (arrows)

Pathophysiology

Pulmonary oedema is the accumulation of fluid within the lung parenchyma and alveoli. The most common mechanism is raised pulmonary capillary failure secondary to left-sided heart failure. The increase in pressure leads to leakage of fluid into the interstitium and, with continuing rises in pressure, into the alveoli. If there is hypoalbuminaemia, pulmonary oedema will occur at a lower capillary pressure.

History/examination

History	• Severe shortness of breath • Orthopnoea • Paroxysmal nocturnal dyspnea • Cough +/- pink frothy sputum • Chest pain • Past medical history of relevant conditions • Drug history
Exam	• Pale and sweaty • Respiratory distress • Hypoxia • Tachycardia • Hypotension (cardiogenic shock) • Raised JVP • Gallop rhythm • Valvular murmurs • Bibasal chest crackles • Hepatomegaly • Peripheral oedema

Table 3.18: History/examination findings in a patient with pulmonary oedema

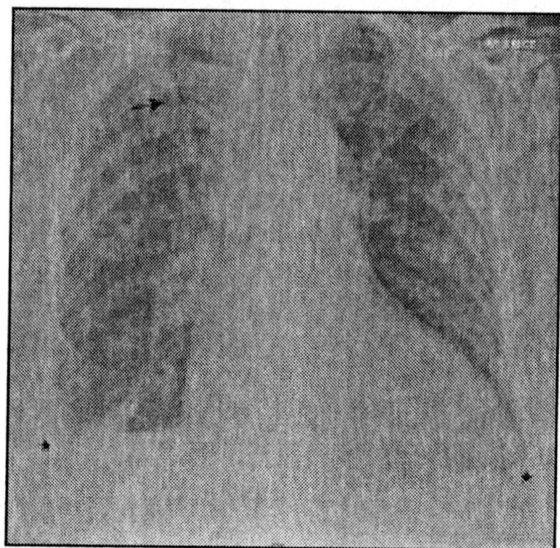

Figure 3.13: Chest X-ray showing bilateral pulmonary oedema with upper lobe diversion, Kerley B lines, fluid in the horizontal fissure and blunting of the costophrenic angles due to pulmonary oedema

Investigations

Blood tests:

- FBC
- U&Es
- LFTs
- Troponin: to exclude acute MI
- ABG: hypoxaemia, hypocapnia due to tachypnoea, hypercapnia and acidosis due to impaired gas exchange (later sign)
- BNP if available

Imaging:

- Chest X-ray: to confirm oedema and exclude other causes of symptoms. Features such as cardiomegaly, upper lobe diversion, bilateral perihilar shadowing (bat's wing distribution), Kerley B lines and fluid in the horizontal fissure may be seen.

Other:

- ECG: to look for evidence of myocardial infarction, arrhythmia or other cardiac disease
- Echocardiogram

Management

Initial therapy:

- Sit the patient up
- Correct hypoxia
- Treatment of any identified underlying cause
- IV loop diuretic
  - 20-40 mg furosemide is suitable in a diuretic-naïve patient.
  - Patients already on diuretic therapy may require higher doses.
  - Renal function, weight and urine output should be monitored closely.

Top tip:

For patients taking bumetanide regularly, 1 mg of bumetanide is equivalent to 40 mg furosemide.

- Opiates
  - Consider IV morphine if the patient is very anxious or distressed.
  - There is some evidence that opiates may increase mortality in acute pulmonary oedema so it is not recommended routinely.
- Nitrates
  - Consider a nitrate infusion in patients with a systolic blood pressure >110 mmHg and no history of severe aortic or mitral stenosis.

Further acute management:

- Inotropes and vasopressors
  - May be useful if there is potentially reversible cardiogenic shock.
- Non-invasive ventilation
  - CPAP should be considered in dyspnoeic patients with a respiratory rate of >20 to improve symptoms and reduce hypercapnia and acidosis.
- Invasive ventilation
  - Consider invasive ventilation if there is respiratory failure, decreased GCS or physical exhaustion.
- Intra-aortic balloon pumping

Ongoing management:

- VTE prophylaxis
- Consider starting an ACE inhibitor and/or a beta-blocker once stable

Prognosis

In-hospital mortality ranges from 2% to 20% depending on clinical factors.

Pulmonary embolism (PE)

Epidemiology

PE is one of the most common cardiovascular diseases, with 47,594 cases reported in the UK between 2013 and 2014.

Aetiology

Virchow's triad describes the three broad categories of factors that lead to thrombosis (hypercoaguability, vessel wall injury and venous stasis). This is illustrated for PE in Figure 3.14.

Pathophysiology

PE occurs when a thrombus lodges in the pulmonary vasculature. It is most commonly caused by an embolus from a pre-existing venous thrombus in the femoral or pelvic veins. There are several different types of emboli, including clot, amniotic fluid, air and fat.

The embolus obstructs the vasculature and leads to increased pulmonary vascular resistance and increased right ventricular workload. The heart rate increases to compensate.

If the embolus is sufficiently large, the increasing pulmonary pressure overcomes the compensatory tachycardia, leading to right ventricular distension and decreased right ventricular output. This reduces the left ventricular preload and therefore the left ventricular output. This can lead to hypotension and cardiogenic shock. This is sometimes termed 'massive PE'.

Case Study: Iatrogenic overload

You are called to see an 88-year-old woman who is being treated for pneumonia, as she is acutely breathless. On arrival, she is pale, sweaty and distressed. She has bibasal crackles on auscultation and peripheral oedema to her mid-thighs. She has been given aggressive fluid resuscitation over the past 24 hours for oliguria and hypotension (fluid balance +4.5L). Her usual dose of furosemide has been withheld due to AKI.

Learning Points

- Advanced age, renal impairment and cardiac impairment increase the risk of fluid overload. Fluid resuscitation is necessary in sepsis, but all patients should have careful monitoring of fluid balance.
- Patients with pulmonary oedema are often very unwell and fluid balance can be complex when there are multiple co-morbidities. Don't be afraid to escalate early.

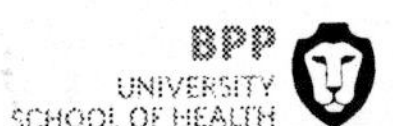

History/examination

History	• Pleuritic/retrosternal chest pain • Shortness of breath • Cough • Haemoptysis • Swollen/painful limb • Dizziness • Collapse and loss of consciousness • Presence of risk factors
Exam	• Tachypnoea • Tachycardia • Hypoxia • Hypotension • Low grade pyrexia • Cyanosis • Raised JVP • Pleural rub or crackles on auscultation • Unilateral limb swelling

Table 3.19: History and examination findings in pulmonary embolism

Investigations

Calculate the Wells score to determine the probability of PE.

Factor	Score
Clinically suspected DVT	3.0
Alternative diagnosis less likely	3.0
Tachycardia >100 bpm	1.5
Immobilisation for >3 days or surgery in past 4 weeks	1.5
History of DVT/PE	1.5
Haemoptysis	1.0
Malignancy (on treatment, treated in last 6 months or palliative)	1.0

Note. PE is considered likely if the Wells score is greater than four and unlikely if it is four or less.

Table 3.20: The Wells score for patients with suspected pulmonary embolism

Blood tests:

- FBC: to exclude infection
- U&Es: to get baseline levels
- Coagulation screen
- Troponin: raised troponin may be indicative of right heart strain
- D-dimer: **only if PE unlikely** based on Wells score (scoring four or less). False positives are seen in pregnancy, sepsis, DIC, malignancy and post-operatively
- ABG: if significantly hypoxic

Imaging:

- CXR: mainly to exclude other causes. The classical finding is a wedge-shaped shadow representing an area of infarction.
- CT Pulmonary Angiogram: should be offered immediately if the Wells score is greater than 4 or the D-dimer is positive.
- V/Q SPECT/planar scan: should be offered if CTPA cannot be performed due to renal impairment or concerns around radiation dose.

Other:

- ECG: a wide range of changes may be present, from sinus tachycardia to the classical S1 Q3 T3 pattern (deep S waves in lead 1, Q waves and T-wave inversion lead 3).
- Echocardiography: to assess for the presence of right heart strain.

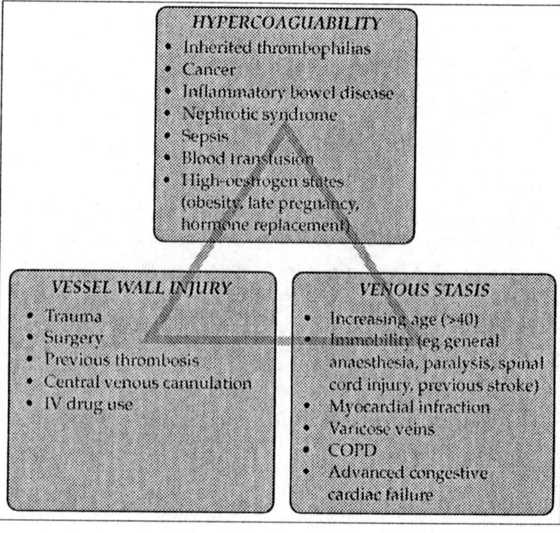

Figure 3.14: Virchow's Triad for determining the likelihood of coagulation

Management

General:

- Oxygen to correct hypoxia.
- Analgesia.
- Anticoagulation: usually LMWH. Other options include fondaparinux and unfractionated heparin. This should be started whilst awaiting definitive imaging.

PE with haemodynamic compromise:

- Haemodynamic support with fluid resuscitation +/- inotropes
- Thrombolysis is indicated if systolic blood pressure is less than 90 mmHg or there is a fall of over 40 mmHg from baseline blood pressure
- Surgical embolectomy

Ongoing anticoagulation:

- In patients with cancer, at least six months of treatment with LMWH is recommended.
- All other patients should have three months' treatment with warfarin, or rivaroxaban.
- Extending the duration of anticoagulation should be considered in patients with unprovoked PEs.
- A second episode of unprovoked PE is an indication for indefinite anticoagulation therapy.

Further investigation of unprovoked PE:

- Patients with unprovoked PE should undergo full history and examination, urinalysis and venepuncture for FBC, LFTs and calcium.
- Consider CT Abdomen/Pelvis (plus a mammogram if female) in patients over the age of 40 with their first unprovoked PE.

Prognosis

PE is the second commonest cause of unexpected death in all age groups. Its untreated mortality is 30%. Even when treated, some patients will develop chronic thromboembolic pulmonary hypertension.

Asthma

Epidemiology

Currently around 5.4 million people are receiving treatment for asthma in the UK. The peak hospital attendances in the UK are between September and October. On average, 3 people per day die from asthma.

Aetiology

Numerous risk factors for developing asthma have been identified, including:

- Family history of asthma or atopy
- Personal history of atopy
- Obesity
- Maternal smoking
- Personal smoking
- Prematurity and low birth weight
- Socioeconomic deprivation
- Early exposure to broad spectrum antibiotics
- Viral infections in early childhood
- Several genes have been associated with asthma

Common triggers for asthma exacerbations include allergens (eg house dust mite, cat hair, occupational exposures), use of NSAIDs or beta-blockers, infections, cold air, exercise and stress.

Pathophysiology

Asthma is a chronic condition where there is paroxysmal and reversible airway obstruction secondary to bronchial inflammation and airway hyper-responsiveness in response to a specific stimulus. Its development is thought to be due to a combination of environmental and genetic risk factors.

In patients with asthma, triggers provoke an exaggerated inflammatory response within the bronchial tree. Inflammatory cells move into the airways, causing changes to the airway epithelium and airway tone and leading to:

- Smooth muscle contraction
- Thickening of the airway wall
- Increased mucus secretion
- Ciliary dysfunction

Over time, there is remodelling of the airways, with destruction of cilia, an increased proportion of mucous-secreting goblets cells and hypertrophy and hyperplasia of smooth muscle.

History/examination

History	• Wheeze • Dyspnoea • Chest tightness • Cough • Symptoms worse at night/early morning • Symptoms of infection • Potential triggers • History of atopy • Previous hospital or ITU admissions due to asthma • Current medication • Use of beta agonists
Exam	• Tachypnoea • Accessory muscle use • Cyanosis • Tachycardia • Reduced chest expansion • Wheeze on auscultation • Low FEV1/peak expiratory flow rate (PEFR) readings

Table 3.21: History and examination findings in a patient with asthma

Acute severe asthma	Life-threatening asthma
Any one of:	
PEFR 33–50% of best or predicted	PEFR <33% of best or predicted
Respiratory rate ≥25	SpO_2 <92%
Pulse rate ≥110 bpm	PaO_2 <8 kPa
Unable to complete full sentences in one breath	$PaCO_2$ normal or raised
	Exhaustion
	Altered conscious level
	Silent chest
	Poor respiratory effort
	Cyanosis
	Hypotension
	Arrhythmia

Table 3.22: Features of acute severe asthma and life-threatening asthma

Investigations

Acute asthma:

If an acute exacerbation of asthma is suspected, treatment should be commenced immediately.

Blood tests:

- FBC: may show evidence of infection
- U&Es: salbutamol may cause hypokalaemia
- CRP
- ABG

Imaging:

- CXR: required if there is suspicion of pneumothorax or pneumonia, presence of life-threatening features, poor response to treatment or prior to mechanical ventilation

Others:

- PEFR: more convenient than FEV1 in the acute setting

Chronic asthma:

In adults, initial diagnosis should be made on a basis of a characteristic history and measurement of airflow obstruction (preferably with spirometry). This is used to stratify probability of asthma into low, intermediate and high probability. Those with a high probability of asthma or evidence of airway obstruction on spirometry (FEV1/FVC <0.7) can progress to a trial of treatment. Further investigations are required (eg chest X-ray, full lung function tests, blood eosinophil count, IgE serology and skin prick testing) in those with a low probability of asthma, an intermediate probability with no evidence of airway obstruction, or where a trial of treatment is unsuccessful.

Management

Acute asthma:

- High flow oxygen to achieve SpO_2 94–98%
- High dose inhaled β_2-agonist via inhaler or nebuliser
- Nebulised ipratropium (500 mcg) every 4–6 hours if poor response or acute severe asthma

- 40–50 mg prednisolone for at least 4–5 days (200 mg IV hydrocortisone if unable to take tablets orally)
- IV magnesium 1.2–2 g can be considered if there is poor response to initial therapy or in acute severe asthma
- IV aminophylline can also be considered
- Consider ITU referral early, particularly if there are any features of acute severe or life-threatening asthma – patients may require intubation and ventilation

Chronic asthma:

General measures include:

- Patient education and development of an asthma action plan
- Smoking cessation
- Weight reduction in obese patients
- Primary care asthma review at least annually

The British Thoracic Society recommends a stepwise approach to asthma therapy, with treatment commencing at the most appropriate step for the severity of symptoms and stepped up or down respectively to optimise good control and minimise side effects.

Top tip:

Magnesium and aminophylline should only be started after discussion with senior medical staff. Failure to respond to bronchodilators is a concerning feature.

Prognosis

The mortality rate of acute severe asthma is significant. About two-thirds of deaths are felt to be preventable.

Complications include aspiration pneumonia, pneumomediastinum, pneumothorax, rhabdomyolysis, respiratory failure and hypoxic brain injury.

There is a good prognosis where asthma is adequately treated.

Inhaled short acting b2 agonist	Add inhaled steroid 200-800mcg/day (start at dose appropriate to disease severity	Add inhaled long-acting b2 agonist (LABA) Assess control: 1. If good, continue LABA 2. If better, continue LABA and increase inhaled steroid 3. If no response, stop LABA, increase steroid and add trials of alternative treatments	Consider trials of: 1. Increasing inhaled steroid upto 2000mcg/day 2. adding leukotriene receptor antagonist, SR theophylline or b2 agonist tablet	Daily steroid tablet at lowest possible dose Maintain maximum inhaled steroid Ensure steroid-sparing treatments continue Refer to specialist care

Note. Patients should begin at the most appropriate step for the severity of their disease and move up and down as required

Figure 3.15: Stepwise management of asthma based on the British Thoracic Society Guidelines

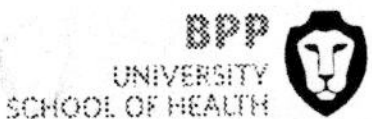

Chronic obstructive pulmonary disease (COPD)

Epidemiology

One million people in the UK have a diagnosis of COPD, with an extra two million thought to be undiagnosed. Around 18% and 14% of male and female smokers are affected respectively.

Aetiology

The chronic inflammatory changes are usually the result of tobacco smoke. Other factors such as air pollution and occupational exposures can contribute.

Alpha-1 antitrypsin deficiency is a rare cause (<1% of cases) and should be considered where there is early onset of symptoms. Alpha-1 antitrypsin is a protease inhibitor. Deficiency leads to uninhibited protease activity and chronic lung damage.

Common precipitants of exacerbations include bacterial infection (*S. pneumonia, H. influenzae*), viral infections and pollutants.

Pathophysiology

COPD is characterised by progressive airway obstruction that is poorly reversible. It is associated with an abnormal inflammatory response of the lungs to noxious particles or gases. The particles activate macrophages and epithelial cells, leading to a release of neutrophils and proteases. The chronic inflammation leads to:

- Narrowing and remodelling of airways
- Enlargement of mucus-secreting glands and increased goblet cells in the central airways
- Subsequent vascular bed changes

These changes lead to increased airway resistance which results in expiratory flow limitation and therefore hyperinflation. Hyperinflation and destruction of lung parenchyma causes hypoxia. This progressive hypoxia causes thickening of vascular smooth muscle and, ultimately, pulmonary hypertension and cor pulmonale.

Exacerbations can occur, where there is rapid and sustained worsening of symptoms. These increase with the severity of underlying COPD.

History/examination

History	• Dyspnoea • Cough • Sputum • Wheeze • Weight loss • Ankle oedema • Fatigue • Symptoms of infection • Confusion/drowsiness if acute hypercapnia or hypoxia • Exercise tolerance • Smoking history • History of exacerbations or ICU admissions for COPD • Home oxygen or nebulisers
Exam	• Tachypnoea • Accessory muscle use • Pursed lip breathing • Cyanosis • Hypoxia • Asterixis if hypercapnic • Reduced BMI • Hyperinflated chest • Wheeze on ausculation • Ankle oedema

Table 3.23: History and examination findings in COPD

Top tip:

Ask about exercise tolerance – this is often a key factor in deciding escalation of treatment to non-invasive ventilation and ITU.

Grade	Description
I	Not troubled by breathlessness except on strenuous exercise
II	Short of breath when hurrying or walking up a slight incline
III	Walks slower than contemporaries because of breathlessness or has to stop for breath when walking at own pace
IV	Stops for breath after walking 100 m or for a few minutes on level ground
V	Too breathless to leave the house or breathless when dressing or undressing

Table 3.24: The Medical Research Council (MRC) dyspnoea scale used to grade breathlessness

Investigations

Acute exacerbation of COPD:

Blood tests:

- FBC: may show increased white cell count in infective exacerbations, or polycythemia due to chronic hypoxia
- U&Es
- ABG: may show type 1 or 2 respiratory failure. In severe cases, respiratory acidosis may develop

Microbiology:

- Blood cultures: if the patient is pyrexial
- Sputum cultures: if there is purulent sputum

Imaging:

- Chest X-ray: to rule out other causes for symptoms. May show hyperinflation, flattened hemidiaphragms, increased intercostal spacing or signs of pulmonary hypertension.

Others:

- ECG: may show right ventricular hypertrophy, ischaemia or arrhythmia

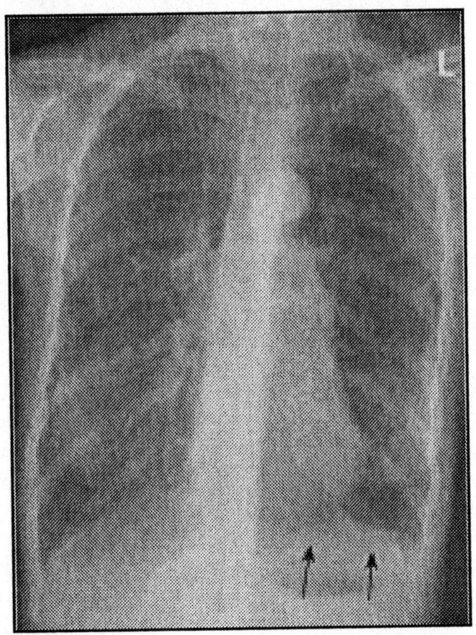

Figure 3.16: Chest X-ray showing bilateral, flattened hemidiaphragms, indicative of chronic respiratory disease

Chronic COPD:

Blood tests:

- FBC: to identify anaemia or polycythaemia
- Serum alpha-1-antitrypsin: if early onset, family history or minimal smoking history

Imaging:

- Chest X-ray: to rule out other causes for symptoms
- CT chest: if suspicious abnormalities on CXR, symptoms are out of proportion to spirometry results or if considering surgery

Others:

- Spirometry: a diagnosis of COPD is confirmed by post-bronchodilator spirometry. A FEV1/FVC ratio is required for diagnosis. The severity of airflow obstruction can be graded as per Table 3.25.
- Echocardiogram: if features of cor pulmonale.

Post-broncho-dilator FEV1/FVC	FEV1 % predicted	Stage
<0.7	≥80%*	Stage 1 – Mild
<0.7	50–79%	Stage 2 – Moderate
<0.7	30–49%	Stage 3 – Severe
<0.7	<30% or <50% with respiratory failure	Stage 4 – Very severe

Table 3.25: NICE classification of severity of airflow obstruction in COPD

***Note.** Patients with Stage 1 spirometry results must have symptoms consistent with the diagnosis of COPD.

Management

Acute exacerbation of COPD:

- Controlled oxygen therapy (ie via Venturi mask) to achieve SpO2 of 88–92%
- High dose short-acting bronchodilators (eg salbutamol or ipratropium via nebuliser or inhaler with spacer device)
- 30 mg prednisolone for 7–14 days
- Antibiotic therapy if symptoms consistent with infective exacerbation
- IV theophylline can be used if there is an inadequate response to bronchodilators

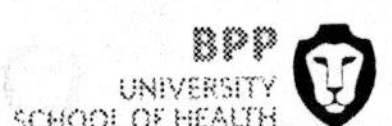

- Non-invasive ventilation (NIV)
- Chest physiotherapy if struggling to clear secretions
- Consider whether ICU referral and invasive ventilation would be appropriate

Chronic COPD:

General measures for the long-term management of COPD include:

- Smoking cessation – the single most important intervention in COPD
- Yearly influenza vaccination
- Pneumococcal vaccination
- Assessment of osteoporosis risk if multiple courses of steroids
- At least yearly primary care review
- Dietician review if low or reducing BMI

Pulmonary rehabilitation should be offered to all patients who have had a recent COPD-related hospital admission or who have symptomatic and disabling breathlessness.

SABA – short-acting β2 agonist
SAMA – short-acting muscarinic antagonist
LABA – long-acting β2 agonist
LAMA – long-acting muscarinic antagonist
ICS – inhaled corticosteroids

- Mucolytic therapy can also be given for patients with chronic productive cough. These patients might also benefit from chest physiotherapy.
- Patients with distressing breathlessness despite inhaler therapy should be considered for home nebuliser therapy.
- Selected patients with chronic hypercapnia may benefit from long-term NIV.

Long-term oxygen therapy (LTOT):

LTOT has been shown to improve both quality of life and survival in patients with severe chronic hypoxia. It is indicated in patients with:

- PaO2 ≤7.3kPa when stable
- PaO2 between 7.3kPa and 8.0kPA when stable, and one of:
  - Secondary polycythaemia
  - Nocturnal hypoxaemia
  - Peripheral oedema
  - Pulmonary hypertension

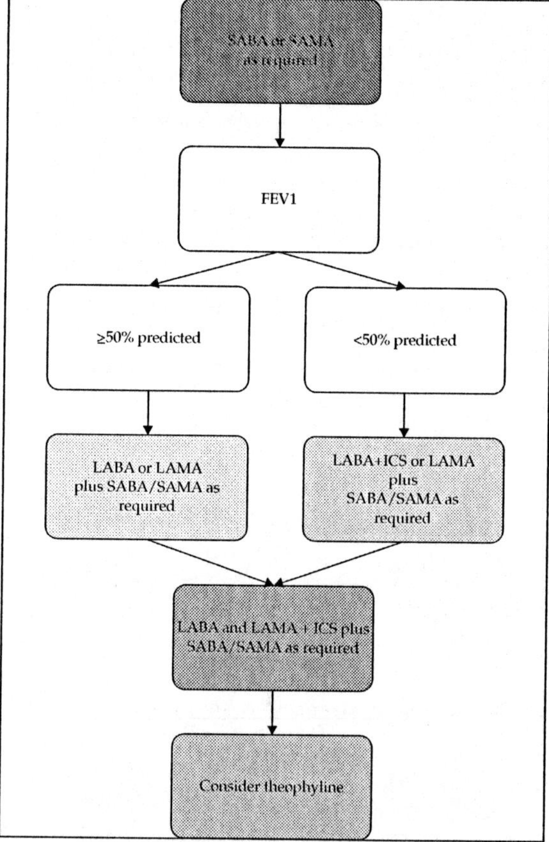

Figure 3.17: Stepwise management of COPD

The PaO2 must be assessed on two occasions at least three weeks apart.

Surgical intervention:

- Bullectomy is indicated if the patient is breathless, has an FEV1 less than 50% and has a single large bulla on CT scan.
- Lung volume reduction therapy should be considered in selected patients with upper lobe predominant emphysema, who are unable to complete activities of daily living despite maximal medical therapy.
- Lung transplantation can improve function and quality of life but does not appear to increase survival.

Prognosis

COPD is a progressive condition and patients will deteriorate, although the course is variable. It is the fifth most common cause of death in the UK. Five-year survival from diagnosis is 78% in men and 72% in women with mild disease, falling to 30% in men and 24% in women requiring oxygen or nebulised therapy. Acute exacerbations are associated with a rapid decline in lung function, reduced quality of life and higher mortality.

A Brief Guide to Bi-level NIV

Bi-level ventilation gives pressure support with differing inspiratory and expiratory pressures. The inspiratory positive airway pressure (IPAP) helps the air flow into the lungs, whilst the expiratory positive airway pressure (EPAP) helps overcome the lungs' intrinsic end-expiratory pressure.

NIV is indicated in acute exacerbations of COPD where there is persisting type 2 respiratory failure with acidosis ($pH < 7.35$) **despite optimal medical therapy**. Relative contraindications to NIV include facial trauma, vomiting, confusion/agitation, undrained pneumothorax, respiratory secretions, reduced consciousness and severe co-morbidity.

NIV should be initiated by a senior doctor (ST2 or above), with a **clear treatment escalation plan** in place – is the patient suitable for ITU and invasive ventilation if they deteriorate?

NIV can be an uncomfortable experience for the patient, so the initial pressures are set at a tolerable level (the British Thoracic Society recommends an IPAP of 10 cm H2O and EPAP of 4-5cm H2O). The IPAP is gradually increased at a rate of around 5 cm H2O/10 minutes until either there is a clinical response, the patient is unable to tolerate higher pressures or the IPAP reaches 20 cm H2O. Oxygen should be continued at a rate that maintains SpO_2 between 88% and 92%.

A repeat ABG should be done 1 hour after initiating NIV and after every subsequent change in setting. Further ABGs should be performed at 4 and 12 hours following initiation, or sooner if the patient deteriorates.

The patient and their ventilator should be reviewed if there is insufficient improvement on NIV. The ventilator should be checked to ensure there are no air leaks, the face mask is fitting well and it is synchronising with the patient's breathing. The patient should be examined to look for signs of general deterioration or of respiratory pathology (eg pneumothorax, mucus plugging).

Patients who improve on NIV should remain on NIV for as much as possible over the first 24 hours, with breaks for meals and medication. A plan for weaning off NIV should be in place and documented in the notes.

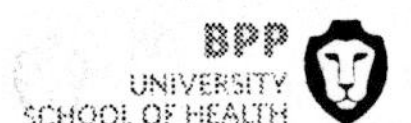

Further reading and references

1. Arnold, A., Harvey, J., and MacDuff, A. on behalf of the BTS Pleural Disease Guideline Group. (2010) BTS Pleural Disease Guideline. *Thorax* 2010; 65 (Supplement 2), ii18-ii31.
2. British Thoracic Society Guideline Development Group. (2008) *The use of non-invasive ventilation in the management of patients with chronic obstructive pulmonary disease admitted to hospital with acute type II respiratory failure (with particular reference to Bilevel positive pressure ventilation)*. London, British Thoracic Society.
3. Eraso, L.H., Galanis, T., Merli, G., et al. (2015) *Pulmonary embolism*. BMJ Best Practice. [Online] Available from: http://bestpractice.bmj.com/best-practice/monograph/116.html [Accessed 8 April 2016].
4. National Clinical Guideline Centre. (2010) *Chronic obstructive pulmonary disease: management of chronic obstructive pulmonary disease in adults in primary and secondary care* (CG101). London, NCGC.
5. National Clinical Guideline Centre. (2012) *Venous thromboembolic disease: the management of venous thromboembolic diseases and the role of thrombophilia testing* (CG144). London, NCGC.
6. National Institute for Health and Care Excellence. (2014) *Acute heart failure: diagnosing and managing acute heart failure in adults* (CG187). London, NICE.
7. Scottish Intercollegiate Guidelines Network and the British Thoracic Society. (2014) *British guideline on the management of asthma*. 141. Edinburgh/London, SIGN and BTS.

Chest pain

Differential diagnosis

System/Causes	Disease
Cardiac	**Acute coronary syndrome** **Aortis stenosis** **Aortic dissection** **Pericarditis** Hypertrophic cardiomyopathy **Myocarditis** Takotsubo cardiomyopathy
Respiratory	Pneumonia Pneumothorax Pulmonary embolism Lung cancer
GI	Gastro-oesophageal reflux disease Oesophagitis Peptic ulcer disease
Musculoskeletal	Costocondritis Rib pain Trauma Radiculopathy Mon-specific musculoskeletal pain
Other	Breast disease Herpes zoster infection Anxiety/panic disorder

Table 3.26: Differential diagnosis of chest pain

Acute coronary syndrome (ACS)

Epidemiology

In the UK, around 114,000 patients with acute coronary syndromes are admitted to hospital each year. The average incidence for MI in those aged 30–69 is about 600 per 100,000 in males and 200 per 100,000 in females. Incidence rates are comparatively higher in Scotland, Northern Ireland and the North of England.

Aetiology

Non-atherosclerotic causes of myocardial ischaemia and infarction include coronary emboli from endocarditis, vasculitis-related arterial occlusion, coronary artery spasm, cocaine use, trauma, increased oxygen requirement (eg hyperthyroidism) and decreased oxygen delivery (eg severe anaemia).

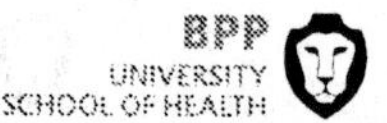

Non-modifiable	Modifiable
• Increasing age • Male sex • Family history of CAD • Premature menopause • South Asian ethnicity • Lower socioeconomic status	• **Smoking** • **Diabetes mellitus** • **Impaired glucose tolerance** • **Hypertension** • **Dyslipidaemia** • **Obesity** • **Physical inactivity**

Table 3.27: Risk factors for atherosclerosis

Pathophysiology

ACS is used to describe a spectrum of acute myocardial ischaemia ± infarction. The majority of cases of ACS are caused by coronary artery atherosclerosis.

Coronary artery atherosclerosis begins as a 'fatty streak', an accumulation of oxidised cholesterol in the intimal layer of the arterial wall. Endothelial damage leads to localised release of inflammatory markers, which stimulate smooth muscle and fibroplast proliferation. This leads to the formation of an atherosclerotic plaque, with a lipid core and a fibrous cap.

The lipid core of an atherosclerotic plaque is highly thrombogenic, and is prone to rupture as the plaque increases in size. Plaque rupture causes thrombus formation, which can embolise and block the distal coronary artery. This results in an acute reduction of blood flow to the distal myocardium. The myocardium becomes ischaemic and eventually may become infarcted.

There are three possible categories of ACS:

1. **ST-elevation myocardial infarction (STEMI):** ST elevation or new left bundle branch block (LBBB) on electrocardiogram (ECG) with accompanying troponin rise.
2. **Non-ST elevation myocardial infarction (NSTEMI):** No ST elevation or new LBBB seen on ECG but troponin rise detected.
3. **Unstable angina:** Symptoms of ischaemia but no ST elevation and a normal troponin.

History/examination

History	• Acute onset • Central/epigastric chest pain • Radiation to the arms, shoulders, neck or jaw • Described as a pressure, crushing or squeezing pain • Sweating • Nausea and vomiting • Breathlessness • Palpitations • Abdominal pain • Confusion • Presence of risk factors • Past cardiac history
Exam	• Patient looks pale and clammy • Altered mental state • Low grade pyrexia • Brady/tachycardia • Cool peripheries • Hyper- or hypotension • Third and fourth heart sound • Systolic heart murmur (mitral regurgitation or ventricular septal defect) • Signs of congestive heart failure

Table 3.28: History and examination findings in a patient with chest pain

Atypical presentations are more common in females, the elderly, diabetes mellitus and in ethnic minorities.

Investigations

Blood tests:

- FBC: to check for anaemia
- U&Es: electrolyte imbalances may cause arrhythmia (particularly potassium and magnesium)
- Lipid profile
- Glucose: hyperglycaemia is associated with an increased risk of complications and higher mortality
- TSH: to exclude hyperthyroidism
- Cardiac enzymes: typically serum troponin – the type of troponin used will vary between hospital trust

ECG:

- Serial ECGs should be performed to assess for dynamic changes.

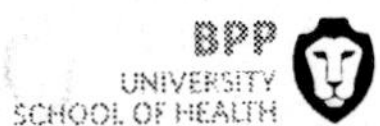

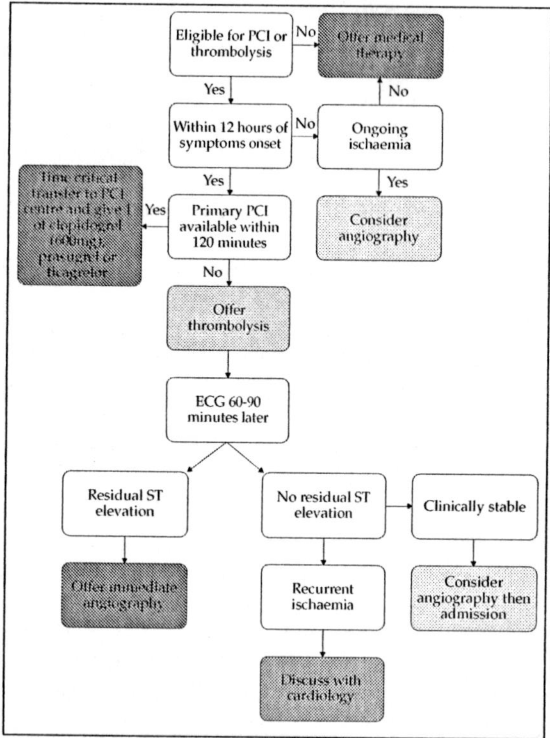

Figure 3.18: Investigation and management schema for a suspected STEMI/NSTEMI

- STEMI: ST segment elevation in at least two consecutive leads of at least 1 mm in the limb leads and 2 mm in the chest leads. Reciprocal ST depression may be present. New LBBB with ischaemic chest pain should be treated as STEMI.
- NSTEMI/unstable angina: T-wave flatting or inversion and ST depression may be seen. The ECG may be normal. The area of infarction in STEMI can be localised by the pattern of ECG changes.

Imaging:

- Chest X-ray: to aid differential diagnosis. May show signs of heart failure, consolidation or mediastinal widening.

Management

Initial management:

- ABCDE and resuscitate as necessary
- Cardiac monitor
- High flow oxygen to achieve SpO2 of 94–98% 300 mg oral aspirin
- Sublingual glyceryl trinitrate (GTN)
- Morphine 2.5–5 mg IV (+ anti-emetic)
- Beta-blocker unless contraindicated
- Sliding scale insulin if blood glucose is over 11 mmol/l

NSTEMI/unstable angina:

- 300 mg clopidogrel
- Fondaparinux 2.5 mg SC or unfractionated heparin
- GRACE score to risk stratify patients
- Indications for angiography:
  - As soon as possible if clinically unstable or high ischaemic risk
  - Within 72 hours of admission if the GRACE score indicates >3.0% 6 month mortality
  - Ischaemia demonstrated on ischaemia testing

STEMI:

- The initial management for STEMI is summarised in Figure 3.18.

Ongoing management:

- An ACE inhibitor should be started as soon as the patient is haemodynamically stable.
- Dual antiplatelet therapy for 12 months, followed by long-term aspirin:
  - Patients with STEMI, who did not undergo stenting, should either have aspirin and ticagrelor for at least 12 months or aspirin and clopidogrel for at least 1 month.
- A beta-blocker should be started as soon as possible after an MI, and continued for 12 months, or indefinitely if there is evidence of left ventricular systolic dysfunction.
- All patients should be offered a cardiac rehabilitation programme with an exercise component.
- Risk factor reduction: Mediterranean-style diet, regular physical activity, smoking cessation, weight loss, statin therapy, good blood pressure control and good glycaemic control.

Prognosis

Up to 50% of those who have an acute MI die within 30 days of the event. Half of these are before medical assistance arrives or the patient reaches hospital.

Prognosis strongly correlates with the degree of necrosis and the timing and nature of the intervention.

Complications of an acute MI include:

- **Ischaemic**: failure of reperfusion, infarction extension, postinfarction angina
- **Mechanical:** heart failure, cardiogenic shock, acute mitral regurgitation, ventricular septal rupture, free wall rupture, left ventricular aneurysm
- **Arrhythmias**
- **Thrombosis and embolic:** deep vein thrombosis, pulmonary embolism, ischaemic stroke
- **Inflammatory:** pericarditis
- **Psychosocial:** anxiety, depression

Aortic stenosis (AS)

Epidemiology

AS is the most common valvular disease in the Western world. It largely affects older people, with patients typically presenting in the seventh or eighth decade.

Aetiology

There are three main causes of valvular AS.

1. **Degenerative**
   This accounts for around 80% of AS in the US and Europe. Arteriosclerotic changes involving the valve lead to calcification (sclerosis) and degeneration, resulting in loss of function. Risk factors include smoking, hypertension, diabetes, increased LDL cholesterol and CKD.

2. **Congenital bicuspid aortic valve**
   Turbulent blood flow and mechanical stresses through the deformed valve result in a gradual stenosis and calcification. The mean age of symptom onset is 40–50 years.

3. **Rheumatic fever**
   AS due to rheumatic fever is rare in industrialised countries, but is still present in the developing world. The streptococcal infection triggers an autoimmune reaction against the valvular epithelium. There is gradual thickening and calcification, which result in the fusion of the aortic valve.

Other causes of LV obstruction can mimic the symptoms of AS. These include hypertrophic obstructive cardiomyopathy, supravalvular obstruction in Williams syndrome and congenital subvalvular AS.

Pathophysiology

Aortic stenosis occurs when there is obstruction to blood flow across the aortic valve due to pathological narrowing. The obstruction leads to chronic elevation in left ventricular pressure and left ventricular hypertrophy. The hypertrophied left ventricle has a smaller volume and is less compliant, resulting in an increased end-diastolic pressure and diastolic dysfunction. The left atrial and pulmonary venous pressures increase to compensate for this.

With increasing stenosis, systolic function also reduces. Increase in cardiac output is limited due to fixed outflow obstruction. This, combined with increased myocardial demand secondary to hypertrophy, leads to ischaemic symptoms on exertion.

Infarct site	Artery occluded	ECG changes
Anterior	LAD	ST elevation in V1-V6 (maximal elevation in V3-4) ST depression in II, III and aVF
Septal	LAD	ST elevation in V1-V4
Lateral	LCX or marginalis obtusis	ST elevation in I, aVL, V5 and V6 Reciprocal ST depression in II, III and aVF
Inferior	RCA (80%) or RCX	ST elevation in II, III and aVF ST depression in I and aVL Bradycardia and heart block
Posterior	RCX	ST elevation in V7-9 High R-waves and ST depression in V1-V3
Right ventricle	RCA	ST elevation in V1 and V4R ST depression in I and AVL

Table 3.29: ECG patterns with different areas of cardiac ischaemia

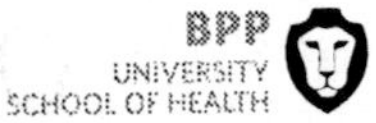

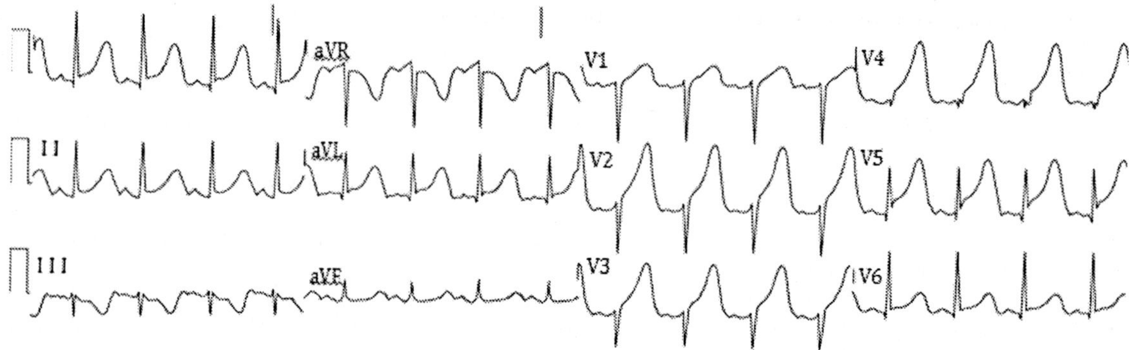

Figure 3.19: ECG pattern showing acute antero-lateral MI

History/examination

History	• Shortness of breath on exertion • Angina • Syncope/dizziness • Sudden death • Presence of risk factors (eg rheumatic fever, arteriosclerotic risk factors)
Exam	• Ejection systolic murmur with radiation to the carotids and heard best at the left sternal edge or aortic region • Soft S2 • Slow rising pulse • Narrow pulse pressure • Left ventricular heave at the apex • S4 (due to left ventricular hypertrophy) • Paradoxically split S2 in severe AS

Table 3.30: History and examination findings in aortic stenosis

Investigations

Imaging:

- CXR: typically will show a prominent enlarged ascending aorta and left ventricular border of the heart. Calcification of the aortic valve may also be seen. Signs of heart failure should be looked for.

ECG:

- Left ventricular hypertrophy
- Left atrial enlargement
- Left axis deviation
- Left ventricular strain (ST depression and T wave inversion in I, aVL, V5 and V6)
- AV nodal conduction disease
- Left bundle branch block

Echocardiogram:

- Thickened, calcified and immobile aortic valve cusps
- Increased aortic pressure gradient
- Reduced aortic valve area
- Reduced left ventricular ejection fraction
- Left ventricular hypertrophy

Second-line investigations include cardiac MRI, exercise stress testing, dobutamine stress echocardiography and cardiac catherisation.

Management

General/conservative:

- Patients should be advised to avoid heavy exertion.

Medical:

- Beta-blockers for angina
- Anti-arrhythmics to maintain sinus rhythm
- Anti-hypertensives (caution as hypotension may precipitate symptoms)
- Statins if hyperlipidaemia
- Treatment of underlying coronary artery disease
- Symptomatic treatment of heart failure with diuretics, an ACE inhibitor and/or digoxin

Surgical:

Patients with symptomatic AS require early surgical intervention.

- Aortic valve replacement
- Transcatheter aortic valve implantation (TAVI)

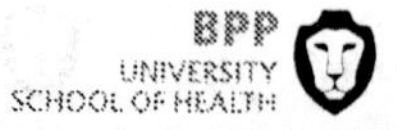

  - For patients who are unsuitable for aortic valve replacement
- Balloon valvuloplasty
  - Usually used as a bridging therapy for patients who are too unwell for valve replacement, as there is a high stenosis recurrence rate

Prognosis

Adults with AS have a mortality rate of 9% per year. Sudden death occurs in 3–5% of patients, rising to 8–34% in symptomatic patients.

The approximate interval from onset of symptoms to death is:

- Two years for heart failure
- Three years for syncope
- Five years for angina

Surgical replacement of the valve results in near-normal life expectancy.

Aortic dissection

Epidemiology

3–4 cases per 100,000 per year occur in the UK. It most commonly occurs in males aged 50–70.

Aetiology

- Hypertension
- Atherosclerosis
- Connective tissue disorders (cause weakening of the media)
- Turner's syndrome
- Vascular inflammation (eg giant cell arteritis)
- Deceleration trauma
- Pre-existing aneurysm
- Coarctation of the aorta
- Pregnancy (most commonly in the third trimester)
- Iatrogenic (during endovascular interventions or aortic surgery)

Pathophysiology

Aortic dissection results from a tear in the intimal layer of the aorta wall, which extends into the media. Blood then passes through the media, creating a false lumen. The dissection may occlude arteries that branch off the aorta, including the coronary arteries, and can cause acute aortic regurgitation. If the dissection breaches the full thickness of the aortic wall, haemothorax and haemopericardium can occur.

History/examination

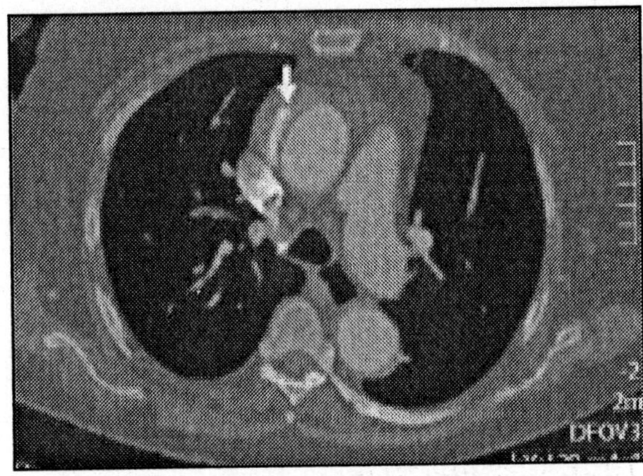

Figure 3.20: CT scan showing an aortic dissection (white arrow)

History	• Sudden onset chest pain • 'Ripping' or 'tearing' pain • Radiation to the back or between the scapula • Migrating pain as the dissection progresses • Syncope • Dyspnoea • Family history • Presence of risk factors • Symptoms depending on artery branch occluded by dissection: – Stroke (carotid) – Angina (coronary) – Paraplegia (spinal) – Abdominal pain (superior mesenteric) – Limb pain (distal aorta)
Exam	• Features of Marfan or Ehlors Danlos syndromes • Left/right blood pressure differential • Aortic regurgitation • Hyper- or hypotension • Hypovolaemic shock • Pulse differential or deficit in the legs

Table 3.31: History and examination findings in aortic dissection

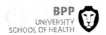

Investigations

Blood tests:

- FBC
- Coagulation screen
- Renal function: AKI may result from renal artery occlusion
- Liver function tests: liver ischaemia
- Cardiac enzymes: to exclude ACS
- Group and save

Imaging:

- CXR: may show a widened mediastinum
- CT angiography: this will demonstrate the intimal flap within the dissected aorta
- MRI: can confirm diagnosis and is better than CT for identifying the involvement of other vessels, but is not as widely available

Others:

- ECG: to look for evidence of myocardial ischaemia
- Echocardiogram: useful in patients who cannot undergo IV contrast

Management

- ABCDE and resuscitate as necessary
- Beta-blockers ± vasodilators to maintain a heart rate of less than 80 and a systolic blood pressure of 100–120
- Adequate analgesia
- Transfer to HDU/ITU

The Stanford classification for aortic dissection is used to guide management. It classifies dissections by whether the ascending aorta is involved – Type A dissections involve the ascending aorta, whereas Type B dissections do not.

- **Type A dissection**: urgent cardiothoracic referral for open aortic replacement ± aortic valve repair/ replacement.
- **Uncomplicated Type B dissection, patient stable**: medical therapy to control pain, heart rate and blood pressure, with close monitoring. Thoracic endovascular aortic repair should be considered.
- **Complicated Type B dissection**: thoracic endovascular aortic repair is the treatment of choice, although open surgery may be necessary in more complex cases.

Prognosis

50–60% will die within 24 hours if untreated. For Type A dissections, surgery reduces mortality at 1 month from 90% to 30%.

Pericarditis

Pathophysiology

Pericarditis is an inflammatory response of the pericardium associated with fibrin deposition and pericardial effusion. The inflammation irritates the underlying myocardium and causes a systemic inflammatory response.

Epidemiology

Pericarditis may account for up to 5% of A&E presentations for chest pain, but a large number go undiagnosed. It is more common in men between the ages of 20 and 50.

Aetiology

- Idiopathic (most common)
- Infections: viral, bacterial, fungal, parasitic
- Systemic autoimmune disorders: SLE, RA, scleroderma
- Secondary to an immune process: rheumatic fever, Dressler's syndrome
- Disease of surrounding organs: acute MI, myocarditis, paraneoplastic syndrome
- Metabolic: uraemia, myxedema
- Traumatic
- Neoplastic: sarcoma, mesothelioma, breast, lung, haematological malignancies, melanoma

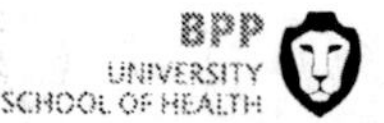

History/examination

History	• Chest pain • Constant • Radiation to the trapezius ridges • Worsened by inspiration, swallowing, coughing and lying flat • Relieved by sitting forwards • Cough • Chills and rigors • Weakness • Risk factors (eg MI, cardiac surgery, infection)
Exam	• Tachypnoea • Tachycardia • Fever • Pericardial rub (best heard at the left lower sternal edge with the patient leading forward in full expiration) • Beck's triad in cases of tamponade – hypotension, increased JVP and quiet heart sounds

Table 3.32: History and examination findings in pericarditis

Investigations

Blood tests:

- FBC: may show raised WCC
- U&Es
- Inflammatory markers: CRP/ESR
- Troponin: to rule out acute MI

Imaging:

- CXR: an enlarged cardiac silhouette may indicate pericardial effusion
- CT/MRI: used where there is diagnostic doubt or in atypical or complicated cases

Others:

- ECG: saddle-shaped widespread ST elevation and PR depression
- Echocardiogram: detects pericardial effusions and left ventricular wall motion abnormalities
- Investigation of the underlying cause is usually not necessary unless TB is suspected or if symptoms don't improve after one week. Further investigations include:
  - Blood cultures
  - Testing for tuberculosis
  - Rheumatoid factor, antinuclear antibody and anti-DNA
  - Thyroid function
  - Viral serology for HIV, influenza virus, echovirus and Coxsackievirus
  - Pericardiocentesis/pericardial biopsy

Management

- NSAID ± colchicine
- Restriction of physical activity
- Avoidance of anticoagulation
- Treatment of underlying cause if identified
- Cardiac tamponade may require pericardiocentesis
- Surgical management may be required in recurrent pericarditis

Patients with any of the following features are considered high risk, and should be admitted to hospital:

- Pyrexia >38.0°C and raised WCC
- Evidence of cardiac tamponade
- A large pericardial effusion
- Immunosuppression
- Oral anticoagulant therapy
- Acute trauma
- Lack of response to NSAIDs after one week
- Elevated troponin (suggests myopericarditis)

Prognosis

20% to 50% will experience one or more recurrences.

Myocarditis

Epidemiology

The mean age of presentation is around 40 years old. It accounts for around 10% of sudden cardiac death in young adults.

Aetiology

- Infection: viral (most common cause in the developed world), bacterial, spirochetal, fungal, parasitic, protozoal, rickettsial
- Immune-mediated: sarcoidosis, SLE, scleroderma, IBD, Kawasaki disease, myasthenia gravis, polymyositis, thyrotoxicosis, heart transplant rejection
- Drug hypersensitivity: clozapine, paracetamol, amitriptyline, furosemide, methyldopa, penicillin, phenytoin
- Toxic: drug-related, heavy metal poisoning, arsenic, insect stings and bites, carbon monoxide
- Physical: electric shock, hyperpyrexia, radiation

Pathophysiology

Myocarditis is defined as inflammation of the myocardium in the absence of ischaemia. The pathogenesis is not completely understood. In viral myocarditis, it is thought that direct invasion of the myocardium by the infectious organism leads to activation of local and systemic immunological processes.

History/examination

Presentation can be variable and myocarditis can be very difficult to diagnose.

History	• May be asymptomatic • Fatigue • Chest pain • Fever • Viral prodrome • Dyspnoea and orthopnea • Palpitations • PMH of autoimmune or infectio[u]s disease • Exposure to relevant drugs or toxins
Exam	• Tachycardia • Pyrexia • Raised JVP • Presence of 3rd and/or 4th heart sound • Bibasal crackles on chest auscultation

Table 3.33: History and examination findings in myocarditis

Investigations

Blood tests:

- FBC: leukocytosis in 25%
- U&Es
- Creatinine kinase
- Troponin
- CRP/ESR
- LFTs

Imaging:

- CXR: may show signs of heart failure
- Cardiac MRI: should be considered in clinically stable patients prior to biopsy

Histology:

- Endomyocardial biopsy: the gold standard diagnostic test. Samples should be sent for histology, viral PCR and immunohistochemistry.

Others:

- EC... T wave changes, conduction disturbances
- E... hy: may show ventricular ... ll motion abnormalities

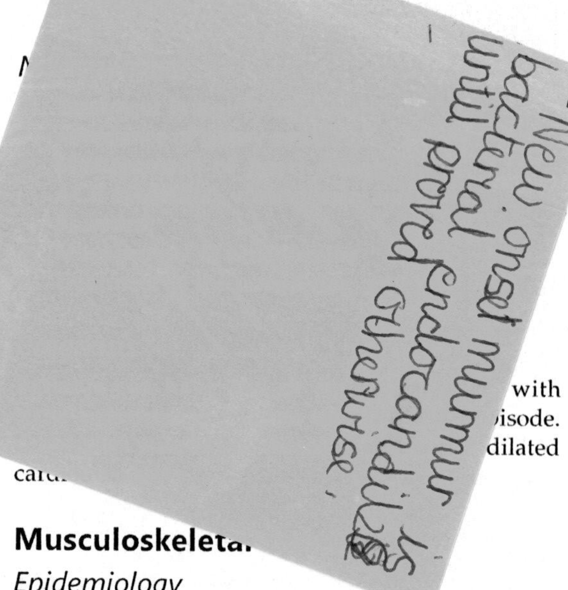

- New onset murmur
bacterial endocarditis
until proved otherwise,

... with ... isode. ... dilated car...

Musculoskeleta...

Epidemiology

Musculoskeletal chest pain is common, and is a more likely cause of chest pain in young patients with no or little cardiac risk factors.

Aetiology

- Inflammation of cartilage: costochondritis, Tietze's syndrome
- Muscular strain
- Bony injury: rib fracture, neoplasm
- Breast disease
- Inflammatory joint disease

Pathophysiology

There are many bony and soft tissue structures in the chest wall that may lead to musculoskeletal chest pain. Mechanisms of pain include acute trauma, muscular strain and inflammatory joint disease.

History/examination

History	• Sharp stabbing chest pain • Localised pain • No radiation • No autonomic symptoms • May be pleuritic or worse on movement • History of preceding trauma or repetitive microtrauma (eg coughing)
Exam	• Tenderness on chest wall palpation • Stable observations

Table 3.34: History and examination findings in musculoskeletal chest pain

Investigations

Investigations are mainly carried out to exclude more serious pathology.

Blood tests:

- Troponin: to exclude cardiac event

ECG:

- No acute or dynamic ischaemic changes

Imaging:

- CXR: to exclude cardiac or pulmonary pathology. Rib fractures may be seen.

Management

Treatment is usually with analgesia and reassurance. Pain must be sufficiently controlled to allow the patient to take deep breaths.

Prognosis

Prognosis depends on the underlying cause. Most causes of musculoskeletal chest pain are self-limiting and carry an excellent prognosis. Complications of chest wall trauma include pneumothorax, haemothorax, surgical emphysema and pneumonia.

Further reading and references

1. Aboyans, V., Boileau, C., Bossone, E. et al. (2014) 2014 ESC Guidelines on the diagnosis and treatment of aortic diseases. European Heart Journal 2014; 35(35), pp.2873-2926.
2. Adler, Y., Badano, L, Barón-Esquivias G., et al. (2015) 2015 ESC Guidelines for the diagnosis and management of pericardial diseases. European Heart Journal 2015; 36(42), pp.2921-2964.
3. Babaliaros, V., Kalra, G.L., and Parker, R.M. (2015) Aortic stenosis. BMJ Best Practice. [Online]. Available from: http://bestpractice.bmj.com/best-practice/monograph/325.html [Accessed 27 April 2016].
4. Arbustini, E., Basso, C., Caforio, A.L.P., et al. (2013) Current state of knowledge on aetiology, diagnosis, management, and therapy of myocarditis. European Heart Journal 2013; 34 (22), pp.2636-2648.
5. National Clinical Guideline Centre. (2013) Myocardial infarction with ST-segment elevation (CG167). London, NCGC.
6. National Clinical Guideline Centre. (2013) MI – secondary prevention (CG48). London, NCGC.
7. National Clinical Guideline Centre. (2010) Unstable angina and NSTEMI: the early management of unstable angina and non-ST-segment-elevation myocardial infarction (CG94). London, NCGC.

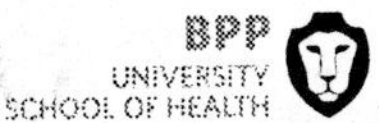

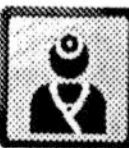

Cough

Differential diagnosis

System/Causes	Disease
Respiratory	**Upper respiratory tract infection** **Pneumonia** Acute bronchitis Asthma Chronic obstructive pulmonary disease **Lung cancer** **Tuberculosis** Cystic fibrosis **Bronchiectasis** Interstitial lung disease
Other	Post-viral airway hyper-responsiveness Gastro-oesophageal reflux Drug-related (eg ACE inhibitors) Foreign body ingestion Upper airway cough syndrome

Table 3.35: Differential diagnosis of cough

Pneumonia

Pathophysiology

Pneumonia refers to acute lung inflammation, with infiltration of the alveoli and bronchioles by inflammatory cells in response to infection. Transmission is usually via droplet inhalation.

Infection can either be confined to one lobe (lobar pneumonia) or occur in a patchy distribution throughout the lung fields (bronchopneumonia).

Community-Acquired Pneumonia (CAP)

Epidemiology

0.5–1% of people will develop a CAP each year, with most cases occurring in the autumn and winter months.

Aetiology

Risk factors for CAP include extremes of age, smoking, alcohol excess, preceding viral infection, underlying respiratory disease, immunosuppression and IV drug use.

Important causative organisms include:

- **Streptococcus pneumoniae**: the most common causative organism across all age groups.
- **Mycoplasma pneumoniae**: common around the winter period, with episodes around every three to four years.
- **Haemophilus influenzae**: particularly common in patients with COPD.
- **Legionella pneumophilia**: found in man-made water-containing systems (eg cooling towers, air conditioning). Around 50% of UK cases are related to foreign travel.
- **Viruses**: influenza, parainfluenza and the Adenoviruses can cause pneumonia at the extremes of age. Rare in the immunocompetent.
- **Staphylococcus aureus**: a rare cause of pneumonia that can complicate viral pneumonia. More common in IV drug users.

History/examination

History	• Cough • Purulent sputum • Shortness of breath • Pleuritic chest pain • Fever • Malaise • Confusion • Recent foreign travel • IV drug use
Exam	• Tachypnoea • Hypoxia • Tachycardia • Pyrexia • Bronchial breathing and/or crackles on chest auscultation • Dullness on percussion over the affected area

Table 3.36: History/examination findings in a patient with CAP

Investigations

Blood tests:

- FBC: raised white cell count
- U&Es: may show acute kidney injury. Hyponatraemia is seen in Legionella pneumonia
- LFTs: may be deranged in Legionella pneumonia

- CRP
- ABG if hypoxic
- Lactate if signs of sepsis

Urine:

- Pneumococcal antigen for moderate to severe CAP (CURB65 of 2 or more)
- Legionella antigen if severe CAP (CURB65 of 3 or more), risk factors or clinical suspicion

Microbiology:

- Sputum culture
- Blood cultures

Imaging:

- Chest X-ray: will show consolidation

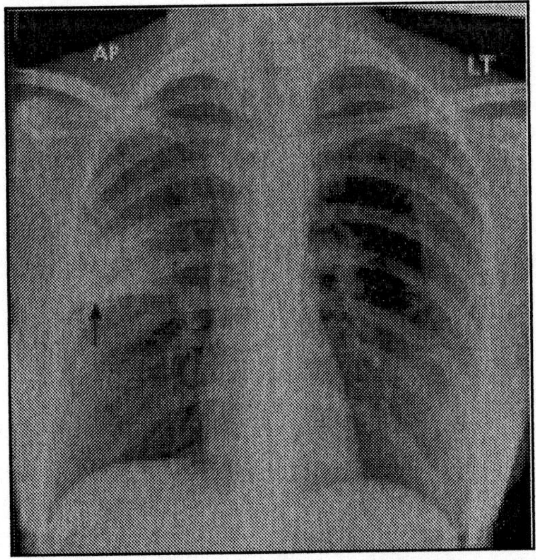

Figure 3.21: Chest X-ray showing consolidation in right middle zone

Management

- Oxygen therapy (target 94–98% unless underlying respiratory disease)
- IV fluids if required
- Some patients with severe CAP may require HDU/ITU involvement

The severity of the pneumonia should be assessed using the CURB65 scoring system below:

C	New onset confusion
U	Urea >7 mmol/l
R	Respiratory rate ≥30
B	Blood pressure <90 systolic or ≤60 diastolic
65	Age ≥65

Top tip:

The CURB65 score tends to underestimate severity in younger patients – it should always be used in conjunction with clinical judgement.

The following table illustrates the British Thoracic Society's recommended empirical antibiotic therapy for CAP. Local antimicrobial guidelines may differ.

Low severity (eg CURB65 0 or 1)	• <3% mortality • 1st line: oral amoxicillin • 2nd line: oral doxycycline or clarithromycin
Moderate severity (eg CURB65 2)	• 9% mortality • 1st line: oral amoxicillin and clarithromycin • 2nd line: oral doxycycline or levofloxacin or moxifloxacin
High severity (eg CURB65 3–5)	• 15–40% mortality • 1st line: IV co-amoxiclav and clarithromycin • 2nd line: IV benzylpenicillin and levofloxacin or ciprofloxacin or IV cefuroxime/cefotaxime/ceftriaxone and clarithromycin • Add levofloxacin if Legionella suspected

Table 3.37: Features of CURB65 score graded CAP

Patients with low severity CAP may be able to be managed in the community setting.

Prognosis

Mortality varies from <3% in low severity CAP to up to 40% in high severity CAP.

Complications include:

- Pleural effusion
- Empyema
- Lung abscess
- Pneumothorax
- Septicaemia and multi-organ failure

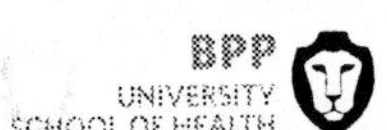

A repeat chest X-ray should be performed four to six weeks later to ensure resolution in changes, particularly in older patients, or those with a smoking history.

Hospital-Acquired Pneumonia (HAP)

Epidemiology

HAP (defined as development of a new pneumonia after 48 hours in hospital) occurs in around 5% of inpatients.

Aetiology

Risk factors for HAP include extremes of age, immunocompromise, underlying lung disease, recent surgery, mechanical ventilation, antacid therapy, poor hygiene from healthcare workers and supine position.

HAP is usually caused by gram-negative bacteria (eg *E.coli* and *Proteus*). Other organisms include *Pseudomonas* (particularly in mechanically ventilated patients and patients with bronchiectasis) and *Klebsiella pneumoniae*.

Management

- Empirical antibiotics are per local microbiology guidelines. Broad spectrum antibiotics that have good gram negative cover are generally used.
- Supportive treatment (eg oxygen, IV fluids) as per CAP.
- Chest physiotherapy may be required.

Prevention:

- Hand hygiene and infection control measures
- Adequate analgesia
- Early mobilisation
- Early chest physiotherapy if required
- Avoidance of stomach pH lowering medication where possible
- Appropriate antimicrobial prescribing

Prognosis

Development of HAP extends hospital stay by 7 to 9 days on average. All-cause mortality for HAP is between 30% and 70%, with an attributable mortality of 10%.

Aspiration pneumonia

Epidemiology

Aspiration may account for up to 15% of community-acquired pneumonia. It is also common in hospitalised patients.

Aetiology

Risk factors for aspiration pneumonia include impaired consciousness, poor oral hygiene, dental disease, swallowing disorders, gastro-oesophageal reflux and cognitive impairment.

Anaerobic organisms are more likely to be implicated than in CAP.

Pathophysiology

Aspiration pneumonia occurs as a result of inhalation of stomach contents or oropharyngeal secretions. Aspiration of small volumes is common even in healthy people – however, normal defence mechanisms mean that usually there is no ill effect. Aspiration has the potential to cause a chemical pneumonitis, obstruct the respiratory tract or lead to lower airways infection.

The usual site for aspiration pneumonia is the right lower lobe due to the anatomy of the bronchial tree.

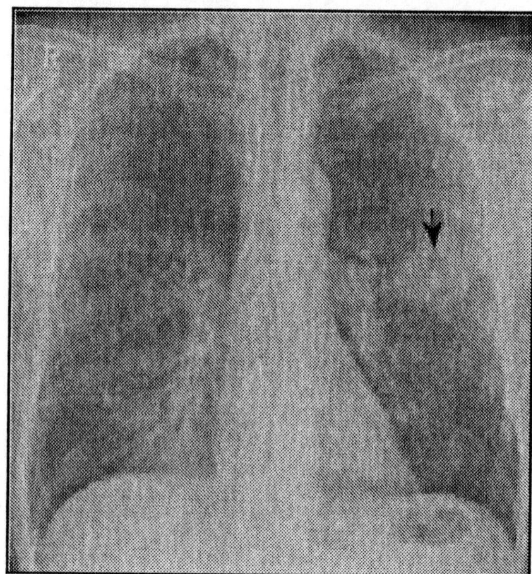

Figure 3.22: Chest X-ray showing a mass in the left middle zone

Management

- Supportive treatment as per CAP/HAP
- Empirical antibiotic therapy, including cover for anaerobic organisms (eg metronidazole)
- Speech and language therapy assessment

Lung cancer

Pathophysiology

A complex combination of genetic and environmental factors leads to activation of oncogenes and inactivation of tumour-suppressor genes. This results in unregulated cell division and tumour growth. The tumour can invade into surrounding tissues and spread to other parts of the body via the bloodstream or the lymphatic system. The excretion of hormones and cytokines by the tumour and the immune response against the tumour can lead to a variety of paraneoplastic syndromes.

Small cell	Around 18% of cases. Generally affects the central lung with mediastinal involvement. It metastasises early, with 75% having metastatic disease by time of diagnosis.
Squamous cell	Around 25% of cases. It predominantly affects central airways. Local invasion is common, with metastasis occurring late.
Adenocarcinoma	Around 21% of cases. A relatively slow growing tumour, which metastasises late. It is often found peripherally. Most common type in non-smokers.
Large cell	Around 3% of cases. It is a central tumour with features of squamous cell and adenocarcinoma. It metastasises early.

Table 3.38: The main histological types of lung cancer

Other less common histological types include bronchoalveolar cell carcinoma and carcinoid tumours.

History/examination

History	• Chronic cough • Dyspnoea • Weight loss • Haemoptysis • Chest pain • Recurrent or persistent chest infections • Fatigue • Hoarseness (laryngeal nerve palsy) • Upper limb and facial swelling (SVC obstruction) • Features of metastasis – bone pain, headache, seizures, weakness, altered sensation, confusion, jaundice, abdominal pain • Family/personal history of cancer • Smoking history
Exam	• Cachexia • Finger clubbing • Horner's syndrome (Pancoast's tumour) • Supraclavicular lymphadenopathy • Upper limb and facial swelling and dilated veins (SVC obstruction) • Signs of pleural effusion or lung collapse • Hepatomegaly and jaundice • Focal neurology

Table 3.39: History and examination findings in patients with lung cancer

Other signs and symptoms may arise from paraneoplastic syndromes, examples of which include:

- Endocrine: SIADH, hypercalcaemia, Cushing's syndrome
- Neuromuscular: neuropathy, Lambert-Eaton syndrome, encephalomyelitis
- Skeletal: hypertrophic pulmonary osteoarthropathy
- Renal: glomerulonephritis, nephrotic syndrome
- Collagen/vascular: SLE, endocarditis, myositis, vasculitis
- Cutaneous: erythema multiforme, urticaria, dermatomyositis
- Haematological: anaemia, acidosis, thrombotic thrombocytopenic purpura, disseminated intravascular coagulation
- Paraneoplastic syndromes are particularly common in small cell lung cancer

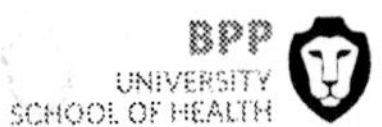

Investigations

Blood tests:

- FBC
- U&Es
- LFTs
- Calcium
- Coagulation screen pre-biopsy

Imaging:

- Chest X-ray: should be requested for all patients with haemoptysis or unexplained or persistent respiratory symptoms
- CT chest/abdomen/pelvis: essential for staging
- PET-CT: offer to patients who are suitable for curative treatment and have a low probability of mediastinal involvement
- Neck ultrasound: offer to patients with a high chance of mediastinal malignancy on CT
- CT/MRI brain if suspicion of brain metastasis

Cytology:

- Aspiration of pleural effusion if present
- Sputum cytology for patients with central masses who are unable to undergo more invasive testing

Histology:

- Transbronchial needle aspiration (endobronchial ultrasound-guided/non-ultrasound-guided)
- Endoscopic ultrasound fine needle aspiration
- Bronchoscopy: for central lesions where nodal staging will not influence treatment
- CT/USS-guided transthoracic needle biopsy: peripheral lung lesions and superficial lymph nodes
- Surgical biopsy: where less invasive methods of biopsy have been unsuccessful

Other:

- Spirometry: this is particularly important if surgery is an option.
- Assessment of performance status (see table below): this will influence treatment decisions.

0	Fully active, no restrictions on activity.
1	Restricted in physically strenuous activity but capable of light work (eg light housework).
2	Self-caring and active for more than 50% of waking hours but unable to carry out work activities.
3	Confined to bed or chair for more than 50% of waking hours. Limited ability to self-care.
4	Confined to bed or chair. Unable to self-care.
5	Dead.

Table 3.40: WHO performance status score

Management

All patients with suspected or diagnosed lung cancer should be referred to a Lung Cancer MDT. NSCLC is staged using the TNM system, whilst SCLC is split into limited- and extensive-stage disease.

Smoking cessation should be encouraged where applicable, particularly in those with a more favourable prognosis.

Case Study: An unusual presentation

A 71-year-old woman with a history of COPD presents with a 4 week history of increasing short-term memory loss, confusion and hallucinations. CT head shows small vessel ischaemia. CXR shows only non-specific ground glass changes – her only respiratory symptom is an occasionally productive cough. She is treated for UTI and SIADH secondary to recent SSRI use. However, her symptoms persist. A CT CAP is performed, showing a paratracheal mass in the right lung and a lesion in the liver. Biopsy leads to a diagnosis of SCLC. Anti-neuronal antibodies are detected in her blood, suggestive of a neurological paraneoplastic syndrome. Due to her performance status, she is treated palliatively.

Learning Points

- SIADH in a patient with a significant smoking history is suspicious for malignancy.
- SCLC can present in a wide variety of ways, and is often metastatic at diagnosis.
- Centrally located lung masses can be difficult to detect on chest X-ray.

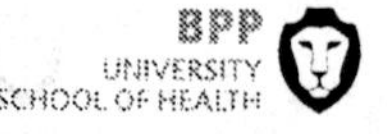

NSCLC:

- Surgery
  - Lobectomy is the treatment of choice for patients with no mediastinal involvement or distant metastases (stages I and II).
  - More extensive surgery might be required to obtain tumour-free margins.
- Radiotherapy
  - Radical radiotherapy should be considered in all patients without metastatic disease (stages I to III) who are not suitable for surgery.
  - Post-operative radiotherapy should be considered if there is incomplete resection of the tumour.
- Chemotherapy
  - Chemotherapy should be offered to patients with mediastinal and metastatic disease (stages III and IV) and good performance status.
  - Can be used as an adjuvant following tumour resection.

SCLC:

- Chemotherapy
  - Multidrug chemotherapy regimens are the treatment of choice.
- Radiotherapy
  - Patients with limited-stage disease should be offered thoracic irradiation if there has been a good response to chemotherapy.
  - Prophylactic cranial irradiation should also be considered.
  - In extensive-stage disease, thoracic irradiation should be considered if there has been a full response at distal sites and a good response in the thorax.
- Surgery
  - Surgery may be an option for those presenting at an early stage, although this is rare.

Palliative care:

- Opiate medication to control breathlessness, cough and pain.
- Palliative radiotherapy can improve symptoms due to bronchial obstruction, haemoptysis, SVC obstruction, bone pain, cerebral metastases and spinal cord compression.
- Bronchoscopic debulking for haemoptysis and bronchial obstruction.
- Stent insertion for bronchial obstruction or SVC obstruction.
- Pleural aspiration or drainage for pleural effusion +/- talc pleurodesis.
- Corticosteroids for cerebral metastases.
- Spinal cord compression can be treated with corticosteroids, radiotherapy and/or surgery.

Prognosis

Prognosis is poor as patients tend to present late and with metastatic disease. The median survival in England is 203 days from diagnosis.

Upper respiratory tract infection

The main categories of upper respiratory tract infection are outlined below.

Common cold

- Acute self-limiting inflammation of the upper respiratory tract mucosa.
- Commonly caused by Rhinoviruses and Coronoviruses.
- Spread via the aerosol route (highly infectious).
- Symptoms develop over one to two days.
- Sneezing and rhinorrhoea are the most common symptoms. Swelling of mucosal passages causes the sensation of a blocked nose. Other symptoms include a sore throat, rhinitis and cough.
- Occasionally secondary bacterial infection can cause sinusitis.
- No investigations are required.
- Treatment is symptomatic, with paracetamol, fluids and decongestants.

Pharyngitis

- Infection of the pharynx (including the tonsils and adenoids).
- Mostly caused by viruses or Group A streptococci.
- There is an acute onset of sore throat and pharyngeal inflammation without nasal congestion. Systemic features such as fever may occur.
- The tonsils may appear enlarged with visible pus. There may be cervical lymphadenopathy.
- The Centor score can be used to calculate the probability of bacterial infection. If the probability is high, consider throat swab and rapid antigen testing for Group A streptococci.
- Pharyngitis is generally self-limiting with supportive treatment only.
- Antibiotics should be given if there is systemic upset, peritonsillar abscess or a significant comorbidity.
- Offer a reassessment or delayed antibiotic prescription in case symptoms are not resolving after one week.

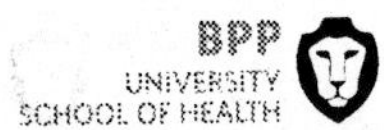

Age range	3–14 years	+1
	15–44 years	0
	>45 years	-1
Exudate or swelling of tonsils	Present	+1
Tender/swollen anterior cervical lymph nodes	Present	+1
Fever >38°C	Present	+1
Cough	Absent	+1

Table 3.41: Centor Criteria used to determine likelihood of bacterial infection in sore throat

Sinusitis

- Inflammation of the nasal sinuses secondary to a virus or bacteria.
- Symptoms include a frontal headache, facial pain, blocked nose and nasal discharge.
- Viral sinusitis is self-limiting.
- Bacterial sinusitis may not require treatment if the patient is well and immunocompetent. Otherwise, antibiotics are indicated.
- If symptoms worsen after an initial improvement, suspect a secondary bacterial infection.

Laryngitis

- Inflammation and infection of the larynx.
- It is mostly viral in nature but can be bacterial.
- Symptoms include hoarseness, odynophagia, cough, malaise and fever.
- Any tissue swelling around the larynx has the potential to compromise the airway, particularly in children.
- Throat swabs should be taken.
- Symptoms usually resolve with supportive care and vocal hygiene.
- Antibiotics are used if a bacterial source is found.

Pulmonary tuberculosis (TB)

Epidemiology

8,751 cases of TB were reported in the UK in 2012. The majority of these cases occurred in large urban areas and in those who were born outside of the UK. Around one-third of the world's population are thought to have latent TB infection.

Aetiology

Primary infection is caused by inhalation of *Mycobacterium*. Risk factors for inhalation include close contact with a person with active TB and being born in or recent visit (five years) to a high prevalence area. Homelessness and poor housing conditions encourage the spread of TB.

Immunocompromise increases risk of both primary infection and reactivation. Risk factors include the extremes of age, malnutrition, HIV, immunosuppressant drugs, haematological malignancy and diabetes.

Pathophysiology

The bacterium *Mycobacterium tuberculosis* is transmitted via inhalation. Host macrophages in the lung engulf the organism and attempt to kill the bacterium by phagocytosis. However, the thick capsule of *M. tuberculosis* protects it, and the bacterium is able to replicate within the macrophage. Eventually this leads to the macrophage's death, and the bacilli are released. The cellular immune system responds by forming a granuloma to prevent further growth and spread. The potential outcomes of primary TB infection are:

- Clearance of the bacterium
- Persistent latent infection
- Progression to primary disease

In severe cases, the bacterium can spread into the bloodstream and result in multiple foci of infection – this is known as military tuberculosis.

Secondary TB occurs due to reactivation of latent infection. It is usually precipitated by impaired immune function.

History/examination

History	• Insidious onset • Malaise • Fever • Weight loss and anorexia • Chronic cough (often purulent) • Haemoptysis • Breathlessness • Chest pain • Night sweats • Presence of risk factors
Exam	• Fever • Cachexia • Finger clubbing • Abnormal chest auscultation • Erythema nodosum

Table 3.42: History and examination findings in pulmonary tuberculosis

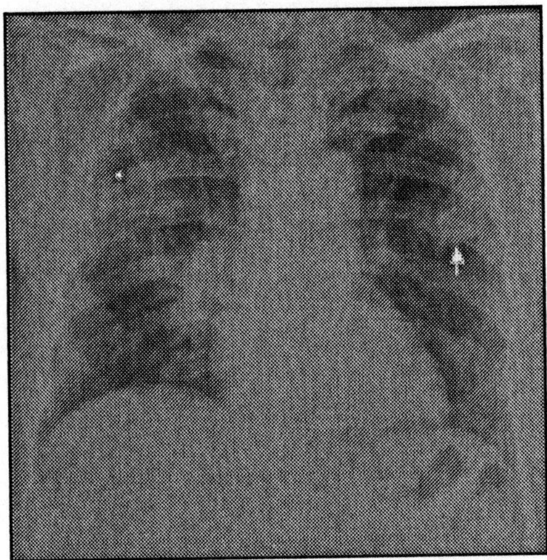

Figure 3.23: CXR showing numerous well-defined tiny nodules throughout the lung in keeping with miliary spread of TB

Investigations

Blood tests:

- FBC: may show anaemia and leukocytosis
- U&Es: prior to starting antibiotic therapy
- LFTs: prior to starting antibiotic therapy

Imaging:

- CXR (see Figures 3.23 and 3.24): the first-line test. TB typically affects the apices of the lungs. Cavitation may be seen. Focal consolidation and pleural effusion can also occur. In military TB, there are widespread tiny nodules throughout the lung fields.

Microbiology:

- Sputum: at least three spontaneous sputum samples (including one early morning sample) should be sent for MC&S, including Ziehl-Nielsen staining and acid fast bacilli testing. These should be sent before or within seven days of starting treatment.
- Induced sputum samples.
- Bronchoscopy and lavage: if unable to obtain spontaneous samples.

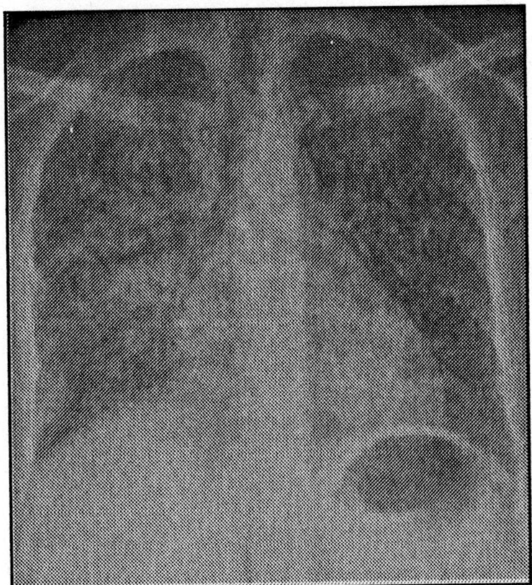

Figure 3.24: Cavitating mass in the RUL in keeping with a TB cavity (star) also note further focal consolidation in left lung (arrow)

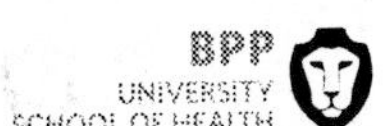

Other:

- Consider testing for blood borne viruses.
- If high risk of multi-drug resistant TB, perform rapid diagnostic tests for rifampicin resistance.
- Pleural effusion sample if applicable.

Management

General measures:

- Any patient with suspected pulmonary TB should be isolated in a negative pressure side room until proven to be non-infectious (usually around 14 days), or treated at home where possible.
- Masks should be worn within the side room.
- All cases of TB must be notified for surveillance data and to allow contact tracing.
  - Contacts should be offered a Mantoux test first line, with interferon gamma testing if this is positive.
- Cases of TB should be managed by a specialist multidisciplinary team.

Medication:

- A multi-drug regimen should be used to reduce the risk of resistance.
- The standard first-line treatment is six months of isoniazid, pyridoxine and rifampicin, with pyrazinamide and ethambutol for the first two months.
- Important side effects of TB therapy include:
  - Liver toxicity
  - Rash
  - Isoniazid: peripheral neuropathy
  - Rifampicin: orange discolouration of body fluids
  - Pyrazinamide: arthralgia, gout
  - Ethambutol: visual disturbances
- Concordance with drug therapy can be improved by patient education, home visits, specialist nurse support and in some cases, DOT.
- Antibiotic therapy for suspected or confirmed multi-drug resistant TB should be decided by a specialist MDT.

Prognosis

TB is a treatable disease, with most patients experiencing minimal or no long-lasting effects. Those who are immunocompromised or who have a multi-drug resistant strain of TB have a worse prognosis.

Bronchiectasis

Epidemiology

Around 1 in 1,000 individuals are affected by bronchiectasis. Prevalence is higher in women, the older age groups and those with underlying lung disease.

Aetiology

A number of pathologies can result in bronchiectasis, including:

- Respiratory: cystic fibrosis, COPD, asthma
- Post-infectious: pneumonia, TB, aspergillosis, childhood respiratory viral conditions
- Distal to bronchial obstruction
- Connective tissue disorders: SLE, RA, systemic sclerosis
- Primary ciliary dyskinesia
- Immunodeficiency
- Other: idiopathic, ulcerative colitis, post-radiation therapy, gastric aspiration

Infective exacerbations of bronchiectasis are often caused by *Staphylococcus, S. pneumoniae, H. influenzae* and *Pseduomonas aeruginosa*.

Pathophysiology

Bronchiectasis is a condition caused by chronic inflammation, either due to infection or underlying disease process. The inflammation damages the elastic and muscular layers of the bronchial wall, resulting in dilatation and thickening of the airways.

This damages the ciliary transport mechanism, allowing accumulation of mucus and secretions in the bronchi. This predisposes to bacterial infections, and further inflammation and damage to the bronchial wall and ciliary system. Bacterial colonisation eventually results.

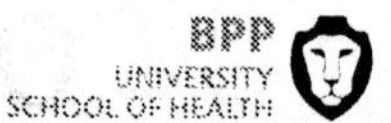

History/examination

History	• Chronic productive cough • Large volumes of purulent sputum • Breathlessness • Chest pain • Haemoptysis • Recurrent episodes of fever • Fatigue • Number of infective exacerbations per year • Relevant past medical history
Exam	• Finger clubbing • Coarse crackles on auscultation • Wheeze

Table 3.43: History and examination findings in bronchiectasis

Investigations

Blood tests:

- FBC: may show raised WCC or polycythaemia/anaemia

Imaging:

- CXR: may show an obscured hemidiaphragm, thickening of the bronchial wall and cystic changes, but can also be normal.
- High resolution chest CT: the gold standard for diagnosis. Will show dilated bronchi +/- bronchial thickening.

Microbiological:

- Respiratory tract samples should be obtained from all patients with bronchiectasis, and should ideally reach the laboratory within three hours.
- Sputum samples should be sent before starting antibiotics for infective exacerbations.

Immunological:

- Serum immunoglobulin and electrophoresis
- Serum IgE to *Aspergillus fumigatus* and aspergillus precipitins

Other:

- Spirometry: all adults should have at least annual assessment of FEV1, FVC and PEF.
- Consider tests for underlying causes (eg CF) if indicated.

Management

The main principle of management is to prevent or slow down further deterioration in lung function.

General measures:

- Smoking cessation
- Influenza and pneumococcal vaccination
- Dietician review to optimise nutrition

Physiotherapy:

- Chest physiotherapy: airway clearance techniques
- Pulmonary rehabilitation

Medical:

- Antibiotic treatment for infective exacerbations:
  - Depends on local microbiology protocols and results of sputum cultures
  - Antibiotic courses usually last at least two weeks
- Long-term antibiotics in patients with frequent exacerbations or significant morbidity due to exacerbations
- Bronchodilators: useful in patients with reversible airflow obstruction
- Long-term oxygen therapy in selected patients
- Non-invasive ventilation in those with chronic respiratory failure

Surgical:

- Surgical lobectomy for localised disease
- Bronchial artery embolisation and/or surgery for massive haemoptysis
- Lung transplantation

Prognosis

Patients with bronchiectasis have a significant reduction in life expectancy, despite advances in treatment. 10% of adults with non-CF bronchiectasis die within 8 years of diagnosis. Prognosis is worse in those with frequent exacerbations, malnutrition and chronic *Pseudomonas* colonisation.

Complications include empyema, abscess, pneumothorax, severe haemoptysis, respiratory failure and cor pulmonale.

Further reading and references

1. British Thoracic Society Community Acquired Pneumonia in Adults Guideline Group (2009). Guidelines for the management of community acquired pneumonia in adults: update 2009. *Thorax*, 64 (supplement III), iii1-iii55.
2. National Clinical Guideline Centre (2014). *Pneumonia: Diagnosis and management of community- and hospital-acquired pneumonia in adults*. NICE Clinical Guideline 191, London: NCGC.
3. National Collaborating Centre for Cancer (2011). *The diagnosis and treatment of lung cancer (update)*.NICE Clinical Guideline 121, Cardiff: NCC-C.
4. National Institute for Health and Care Excellence (2016). *Tuberculosis: Prevention, diagnosis, management and service organization*. NICE Clinical Guideline 33, London: NICE.
5. Pasteur MC., Bilton D. and Hill AT., on behalf of the British Thoracic Society Bronchiectasis (non-CF) Guideline Group (2010). Guideline for non-CF Bronchiectasis. *Thorax*, 65 (Supplement 1), i1-i58)

Top tip:

Always review the patient first – regardless of how terrible a referral, you should always review the patient personally before pronouncing decisions. Then you're going on your own judgement rather than someone else's.

Diarrhoea

Differential diagnosis

System/ Organ	Disease
Intestinal	Inflammatory (ulcerative colitis and Crohn's disease) **Coeliac disease** Colonic carcinoma Diverticular disease **Gastroenteritis** Irritable bowel disease Faecal impaction (overflow diarrhoea)
Infective	**Campylobacter jejuni** **Salmonella spp** **Escherichia coli** Yersinia enterocolitica **Clostridium difficile**
Pancreatic	Chronic pancreatitis Pancreatic cancer Cystic fibrosis
Other	Thyrotoxicosis **Carcinoid syndrome** Drugs such as antibiotics and laxatives Artificial enteral feeding

Table 3.44: Differential diagnosis of diarrhoea

Coeliac disease

Epidemiology

The main cause of malabsorption involving the small intestine in the developed world. Affects 1 in 100 to 1 in 300 of the population in the UK and is slightly more common in the Irish population. The disease can remain subclinical for many years, so although the most common presentation is in early childhood it can present at any time from weaning to old age.

Aetiology

Also known as gluten-induced enteropathy, a malabsorption disorder in which there is damage to the enterocytes of the small intestine as a result of intolerance to dietary gluten.

Abnormalities develop within the proximal small bowel mucosa, which are reversible with the withdrawal of gluten from the patient's diet.

Genetics plays an important role and there is a 10–20% risk of disease development in first degree relatives. 85% of coeliac sufferers possess the HLA B8 antigen, an association also seen with dermatitis herpetiformis,

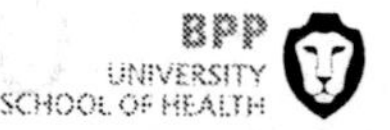

Process 1	Direct toxic effect of the breakdown products of gluten upon enterocytes in genetically susceptible individuals.
Process 2	A possible enzyme defect within the enterocytes: also genetically associated, which results in reduced production of peptidase and therefore impaired breakdown of gluten resulting in potentially toxic products available to cause damage to enterocytes.
Process 3	An immune mediated response of mucosa exposed to gluten. There may be deficient IgA production and hence reduced antibody coverage which permits potentially toxic products of gluten to have access to the mucosa. Therefore, patients with hyposplenism and related impairments within the immune system are more susceptible to development of coeliac disease.
Process 4	There may be an association with human adenovirus type 12. Onset of disease may be preceded by an episode of gastroenteritis in susceptible individuals. This accounts for the unpredictable age of onset of disease and newly diagnosed cases in middle-aged and even elderly individuals.

Table 3.45: The four main proposed pathological processes involved in coeliac disease

a skin disease found in up to 20% of coeliac patients. In those who are genetically susceptible, there is a specific immune reaction to a breakdown product of gluten, triggered by the ingestion of relevant foods.

The specific genes involved in coeliac disease have not yet been identified; however, certain MHC class II gene alleles have been found to have a strong association: DR3/DQW 2 and DR7/DQW. Patients with Down's and Turner's syndromes are at increased risk of developing coeliac disease.

Pathophysiology

Gluten refers to a number of water-insoluble proteins contained in cereal grains. Gliadin is the alcohol-insoluble fraction of this protein in wheat which is responsible for the toxicity to the small intestine (the equivalent in rye is secalin and in barley is hardein).

There are four main processes thought to be responsible for the underlying pathology of coeliac disease (see Table 3.45).

The proximal small bowel mucosa (duodenum and proximal jejunum) is predominantly involved with progressive reduction in severity towards the ileum. The result is malabsorption, particularly in the proximal small intestine:

- Sugars, fatty acids, monoglycerides and amino acids.
- Iron and calcium absorption are particularly affected since their absorption is predominantly in the proximal small intestine.
- Folic acid, vitamin C and B12 are mainly absorbed in the jejunum and ileum and so their absorption is only affected in advanced disease.

Production of hormones from the small intestine may be deficient and hence there is a decrease in pancreatic secretion and bile flow, which accounts for the malabsorption of fat.

There is an increased risk of lymphoma (100 fold) or carcinoma, greatest in those who are non-compliant or present late in life, in particular small bowel T-cell lymphoma (very rare in non-coeliac patients). Metabolic bone disease (osteomalacia and osteoporosis) is found in up to 25% of patients. Calcium malabsorption results in increased parathyroid hormone secretion, causing an increase in bone turnover and cortical bone loss.

History/examination

- May be asymptomatic
- Diarrhoea – ask specifically about steatorrhoea
- Abdominal discomfort/pain
- Flatulence and bloating
- Weight loss
- Look for dermatitis herpetiformis – highly pruritic subepidermal bullous eruption typically affecting the extensors such as the elbow and the buttocks
- Menstrual disturbances
- In children there may be failure to thrive
- Symptoms of anaemia – either iron deficiency or folate deficiency (fatigue, pallor, glossitis, aphthous ulceration)
- Rarely vitamin D deficiency may cause fractures

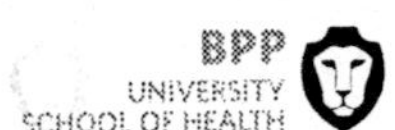

- Past or family history of atopy or autoimmune conditions such as thyroid disease, type 1 diabetes, Sjögren syndrome and primary biliary cirrhosis
- Family history of coeliac disease
- Neurological symptoms are rare and include seizures, ataxia and peripheral neuropathy

On examination:

- Oedema
- Bruising
- Evidence of weight loss
- Abdominal examination: pain, distension and bloating
- Neurological examination: peripheral neuropathy and ataxia
- Dermatitis herpetiformis

Investigations

Blood tests:

- FBC and blood film: iron deficient/megaloblastic anaemia due to folate deficiency.
- Prothrombin time: may be prolonged with vitamin K deficiency.
- Biochemistry: calcium and phosphate may be low and ALP raised, indicative of osteomalacia. Hypoalbuminaemia from protein malabsorption. Low folate and vitamin B12.
- Tissue transglutaminase (tTGA): this is the primary diagnostic blood test for coeliac disease. It has a 90% sensitivity and 97% specificity. There is a false negative result with IgA deficiency, so IgA levels must be measured concurrently.
- Endomyseal antibodies (IgA): high specificity (~100%) and sensitivity (~90%) for the diagnosis of untreated coeliac disease. Used if the tTGA test is equivocal.

Endoscopy:

- Lesions are diagnostic and can range from increased intra-epithelial lymphocytes to total villous atrophy.
- To confirm the mucosal lesion is gluten-induced, three biopsies may sometimes be required – before treatment, after gluten withdrawal, and after re-challenge.

Imaging:

- Small bowel barium follow-through: evidence of dilatation of bowel loops as well as changes in the intestinal mucosa, such as coarsening. It is useful in terms of excluding other causes of malabsorption, for instance terminal ileum Crohn's disease. It is also helpful to detect the development of any complications such as bowel strictures.
- DEXA scan: If osteoporosis is suspected.

Management

Patients require a detailed explanation of their diagnosis and its implications. This includes the implications for family members of a positive test. Patients should also be given information regarding support groups such as the Coeliac Society.

The mainstay of management is adherence to a strict gluten-free diet (see below), which must be emphasised to patients. This results in rapid improvement in clinical features (within days/weeks) and intestinal morphology (3–12 months).

A dietician should be involved in advising and supporting dietary requirements.

Non-compliance is the main cause of treatment failure.

Other:

Dermatitis herpetiformis usually resolves upon withdrawal of gluten from the diet. If there is no clinical improvement, treatment with Dapsone (50–200 mg daily) or sulphonamides may be commenced – this treats the skin symptoms and not the bowel.

Small bowel T cell lymphoma. Treatment is usually with surgery and resection, followed by chemotherapy and radiotherapy.

'Unresponsive' coeliac disease:

Occurs in some patients despite adherence to a strict diet. Treatment with corticosteroids or immuno-suppressants may induce remission.

Prognosis

In most patients, prognosis is excellent with compliance to a strict gluten-free diet. The presence of lymphoma significantly increases the mortality.

Chronic pancreatitis

A chronic inflammatory condition of the pancreas associated with irreversible destruction of pancreatic structure and function.

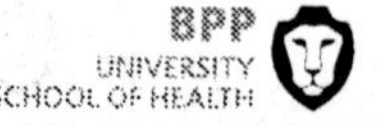

Epidemiology

It is estimated that around 0.04% of the UK population are affected, with a strong male predominance.

Aetiology

Most common causes are remembered with the following mnemonic: I GET SMASHED.

I – IDIOPATHIC
G – GALLSTONES
E – EtOH (alcohol excess)
T – TRAUMA
S – STEROIDS
M – MUMPS (Coxsackie virus)/MALIGNANCY
A – AUTOIMMUNE
S – SCORPION STING (Tityinae family)/ SPIDER BITE
H – HYPERCALCAEMIA/PARATHYROIDISM/ LIPIDAEMIA
E – ERCP (Endoscopic Retrograde Cholangiopancreatogram)
D – DRUGS (Azathioprine, Sulphonamides, Tetracycline etc)

Pathophysiology

A number of processes are proposed, each of which leads on to the chronic disease:

- Protein plugs deposit within the ducts of the pancreas
- Mechanical obstruction by intra-ductal stones
- Toxins or recurrent episodes of acute pancreatitis causing inflammation and fibrosis

There is resultant duct dilatation and atrophy of the acinar cells. Widespread fibrosis surrounds the pancreatic ducts and eventually there are few functioning acinar and islet cells. The pancreatic ducts are significantly dilated. The protein plugs become calcified and there is resultant formation of calculi.

Complications of chronic pancreatitis result from this inflammatory process and destruction of pancreatic function, and include:

- Chronic abdominal pain
- Malabsorption
- Diabetes mellitus
- Pseudocyst formation
- Stricture of the common bile duct
- Bowel obstruction
- Ascites
- Aneurysm of the arteries which surround the pancreas
- Thrombosis of splenic vein causing portal hypertension

History/examination

- Recurrent epigastric pain which radiates to the back, is often severe and described as 'deep'
- Obstructive jaundice or diabetes
- Bloating
- Anorexia and weight loss
- Steatorrhoea (results when the pancreatic lipase production is reduced by more than 90%)
- Past history of acute pancreatitis, gallstones or autoimmune diseases
- Alcohol consumption

On examination:

- Epigastric or general abdominal tenderness
- The patient may appear thin and wasted
- Signs of anaemia and jaundice

Investigations

Blood tests:

- Protein and albumin may be reduced.
- Serum amylase is normal or slightly raised.
- LFTs may be in keeping with obstructive jaundice.
- Calcium (and PTH if indicated).
- Fasting glucose or glucose tolerance test if diabetes is suspected.
- IgG levels if autoimmune cause suspected (will be raised).

Imaging:

- AXR: may reveal pancreatic calcification.
- CT abdomen: will illustrate an irregular, calcified and fibrosed gland. May show complications eg pseudocyst.

Other:

- **Stool fat test**: rarely performed (if fat >6 g in 72 hours = steatorrhoea)
- **Endoscopic retrograde cholangio-pancreatography (ERCP) or magnetic retrograde cholangio-pancreatography (MRCP)**: outlines the pancreatic ducts and may show dilatation and strictures as well as pancreatic duct stones
- **Endoscopic ultrasound**: the best way to visualise the pancreas in skilled hands

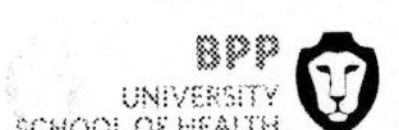

Management

Nocurative treatment – usually supportive only.

Patients are advised to avoid alcohol, in conjunction with a multidisciplinary approach to assist with abstinence.

Pain control tends to be very difficult:

- WHO pain ladder
- Consider specialist pain team referral
- Pancreatic duct stenting or coeliac-plexus block may help with symptom management
- Surgery may be required for partial or complete pancreatic resection

Complications:

- Pancreatic pseudocysts:
  - Occur in 10% of patients
  - Only require treatment if large
  - Increase pain, nausea and vomiting
  - Can be managed conservatively with aspiration and follow-up with ultrasound examination or definitively with surgical resection
- Pancreatic ascites or pleural effusions:
  - Disruption of the pancreatic duct causes a communication between the pancreatic duct and peritoneal cavity
  - The fluid will have a high level of amylase
- Pancreatic insufficiency:
  - Pancreatic enzyme replacements such as Creon or Pancrex V will aid in control of the symptoms which result from the inadequate exocrine function of the pancreas
  - Dietician to advise on diet and supplementation: a low-fat diet (limit fat intake to 45 g per day); high protein and calorie intake; fat soluble vitamin supplements
- Diabetes:
  - Treatment with oral antiglycaemic agents or insulin
- Gallstone removal if it is recognised as the causative factor

Surgical treatment is indicated to treat obstruction of the duodenum or biliary tree or to remove pseudocysts.

Prognosis

Improved in those who abstain from alcohol, but overall there is a 30% 10-year mortality.

Carcinoid syndrome

Epidemiology

Around 2 in 100,000 individuals are affected by a carcinoid tumour. Around 10% of small bowel carcinoid tumours result in carcinoid syndrome. It usually affects individuals from middle age onwards, with the median onset in the 6th decade.

Aetiology

The precise aetiology of carcinoid tumours is unknown. It can form a part of multiple endocrine neoplasia type 1, an autosomal dominant condition which results in the tendency to form tumours involving the endocrine organs.

Pathophysiology

Carcinoid tumours are derived from the enterochromaffin (APUD) cells in the bowel. The most common sites are the distal small bowel and the appendix. The next most common site for carcinoid tumours is the bronchus, but less than 5% of bronchial carcinomas are carcinoid.

Only 2% of bronchial carcinoid tumours result in carcinoid syndrome. The tumour cells produce serotonin (5-hydroxytryptamine (5 HT)), bradykinin, histamine and tachykinins in addition to prostaglandins. Serotonin causes the symptoms of diarrhoea and cardiac abnormalities and bradykinin results in skin flushing as it causes vasodilatation, bronchospasm and increased bowel motility.

These agents, when released from the primary tumour in the bowel, are inactivated by first pass metabolism in the liver. The symptoms of carcinoid syndrome only become apparent when this metabolism is compromised, for example when a carcinoid tumour metastasises to the liver.

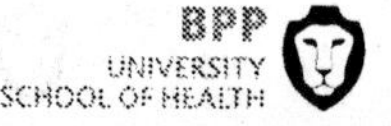

History/examination

It is often asymptomatic, found incidentally in an excised appendix. The following are the most frequently encountered features:

- Flushing is the most frequent symptom. Caused by a transient vasodilation, it results in reddening of the face, head and neck, initially for only a few minutes, but it can last significantly longer as the disease progresses. It can be precipitated by exertion, excitement or alcohol. If this occurs chronically then telangectasia can form in the affected areas.
- Recurrent abdominal pain and watery diarrhoea.
- Bronchospasm causing dyspnoea and wheezing.
- May present with a complication such as intestinal obstruction, perforation or haemorrhage.
- Palpitations, hypotension, fever, fatigue, dizziness and nausea and vomiting.
- Weight loss.
- Symptoms from the primary tumour, such as recurrent haemoptysis or intermittent diarrhoea.
- 50% have cardiac abnormalities involving the right side of the heart, particularly tricuspid regurgitation. This may result in right ventricular hypertrophy and failure.
- Bronchial carcinoid affects the left side of the heart.
- Irregular hepatomegaly.

Investigations

Blood tests:

- FBC
- U&Es
- LFTs
- Clotting screen

Imaging:

- **Ultrasound scan**: will reveal any liver metastases.
- **CXR and/or CT scan of the chest/abdo/pelvis**: can reveal the primary tumour.

Histopathology:

- Biopsy of the primary tumour
- A liver biopsy to confirm the presence of metastases

Other:

- **ECG and echocardiogram**: to reveal cardiac involvement
- **Barium studies**: to delineate the tumour
- **Radioisotope scanning with radio-labelled Octreotide:** to localise carcinoid tumours
- **Urine:** the metabolism of serotonin results in the production of 5-hydroxyindoleacetic acid (5 HIAA). It is measured over a 24-hour period whilst the patient is kept on a low serotonin diet

Management

Medical management:

- ABC assessment, fluid resuscitation and electrolyte correction for severe diarrhoea
- Octreotide (a somatostatin analogue)
  - Prevents the production of a number of hormones from the bowel
  - Relieves symptoms of flushing and diarrhoea
  - May also inhibit tumour growth
- Methysergide (serotonin antagonist)
- Anti-diarrhoeal agents
- Methyldopa and corticosteroids can provide relief from flushing
- Chemotherapy has a limited role in management – usually advanced disease

Surgical management:

Surgical resection of a localised carcinoid tumour is occasionally performed, but is only an option if the tumour is detected prior to the development of the syndrome. Resection of hepatic metastases may be beneficial.

Prognosis

Carcinoid tumours tend to be slow-growing. Despite having metastases in carcinoid syndrome, the 5-year survival is estimated at 40% and the 10-year survival is 15%.

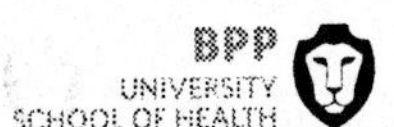

Gastroenteritis

Epidemiology

Gastroenteritis is a common condition affecting 20% of the population in the UK. Groups at increased risk include the immunocompromised and those at the extremes of age, as well as travellers. Infective diarrhoea is a major cause of mortality in the developing world with an estimated 2–3 million deaths per year in the under-5s.

Aetiology

Bacteria and viruses account for the majority of cases. Infection is commonly through contaminated food (such as meat, milk or egg) and water. Ingestion of organic or inorganic toxins can also cause symptoms.

Pathophysiology

The effects of infection within the gut depend largely on the following factors:

- The extent of adherence of organisms to enterocytes
- Production of enterotoxins, which cause secretion of water and electrolytes from the small bowel, resulting in watery diarrhoea
- Invasion of organisms through the intestinal mucosa causing bloody diarrhoea
- Organisms such as *clostridium difficile* and *shigella* multiply within the bowel lumen and directly invade colonic epithelial cells, producing cytotoxins that damage the mucosa and cause inflammation

History/examination

- Sudden onset of diarrhoea with or without vomiting as well as general malaise and cramping abdominal pain
- Watery or bloody diarrhoea
- Duration of symptoms, as well as the frequency and description of the vomitus and stool is important in diagnosis
- Recent food and fluid intake of the patient as well as how it was cooked, the time until onset of symptoms
- Any medication
- Other affected household members
- Travel history and occupation
- Any activities such as swimming, canoeing, diving
- Any signs of systemic illness
- Fevers, sweating, and tenderness on examination of the abdomen
- Assess dehydration and look for shock (see Chapter 5)

Investigations

Blood tests:

- FBC, U&E, LFT, CRP, Amylase. There may be an increased WCC and CRP, but this will not distinguish infective diarrhoea from an inflammatory cause. Reduced renal function will be seen if the patient is dehydrated.

Imaging:

- AXR – to exclude another cause of symptoms

Other:

- Stool sample: microscopy and culture, *C. difficile* toxin and ova, cysts and parasites if indicated.
- If the patient is from an institution or day care or an outbreak is suspected the food source can be cultured to identify the causative organism.

Management

Supportive care is the mainstay as most cases resolve spontaneously within one to six days and is based around symptom control and ensuring adequate hydration.

- Isolation in a side room and barrier nursing to minimise risk of transmission to other patients and staff.
- Good hand hygiene!
- Small and frequent volumes of oral fluids (such as Dioralyte) should be encouraged if possible.
- IV fluids if the patient cannot tolerate oral intake or has significant dehydration.
- Anti-emetics.
- Antibiotics should only be prescribed as per hospital protocol or in discussion with the microbiologist. For example oral Metronidazole or Vancomycin for *C. difficile* and Ciprofloxacin (for travellers) with *campylobacter* and *shigella*.
- If the symptoms are persistent consider further differentials of diarrhoea.
- Local notification procedures should be activated, with contact tracing and investigation of outbreaks.

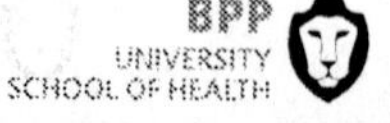

Complications

- Haemolytic-ureamic syndrome (HUS) after *enterohaemorrhagic E Coli*
- Guillain-Barré syndrome after campylobacter
- Aseptic arthritis after *salmonella, shigella* and *yersinia*
- Irritable bowel syndrome is increasingly recognised as a post-infective complication

Prevention

Typhoid and cholera vaccination is recommended if visiting endemic areas.

Good food and hand hygiene should be emphasised, especially when travelling abroad, avoiding unboiled or unbottled water, ice cubes and fresh salads.

Organism	Source	Incubation period	Symptoms	Diagnosis	Recovery time
Clostridium difficile	Release of spores from the bacteria found on contaminated toilets and floor – person to person spread or via hands of healthcare workers	1–10 days	Bloating, constipation, severe diarrhoea and abdominal pain	Stool culture for the C.diff toxin	Up to 30 days
Norovirus	Spread by aerosol route, person to person, or faecally contaminated food/water	24–48 hrs	Nausea, vomiting, diarrhoea and abdominal pain. Lethargy, weakness, myalgia and headache may occur	Norovirus RNA in stool	Up to 60 hours
Staphylo-coccus aureus	Contaminated food, eg meat	2–6 hrs	Abdominal pain, diarrhoea, vomiting, dehydration	Culture the organism in stool or food	Usually a few hours
Bacillus cereus spores	Found in food eg rice	1–6 hrs	Diarrhoea, vomiting, dehydration	Culture the organism in stool or food	Usually rapid
E. coli	Uncooked beef and raw cow's milk	12–48 hrs	Watery diarrhoea, +/– haemorrhagic colitis, haemolytic uraemic syndrome	Stool culture	10–12 days
Salmonella	Found in meat, eggs, poultry	12–24 hrs	Abrupt onset of diarrhoea, vomiting, fever, septicaemia	Stool culture	From 2–14 days
Campylobacter jejuni	Found in milk, poultry and water	2–5 days	Bloody diarrhoea, abdominal pain, malaise and fever	Stool culture	3–5 days
Shigella	Found in contaminated food	2–3 days	Sudden onset of watery, bloody diarrhoea	Stool culture	3–4 days
Rotavirus	Found in food or water	1–7 days	Diarrhoea, vomiting, fever, malaise	Stool culture	3–5 days
Clostridium perfringens spores	Found in food and survive boiling	8–22 hrs	Watery diarrhoea and cramping abdominal pain	Culture the organism in stool or food	2–3 days
Clostridium botulinum	Found in canned or bottled food and survive boiling	18–36 hrs	Brief episode of diarrhoea/ vomiting and paralysis due to neuromuscular blockade	Toxin found in food or faeces	10–14 days

Table 3.46: Causes of gastroenteritis and associated symptoms

Further reading and references

1. Coeliac UK, www.coeliac.org.uk.
2. British Society of Gastroenterology. (2007) *Guidelines for osteoporosis in inflammatory bowel disease and coeliac disease*. [Online]. Available from: www.bsg.org.uk/pdf_word_docs/ost_coe_ibd.pdf [Accessed 7 November 2016].
3. National Centre for Health and Clinical Excellence. (2009) *Coeliac Disease* (CG061).
4. Heaton, K.W. and Lewis, S.J. (1997) Stool form scale as a useful guide to intestinal transit time. *Scand. J Gastroenterol* 1997; 32(9): 920–4.

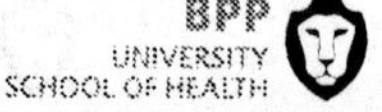

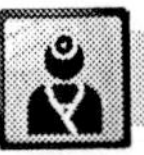

Falls

Differential diagnosis

Cause
Drugs
Acute medical illness
Cardiac syncope
Neurally mediated syncope
Orthostatic (postural) hypotension
Carotid sinus hypersensitivity
Neurological
Musculoskeletal
Environmental
Urinary incontinence
Accidental 'mechanical' fall

Table 3.47: Differential diagnosis of falls

General principles of falls assessment

Falls are a very common occurrence, especially in the elderly population. They are one of the four 'geriatric giants' (falls, immobility, incontinence, confusion) and require a careful and thoughtful assessment.

The definition of a fall, as used by the National Institute for Health and Clinical Excellence, is 'an event whereby an individual comes to rest on the ground or another lower level with or without loss of consciousness'.

Falls often occur in hospital and foundation doctors are often asked to review patients who have fallen. All patients deemed to be at risk of falling should have a falls risk assessment completed on admission. These should be reviewed regularly and updated should the patient's conditions alter. Such a review should include a thorough assessment of the patient's current medical state, as well as looking for (and removing) any precipitating causes. Document your findings and complete any trust incident paperwork as required (the nurses will make sure you do!).

Epidemiology

The incidence increases with age. Approximately 30% of the over-60 age group experience falls each year, rising to 50% of the over-80s. Hospital inpatients and those living in institutional care are at increased risk.

Falls have a number of consequences. The most common is physical injury directly relating to the falls. Around 40–60% of falls lead to an injury. The majority are only minor, but 5% of falls result in fractures (1% leading to hip fracture) and an additional 5% result in a non-fracture major injury.

Falls are frightening and can therefore impact on an individual's self-confidence, resulting in an increased level of dependency.

Aetiology

Falls are often due to multiple factors, which must all be addressed if possible to prevent another occurring.

DRUGS – a massive contributing factor in many falls:

- Polypharmacy (four or more medications)
- Antihypertensives
- Analgesics with sedating side effects
- Sedatives or antidepressant/anxiolytics
- Psychoactive medications
- Alcohol

Acute medical illness:

- Sepsis – high suspicion for UTI, but don't assume it's the source
- Delirium – secondary to whatever cause
- Acute MI
- Pulmonary embolus
- Aortic dissection

Syncope:

- Cardiac causes
  - Structural
  - Arrhythmic
- Orthostatic hypotension
- Neurally mediated
- Carotid sinus hypersensitivity

Orthostatic hypotension:

- Defined as a drop in systolic bBP >20mmHg or diastolic >10mmHg on adopting a standing position

Musculoskeletal:

- Arthritis
- Muscular deconditioning

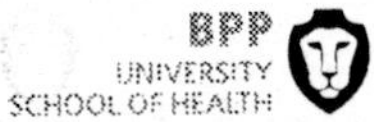

Urinary incontinence:

- Any cause may lead to falls trying to access the toilet in a hurry, particularly in dim light at night

Neurological:

- Seizures
- Dementia or delirium
- TIA (focal neurological symptoms at the time of fall)
- Previous stroke with residual weakness
- Visual impairment (eg cataract, macular degeneration)
- Reduced vestibulo-ocular reflexes
- Vestibular dysfunction
- Peripheral neuropathy (eg diabetes)
- Normal pressure hydrocephalus

Environmental:

- Loose carpet/rugs
- Poor lighting
- Poor footwear
- Poor vision and/or glasses
- Elderly and living alone

Accidental 'mechanical' fall

- Beware the 'I just tripped' statement – this is rarely the only cause of a fall

Pathophysiology

The pathophysiology is dependent on the aetiology.

History/examination

- **Circumstances leading up to the fall:**
  - Where was it?
  - What **exactly** was the patient doing/had they just done at the time?
  - Was there any warning?
  - What preceding symptoms were felt?
  - Did the patient become pale?
- **The fall:**
  - Was the fall witnessed?
  - Any loss of consciousness? If so, for how long?
  - Any evidence of seizure activity – incontinence/tongue biting if unwitnessed
  - Any injuries sustained?
- **After the fall?**
  - How were they afterwards?
  - Confused/disorientated?
  - Any focal weakness?
  - How long did these symptoms last?
  - How long were they on the floor?
- A witness account is invaluable
- Previous falls
- Previous cardiac history
- Past medical, drug and social history:
  - Night-time sedatives
  - Number of episodes of nocturia
  - Previous fractures or risk factors for fracture (eg steroid use)
- Family history
- MMSE if evidence of cognitive impairment
- A full examination is required, but especially detailed cardiac, neurological (cranial and peripheral nerves) and musculoskeletal examinations
- Check for and document any pressure sores
- Postural bBP measurement:
  - Patient is relaxed and supine for at least five minutes
  - Measure BP
  - Stand patient
  - Measure BP at one, three and five minutes after standing and note the greatest BP drop (both SBP and DBP)
  - Record any concurrent symptoms
- Level of consciousness
- Examine gait
- Timed Get up and Go Test: time the patient standing up from a chair, walking 3 m, turning around, walking back to chair and sitting down. Less than 10 seconds is considered normal and greater than 20 seconds is considered abnormal

Investigations

Blood tests:

- FBC, U&Es, LFTs
- Bone profile
- TFT
- Clotting
- Creatinine kinase: to exclude rhabdomyolysis if there has been a long lie
- Troponin: if MI suspected
- B12/folate

Imaging:

- CXR – to look for intercurrent chest infection

Others:

- ECG

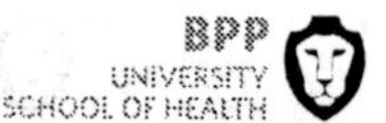

Further investigations may include:

Imaging:

- CT brain – in the acute setting this may be required if a head injury has been sustained. The NICE head injury guidelines are detailed about who should receive this
- DEXA scan

Other:

- 24 hour tape/7 day event recorder/Loop recorder: if arrhythmia considered likely
- Tilt test
- Carotid sinus massage
- Echocardiograph: if clinical evidence of valvular disease or signs of cardiac failure
- EEG

Management

Acute management consists of identification and treatment of physical injuries.

- A to E assessment
- Close attention to potential fractures, especially C-spine and neck of femur – all fractures should be discussed with the orthopaedic surgeons
- Medication review and rationalisation if possible
- Correction of any underlying metabolic/electrolyte imbalance
- Further management depends on the exact cause
- Most acute NHS Trusts have a falls clinic. Patients who meet the criteria should be referred to this clinic on discharge if they meet the referral criteria
- Physiotherapy to improve strength, mobility and balance
- Occupational Therapy if environmental risk factors are found
- Consider need for primary or secondary osteoporosis prevention (see section above on osteoporosis)

Prognosis

The majority of falls do not cause significant immediate or long-term consequences. However, there are a number of serious sequelae:

- Falls are the commonest cause of injury-related death in the elderly.
- Injuries can result in permanent reduction in mobility, leading to:
  - Loss of independence
  - Social isolation with concomitant increase in loneliness and depression
  - Increased risk of institutionalised care
  - Anxiety and fear of falling

Syncope

Syncope is a symptom and not a diagnosis. It is a transient loss of consciousness, with a rapid onset and rapid recovery, due to transient cerebral hypoperfusion.

Epidemiology

Syncope accounts for 3–5% of Accident and Emergency (A&E) attendances and incidence increases with age.

Aetiology

- Cardiac causes
  - Structural (eg valvular heart disease, atrial myxoma or cardiac tamponade)
  - Arrhythmia (eg tachyarrhythmia, bradyarrhythmias, tachy-Brady or sick sinus syndrome, AV nodal conduction delay, long QT interval or pacemaker malfunction)
- Orthostatic hypotension
- Neurally mediated causes
  - Vasovagal (faint)
  - Situational – eg cough, micturition syncope
- Carotid sinus hypersensitivity

Pathophysiology

Cardiac causes for syncope are due to a reduction in cardiac output. Neurally mediated causes lead to inappropriate vasodilatation.

History/examination

- Short prodrome with the patient becoming pale.
- Short period of loss of consciousness.
- Beware 'convulsive syncope' when a short burst of myoclonic jerks is witnessed. This is commonly misdiagnosed as epilepsy.
- An eyewitness account should be sought if at all possible.

Investigations

See investigations under 'general principles' section. If the syncope remains unexplained after initial investigations, it is important to perform tilt table testing and carotid sinus massage.

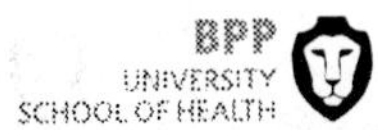

Tilt test:

1. The patient lies on the table and is strapped in place.
2. Non-invasive pulse and BP monitoring is attached.
3. The patient lies horizontal for at least 10 minutes.
4. A head-up tilt, usually of 60 degrees, is applied and the patient monitored for at least 20–40 minutes.
5. Sublingual GTN may be given to try to stimulate symptoms.

A drop in pulse or BP (or both) associated with symptoms is considered a positive test

Carotid sinus massage:

Used to diagnose carotid sinus hypersensitivity

1. A firm massage of each side of the neck over the carotid sinus for five seconds
2. Performed supine and in the head-up tilt position
3. Contra-indicated if a carotid bruit is heard or has had a recent stroke

Cardioinhibitory response: More than three seconds of asystole

Vasodepressor response: Drop of more than 50 mmHg BP (a mixed response is also possible)

Management

Will depend on the cause.

Structural heart disease and arrhythmias may need cardiology referral and a symptomatic three-second asystole on cardiac monitoring warrants referral for consideration of cardiac pacemaker insertion.

Avoiding known triggers of vasovagal syncope. There are driving restrictions on patients with syncope and patients should be advised of these. The exact nature of these restrictions varies with cause (see further reading).

Orthostatic (postural) hypotension

Orthostatic (postural) hypotension is defined as drop of 20 mmHg or more in standing systolic BP or 10 mmHg or more in standing diastolic BP.

Epidemiology

Prevalence increases with age and is reported to be between 5% and 30% in the elderly. This wide variation reflects differences in evaluation methods, definitions and populations studied.

Aetiology

1. **Drug therapy:**
   This is the commonest cause of orthostatic hypotension.
   i) Anti-hypertensives
   ii) Diuretics
   iii) Vasodilators
   iv) Antidepressants
   v) Anti-parkinsonian medication
2. **Neurogenic causes:**
   i) **Primary autonomic failure:** Parkinson's disease, Shy-Drager syndrome (combination of multisystem atrophy with autonomic failure)
   ii) **Secondary autonomic failure:** Diabetes mellitus
   iii) **Spinal cord lesions:** syringobulbia, syringomyelia, cord transection, transverse myelitis, amyloid
3. **Volume depletion causes:**
   i) Fluid loss: acute haemorrhage, diarrhoea
   ii) Sepsis
   iii) Addison's disease

Pathophysiology

On standing there is rapid displacement of about 10% of the blood volume from the thorax to the lower body. The normal physiological response to maintain BP involves the neuroendocrine system, baroreflex function and beta-adrenergic responses. With increasing age these responses are decreased resulting in a fall in BP on standing.

Progressive orthostatic hypotension is characterised by a slow progressive decrease in systolic BP with a compensatory increase in heart rate on assuming the upright posture. Symptoms tend to occur after a few minutes of standing rather than immediately. It is mainly seen in the elderly and is associated with other co-morbidities and vasoactive drugs.

History/examination

- May be asymptomatic
- Symptoms on, or soon after, standing including dizziness, visual disturbances and feeling light-headed

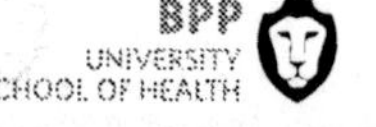

- Unexplained falls
- Drug history, especially those listed above and any recent changes
- Correctly perform postural BP measurement (as above)

Investigations

- As for syncope

Management

- Stop any predisposing drugs
- Ensure adequate hydration
- **Pharmacological therapy**
  - Fludrocortisone (a mineralocorticoid). Fluid retention and hypertension are side effects.
  - Midrodine (an alpha agonist) has shown promising results in small studies but its use is limited by systemic vasoconstriction and hypertension.
  - Desmopressin (DDAVP) may be useful in patients with autonomic failure but hyponatraemia may limit its use.
- **Non-pharmacological treatment**
  - Encourage fluid intake
  - Encourage caffeine intake
  - Head-up tilt on the bed
  - Physiotherapy with balance classes
  - Advise the patients to avoid suddenly standing up, alcohol or hot baths

Further reading and references

1. Drivers Medical Group. (2009) *For Medical Practitioners: At a glance guide to the current medical standards of fitness to drive.* Swansea, DVLA.
2. Drivers Medical Group. (2009) *For Medical Practitioners: At a glance guide to the current medical standards of fitness to drive.* Swansea, DVLA.
3. European Society of Cardiology. (2004) Task Force Report. Guidelines on Management (Diagnosis and Treatment) of Syncope – Update 2004. *Europace* 2004; 6: 467–537.
4. National Institute for Health and Clinical Excellence. (2004) *Falls: the assessment and prevention of falls in older people* (CG021). [Online]. Available from: www.nice.org.uk/guidance/cg161 [Accessed 7 November 2016].
5. National Institute for Health and Clinical Excellence. (2007) *Head injury: triage, assessment, investigation and early management of head injury in infants, children and adults: partial update of clinical guideline 4* (CG056). [Online]. Available from: www.nice.org.uk/guidance/cg56 [Accessed 7 November 2016].
6. Britton, M., Oliver, D., Seed, P., et al. (1997) Development and evaluation of evidence-based risk assessment tool (STRATIFY) to predict which elderly patients will fall. *BMJ* 1997; 315: 1049–53.
7. World Health Organization. (2004) *WHO Scientific Group on the Assessment of Osteoporosis at Primary Health Care Level.* [Online]. Available from: www.who.int/chp/topics/Osteoporosis.pdf [Accessed 7 November 2016].
8. Collaborating Centre for Metabolic Bone Diseases. *WHO Fracture Risk Assessment Tool.* [Online]. Available from: www.shef.ac.uk/FRAX [Accessed 7 November 2016].

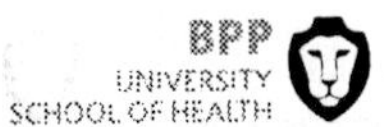

Fever

Differential diagnosis

Cause	Disease
Bacterial infection	Meningitis Pneumonia Urinary sepsis **Infective endocarditis** **Staphylococcal toxic shock syndrome**
Viral infection	Influenza **Glandular fever**
Fungal infection	Aspergillosis *Candida albicans Cryptococcus neoformans* *Pneumocystis jiroveci*
Immunocompromised	**Brucellosis** **Cryptosporidium** *Toxoplasma gondii*
Non-infective	Rheumatological diseases Malignancy (eg lymphoma) Transfusion reaction Rarer causes eg familial Mediterranean fever
Other	**Malaria**

Table 3.48: Differential diagnosis of fever

A general approach to sepsis

Epidemiology

Sepsis is the body's response to infection and can range greatly in severity. Severe sepsis is still a leading cause of mortality, but good evidence shows that early goal-directed therapy can be instrumental in reducing this. In 2002 the Surviving Sepsis Campaign was launched to highlight this and many resources are available at www.survivingsepsis.org.

Sepsis is very common in inpatients and severe sepsis has an incidence of 1 in 200,000 per year. Mortality in severe sepsis varies widely (25–80%) with the greatest mortality in the elderly as well as those who are immunocompromised and have a chronic underlying disease.

Definitions

Bacteraemia:

- A 'positive' blood culture

Systemic inflammatory response syndrome (SIRS):

- At least two of:
  - Temp >38 or <36°C
  - Heart rate (HR) >90 beats per minute
  - Respiratory rate (RR) >20 or pCO2 <4.3 kPa
  - WCC >11x109/L or <3.5x109/L
- **Sepsis:**
  - SIRS plus suspicion or evidence of microbial infection
- **Severe sepsis:**
  - Sepsis plus organ dysfunction
- **Septic shock:**
  - Severe sepsis with hypotension despite adequate volume resuscitation

Aetiology

The infecting organisms relate to the age and health of the patient. The most common organisms are:

- Gram-negative coliforms (40%)
- *Staphylococcus aureus* (12%)
- *Streptococcus pneumoniae* (10%)

Pathophysiology

Gram-negative organisms in particular more commonly cause septic shock as they possess a lipopolysaccharide on their surface which triggers the release of TNF and interleukin-1 into the circulation which potentiate the features of shock and tissue damage via the release of agents such as prostaglandins and nitrous oxide.

History/examination

- Any recent illnesses or symptoms indicative of infection are significant, such as dysuria, diarrhoea, and a productive cough
- Recent surgery or procedures in particular involving the gastrointestinal or urinary tract
- Any implants or prosthetic devices
- Immunosuppression eg diabetes, medication

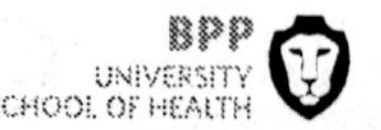

- Early features on examination include fever, rigors, nausea and confusion as well as signs such as tachycardia and warm peripheries
- A later sign is hypotension with cold and clammy peripheries, followed by acute renal failure, metabolic acidosis and adult respiratory distress syndrome
- The elderly may not mount an obvious septic response and thus may present late
- Any immune compromise must be recognised and sepsis treated aggressively in these patients
- **Cardiovascular:** murmurs – think endocarditis
- **Respiratory:** consolidation or crepitations – CAP/HAP
- **Abdominal:** any signs of urinary tract or gastroenterological infections
- **Neurological:** any focal neurology, confusion, neck stiffness or photophobia
- **Skin:** cellulitis, rash or other lesions such as erythema gangrenosum (associated with Gram negative infection)
- **Musculoskeletal:** septic arthritis
- **Gynaecological** (if female): exclude a retained tampon if suspected

Investigations and management

In 2002, the the Surviving Sepsis Campaign was set up. A joint collaboration between the Society of Critical Care Medicine and the European Society of Intensive Care Medicine, it aimed to produce simple guidelines to reduce mortality and morbidity from sepsis.

The 'Sepsis 6' bundle:

Within three hours of presentation:

1. Measure lactate level – ideally on an ABG, start high flow oxygen (and send off FBC, inflammatory markers, U&Es, LFTs)
2. Obtain blood cultures prior to administration of antibiotics (and culture any other possible sources – eg urine/aspirate MC&S, wound swabs, line tips)
3. Administer broad spectrum antibiotics as per local guidelines
4. Administer 30 ml/kg crystalloid for hypotension or lactate ≥ 4 mmol/L (insert a catheter for accurate fluid balance)

Within six hours of presentation:

5. Apply vasopressors (for hypotension that does not respond to initial fluid resuscitation) to maintain a mean arterial pressure (MAP) ≥65 mmHg
6. In the event of persistent hypotension after initial fluid administration (MAP < 65 mmHg) or if initial lactate was ≥4 mmol/L, reassess volume status and tissue perfusion. Remeasure lactate if initial lactate elevated

A CXR should also be perfomed as part of the septic screen and any other imaging as indicated by the history and clinical findings.

Prognosis

The risk of mortality is related to the general health of the patient. It is much higher (at least four times) in those with an underlying pre-existing illness.

The overall mortality rate is as high as 20–50% which is why prompt recognition and treatment is essential and effective implementation of the 'Sepsis 6' bundle has been associated with a significant reduction in mortality.

Staphylococcal toxic shock syndrome

Epidemiology

It is a rare condition with up to 40 cases nationally per year; approximately 50% are related to a retained tampon. It occurs predominantly in younger adults.

Aetiology

Staphylococcal toxic shock syndrome is caused by exotoxins released from a localised staphylococcal infection – commonly *Staphyloccus aureus*. The most common exotoxins are toxic shock syndrome toxin-1 (75%) and staphylococcal enterotoxin B (20–25%). Staphylococcal toxic shock syndrome can follow burns, boils, insect bites, post-operative infections and retained tampons.

Pathophysiology

Pathophysiology is dependent on the aetiology.

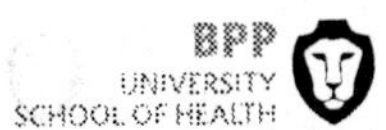

History/examination

- Fever, headache, abdominal pain, vomiting, myalgia and postural dizziness followed by profuse watery diarrhoea
- Systemic upset, tachycardia and hypotension
- There is an associated macular erythroderma which resembles sun burn
- Evidence of multi-organ dysfunction
- Desquamation of the hands and feet

Investigations

Blood tests:

- FBC: elevated WCC
- Raised inflammatory markers
- Coagulation: elevated prothombin time
- U&Es: evidence of renal failure
- Bone profile: evidence of renal failure
- LFTs: hypoalbuminaemia is likely to be present (70%)

Microbiology:

- Blood cultures
- Urinalysis
- Swabs if indicated

Management

1. Identify and decontaminate the site of toxin production.
   i) Drain abscesses
   ii) Debride lesions
   iii) Remove foreign material
2. Aggressive fluid resuscitation: up to 10 litres can be required in 24 hours.
   i) Drain abscesses
   ii) Debride lesions
   iii) Remove foreign material
3. Anti-staphyloccocal antibiotics: as per local policy (penicillin or clindamycin/gentamicin) – if caused by MRSA will need effective antibiotic such as vancomycin.
4. Supportive care – likely HDU/ITU.

Prognosis

2–3 people die per year.

Mortality rate for menstrual cases is 2.5%, the incidence being 2–3 times higher for non-menstrual cases.

Between 5% and 40% will be recurrent.

Pyrexia of unknown origin

Epidemiology

Classification:

- Classic: temperature of 38.3°C with no diagnosis after 3 outpatient visits, 3 days as an inpatient or one week of 'intelligent and invasive' ambulatory investigation
- Nosocomial: at least 24 hours as an inpatient prior to onset of temperature of 38.3°C and no obvious source
- Immune deficient (neutropenic): temperature of 38.3°C, neutrophils of <1 with negative cultures and no diagnosis after 3 days
- HIV related: temperature of 38.3°C for 4 weeks as an outpatient or 3 days as an inpatient with no diagnosis after 3 days of investigation

Aetiology

The causes tend to be unusual presentations of common diseases. There are five main categories of causes:

- Infections
- Neoplasms
- Connective tissue diseases
- Miscellaneous ie alcoholic hepatitis
- Undiagnosed

Between 50% and 80% of cases are attributable to infections and neoplasm.

Around 10–20% are caused by autoimmune disorders. The diagnosis is one of exclusion.

Pathophysiology

Pathophysiology is dependent on the aetiology.

History and examination

- Occupation ie farmers, sewage workers, vets, doctors, nurses and foresters
- History of travel and recreational activities
- Contact with animals including pets such as dogs, cats and birds
- Sexual history and activity
- Any ingestion of any unpasteurised milk or cheese or poorly cooked meat or eggs
- Drug history – both prescribed and non-prescribed medications eg certain antibiotics and phenytoin

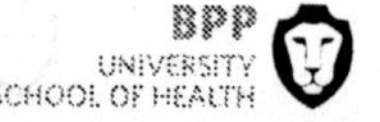

Type	Disease
Bacterial	Abscesses TB Hepatobillary infection Osteomyelitis Brucellosis Borrelia Chlamydophila (Psittacosis)
Viral	Cytomegalovirus (CMV) Epstein-Barr Virus (EBV) HIV
Parasites	Toxoplasmosis Trypanosoma Leishmania
Neoplasms	Hodgkins and Non-Hodgkins Lymphoma Leukaemia Renal cell carcinoma
Collagen vascular and autoimmune disease	Juvenile rheumatoid arthritis (Still's disease) Polyarthritis nodosa Rheumatoid arthritis
Granulomatous disease	Sarcoidosis Crohn's disease
Vasculitides	Giant cell arteritis Polymyalgia rheumatica Behcet's disease
Inherited disease	Familial Mediterranean fever
Endocrine disorders	Hyperthyroidism Subacute thyroiditis Adrenal insufficiency
Drugs	Beta-lactam antibiotics Isoniazid

Table 3.49: Causes of pyrexia of unknown origin

- A full physical examination to identify any likely cause and daily examination to reveal any features which have developed with progression of the fever
- **Cardiovascular:** murmurs, whether new or changing in nature, and any tenderness of the temporal arteries
- **Respiratory:** any crepitations or crackles indicative of early pneumonia
- Focal abscesses can occur in respiratory conditions such as tuberculosis (TB) and bronchial carcinoma
- **CNS:** it is very difficult to detect intracranial abscesses clinically. Look for signs of raised intracranial pressure or focal neurological deficit on examination
- **Abdominal:** any organomegaly – inflammatory bowel disease in particular is associated with abscess formation
- **Musculoskeletal:** any muscle stiffness or tenderness on examination
- Any lymph gland enlargement
- Inspect any lines or catheters for signs of infection

Investigations

Blood tests:

- Inflammatory markers, FBC – any neutrophilia or lymphocytosis associated with bacterial or viral infection respectively.
- A raised ESR may be indicative of myeloma, temporal arteritis or metastases.
- LFTs may be deranged due to a primary tumour or metastases.

Microbiology:

- Urine dipstick can reveal microscopic haematuria which may accompany endocarditis and renal carcinoma.
- Sputum sample for microscopy and culture and any organisms such as acid fast bacilli.
- Three sets of blood cultures from separate sites at different times.
- Swabs from any suspected sources of infection such as lines or catheters, for microscopy and culture.
- Lumbar puncture if CNS infection is suspected.

Imaging:

- CXR: primary lung tumours, metastases, an aspergilloma etc
- Ultrasound/CT/MRI (based on clinical suspicion): to detect any abdominal lesions or masses or lymphadenopathy
- Echocardiogram (to exclude vegetations as endocarditis may be a cause but not be clinically obvious)
- Imaging-guided lymph node biopsy or bone marrow aspiration

Other:

Further investigations based on history, examination findings and results of investigations. In immunocompromised patients, particularly consider and investigate for fungal infections such as:

- *Candida albicans*: oral or genital white plaques
- *Cryptococcus neoformans*: symptoms of meningitis

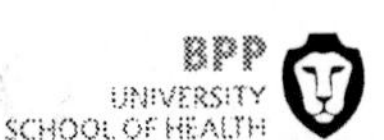

- *Aspergillus fumigatus*: asthma, wheezing and haemoptysis
- *Pneumocystis jiroveci*: severe pneumonia

Management

Immune deficient neutropenic cases should be treated aggressively with broad spectrum antibiotics immediately according to local microbiology guidelines. Cultures must be obtained, preferably prior to antibiotic administration.

Treat empirically if case suggestive of:

- Culture negative endocarditis
- Cryptic disseminated tuberculosis (or other granulomatous infections)
- Temporal arteritis (with vision loss)

Infectious mononucleosis (glandular fever)

Epidemiology

Over 50% of all children have been exposed to the Epstein Barr Virus (EBV) and over three-quarters will have developed antibodies. The infection tends to be milder in children and adolescents and may even be asymptomatic.

Aetiology

The causative organism is EBV (*Human herpes virus 4*). The virus is present in saliva and is spread via close contact ('kissing disease').

Pathophysiology

EBV preferentially infects B lymphocytes.

History/examination

There are two types of presentation:

1. **Anginose** type:
   i) Production of tonsillar exudate
   ii) Hard palate petechiae
   iii) Tonsilar and facial oedema
   iv) Splenomegaly
   v) Nasal vocal changes
   vi) Cervical lymph node enlargement
   vii) Maculo-papular rash
2. **Juvenile** type:
   i) Generalised lymphadenopathy and malaise
   ii) Mild sore throat
   iii) Myalgia and arthralgia
   iv) Low-grade fever
   v) Complications include dysphagia and threatened obstruction of the pharynx due to tonsillar enlargement
   vi) Rarely: secondary bacterial infection, splenic rupture, hepatitis or pancreatitis and meningoencephalitis

Investigations

Blood tests:

- FBC: lymphocytosis and usually thrombo cytopenia
- LFTs: mildly deranged and inflammatory markers raised
- Specific immunoglobulin M (IgM) antibodies indicate acute infection
- The monospot (heterophil antibody) test
- Blood film: atypical lymphocytes may be present

Management

- Mostly symptomatic management.
- Bed rest, gargling and anaesthetic lozenges.
- If there is impending obstruction of the airway due to enlarged tonsils, steroids are effective in reducing the oedema.
- Ampicillin should be avoided as it results in a florid skin rash.

Prognosis

Generally good with the majority of patients making a full recovery. Complications are rare, but include chronic fatigue and Guillain-Barré syndrome.

Malaria

Epidemiology

Predominantly seen in subtropical regions, where more than 1.5 billion people are exposed every year. It is endemic in Africa, Central and South America and Asia. Although malaria is no longer a problem in Europe and North America, there is a risk of imported cases, with over 2,000 cases being reported per year in the UK.

Individuals of all ages are at risk. It has been found that individuals who carry the sickle cell trait are at reduced risk of disease, but those with sickle cell disease fare worse when infected.

Aetiology

- *Plasmodium falciparum*, mostly found in Sub-Saharan Africa and Papua New Guinea, is particularly implicated in the imported cases, probably as a result of an increase in tourists travelling to Africa and the persistence of malaria in this region.
- *Plasmodium vivax* also commonly infects humans and is more common in South America and India.
- *Plasmodium ovale* is less common, found only in West Africa.
- *Plasmodium malariae* is much less common and occurs mainly in Africa.

A number of factors influence the transmission of malaria:

- Environment
- Host
  - Pregnant women and patients with a splenectomy will be affected more severely.
  - Children who are better nourished develop more severe disease when infected.
  - Sickle cell trait, alpha and beta thalassaemia trait, glucose-6-phosphate dehydrogenase (G6PD) deficiency and malnutrition all reduce the risk of disease and its severity if it is transmitted.
- Vector – the female anopheles mosquito

Pathophysiology

The malarial sporozoites enter the blood stream when a mosquito bites. They reach the hepatocytes and undergo multiple divisions over one to two weeks. The merozoites enter the blood stream and host erythrocytes, and a cycle of division within the erythrocyte, subsequent rupture with further merozoite release and infection of new red cells begins, resulting in a rapid increase in parasitaemia.

Incubation periods:

- *P. falciparum* is about one month, but rarely presents up to one year after exposure.
- *P. vivax* and *P. ovale* are longer but additionally have a hypnozoite form which lies dormant in the liver, and can induce recurrence many months following the initial infection.

History/examination

- 'Flu-like' symptoms – persistent fever, sweats, rigors, malaise, headache and myalgia following travel to an endemic area.
- Good concordance with prophylaxis does not exclude infection.
- Diarrhoea, mild jaundice, confusion and seizures.
- Hepatosplenomegaly and herpes of the labia are common.
- Periods of fever indicate a rupture of the red cells infected with parasite - there may be a classical tertian (three-day) or quartan (four-day) cycle of fever.

Complications

Complications are more common when there is a high parasite count and hence are more likely to occur in patients with no immunity, young children and travellers. They are more commonly seen in falciparum malaria.

- Hypovolaemic shock
- Cerebral malaria
- Pulmonary oedema (frequently seen)
- Renal failure
- Severe anaemia
- Blackwater fever:
  - Haemoglobinuria due to severe haemolysis secondary to a high parasite count in the blood.
  - Where red cells infected with parasites obstruct the cerebral capillaries, there is a reducing level of consciousness ranging from mildly drowsy to coma, seizures and psychosis.

Investigations

Blood tests:

- WCC: classically normal with a relative lymphopenia. A low platelet count is usual.
- U&Es: hyponatraemia, hypocalcaemia and hypoalbuminaemia.
- Increased bilirubin secondary to haemolysis or generally raised LFTs.
- Glucose: low from the infection or quinine treatment.
- Blood film: confirms the presence of parasites. Parasitaemia of >2% is considered severe in patients with no immunocompromise. At least 3 films are required and should be taken when the fever peaks and a short period afterwards.

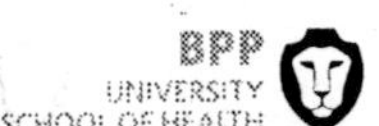

Microbiology:

- Blood cultures: supra-added bacterial infection

Imaging:

- CXR: pneumonia and pulmonary oedema

Others:

- Urinalysis: haematuria
- Pregnancy test (in appropriate individuals): as pregnancy increases the risk associated with malaria

Management

If the clinical suspicion of malaria is high after an initial negative blood film, admit for ongoing investigations. Cases should be notified to the local health protection agency.

Falciparum malaria:

- Admit and assess for severity and complications:
  - Parasitaemia greater than 2%
  - Acidosis (pH <7.3) or lactate >4.0
  - Shock
  - Reduced GCS
  - Hypoglycaemia (<2.2 mmol/L)
  - Fits
  - Renal impairment
  - Respiratory distress or pulmonary oedema
  - Haemoglobin less than 8.0 g/dL
  - Haemoglobinuria
- Artemesinin derivatives in a combination therapy are recommended as first-line therapies.
- Artesunate is recommended in severe or complicated malaria, along with ICU/HDU admission for supportive management.
- Exchange transfusions may be indicated when patients are extremely ill and have a parasitaemia above 10%.

Infective endocarditis

Epidemiology

Infection of the cardiac valves or the endocardium. It is commonly caused by streptococcal infections. Previously found to be more common in young individuals with rheumatic heart disease. It mostly affects those aged 50 or over with degenerative disease of the aortic and mitral valves. The prevalence is twice as high in men than women.

Aetiology

The usual causative organisms are:

- *Streptococcus viridans* accounts for 50% of cases.
- *Staphylococcus aureus* (20% of cases) can result in rapid destruction of the cardiac valves.
- *Staphylococcus epidermis* is more common following valve replacement.
- Gram-negative organisms found rarely in patients following heart valve surgery or in IV drug users.
- Fungal organisms (candida, aspergillus) are very rarely encountered.

Pathophysiology

The organisms generally arise from sources including the teeth, tonsils, urinary tract, central venous catheterisation and the skin. Occasionally, the infection may be caused by a sexually transmitted disease (chlamydia or gonorrhoea).

IV drug use has resulted in a higher incidence of right sided endocarditis, in particular involving the tricuspid valve, over the past few years. Patients with prosthetic heart valves are particularly at risk and once infection ensues, it is extremely difficult to resolve. Permanent pacemakers also increase the risk of endocarditis.

Clusters of organisms form on a valve, with fibrin and platelets aggregating to form vegetations. The valves are usually destroyed with resultant regurgitation or stenosis, systemic embolisation of emboli/clots and potentially formation of myocardial abscesses.

History/examination

- New or different character to an existing heart murmur and a swinging fever.
- Symptoms similar to influenza, anaemia and weight loss.
- Extra-cardiovascular features, resulting from systemic embolisation and deposition of immune complexes:
  - Emboli may result in splenic, gastrointestinal or renal infarction, MI ischaemic stroke, and loss of peripheral pulses.
  - Deposition of immune complexes can result in vasculitis. There may be small haemorrhages within the skin, mucosa, retina (Roth's spots) or nail beds (splinter haemorrhages).
  - Other features include erythematous macules in the palms (Janeway lesions) and small,

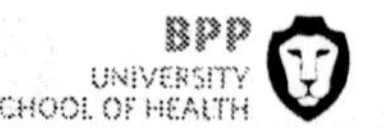

tender, subcutaneous swellings in the digits (Osler's nodes).

- Haematuria is a common feature and may be microscopic or macroscopic.
- Splenomegaly may occur as with any chronic infection, and splenic infarction will give symptoms of left sided abdominal pain.
- Finger clubbing is a late feature.
- When there is right heart involvement, embolisation to the lungs can result in pleuritic-type chest pain with haemoptysis.

Investigations

Blood tests:

- FBC: raised WCC and a normochromic normocytic anaemia
- Inflammatory markers: elevated ESR (present in 90% of cases) and CRP
- U&Es: elevated
- LFTs: deranged

Microbiology:

- Blood cultures: must be taken over a 12 to 24 hour period and at least 3 sets from 3 different sites in the body (prior to antibiotics) – negative cultures are associated with a poorer prognosis.

Imaging:

- CXR: may illustrate features of cardiac failure.
- If there is right-sided heart involvement, there may be evidence of a pulmonary emboli or lung abscess.
- CT/MRI: to check for myocardial abscesses.

Others:

- ECG: usually nothing to note; however, if the conducting tissue is involved, there may be a prolonged PR interval, which is indicative of severe infection. Should be repeated daily to assess for progression of cardiac disease.
- Echocardiogram: may confirm the presence of vegetations (but only those >2 mm in size).
- A transoesophageal echocardiogram is more sensitive in identifying vegetations.
- Urine dipstick: may be positive for both blood and protein.

Management

It is essential to identify the underlying source of infection and treat that cause.

Pharmacological management:

- There will be local microbiology guidelines; however, a common regime is IV Benzylpenicillin (Vancomycin if Penicillin allergy) and Gentamicin (with appropriate monitoring) – altered when culture results are known.
- IV antibiotic therapy is required for at least two weeks and then oral antibiotics for a further four weeks (unless complications arise).

Surgical management:

One in four patients will require surgical intervention. Main indications are:

- Worsening cardiac failure
- Persistent infection with fever or worsening renal failure that is not responding to antibiotics or antifungals
- Prosthetic heart valves – antibiotics are rarely effective in eradicating infection of prosthetic material
- Evidence of myocardial abscesses which are suspected when there is a prolonged PR interval on ECG; if this is detected a temporary pacing wire is indicated as there is a high risk of complete heart block or even death
- Regurgitation of heart valve

Types of surgical intervention:

- Valve repair
- Valve replacement
- Abscess drainage

Prognosis

The mortality rate is 20% mostly as a result of the increase in the number of prosthetic heart valve replacements, IV drug users and antibiotic resistance of the most virulent organisms. Without appropriate treatment, the mortality rate is as high as 95% – usually from cardiac failure or valve destruction.

Prophylaxis:

Recent National Institute for Health and Clinical Excellence (NICE) guidance recommends the administration of prophylactic antibiotics for patients with known valvular disease or a prosthetic heart valve, only when there is going to be a medical or surgical intervention at a site where there is a suspected infection in gullet, stomach, intestines, reproductive tract or urinary tract. Good oral and dental hygiene is imperative for those at risk.

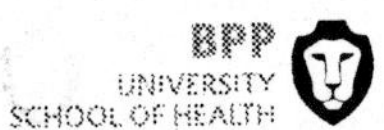

Further reading and references

1. British Infection Society. (2007) Malaria – algorithm for initial assessment and management in adults.
2. Daniels, R., Galvin, C., McNamara, G., et al. (2011) The sepsis six and the severe sepsis resuscitation bundle: a prospective observational cohort study. *Emerg Med J* 2011; 28(6):507-12.
3. Angus, D.C., Annane, D., Beale, R.J., et al. (2008) Surviving Sepsis Campaign: International guidelines for management of severe sepsis and septic shock. *Intensive Care Med* 2008; 34(1): 17–60, 2008.
4. Promed, www.healthmap.org/promed – a useful website giving worldwide locations of disease outbreaks.
5. National Institute for Health and Clinical Excellence. (2008) *Prophylaxis against infective endocarditis* (CG064). [Online]. Available from: www.nice.org.uk/guidance/cg64 [Accessed 7 November 2016].
6. Surviving Sepsis Campaign, www.survivingsepsis.org.
7. Tidy, H. (1952) Glandular Fever. *Br Med J* 1952; 2: 436–439.
8. Toxic Shock Syndrome Information Service, www.toxicshock.com.

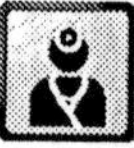

Haematemesis and melaena

Differential diagnosis

System/Organ	Disease
Gastrointestinal	**Peptic ulcer disease** **Oesophageal varices** **Mallory-Weiss tear** **Oesophagitis** Dieulafoy lesion Upper gastrointestinal (GI) tract tumours Vascular malformations Angiodysplasia Hereditary haemorrhagic telangiectasia Aortoenteric fistula

Table 3.50: Differential diagnosis of haematemesis and melaena

Other causes include:

- Primary biliary cirrhosis
- Budd-Chiari syndrome
- Sarcoidosis
- Schistosomiasis (important worldwide)
- Congenital hepatic fibrosis
- Idiopathic portal hypertension

Variceal bleeding

Epidemiology

Variceal bleeding is responsible for 50–60% of bleeding in patients with cirrhosis, 5% of acute upper gastrointestinal bleeds in the UK. The risk of bleeding in patients rises to 15% per year with large varices.

Aetiology

Portal hypertension, and subsequent variceal formation, has a number of causes but the most common is cirrhosis caused by alcoholic liver disease.

Pathophysiology

Cirrhosis causes portal hypertension due to the distortion of hepatic architecture causing increased resistance to blood flow though the liver. In addition to the portal vein, the portal circulation also anastomoses with the systemic venous circulation at several other sites – the oesophagus, umbilicus and rectum.

In portal hypertension, increased flow at the sites of these anastomoses may lead to dilatation and the formation of dilated tortuous veins known as varices.

History/examination

- Haematemesis: amount, frequency and any previous episodes. Copious fresh bleeding may raise the suspicion of a variceal source but does not rule out other causes.
- Melaena: loose, black, tar-like, foul-smelling stool. Ask about amount and frequency. When did it begin? Is there any associated bleeding per rectum?

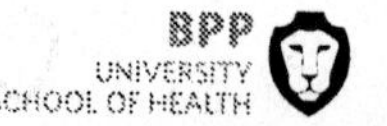

- Alcohol: amount and frequency. Find out when last drank as a withdrawal regime may be necessary.
- Past medical history: known chronic liver disease and cirrhosis. Results of previous endoscopies. Exacerbating factors such as coagulopathies.
- Signs of hypovolaemic shock: tachycardia, tachypnoea, cool peripheries, prolonged capillary refill time, pallor, hypotension (or significant postural bBP drop).
- Signs of chronic anaemia: pale conjunctivae, pale palmar creases.
- Signs of chronic liver disease: jaundice, encephalopathy, leuconychia, clubbing, palmar erythema, asterixis, spider naevi, gynaecomastia.
- Abdomen: tenderness, guarding, hepatomegaly, splenomegaly, ascites, epigastric mass.
- Digital rectal examination: blood or melaena.

Investigations

Blood tests:

- FBC: low Hb, microcytic indices if chronic bleeding. Note, initial Hb may not be a true reflection of extent of blood loss and should be frequently rechecked. Platelets may be low in alcoholism and may be contributing to the bleeding.
- U&Es: urea may be disproportionately raised compared to creatinine owing to breakdown of haemoglobin in the upper GI tract.
- LFTs: may indicate chronic liver disease. If so, consider variceal bleeding as a possible cause of bleeding.
- Coagulation screen: PT may be prolonged in chronic liver disease.
- Cross-match.

Imaging:

- Erect CXR and AXR: To look for free air under the diaphragm which may indicate perforation.

Urgent endoscopy:

- Oesophagogastroduodenoscopy (OGD) is a diagnostic and therapeutic procedure which involves passing a flexible fibre-optic endoscope through the mouth and into the oesophagus, stomach and duodenum.

Management

Initial management:

- A to E assessment and urgent resuscitation
- High flow oxygen
- Consider early ICU review if haemodynamically compromised
- Large-bore IV access and IV fluids
- Blood transfusion if Hb less than 10 g/dl
- Platelet transfusion if less than 50 ¥ 109/L
- Reverse any coagulopathy: Vitamin K/FFP
- Urinary catheter to monitor fluid balance
- Terlipressin (2 mg stat then 1–2 mg 6 hourly)
- Antibiotics
- Urgent referral to the endoscopist on-call/general surgeons
- Endoscopic banding of varices – if bleeding not controlled may need to tamponade with a Sengstaken-Blakemore tube under GA

Ongoing management:

- Continue Terlipressin
- Beta-blocker (usually Propranolol)
- Alcohol withdrawal regime – pabrinex and benzodiazepine
- Consider a Tranjugular Intrahepatic Portosystemic Shunting (TIPSS) procedure (creation of a shunt between the portal and hepatic veins to release some pressure)

Prognosis

A variceal bleed has a high mortality rate – up to 30–50% in some series. The Rockall Score (see below) gives an indication of likely mortality risk.

Patients with a score of 0 can be managed as outpatients; scores of 6 or greater are associated with a 50% risk of needing an intervention.

A score of less than 3 is associated with a good prognosis, whereas a score of 8 is associated with a high risk of rebleeding and mortality.

Variable	Score
Urea (mmol/L)	
6.5–8.0	2
8.0–10.0	3
10.0–25.0	4
>25.0	6
Hb (g/L) men (women)	
12.0–12.9 (10.0–11.9)	1 (1)
10.0–11.9	3
<10.0 (<10.0)	6 (1)
SBP (mmHg)	
100–109	1
90-99	2
<90	3
Other	
HR >100 bpm	1
Melaena	1
Syncope	2
Hepatic failure	2
Cardiac Failure	2

Table 3.51: Glasgow-Blatchford Score: for use on admission, pre-endoscopy, to guide inpatient/ outpatient management

	Score 0	Score 1	Score 2	Score 3
Age	<60	60–79	>80	
Shock	nil	HR >100 SBP >100	SBP <100	
Co-morbidity	Nil		IHD/CHD/ other	Liver/renal failure or metastatic cancer
Diagnosis	Mallory-Weiss	Other	GI malignancy	
Bleeding	nil		Clot/ spurting vessel	

Table 3.52: Rockall Score: for use post-endoscopy to stratify patients for risk of rebleeding and mortality

Non-variceal bleeding

Epidemiology

The incidence of non-variceal bleeds ranges between 50 and 125 per 100,000 and causes 2,500 hospital admissions per year in the UK. Peptic ulcer disease is the most common, accounting for 50% of cases.

Aetiology

The commonest causes are:

- Peptic ulcer disease
- Oesophagitis/gastritis/duodenitis
- Mallory-Weiss tear

Pathophysiology

- **Peptic ulcer disease:** see earlier section on PUD.
- **Mallory-Weiss tear:** forceful/repeated retching, vomiting or coughing causes a small tear in the oesophageal mucosa. Rarely, perforation may occur (Boerhaave syndrome).
- **Oesophagitis:** GORD is the most common cause of oesophagitis. Other causes include candidiasis, chemical corrosion and exposure to ionising radiation.
- **Gastritis/duodenitis:** Epithelial damage caused by a similar process to PUD.

History/examination, investigations and management

– as per variceal bleeding

Prognosis

An overall unselected mortality rate of 10%.

Further reading and references

1. Devlin, H.B., Logan, R.F., Rockall, T.A., et al. (1996) Risk assessment after acute upper gastrointestinal haemorrhage. *Gut* 1996; 38 (3): 316–21.
2. Scottish Intercollegiate Guidelines Network. (2008) *Management of acute upper and lower gastrointestinal bleeding*. 105. Edinburgh, Scottish Intercollegiate Guidelines Network.

Headache

Differential diagnosis

System/Organ	Disease
Primary headache	**Migraine** **Tension-type** **Cluster headache** Hemicranias continua Benign exertional/sex headache
Secondary headaches	Infection **Meningitis/encephalitis** Sinusitis Dental abscess Vascular **SAH**
Subdural haemorrhage (SDH)	Cerebral venous thrombosis Vasculitis
Vasculitis	**Temporal arteritis/Giant cell arteritis**
Other	Carbon monoxide poisoning Tumour **Raised intracranial pressure (ICP)** Primary angle-closure glaucoma

Table 3.53: Differential diagnosis of headache

Headache is a very common medical condition that accounts for approximately 5% of General Practice consultations with 9 out of 10 people likely to suffer from headache at some point.

Almost 30% of neurology outpatient appointments are related to headache.

Primary headaches may carry a heavy morbidity but secondary headaches, ie those with an underlying pathological condition, have a significant mortality, which is a source of much litigation when incorrectly treated.

When investigating headaches an accurate history is important since many significant pathologies can result in few clinical signs and rapid diagnosis and treatment can have a beneficial impact on outcome. Investigations need to be directed and will be dictated by the history.

Red flag features in a 'headache history'

- New onset/change in headache in those over 50
- Thunderclap onset, ie less than five minutes to peak severity
- Focal neurological symptoms
- New cognitive impairment
- Headache changing with posture (worse when flat/early morning)
- Headache precipitated by exertion or Valsalva manoeuvre
- Headache causes sufferer to awake from sleep
- Jaw claudication
- Neck stiffness/fever
- Headache on a background of HIV, infection or cancer

Figure 3.25: Red flag features in a headache history

Migraine

Epidemiology

Migraine is the commonest cause of a recurrent disabling headache and it accounts for 5–20% of those presenting to the emergency department with headache. There is a female preponderance with an annual prevalence of 15% in female and 6% in males. Attacks commonly start with the onset of puberty and there is often a family history of migraine.

Aetiology

Stress, missed sleep and strenuous exercise are well known trigger factors. 20% report a dietary trigger, commonly cheese, chocolate and alcohol. Women are more susceptible to migraines around the time of menses and there is an increased risk of stroke in women with migraine using the combined OCP with a relative risk of 8.7.

Pathophysiology

Aura/prodome is thought to be related to low levels of serotonin causing artery spasm and pain, ie headache caused by subsequent dilation of arteries. It is thought to be linked to hormone level fluctuation but the exact mechanism is unclear.

History/examination

- Headache, usually with gradual onset, classically lasting 4–72 hours.
- Throbbing, usually unilateral.
- The sufferer finds they want to lie down and stay still.

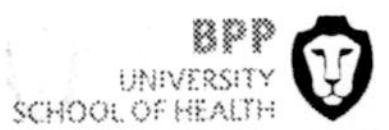

- Nausea and vomiting are common.
- 50% of patients have a prodrome, feeling fatigued, irritable with neck stiffness.
- 15% of patients have an aura, which may include blurring or transient loss of vision, photophobia, zigzag lights and paraesthesia (particularly of the face and hands). This lasts up to an hour before the headache and may last during the migraine.
- The International Headache Society has formulated a diagnostic criteria for migraine without aura.

Diagnostic criteria for 'migraine without aura'
More than 4 headaches lasting 4–72 hours with at least 2 of:
- Unilateral headache (but bilateral in 20%)
- Pulsating
- Moderate or severe
- Worsened by physical activity

And at least one of:
- Nausea/vomiting
- Photophobia

Figure 3.26: International Headache Society's diagnostic criteria for migraine without aura

Investigations

No specific investigations will aid the diagnosis of migraine; however, a secondary cause for the headache may need excluding. Patients should be advised to keep a diary of attacks asking them to note what they were doing at the time and what they had consumed/ any other exacerbating features.

Management

If possible, drug therapies during an attack should be combined with rest. Treatment should begin as soon as possible after the attack starts.

Pharmacological:

- Simple analgesia with anti-emetics. Paracetamol or Ibuprofen is recommended with a prokinetic anti-emetic such as metoclopramide if required.
- Sumitriptan, or other triptans (5-hydroxytryptamine type 1 ($5HT^1$) agonist) administered orally/ subcutaneously or per rectum (caution is needed in uncontrolled hypertension and with concomitant cardiovascular disease).
- Opiates increase nausea and vomiting and should not be used to treat acute migraine.
- Preventative medication can be considered if attacks are frequent. It should be continued for six months and withdrawn slowly:
  - Propranolol or other beta-blocker
  - Tricyclic antidepressants eg Amitriptyline
  - Anti-epileptics eg Valproate
  - Topiramate
  - Methylsergide

Non-pharmacological:

- Rest (in a darkened room if photophobic)
- Prophylaxis-avoidance of trigger factors

Tension-type headache

Epidemiology

Tension-type headaches are the most common type of headache. They affect 78% of the general population.

Aetiology

As with the other primary headache syndromes, the precise aetiology is uncertain. There is an association with stress and musculoskeletal problems in the head or neck. Prolonged usage of analgesia in chronic tension-type headache may lead to medication overuse headache.

Pathophysiology

Pathophysiology is not fully understood but there is a possible link to muscle tension. Recent evidence suggests that could be linked to serotonin levels. Chronic tension-type headache occurs, by definition, on more than 14 days/month. This can be disabling and may not respond well to analgesics.

History/examination

- Bilateral, non-throbbing headache which is not as incapacitating as migraine
- Classically described as a 'pressure' or 'band' around the head
- May spread into the neck
- Usually last a few hours
- There is an association with hHRT
- Examination will be normal

Investigations

– as per migraine

Management

- Reassurance and explanation
- Address stress and musculoskeletal triggers

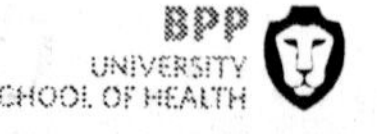

- Simple analgesia (but beware of medication overuse headache – a trial of analgesia withdrawal may help establish if this is the cause)
- Tricyclic antidepressants may be of benefit
- Pain clinic/psychological referral if no improvement and significantly impacting on quality of life

Cluster headache

Epidemiology

Cluster headaches have a prevalence of 0.05%. It more commonly affects middle-aged men and there is a male-to-female ratio of 6:1.

Aetiology

The aetiology is not known but a familial predisposition may exist. It has been linked to a history of head trauma, heavy cigarette smoking and heavy alcohol intake. Sleep apnoea is common in people with the disease, suggesting that hypoxia might trigger attacks, which often occur at night.

Pathophysiology

The pathophysiology is not well understood.

History/examination

- Rapid onset of intense unilateral headache typically lasting 45–90 minutes
- Several attacks per day, usually self-terminating within 2–3 weeks
- Migraine-type symptoms of photophobia, phonophobia, nausea and vomiting
- Prominent ipsilateral autonomic features: conjunctival injection, lacrimation, nasal congestion, rhinorrhea, flushing, sweating – may result in a partial, resolving Horner's syndrome

Investigations

– as per migraine

Management

- Initially simple analgesia, but this rarely achieves adequate relief
- Subcutaneous Sumatriptan can be helpful
- Explanation of the diagnosis
- Avoidance of alcohol during the headache
- Prophylactic drug treatment, starting as soon as possible after the start of the headache
  - Verapamil
  - Prednisolone

Subarachnoid haemorrhage (SAH)

Epidemiology

The incidence of SAH is 8–10/100,000 per year with peak incidence in the 6th decade. It accounts for approximately 3% attendances to ED with headache, but for 10–25% of those presenting with an acute headache.

Aetiology

Up to 75% spontaneous SAH are due to a ruptured berry aneurysm, most commonly found on the anterior communicating artery, followed by the internal carotid artery, middle cerebral artery and finally the vertebrobasilar circulation. The risk is increased by smoking and hypertension. 20% have no identifiable cause but rarer causes include:

- Arteriovenous malformations of the brain or spine
- Arterial dissection
- Sympathomimetic drugs, including cocaine
- Tumours
- Connective tissue disorders and vasculitis

Pathophysiology

Blood in subarachnoid space causes chemical meningitis and subsequent increase in ICP leads to cerebral oedema.

History/examination

- Acute severe headache, maximal immediately or within a few seconds (less than five minutes), which lasts longer than an hour and can continue for days.
- Often described as 'thunderclap' and 'worst ever'.
- In 10% of cases, headache is the only symptom.
- Symptoms of meningism: nausea, vomiting, photophobia and neck stiffness may be present.
- Headaches prior to the SAH have been described, resulting from 'sentinel bleeds' but some evidence suggests that these headaches have other causes, or perhaps are 'missed' SAH.
- Examination may be completely normal.
- Focal neurological symptoms including hemiparesis and cranial nerve palsies.
- Loss of or alteration in consciousness which may be transient or persisting.
- Epileptic seizures in about 6% of cases.

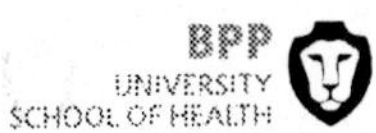

- 10% of cases of spontaneous SAH present with sudden death.
- Pain may be relieved by simple analgesia and sometimes from tripans – beware!

Investigations

Blood tests:

- FBC
- U&Es
- Clotting
- Glucose

Imaging:

CT head: performed as soon as possible as subarachnoid blood is rapidly reabsorbed and the sensitivity of CT decreases with time (almost 100% within 24 hours reducing to 50% at first week and almost 0% at third week).

- Such scans will miss about 2% SAH at 12 hours, rising to 7% at 24 hours, therefore, a negative CT scan should be followed by a lumbar puncture to look for xanthochromia in the CSF.
- CT angiography: will also be necessary if presenting more than two weeks after a bleed.

Others:

- ECG
- LP: as above – mandatory with a history of acute headache and a negative CT brain. Ideally delay until 12 hours post-headache onset as LP may be negative if perfomed too early (unless meningitis suspected):
  - Opening pressure will be raised in 60% SAH cases
  - Assess for protein and glucose, red blood cells and xanthochromia (oxidised haemoglobin – ensure sample protected from light)

Management

- Adequate analgesia
- DVT prophylaxis
- Nimodipine 60 mg every 4 hours to reduce vasospasm
- Ongoing monitoring of neurological status using the GCS

Prognosis

There is 50% mortality with about 25% mortality in the first 24 hours.

20% of survivors have long-term dependency.

If left untreated up to 20% will re-bleed within the first 2 weeks with a long-term re-bleeding risk of 3% per annum. Re-bleeds have a greater mortality, so SAH is an important diagnosis to make. Hydrocephalus is seen in 10–30% which sometimes requires ventriculo-peritoneal shunt placement.

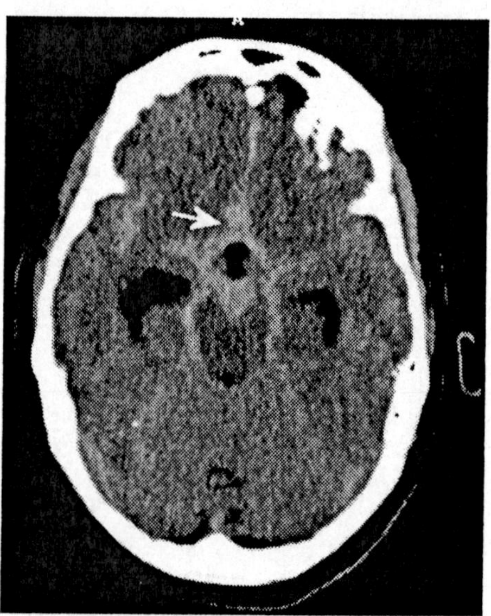

Figure 3.27: Non-contrast enhanced CT brain showing increased density along the circle of Willis (arrow) in keeping with an acute SAH

Cerebral venous thrombosis

Epidemiology

Estimated incidence 3–4 cases per million per year. It is most common in the third decade and 75% are female.

Aetiology

There are various risk factors for cerebral venous sinus thrombosis:

- Infections: meningitis, mastoiditis and sinusitis
- Drugs: OCP, HRT, androgens, and anabolic steroids
- Pregnancy and puerperium

- Coagulopathies: factor V Leiden, protein C, protein S or antithrombin deficiency
- Systemic diseases with pro-coagulant states: nephrotic syndrome, Polycythemia vera and systemic lupus erythematosus
- Head injury
- Intracerebral space occupying lesions

Pathophysiology

Thrombus formation within a venous sinus can create a partial or complete blockage leading to localised congestion within the venous system and the brain. This causes increased ICP, massive ischaemia, and infarction of cerebral tissue. Haemorrhagic conversion can occur in larger infarctions.

History/examination

- Headache (90%) this may be of gradual onset, but can also be 'thunderclap' in presentation
- Nausea and vomiting
- Past medical/family history of thrombophilia
- Drug history of treatment for sinusitis/mastoiditis
- Focal neurology mimicking a stroke
- Seizures
- Signs of raised ICP: papilloedema, nausea/ vominting and reduced level of consciousness
- May have nystagmus, dysphagia, hearing loss, and cerebellar incoordination

Investigations

Blood tests:

- Thrombophilia screen

Imaging:

- Contrast-enhanced CT may show the 'empty delta sign' in the superior sagittal sinus, ie enhancement of the collateral veins surrounding the less dense thrombosed sinus.
- MRV is the investigation of choice.

Management

- Full A to E assessment
- IV access and fluids
- Control any seizures
- Treat any underlying infection
- Stop OCP/HRT
- Anticoagulation with treatment dose heparin in the first instance

Prognosis

- Estimated mortality of 20; however, in survivors the frequency of long-term neurological deficits and epilepsy is low.
- A recurrent thrombosis occurs in about 20% if no treatment is given.

Meningitis/encephalitis

Epidemiology

Bacterial infections have an incidence of 5 per 100,000 while viral encephalitis has an incidence of 5–10 per 100,000.

Aetiology

Risk of meningitis is increased in any condition compromising immunity. Organisms can enter by haematogenous spread or direct invasion from infection in local tissues. The typical causative organism of bacterial meningitis varies according to age.

The causes of viral meningo-encephalitis are HSV, enteroviruses, CMV, Epstein-Barr Virus (EBV) and HIV.

Age	Pathogens
<1 month	Group B Streptococcus, *E. coli*, Klebsiella, *proteus spp*, *L. monocytogenes*
1–3 months	Group B Streptococcus, *E. coli*, *Klebsiella*, *proteus spp*, *L. monocytogenes*, *S. pneumonia*, *N. meningitides*, *H. influenzae type B*
3 months–5 years	*S. pneumonia*, *N. meningitides*, *H. influenzae* type B
5–50 years	*S. pneumonia*, *N. meningitides*
>50 years	*S. pneumonia*, *N. meningitides*, *L. monocytogenes*, Gram negative bacilli

Table 3.54: Microbes usually found to cause meningitis in different age groups

Pathophysiology

Neutrophils are drawn into the CSF by bacterial surface components, complement, and inflammatory cytokines (eg TNF or IL-1). They release metabolites that damage cell membranes, including those of the vascular endothelium leading to vasculitis and thrombophlebitis, which can cause focal ischaemia,

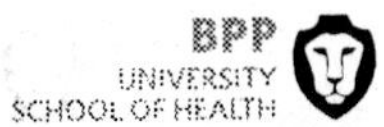

infarction and oedema. Vasculitis also disrupts the blood-brain barrier, further increasing oedema. The purulent exudate in the CSF blocks CSF reabsorption by the arachnoid villi, causing hydrocephalus. Brain oedema and hydrocephalus increase ICP and can cause herniation and death.

History/examination

- Headache, usually of subacute onset, but can be sudden
- Photophobia
- Neck stiffness (absent in 30%)
- Fever
- Encephalitic symptoms eg abnormal behaviour, reduced level of consciousness, focal neurological signs and seizures.
- Meningococcal meningitis and septicaemia give a non-blanching purpuric rash

Investigations

Blood tests:

- FBC
- U&Es
- Inflammatory markers: CRP
- Clotting screen

Microbiology:

- Blood cultures: ideally before antibiotics, but the antibiotics should not be delayed
- A full septic screen (CXR, urinalysis/MC&S and cultures of any other potential source of infection) should also be carried out

Imaging:

- CT following discussion with the radiologist on call. However, if the patient has a normal GCS, neurological examination (including fundoscopy), no history of cancer or intracerebral SOL and no evidence of immunosuppression then CT brain is not usually required prior to LP.

Others:

- LP: for analysis of CSF

Management

- On clinical suspicion of meningitis do not delay giving antibiotics. IV Ceftriaxone 2 g is usually the first-line option, but see local guidelines.

Temporal arteritis/giant cell arteritis

Epidemiology

Prevalence of 18–22/100,000 of population. Predominantly in over-50s and more common in women than men (2.5 times more likely). Rare in Asians and Afro-Caribbeans.

	WBC	Protein	Glucose	Gram Stain	Comments
Normal	<5 cells/mm	0.15–0.45 g/L	>2/3 plasma	–	Opening pressure 10–20 cmH2O
Bacterial	>1,000 neutrophils	Increased (>1.0 g/L)	Decreased (<1/3 plasma)	Positive in 60–90%	–
Partially treated bacterial	100–1,000 neutrophils or lymphocytes	Normal or increased	Normal or decreased	Positive in 40–60%	Listeria will also give this picture
Viral	10–100 lymphocytes	Normal or mild increase	Normal or decreased	Normal	HSV polymerase chain reaction (PCR)
Tuberculous	10–100 lymphocytes	Increased (>1.0 g/L)	Decreased	Normal	AFB on Z-N stain and PCR
Fungal	10–100 lymphocytes	Increased	Increased	Normal	India Ink and Cryptococcal antigen

Table 3.55: Interpretation of CSF results

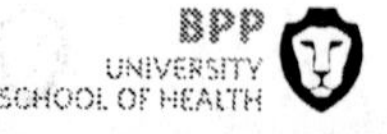

Aetiology

The aetiology is not proven, but is felt to be a maladaptive autoimmune response to an environmental stimulus. These environmental stimuli are either infectious or non-infectious. Infectious causes include human para-influenza virus, parvovirus B19 and *Mycoplasma pneumoniae* while non-infectious causes include smoking.

Pathophysiology

Vasculitis primarily affecting the elastic lamina of medium and large arteries. Typically affects the temporal arteries. Transmural inflammation of the artery is seen with infiltration by multinucleated giant cells. The hyperplasia can result in arterial luminal narrowing, which may cause ischaemia distally. The major complication is irreversible blindness, and consequently is considered a medical and ophthalmological emergency.

History/examination

- Need to exclude in any new headache in the over-50s
- Usually a unilateral headache, but can be bilateral (usually not localised to the temples)
- Associated with jaw claudication and visual disturbances
- Symptoms of polymyalgia rheumatica may be present, including muscle aches and fatigue
- Enlarged, tender temporal arteries
- Scalp tenderness

Investigations

Blood tests:

- Inflammatory markers: ESR is usually raised to more than 50 mm/hr but sometimes normal. CRP is always raised.

Others:

- Temporal artery biopsy

Management

- High dose steroids: 1 mg/kg Prednisolone should be started on clinical grounds before temporal artery biopsy due to the risk of blindness. A rapid improvement in symptoms should be seen.

Raised intracranial pressure

Epidemiology

Varies dependent on the causation.

Aetiology

Raised ICP is caused by a number of pathologies including tumour, encephalitis, hydrocephalus and trauma. It can also be idiopathic in obese young women.

Pathophysiology

The pathophysiology is dependent on the aetiology, but the Munroe-Kelly doctrine dictates the progression. This states that the cranial compartment is incompressible and the cranium is a fixed volume. Therefore, if the volume of brain tissue, CSF or blood increases, it must compress the other two constituents, resulting in increased ICP and possible tonsillar herniation.

History/examination

- Diffuse headache
- Exacerbated by lying down – therefore noticed to be worse in the early morning, valsalva manoeuvre and exertion
- Neurological signs are usually present:
  - Localising: directly from the pathology
  - False: resulting from the raised ICP, classically a cranial nerve VI palsy
- Papilloedema: ensure fundoscopy performed
- As pressure rises, bradycardia and hypertension with a widened pulse pressure and irregular respirations develop (Cushing's Triad)
- As 'coning' begins: unilateral then bilateral fixed, dilated pupil, cranial nerve III palsy

Investigations

Imaging:

- CT of the brain

Others:

- LP with particular emphasis on the opening pressure

Management

- Pressure will be relieved by LP
- Acetazolamide

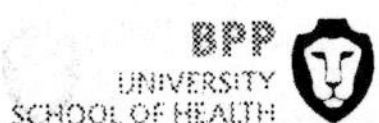

- Treatment of the underlying cause eg abscess drainage or tumour debulking
- Neurosurgical referral for consideration of shunt placement

Trigeminal neuralgia

Epidemiology

There is an annual incidence of about 4–5/100,000. It most commonly occurs after the age of 40 and females are more affected.

Aetiology

Rarely in association with multiple sclerosis (3%) or a tumour compressing the nerve root (6%). There may be a genetic predisposition.

Pathophysiology

The underlying pathology can be due to compression of the trigeminal nerve or degeneration of the nerve. Compression of blood vessels may press on the trigeminal nerve as it leaves the brainstem at the level of the pons. This is more likely as vessels become more ectatic with age. Compression of the nerve leads to demyelination. This results in spontaneous generation of electric impulses.

Some have postulated it to be part of the ageing process as with increasing age the brain atrophies leading to redundant arterial loops which can cause compression. Myelin sheath infiltration eg tumour or amyloidosis.

History/examination

- Usually a disease of the over-50s and more common in women
- Severe knife-like pain lasting a few seconds
- There may be triggers, typically chewing, speaking and touching the affected area
- There may be associated facial spasms
- Confined to the distribution of the trigeminal nerve (CN V) on one side, usually the maxillary or mandibular divisions

Investigations

Imaging:

- MRI of the brain may be indicated to exclude multiple sclerosis or a tumour.
- There are no diagnostic investigations.

Management

- **Pharmacological**
  - Carbamazepine
  - Gabapentin
- **Non-pharmacological**
  - Surgical decompression in intractable cases

Further reading and references

1. Al-Shahi, R., Davenport, R.A., Lindsay, K.W., et al. (2006) Subarachnoid haemorrhage. BMJ *2006*; 333: 235–240.
2. British Association for the Study of Headache, www.bash.org.uk.
3. British Infection Association, www.britishinfection.org.
4. International Headache Society, www.ihs-headache.org.
5. Scottish Intercollegiate Guidelines Network. (2008) *Diagnosis and Management of Headache in Adults*. 107. Edinburgh, Scottish Intercollegiate Guidelines Network.

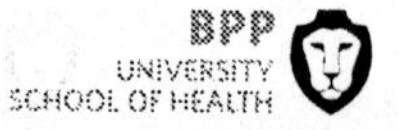

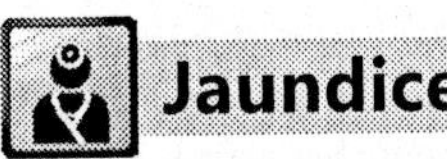

Jaundice

Differential diagnosis

System/Organ	Disease
Pre-hepatic	Hereditary Spherocytosis Sickle cell disease Glucose-6-phosphate dehydrogenase (G6PD) deficiency Malaria Transfusion reaction Hypersplenism
Hepatic	Hepato-cellular carcinoma (refer to insidious onset) **Viral hepatitis** **Fatty liver** **Alcoholic hepatitis** Drug induced hepatitis **Autoimmune hepatitis** Ischaemic hepatitis Infiltrative disease Cirrhosis (covered in medical section) **Primary biliary cirrhosis (PBC)** Haemochromatosis Wilson's disease Gilberts syndrome Crigler-Najjar syndrome
Post-hepatic	Acute cholecystitis Obstructive jaundice Ascending cholangitis (refer to acute abdominal pain) Sclerosing cholangitis Acute pancreatitis (refer to acute abdominal pain) Sclerosing cholangitis Biliary stricture Cholangiocarcinoma (refer to insidious onset) Gallbladder cancer (refer to insidious onset) Pancreatic carcinoma (refer to insidious onset) Pancreatic pseudocyst

Table 3.56: Differential diagnosis of jaundice

Alcoholic liver disease

The incidence of alcoholic liver disease is increasing in the UK as individuals are starting to consume alcohol at a younger age. Traditionally it was men aged 40 to 50 years of age who were affected but this has changed along with the drinking patterns in the UK. Alcohol is the most common cause of liver disease. The risk of developing the disease depends upon the following:

- The amount of alcohol consumed. The recommended safe levels for both men and women in the UK are 14 units weekly.
- Females are more susceptible than males.
- Obesity.
- Co-existing disease affecting the liver such as chronic hepatitis, alpha-1-antitrypsin deficiency and haemochromatosis.

The harmful effects of alcohol are mostly attributable to acetaldehyde, which is the primary product of ethanol metabolism. Alcohol causes three different types of liver damage:

- Fatty liver
- Alcoholic hepatitis
- Alcoholic cirrhosis

Fatty liver

Epidemiology

Incidence is increasing due to increased alcohol consumption.

Aetiology

Fatty liver is caused by chronic excessive alcohol consumption.

Pathophysiology

Fatty liver is the most common finding in alcoholic individuals and an early finding following excessive alcohol intake. Hepatic alcohol metabolism results in fat production and this accumulates in the liver cells. Fat will dissipate with alcohol withdrawal but continued consumption results in progression to fibrosis and cirrhosis.

History/examination

- Increased alcohol intake over a prolonged period of time – beware the 'edited' alcohol consumption history, get a collateral if possible
- Risk factors for hepatotoxicity
- An alcohol 'odour'
- Hepatomegaly is usual and jaundice is sometimes seen
- Signs of alcohol withdrawal eg profuse sweating, shaking, agitation

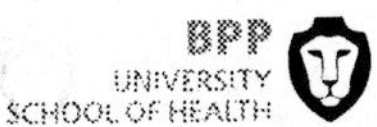

Investigations

Blood tests:

- FBC: Macrocytosis without anaemia.
- Liver biochemistry: AST will be raised more than ALT. GGT will be raised.

Imaging:

- USS: will reveal diffuse areas of high echogenicity within the liver.

Others:

- Liver biopsy: will show fatty infiltration of the liver cells with enlargement of the cells and the nuclei.

Management

- Abstinence from alcohol and weight reduction
- Education about alcohol-related liver damage and the consequences of continuing alcohol consumption
- Referral to or information about local alcohol support services

Prognosis

Usually good if alcohol consumption is curtailed.

Alcoholic hepatitis

Epidemiology

Increasing due to increased alcohol consumption.

Aetiology

Excess alcohol consumption.

Pathophysiology

Alcoholic hepatitis involves necrosis of the hepatocytes and leucocyte infiltration. There is accumulation of dense cytoplasmic material within the liver cells known as Mallory bodies. Continued consumption of alcohol will lead to cirrhosis.

History/examination

- Alcohol intake.
- Risk factors for hepatotoxicity.
- Commonly jaundice and right upper quadrant abdominal pain.
- On examination, milder cases may have no findings. However, more severe cases may have evidence of chronic liver disease and portal hypertension, encephalopathy etc.
- Often accompanied by fever.

Investigations

Blood tests:

- FBC: macrocytosis and a leucocytosis (mainly a neutrophilia). Thrombocytopenia is common.
- Liver biochemistry: The classical picture is of raised AST with normal or mildly raised ALT. Also increased bilirubin, a normal or mildly raised ALP and a markedly raised GGT. Hypoalbuminaemia may be present and a prolonged PT time is a late feature.
- Raised inflammatory markers.

Imaging:

- USS: of the liver will show enlargement with no focal lesions
- CXR: to exclude concurrent sepsis

Others:

- Urinalysis: to exclude concurrent sepsis
- Liver biopsy: necrosis of the liver cells, infiltration with neutrophils, steatosis, as well as features of fibrosis

Management

Mainly supportive and targeted at symptom control, especially during alcohol withdrawal.

- Abstinence from alcohol.
- Nutritional support and dietician advice – vitamin B supplements as well as dietary supplements may be indicated.
- 10 mg vitamin K for 3 days if there is a raised INR.
- Steroids have been shown to reduce the risk of premature death. It is not recommended for use in those with encephalopathy.

Prognosis

Prognosis is worse if individuals continue with excessive alcohol consumption.

In severe disease, there is renal failure, progressive liver failure with resultant complications that lead to death.

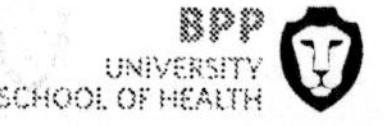

Alcoholic cirrhosis

Epidemiology

Increasing incidence due to alcohol consumption.

Aetiology

Excess alcohol consumption.

Pathophysiology

Alcoholic cirrhosis is the final stage of alcoholic liver disease and an irreversible process. Chronic hepatic injury with regeneration results in fibrosis, nodule formation and distortion of the hepatic architecture. The intra-hepatic changes cause disruption of the sinusoids, increasing vascular resistance and causing portal hypertension.

History/examination

- Full alcohol history
- Risk factors for hepatotoxicity
- Features of chronic liver disease – jaundice, ascites, easy bruising/bleeding, gynaecomastia, spider angiomata, hepato-/splenomegaly, Korsakoff syndrome or Wernicke's encephalopathy

Investigations

Blood tests:

- FBC: anaemia and thrombocytosis
- U&Es: hyponatraemia is common. Exclude renal failure seen in hepatorenal syndrome
- Liver biochemistry: raised transaminases predominate but raised bilirubin will also be seen
- LFTs: decreased albumin
- Coagulopathy

Imaging:

- CXR: exclude sepsis as a cause for decompensation.
- USS of the liver: shows a small, nodular liver with dilation of the portal vein. Hepatocellular carcinoma can be identified.

Others:

- Liver biopsy: shows features including Mallory's hyaline, fibrosis, and fatty infiltration.
- Ascitic tap: positive if the neutrophil count is more than 250/ml.
- Endoscopy may be indicated, especially if variceal bleed suspected. May also show portal hypertensive gastropathy.

Management

Mainly supportive, targeted at symptom control, especially during alcohol withdrawal.

- Counselling and close support for alcohol abstinence.
- Avoidance of other hepatic insults, especially drugs.
- 10 mg of vitamin K for 3 days.
- Treatment of complications:
  - **Varicies:**
    - Variceal banding
    - Propranolol to reduce portal hypertension
  - **Ascites:**
    - Low sodium diet
    - Diuretics
    - Monitor and correct U&Es
  - **Paracentesis:**
    - To drain ascites (acutely in decompensation or planned paracentesis if diuretic-resistant)
    - With IV salt-poor albumin
    - Indications include: diaphragmatic splinting, suspected infection or uncomfortable ascites)
  - **Spontaneous bacterial peritonitis:**
    - Antibiotics
    - Drainage of ascites
  - **Hepatorenal syndrome:**
    - Multispeciality management
    - Fluid replacement with albumin with close monitoring of fluid balance
    - Trans-jugular intra-hepatic portosystemic stent placement

Liver transplant may be considered but strict criteria apply for the six months of abstinence prior to transplantation.

Prognosis

The Child-Pugh score is used to assess prognosis, but this is generally better in those individuals who abstain from alcohol.

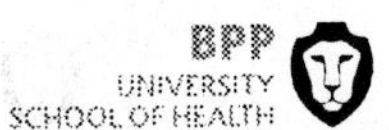

Factor	1 point	2 points	3 points
Bilirubin (micromol/L)	<34	34–50	>50
Albumin (g/L)	>35	28–35	<28
INR	<1.7	1.7–2.2	>2.2
Ascites	None	Present	Refractory
Encephalopathy	None	Grade I-II	Grade III-IV
Child-Pugh Class	Score	1 year survival	
A	5–6	100%	
B	7–9	80%	
C	10–15	45%	

Table 3.57: The Child-Pugh score

Hepatitis A virus (HAV)

Epidemiology

HAV is responsible for 30–40% of acute hepatitis worldwide. It mainly affects children aged 5–14 years and young adults. Infection is much more likely where there is overcrowding and poor sanitary conditions. It is most commonly found in Africa, India and parts of South America.

Aetiology

HAV is an RNA virus transmitted via the faecal-oral route and contaminated water and food products. Rarely is it transmitted via blood. Use of contaminated needles in IVDU and unprotected sexual intercourse are also sources of transmission.

Pathophysiology

HAV has an average incubation period of 28 days and will be found in the faeces up until the stage where jaundice appears.

History/examination

- Assessment of risk factors: travel to an endemic region or close personal contact with a known case
- Pre-icteric prodrome for one week and the icterus peaks at two weeks
- Fever
- Hepatomegaly and right upper quadrant pain
- Nausea and vomiting
- Diarrhoea
- Anorexia
- Headache
- Malaise
- Jaundice (dark urine and pale stools)

Investigations

Blood tests:

- FBC
- U&Es
- Liver biochemistry: a high serum AST and ALT
- Clotting: a marker of disease progression and severity

Serology:

- IgM antibodies to HAV: indicate infection within the last four to six months
- Ig G antibodies to HAV: indicate previous infection

Case Study: A sad consultation

'So just how much do you drink?' the GP trainee asked the man sitting before her. He had a ruddy, weathered complexion with a slight paunch and exuded a gentle odour of unkemptness. 'Oh, not so much really,' he replied, 'a few pints most nights, a few more at the weekend maybe, a couple of glasses of wine sometimes too.' He was uncomfortable and defensive. 'And the rest,' his wife broke in, 'sorry doctor, but I'm the reason we're here. I can't stand finding empty bottles hidden at the back of the wardrobe any more. I can't stand having to clear up vomit or carry him up the stairs at night. We never go out now, he just sits on the sofa and drinks...and drinks...and drinks. He's lost his job and we can't pay the bills on my wages. None of the children will come and visit because they don't like to see him like this and even my friends have stopped coming round because they're too embarrassed. I don't know what to do anymore, I'm worried about what he's doing to his body. I'm worried about what he's doing to us. I can't take it any more and if you don't do something, I'm leaving you.' She addressed the last few words in desperation to the man next to her, who stared blindly at the floor. There was a long silence when the woman finished speaking and her words seemed to resonate around the room. 'Well, we'd better see what we can do to help,' the GP trainee said.

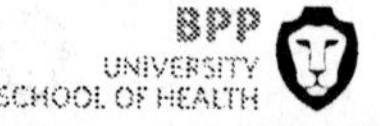

Imaging:

- Abdominal USS: exclude bile duct obstruction, cirrhosis and hepatocellular carcinoma (rare with HAV infection)

Management

- Supportive management with avoidance of excessive alcohol.
- Prevention is key, with public health measures that encourage careful attention to hygiene and adequate sanitation.
- Vaccinate travellers to endemic areas.
- Post-exposure prophylaxis in the form of human immunoglobulin and vaccination can be given.

Prognosis

- Rarely any long-term sequelae – <1% progress to fulminant liver failure.
- Liver function will return to normal within 3 months.

Hepatitis B virus (HBV)

Epidemiology

HBV is responsible for 0.2% of acute hepatitis in the UK. Around 350 million chronic carriers of the virus exist worldwide. It is common in Africa, China and South-East Asia. There is a less than 1% incidence of chronic carriage in the UK.

Aetiology

HBV is spread by blood and any blood products. It is also found in bodily excretions such as saliva, vaginal and menstrual discharges, and seminal fluid. Modes of spread include:

- Horizontal: person to person when there is inoculation of tiny amounts of the contaminated fluid via needles or sexually
- Vertical: from mother to baby

Those at higher risk of infection in the UK include immigrants from endemic regions, IVDU and individuals with multiple sexual partners.

Pathophysiology

HBV is a DNA virus of the hepadnavirus family. The incubation period lasts up to six months. Important antigens are the surface antigen (HBsAg), the core antigen (HBcAg) and the pre-core or 'e' antigen (HBeAg).

The majority of HBV infections are asymptomatic, with only 30% having symptoms. It progresses to chronic disease in around 20%. There is a 15–30% chance of developing cirrhosis with chronic HBV carriage but the risk is greatest in those co-infected by HDV or HIV.

History/examination

- Risk factors: sexual history (number of partners, sexual contact with an infected individual and men who have sex with men), IVDU
- Clinical features in symptomatic individuals:
  - Fever
  - Hepatomegaly and right upper quadrant pain
  - Nausea and vomiting
  - Diarrhoea
  - Anorexia
  - Headache
  - Malaise
  - Jaundice (dark urine and pale stools)

Investigations

Blood tests:

- FBC
- U&Es
- Liver biochemistry: a high serum AST and ALT
- HBV DNA: diagnostic of infection and can also be used to monitor response to treatment
- Clotting: a marker of disease progression and severity

Serology:

- HBsAg: appears six weeks after the initial acute infection and usually disappears by three months. Persistence longer than six months means chronic infection.
- HBcAg: is usually found only in the liver cells.
- HBeAg: is found early in the acute phase and usually undetectable after a few weeks. Positivity at three months indicates increased risk of chronicity. It is an indicator of high infectivity.
- Hepatitis B surface antibody (HBsAb): is detectable post-immunisation or post-infection.

Imaging:

- Abdominal USS: to exclude bile duct obstruction, cirrhosis and hepatocellular carcinoma

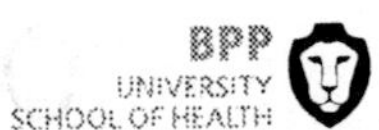

Others:

- Liver biopsy: may show evidence of cirrhosis and certain staining may illustrate the HBcAg and HBsAg in hepatocytes

Management

- Mostly supportive in the acute phase
- Monitoring of HBsAg to ensure clearance of the virus
- If the HBsAg persists for six months, the diagnosis of chronic HBV infection is made
- Chronic HBV is treated with antiviral agents including pegylated interferon alpha and Lamivudine
- Vaccinate at-risk individuals (including healthcare workers)
- Post-exposure prophylaxis in the form of human immunoglobulin and vaccination can be given (eg following a needlestick injury or to babies with infected mothers)

Prognosis

- Infection resolves completely for the majority of people.
- Around 20% of patients may go on to develop chronic infection:
  - Around 5% of patients will seroconvert by the first year compared to up to 50% of individuals who receive treatment.
  - Without treatment the infection will progress to cirrhosis and eventually hepatocellular carcinoma.
  - Those with established chronic disease, higher levels of viral DNA and raised liver have a worse prognosis.

Hepatitis C virus (HCV)

Epidemiology

HCV is responsible for 15–20% of acute hepatitis worldwide. Global prevalence is approaching 3%, but is closer to 0.5% in the UK. It is endemic in many parts of the world, especially in Southern Europe and Japan.

Aetiology

HCV is spread by exposure to contaminated blood, classically via blood transfusions prior to the introduction of screening and sharing needles whilst injecting drugs. It can also be transmitted vertically during childbirth.

Pathophysiology

HCV is a single stranded RNA flavivirus and consists of six genotypes which all respond differently to therapy. The subtype 1b virus of the genotype 1 is the most virulent and the commonest genotypes in the UK are the genotypes 1, 2 and 3. HCV is usually involved in post-transfusion hepatitis and there is a significantly higher risk of becoming chronically infected with HCV than with HBV.

History/examination

- Risk factors: IVDU and previous blood transfusion
- Initially asymptomatic followed by mild jaundice, features of chronic liver disease and cirrhosis

Investigations

Blood tests:

- FBC
- U&Es
- Liver biochemistry: high serum AST and ALT
- Clotting – a marker of disease progression and severity

Serology:

- HCV antibodies
- HCV RNA (the most useful diagnostic test)
- Viral genotyping is useful in predicting response to treatment

Imaging:

- Abdominal USS: to exclude bile duct obstruction, cirrhosis and hepatocellular carcinoma

Others:

- Liver biopsy: In HBV or HCV it may show evidence of cirrhosis.

Management

- Acute infection is treated with interferon-alpha (duration is dependent on viral genotype).
- Chronic infection is treated with pegylated interferon-alpha and Ribavirin for at least 6–12 months tailored according to response to treatment.
- Treatment is associated with reduction in the amount of fibrosis and a lower risk of developing hepatocellular carcinoma.
- Chronic carriers should be advised to abstain from alcohol, advised about safe sex especially

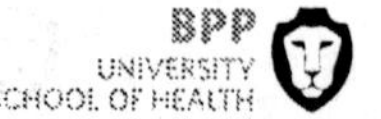

to avoid co-infection with HIV, and should be offered HAV and HBV vaccination.

- Prevention involves awareness of the dangers of sharing needles and unprotected sexual intercourse. Needle exchange programmes have been shown to be successful.
- Advanced liver disease should be managed by a hepatologist and the possibility of liver transplantation should be considered.

Prognosis

- The majority of affected individuals become chronic carriers and of those 20% will eventually develop cirrhosis over a 20-year period.
- Cirrhotic patients should be monitored for complications including hepatocellular carcinoma – there is around a 5% annual risk of developing liver failure or hepatocellular carcinoma.
- Renal function should be monitored for the possibility of glomerulonephritis caused by cryoglobulinaemia.
- Older patients tend to have more aggressive symptoms.
- Very rarely there will be cases of acute liver failure.

Chronic hepatitis

Persistently deranged liver biochemistry for more than three months and evidence of necrosis of the liver cells on liver biopsy indicates chronic hepatitis. Causes of chronic hepatitis include:

- Autoimmune hepatitis
- Chronic HBV and HCV infection
- Wilson's disease
- Haemachromatosis
- Alpha-1-antitrypsin deficiency
- Certain drugs such as methyldopa

Eventually chronic liver disease will follow chronic hepatitis. Generally, the features of chronic liver disease are (with associated conditions):

- Clubbing
- Palmar erythema
- Leukonychia (hypoalbuminaemia)
- Dupytren's contracture (alcohol dependence)
- Asterixis (hepatic encephalopathy)
- Parotidomegaly (alcohol dependence)
- Keiser-Fleisher rings (Wilson's disease)
- Xanthelasmata (PBC)
- Excoriations
- Spider naevi
- Gynaecomastia
- Ascites (portal hypertension and hypoalbuminaemia)
- Small irregular shrunken liver (cirrhosis)
- Distended abdominal veins/caput madusae
- Testicular atrophy
- Reduction in body hair
- Anaemia
- Drowsiness (hepatic encephalopathy)
- Hyperventilation (hepatic encephalopathy)
- Jaundice (excretory dysfunction)
- Peripheral oedema (hypoalbuminaemia)
- Bruising (coagulopathy)
- Peripheral neuropathy (alcohol and certain medications)
- Cerebellar signs (alcohol dependence and Wilson's disease)
- Hepatomegaly (alcohol dependence, non-alcoholic fatty liver disease, haemochromatosis)
- Increased skin pigmentation (haemochromatosis)
- Signs of right heart failure
- Tattoos (HCV infection)
- Signs of COPD (alpha-1 antitrypsin deficiency)

Autoimmune hepatitis

Epidemiology

Incidence is approximately 1 per 100,000 per year. A bimodal distribution exists with peaks at ages 20–30 and 55–65 years. It is more common in females than males with a female to male ratio of 8:1.

Aetiology

The aetiology is unknown.

It is associated with HLA phenotype B8, DR3 and DR4. Environmental triggers are unclear. There are four recognised subtypes of autoimmune hepatitis:

1. Positive for ANA and SMA and raised IgG.
2. Positive for anti-liver/kidney/microsomal (anti-LKM) antibodies. This is typically found in female children and teenagers.
3. Positive for antibodies against soluble liver antigen (anti-SLA). This is clinically similar to group 1.
4. No auto-antibodies detected.

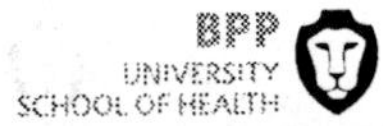

Pathophysiology

Autoimmune hepatitis is a chronic inflammatory disease characterised by autoimmune hepatocyte damage.

History/examination

- Other autoimmune diseases: hyperthyroidism, type 1 diabetes mellitus, UC, coeliac disease and rheumatoid arthritis in the past medial history or family history
- Features of jaundice, pruritis, fatigue, nausea, anorexia, abdominal discomfort and arthralgia
- Hepatomegaly
- Rarely, complications of liver disease – ascites, splenomegaly, portal hypertension, encephalopathy

Investigations

Blood tests:

- FBC
- U&Es
- Coagulation screen
- Liver biochemistry: transaminases are always moderately raised but A LP/GGT may be normal

Serology:

- Auto-antibodies: look for ANA, SMA, anti-SLA and anti-LKM.
- Serum IgG is often found to be raised.

Others:

- Liver biopsy

Management

- Steroid regimen – reducing as transaminases improve.
- Azathioprine can also be first-line or is added when steroids are reducing and the LFTs have returned to normal.
- Life-long treatment with steroids, azathioprine or ciclosporin is required and it can rarely be withdrawn successfully without relapse.
- Osteoporosis prevention is required with long-term steroid use.
- A liver transplant is indicated in patients who do not respond to treatment.

Prognosis

Over 80% of patients enter remission but this may take several years to achieve.

There is a 50% 5-year survival rate without appropriate treatment. Treatment initiated before any features of cirrhosis results in a 90% 10-year survival, but it is considerably lower if cirrhosis is established.

Primary biliary cirrhosis (PBC)

PBC is an autoimmune disease characterised by intra-hepatic duct inflammation, fibrosis and cirrhosis of the liver.

Epidemiology

It affects 1–2 in 5,000 women in Europe and rarely occurs in Africa and India. It mostly affects middle-aged individuals (40–60 years).

Aetiology

PBC has an autoimmune basis and hence may be associated with other autoimmune conditions such as:

- Diabetes
- Sjögren syndrome
- Sicca syndrome
- Thyroid disease eg Grave's disease
- Vitiligo
- Coeliac disease
- Systemic sclerosis

Over 95% of patients are positive for AMA.

Pathophysiology

Progressive immune-mediated damage to the intra-hepatic bile ducts with loss of ducts. Eventually this leads to cholestasis and the consequent damage to the liver itself results in cirrhosis.

Key features in the history/examination

- History/family history of autoimmune disease.
- Presentation may be asymptomatic and only an incidental finding.
- May be progressive symptoms of pruritus, classically associated with PBC, followed by jaundice. Look for excoriation marks.
- Presentation may be with complications such as ascites, jaundice, and gastrointestinal (particularly variceal) bleeding. However, these tend to represent advanced disease.
- Pale stools, dark urine and steatorrhoea.
- Hepato-splenomegaly is common.
- Pigmentation and periorbital xanthomas.

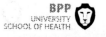

Investigations

Blood tests:

- FBC: check for anaemia and platelet count
- U&Es
- Liver biochemistry: initially increased ALP and GGT and with disease progression, raised bilirubin, reduced albumin and prolonged PT time
- Clotting screen
- Alpha-fetoprotein

Serology:

- Serum immunoglobulins: will be increased – particularly IgM
- Antimitochondrial antibodies: particularly M2 subtype will be present
- ANA: may be present but are less common

Imaging:

- Liver USS to exclude extra-hepatic biliary obstruction

Others:

- Liver biopsy: will show infiltration of lymphocytes in and around the intra-hepatic bile ducts, followed by duct proliferation, fibrosis and eventually cirrhosis

Management

No treatment has been found to improve the prognosis in these patients.

- Ursodeoxycholicacid improves the LFTs and slows deterioration.
- Cholestyramine is effective in reducing symptoms of pruritus as it binds the bile acids in the gut. Antihistamines should be avoided as they are ineffective.
- Fat-soluble vitamin supplements may provide useful nutritional support.
- Patients with decompensated liver disease should be treated symptomatically for ascites, varicies and other complications and referred to a transplant centre for consideration of liver transplant.

Prognosis

- Follow-up should be done at least annually to screen for deteriorating hepatic function. This is achieved by monitoring bilirubin, albumin and prothrombin time.
- Monitor progression of portal hypertension and occurrence of hepatocellular carcinoma too.
- There is a variable survival rate which is inversely proportional to the bilirubin level.

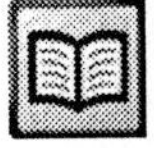

Further reading and references

1. British Society of Gastroenterology. (2003) *Guidance on the Treatment of Hepatitis C incorporating the Use of Pegylated Interferons*. [Online]. Available from: www.bsg.org.uk/clinical-guidelines/liver/guidance-on-the-treatment-of-hepatitis-c-incorporating-the-use-of-pegylated-interferons.html [Accessed 7 November 2016].
2. British Society of Gastroenterology. (2006) *Guidelines on the Management of Ascites in Cirrhosis*. [Online]. Available from: www.bsg.org.uk/clinical-guidelines/liver/guidelines-on-the-management-of-ascites-in-cirrhosis.html [Accessed 7 November 2016].
3. Scottish Intercollegiate Guidelines Network. (2008) *Management of acute upper and lower gastrointestinal bleeding*. 105. Edinburgh, Scottish Intercollegiate Guidelines Network.

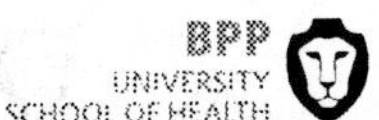

Limb pain and swelling

Differential diagnosis

In an acute mono-arthritis with a painful, red, hot, swollen joint, septic arthritis must be excluded.

	Disease
Musculoskeletal (non-trauma)	Osteoarthritis **Rheumatoid arthritis** **Gout** **Pseudogout** Seronegative arthropathies
Trauma	Fracture Soft tissue injury (eg sprain) Compartment syndrome
Infections	Abscess Cellulitis **Necrotising fasciitis** Septic arthritis
Vascular	**Deep Vein Thrombosis** Venous insufficiency
Other	Lymphoedema Neuropathic pain
Bilateral Leg Swelling	Heart failure Cirrhosis Nephrotic syndrome Hypoalbuminaemia Hypothyroidism Dependent oedema Drug side effects eg calcium channel blockers

Table 3.58: Differential diagnosis of limb pain and swelling

Rheumatoid arthritis (RA)

RA is a chronic inflammatory condition which predominantly affects joints but also has significant multisystem involvement.

Epidemiology

RA affects approximately 1% of the population with a 2:1 female:male ratio. The most common age of onset is in the 5th decade.

Aetiology

RA is an autoimmune disease of multi-factorial origin. There is evidence to suggest that some HLA polymorphisms on chromosome 6 can increase the chance of the disease. The environmental triggers are poorly understood.

Pathophysiology

The synovial tissue proliferates, eroding first the cartilage and then the underlying bone, resulting in joint deformity and joint destruction.

History/examination

The 1988 revised American College of Rheumatology criteria are used for diagnosis (four of the seven criteria must be present, with three existing for at least six weeks):

1. Morning stiffness lasting at least one hour
2. Arthritis of three or more joint areas simultaneously (left and right – PIP, MCP, wrist, elbow, knee, ankle and metatarsophalangeal joints)
3. Hand joint involvement
4. Symmetrical arthritis
5. Rheumatoid nodules (subcutaneous nodules, classically at the elbow)
6. Rheumatoid factor positivity
7. Radiographic changes typical of RA on hand or wrist X-rays

Investigations

Blood tests:

- FBC: anaemia, leucocytosis and thrombocytosis
- Raised ESR and CRP
- Rheumatoid factor
- Joint and extra-articular involvement
- History/family history of other autoimmune diseases

Imaging:

Joint X-rays: typical radiological features are:

1. Joint space narrowing
2. Joint erosions
3. Juxta-articular osteoporosis
4. Cysts
5. Subluxation and deformation

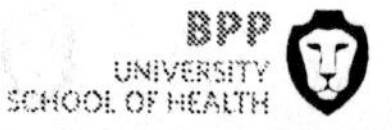

Summary of features to expect on examination:

System	Features
Rheumatoid hands	• Active synovitis, typically at the MCP and PIP joints (with sparing of the DIP joints) and the wrist • Ulnar deviation of the fingers at the MCP joints • Swan-neck/boutonnière finger deformities and Z-thumbs • Dorsal subluxation of the ulna at the carpal joint • Small muscle wasting • Nail-fold infarcts • Palmar erythema • Carpal tunnel syndrome • Functional assessment: writing, combing hair and picking up coins
Lung	• Pleural effusions (exudates) • Fibrosis • Recurrent infections due to parenchymal lung damage and immunosuppression
Cardiac	• Pericardial rub
Neurological	• Mono-neuritis multiplex • Peripheral neuropathy • Cervical myelopathy caused by atlanto-axial subluxation
Skin	• Rheumatoid nodules
Ophthalmic	• Scleritis/episcleritis • Sjögren syndrome
Haematological	• Anaemia of chronic disease • NSAID – related gastrointestinal bleeding • Megaloblastic anaemia associated with pernicious anaemia/methotrexate therapy • Bone marrow suppression from DMARDs • Felty's Syndrome anaemia and splenomegaly

Table 3.59: Summary of features on examination in rheumatoid arthritis

- CXR: evidence of fibrosis, effusions and rheumatoid nodules
- Chest CT (if appropriate) for confirmation or further clarification of X-rays

Others:

- Joint aspiration: typically straw-coloured with a slight neutrophilia. Check for crystals and send to microbiology to exclude infection.

Assessment of cardiovascular risk factors:

- Lipid profile
- Diabetes
- ECG

Management

Pharmacological:

- Analgesia, eg simple analgesia, NSAIDs
- Corticosteroids
- DMARDs – methotrexate, hydroxychloroquine, leflunamide, sulfasalazine
- Anti-cytokine agents eg Infliximab (anti-TNF-a)
- Treatment of extra-articular features as required
- Cardiovascular risk reduction strategies eg statins

Non-pharmacological:

- Patient education – information sources such as Arthritis Research UK
- Physiotherapy
- Surgical: treatment of joint deformities eg arthrodesis/arthroplasty

Gout

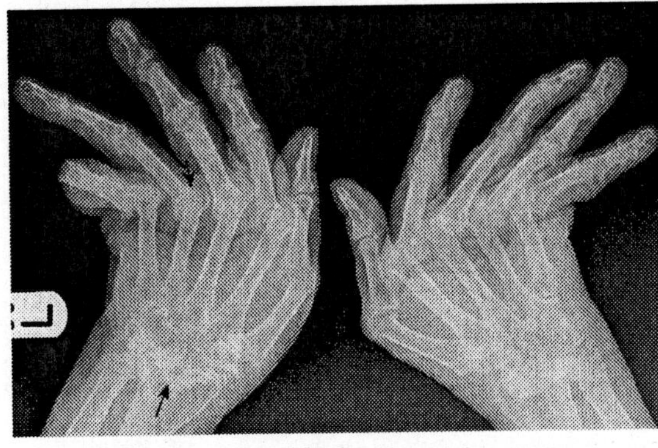

Figure 3.28: Plain X-ray of both hands showing multiple joint subluxations, periarticular cyst formation and erosions (arrow)

Epidemiology

Prevalence of approximately 1%. The prevalence is increasing. The reason for this is not clear but may be connected to rising obesity and diuretic use. Gout is the commonest cause of crystal arthritis and much more common in men. Risk of gout increases with increasing uric acid levels.

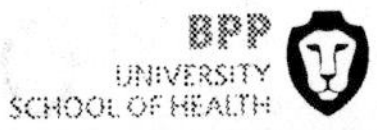

Aetiology

Crystal arthropathy is caused by an inflammatory response to urate crystals in the joint space. Both genetic and environmental causes influence urate levels.

An acute attack may be precipitated by:

- Dietary excess (diets containing high levels of red meat or shellfish)
- Alcohol
- Trauma
- Severe systemic illness
- Surgery
- Drugs (cytotoxic drug therapy, diuretics, commencement of allopurinol, commencement of B12 for pernicious anaemia)

Pathophysiology

Uric acid is produced by purine metabolism. Purines may come from dietary intake or catabolism, especially of purine nucleotides.

Hyperuricaemia may result from reduced renal excretion of urate (90%) or increased urate production (about 10%):

Causes of reduced renal excretion	Causes of increased production
Diuretics (especially thiazide) Aspirin Hypertension Chronic kidney disease	Glucose-6-phosphate deficiency Lymphoproliferative disorders Myeloproliferative disorders Cytotoxic therapy Carcinomatosis Idiopathic

Table 3.60: Causes of hyperuricaemia

History/examination

- Usually an acute mono-arthritis, typically in the first metatarsophalangeal joint
- Polyarticular presentation in about 10% of cases
- Previous episodes of arthritis
- Previous history of renal stones
- Family history of gout
- Sudden onset of hot, red, swollen and exquisitely tender joint(s)
- Chronic hyperuricaemia can result in renal impairment, renal calculi and gouty tophi, ie deposition of urate in the tissues especially in finger tendons and the pinnae

Investigations

Blood tests:

- FBC: Raised WBC in acute gout
- U&E – renal impairment
- CRP
- Clotting
- Glucose
- Uric acid

Imaging:

- X-ray joint: any bony injury needs to be excluded: characteristic changes of punched out periarticular erosions, secondary degenerative change and soft tissue swelling.

Others:

- Joint aspiration: urgent Gram stain and MC&S to exclude septic arthritis and polarised light microscopy. The presence of negatively birefringent (needle shaped) crystals confirms the diagnosis.

Management

- Analgesia: NSAIDs or colchicine
- Allopurinol can be used for long-term prevention but should not be started during an attack as it can exacerbate or prolong symptoms
- Consider a long-acting steroid joint injection if infection excluded
- Physiotherapy

Pseudogout

Epidemiology

Although chondrocalcinosis (intra-articular/soft tissue calcium deposition) is very common in the elderly, attacks of pseudogout are relatively uncommon.

Aetiology

Crystal arthropathy caused by an inflammatory reaction to CPPD in the joint. There may be no clear precipitating factor for an acute attack, but it may follow trauma or be triggered by an acute illness.

Pathophysiology

Risk factors include: old age, osteoarthritis, hyperparathyroidism, haemochromatosis and hypothyroidism.

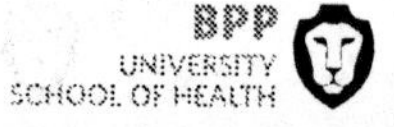

Case Study: More than skin deep

As Mr G entered the room, a sweet, sickly, almost putrid smell accompanied him. 'I have psoriasis,' he said, unnecessarily, as he sat down and indeed, every visible patch of skin was red and flaky, 'I get a bit down now and again, my skin, you know'. It was easy to imagine. Despite the heat of the summer day he was dressed in long, heavy jeans and a hooded sweatshirt so that only his hands and red, raw face were visible. 'My finger's been a bit swollen for a while now, but a few days ago, it suddenly got like this.' He extended the hand towards me. 'I've had gout before, but never like this!' 'A bit swollen' was a grotesque understatement. His middle finger was hideously deformed, protruding above a large, silver ring like some kind of awful monster. He screamed in agony as he caught the swollen joint against his sleeve and beads of sweat appeared on his forehead. 'How much do you drink?' I asked, cautiously probing the offending finger. 'A few cans is all,' he answered, 'Three, maybe four a night. Been drinking a bit more recently, my skin's got worse, you know, I've been a bit down. My doctor was talking about starting a tablet to try and stop my gout from playing up, but I missed the last appointment with him, feel a bit rough in the mornings sometimes.' Despite a normal urate level, Mr G's finger was a classic presentation of gout, so, after failing to remove his titanium ring he was discharged with anti-inflammatories to try his luck with stronger ring cutters at the fire service and advice to contact his GP again to discuss preventative therapy. Of course, none of us were tackling the real problem, which lay hidden, like his scaly, crimson skin.

History/examination

- Usually a mono-arthritis, typically of the knee but also commonly the hip or wrist
- Can be spontaneous but may be precipitated by illness or trauma
- Hot, red, swollen, stiff and exquisitely tender joint(s)

Investigations

Blood tests:

- FBC
- U&E
- CRP
- Clotting
- Glucose
- Uric acid

Imaging:

- X-ray joint: bony injury needs to be excluded. Chondrocalcinosis may be seen.

Other:

- Joint aspiration: Send for urgent Gram stain and MC&S to exclude septic arthritis and polarised light microscopy. The presence of positively birefringent (rhomboid shaped) crystals confirms the diagnosis.

Management

- Usually self-limiting
- NSAID (or Colchicine if gastrointestinal or other contraindications)
- Consider injecting joint with long-acting steroid (if infection excluded)

Cellulitis

Epidemiology

Very common and affects both sexes equally.

Aetiology

An acute dermal infection of the skin usually caused by Gram positive bacteria, ie *Streptococci* and *Staphylococci.*

Risk factors:

- Trauma
- Surgery
- Obesity
- Diabetes
- Peripheral vascular disease
- Peripheral oedema
- Ulcerated skin eg chronic wounds
- Immunosuppression eg medication
- Concomitant skin disorder

Pathophysiology

Often caused by a break in the skin eg due to insect bite. In the hospital it may occur at a site of venepuncture or cannulation. It is associated with

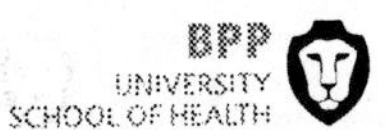

a local inflammatory response with pain, oedema and warmth.

History/examination

- Sudden onset
- History of break in skin integrity
- Past medical history or family history of diabetes or immunocompromised
- Fever
- Erythema, swelling and pain at affected site with peau d'orange dimpling of skin
- Localised lymphadenopathy
- Possible palpable collection if abscess forming

Investigations

Blood tests:

- FBC, CRP & ESR: elevated WCC and inflammatory markers
- U&Es
- LFTs
- Glucose: to exclude a new diagnosis of diabetes mellitus

Microbiology:

- Blood cultures, if there are signs of systemic illness
- Wound swab, if wound is present

Other:

- Mark and date extent of erythema to observe for signs of deterioration or improvement

Management

- Oral or IV antibiotics depending on severity and causation, which should be altered as organisms and sensitivities become known
- Surgical intervention if abscess present
- Elevation of affected limb
- Analgesia

Necrotising fasciitis

Epidemiology

An estimated 500 new cases per year with a mortality rate of 20%.

Aetiology

Progressive, rapidly spreading inflammatory infection of the deep fascia that causes necrosis of the subcutaneous tissue. Causative bacteria can be aerobic, anaerobic or mixed flora. The most common causative organism is *Streptococcus pyogenes*.

Necrotising fasciitis can occur after:

- Trauma
- Intramuscular or IV injection
- Surgical procedures
- Insect bites
- Childbirth

Peripheral vascular disease increases risk. The immunocompromised individuals are at more risk. There is a possible link to NSAID use during a varicella infection.

Pathophysiology

A rapidly spreading infection that causes the release of toxins, leading to tissue hypoxia and death.

Causative organisms	
Gram positive aerobic bacteria	Group A ß haemolytic streptoccoci Group B streptococci Enterococci Coagulase negative staphylococci *Staphylococcus aureus* *Bacillus species*
Gram negative aerobic bacteria	*Escherichia coli Pseudomonas aeruginosa Proteus species* *Serratia species* *Anaerobic* bacteria *Bacteroides species* *Clostridium species* *Peptostreptococcus species*
Fungal	Zygomycetes Aspergillus Candida
Other	*Vibrio species*

Table 3.61: Causative organisms of necrotising fasciitis

Exotoxin A stimulates the release of cytokines, which damage the endothelial lining of vessels and alters the permeability of cell membranes such that fluid leaks into the extravascular space. This reduces perfusion, leading to ischaemia and death.

History/examination

- Trauma or recent surgery
- Sudden onset of pain and swelling at site

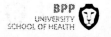

- Severe pain that does not respond to analgesia
- Later loss of sensation
- Possible diarrhoea and vomiting
- Rapidly spreading erythema changing to a dusky pink colouration at site of insult (sometimes no visible skin changes, just a feeling of induration)
- Signs of septic shock: pyrexia, hypotension, tachycardia, confusion
- May have crepitations at the site of infection

Investigations

The diagnosis is clinical and investigations should not delay surgical management.

Blood tests:

- FBC: raised WBC
- U&Es: often elevated urea and creatinine
- Glucose: often raised
- ABG: raised lactate

Microbiology:

- Blood cultures
- Tissue biopsy and culture taken during surgical debridement

Imaging:

- X-ray: localised subcutaneous gas
- MRI: anatomical site and extent of necrosis (oedematous tissues)

Management

- A to E assessment
- IV fluid resuscitation
- Commence urgent broad spectrum antibiotics following local trust policy (usually a combination of penicillin, gentamicin and either metronidazole or clindamycin) changing once sensitivities are known
- Calculate LRINEC score to assess likelihood that diagnosis is necrotising fasciitis
- Urgent aggressive surgical debridement and repeat debridement may be necessary – this is also a diagnostic step
- May require intensive care to manage the septic shock
- Later will require reconstructive surgery depending on extent of debridement and psychological input

CRP	<150	0	>150	+4		
WCC	<15	0	15-25	+1	>25	+2
Hb	>13.5	0	11-13.5	+1	<11	+2
Na	>135	0	<135	+2		
Cr	<1.6	0	>1.6	+2		
Glu	<180	0	>180	+1		

Table 3.62: LRINEC score

Scores <6 = low risk for necrotising fasciitis
Scores of 8 or higher = high risk for necrotising fasciitis

Case Study: Just a small scratch...

JC was 22 when one day she accidentally caught her leg whilst shaving. Thinking no more about it, she covered the scratch with a plaster and carried on normally with life. 24 hours later she went to A&E with a slight temperature feeling a little unwell. She was dismissed with some paracetamol and advice to contact her own GP after the weekend. Six hours later she was intubated on inotropic support and strong antibiotics in intensive care, having had most of the soft tissues debrided from her left leg to control the necrotising infection that had rapidly swept through her body. She required two further operations before the infection was finally tamed and remained in intensive care for a further ten days.

Upon returning to the ward, JC discovered that her recovery had only just begun. Although she had survived, most of her left leg would have to be reconstructed – a process that would take months of surgery and physiotherapy – and those were just the physical scars. Psychologically she remained traumatised for weeks, trying to rationalise and explain the devastating events she had lived through. A simple, insignificant scratch had profound and life-changing consequences.

Prognosis

- Very high mortality if not diagnosed and treated effectively.

Even with good treatment mortality approaches 20%.

Deep vein thrombosis (DVT)

Epidemiology

DVT is a common condition.

Aetiology

A DVT is a thrombus formed within the deep veins of the leg. It can occur anywhere from the deep veins of the calf to the ilio-femoral veins.

Pathophysiology

Virchow's triad dictates that thrombosis results from one or more of: vascular wall injury, circulatory stasis and hypercoaguable state.

History/examination

- Pain and swelling
- Risk factors for DVT, eg cancer, immobility, trauma, surgery, pregnancy and the puerperium, OCP/HRT therapy
- Past/family history of DVT/pulmonary embolism (PE) or hypercoaguability (Antithrombin III, Protein C or S deficiency, antiphospholipid syndrome)
- Classical symptoms of DVT: limb pain, pitting oedema, erythema and dilation of the surface veins; however, these are often not all present
- > 3 cm calf circumference difference
- Evidence of complications, principally pulmonary embolus

Investigations

- Initial clinical examination and blood tests on presentation
- Dose of LMWH (whilst awaiting Duplex Doppler ultrasound)

Blood tests:

- FBC
- U&E
- CRP
- D-dimer (depending on Wells score as may be artificially raised in many other states. Only effective at ruling out DVT if low clinical suspicion, cannot be used for positive diagnosis)

Duplex Doppler ultrasound:

- Identifies presence and extent of clot

Venogram:

- The 'gold standard' test, but rarely performed nowadays

Wells score:

Wells pre-test probability	
Clinical feature	**Score**
Active cancer	1
Paralysis/Plastered leg	1
Bedridden for 3 days in last 4 weeks	1
Localised tenderness along a deep vein	1
Entire leg swollen	1
Calf swollen >3 cm compared to normal	1
Pitting oedema	1
Superficial collateral veins	1
Alternative diagnosis more likely	-2
A score of <1 is low probability A score of 1–2 is medium probability A score of >2 is high probability	

Table 3.63: The Wells score

Management

For a confirmed DVT, the patient will require ongoing anticoagulation, usually with warfarin with additional LMWH until the INR is within the therapeutic range. It may not be necessary to anticoagulate a below-knee DVT as the risk of embolisation is slight.

If no clear cause for the DVT is found, this will need to be investigated. The precise investigations depend on the clinical scenario, but may include:

- Thrombophilia screen (before any anticoagulation)
- Pelvic ultrasound
- CXR to look for lung cancer

Referral will need to be made to the anticoagulant clinic for stabilising the INR and warfarin dose.

If DVT is not confirmed, an alternative diagnosis for the leg swelling must be sought.

Further reading and references

1. Hart, N.B., Hasham, S., Matteucci, P., et al. (2005) Necrotising fasciitis. *BMJ* 2005; 330: 830–833.
2. National Institute for Health and Clinical Excellence. (2009) *Rheumatoid Arthritis* (CG079). [Online]. Available from: www.nice.org.uk/guidance/CG79 [Accessed 7 November 2016].
3. National Institute for Health and Clinical Excellence (2007). *Rheumatoid arthritis – adalimumab, etanercept and infliximab* (TA30). [Online]. Available from: www.nice.org.uk/guidance/ta130?unlid=29220042220162317380 [Accessed 7 November 2016].

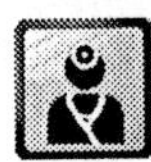

Metabolic disorders

Diabetic ketoacidosis (DKA)

DKA is a common and life-threatening complication of diabetes.

The diagnostic criteria are:

1. Raised serum glucose ≥11.0 mmol/L or known diabetes
2. Ketonaemia ≥3 mmol/L, or ketonuria on dipstick (≥2+ on standard urine dipsticks)
3. Metabolic acidosis with serum bicarbonate <15 mmol/L and/or venous pH <7.3

Epidemiology

DKA is the most common acute hyperglycaemic diabetic emergency. It effects up to 4% of type 1 diabetics per year (although can occur in type 2 diabetics). Of these, 6% of cases are previously undiagnosed diabetics.

Aetiology

- Infection is the most common precipitating cause (pay particular attention to urinary tract infections and pneumonia)
- Inadequate insulin
- Newly diagnosed diabetes
- Myocardial infarction
- Stroke
- Sepsis
- Drugs (eg sympathomimetics, beta-blockers, corticosteroids or diuretics)

Pathophysiology

Inadequate insulin levels lead to insufficient cellular uptake of glucose. There is a subsequent stress response resulting in the release of glucagon, cortisol, adrenaline and growth hormone. This encourages gluconeogenesis and glycogenolysis in the liver, further worsening the hyperglycaemia. Hyperglycaemia causes an osmotic diuresis manifesting as polyuria, with polydipsia occurring in response. Although the patient is hyperglycaemic, there is a lack of intracellular glucose which results in the body switching to the metabolism of fatty acids. The end result of fatty acid metabolism is the production of the ketone bodies, 3-hydroxybutyrate and acetoacetic acids.

The lack of insulin has a second effect in that it leads to an extracellular hyperkalaemia but a reduction in intracellular potassium stores. This is due to insulin's action on promoting potassium uptake by cells.

History

- Polyuria and polydipsia
- Nausea and vomiting
- Weight loss (due to protein and fatty acid catabolism)
- Fatigue and weakness
- Abdominal pain
- Drowsiness and confusion
- Symptoms related to precipitating factors eg fever, productive cough, dysuria, insulin dosing and injection sites, chest pain or recent changes to medication

Examination

- Reduced level of consciousness
- Tachycardia
- Hypotension
- Signs of clinical dehydration: reduced skin turgor, dry mucous membranes, reduced urine output
- Kussmaul's breathing (a deep and laboured breathing pattern)
- Ketone breath (fruity odour similar to nail polish remover)

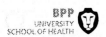

- Evidence of infection may be present – localisation of source is important

Investigations

Blood tests:

- Venous blood gas (glucose, bicarbonate, pH)
- Capillary blood glucose
- Blood ketones
- FBC
- U&Es
- CRP
- ABG: if desaturation or low GCS (VBG is sufficient for diagnosis of DKA)
- Cardiac enzymes: to rule out silent MI

Microbiology:

- Blood cultures if septic
- Sputum culture if signs of pneumonia

Imaging:

- Chest X-ray if clinically indicated: may show evidence of consolidation

Others:

- ECG: may show ischaemic changes.
- Urinalysis: ketones and glucose. May also show leucocytes and nitrites which may indicate UTI. If so, send urine sample for microscopy, culture and sensitivity.

Management

(Guidelines from joint British diabetes societies inpatient care group 2013 for patients aged >18)

General measures:

- A to E assessment.
- Oxygen (high flow for the critically unwell).
- Close monitoring with regular clinical review, hourly blood glucose and hourly ketone measurements. At least two hourly serum potassium and bicarbonate levels for the first six hours.
- Urinary catheter to monitor fluid balance if incontinent or anuric.
- DVT prophylaxis.
- Consider antibiotics if evidence of infection according to trust microbiology policy.
- Sodium bicarbonate is generally not recommended and should only be commenced by a consultant and in a HDU/ITU setting.
- Nil by mouth if vomiting or reduced GCS. May need an NG tube.
- Consider ICU review if haemodynamically compromised or significantly reduced level of consciousness. The guidelines contain specific biochemical parameters which indicate severe DKA.
- Diabetes specialist nurse/diabetologist referral. Their involvement shortens admission time and improves patient satisfaction. This should be within the first 24 hours.
- Resolution of DKA is defined as pH >7.3 units, bicarbonate >15 mmol/L and blood ketone level <0.6 mmol/L.

Specific therapies:

Fluid & electrolyte replacement:

- Rapid fluid replacement is recognised as the most important action in DKA followed by insulin administration
- Patients are often severely dehydrated
- 0.9% saline is the usual fluid choice; however, if blood glucose falls below 14.0 mmol/l then 10% dextrose is recommended alongside 0.9% saline
- Suggested replacement with 0.9% saline (based on a 70 kG man):
  - If SBP < 90 mmHg: 1 litre stat. If remains below 90 mmHg then senior input is required.
  - If SBP > 90 mmHg then:
    - 1L (+/- KCL – potassium required if 1 litre or more of 0.9% saline already given) over 1hr then:
    - 1L + KCL over 2 hrs (x2)
    - 1L + KCL over 4 hrs (x2)
    - 1L + KCL over 6 hrs
- Potassium replacement as below:
  - >5.5mM – nil
  - 3.5-5.5mM – 40 mmol/L
  - <3.5 – senior review
- Hypokalaemia and hyperkalaemia are both life-threatening conditions associated with DKA. Although initial potassium may be normal or high, there is a total body depletion. As acidosis improves and insulin is prescribed, potassium is driven intracellularly and plasma levels fall. Aim to keep potassium 4–5 mmol/L.

Insulin therapy:

- A fixed rate intravenous insulin infusion (FRIII) is used. Dose calculated by 0.1 units/kg/hr.
- Only give a bolus (stat) dose of IM insulin (0.1 unit/kg) if there is a delay in setting up the FRIII.

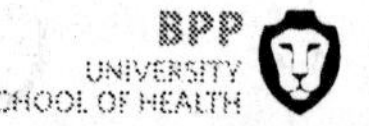

Case Study: A tragic tale

SJ was 17. He lived with his parents in a small house in a small rural town. He had no particular plans for the future, except maybe going to college when he finished school, as he knew this would please his parents. One day, his mother took him to see the local GP. She was concerned that he was becoming more withdrawn and quiet, spending more time alone and losing weight. On further questioning, she had not noticed a decline in his appetite, he seemed fairly happy at school and did not seem to have any particular worries or stresses. The only thing she did mention was that he seemed a little thirstier than usual and would often drink several glasses of water before leaving for school in the mornings. There was no history or family history of diabetes and no other signs to make the GP suspicious. However, she sent SJ away with a bottle to provide a urine sample, arranged to see him alone in a few days to discuss how he was feeling in a bit more depth, and warned his mother that if anything were to change, and he became more unwell, she should call the practice or the emergency services immediately. Unfortunately, that evening, SJ suffered a hypoglycaemic attack, lost consciousness and suffered multiple fits. His parents, unsure about what was happening, delayed sending for an ambulance until after the fourth seizure. SJ was assessed by the acute medical team in the middle of an exceptionally busy 'take' shift, who initially missed the diagnosis of diabetic ketoacidosis and it was only after the consultant saw him an hour or so after admission that fluid resuscitation was started. By this point it was too late. SJ never regained consciousness and he died later that evening. Nobody blamed the GP and indeed SJ's parents continued to request her care. However, his name was ingrained on her memory and whenever she drove past their old address a flood of guilt rushed through her.

- If the patient usually takes long-acting insulin analogues Lantus, Levemir or Degludec then continue this at the usual dose and usual time.
- Transfer to subcutaneous insulin once resolution of DKA and if the patient is eating and drinking normally. Start S/C insulin before stopping the FRIII, ideally around a meal time and discontinue IV insulin one hour later. If patient not ready to eat and drink, then a VRII (also known as a sliding scale) can be commenced until they are ready.

Targets of above treatment:

- Reduce blood ketone level by 0.5 mmol/L/hour
- Increase the venous bicarbonate level by 3.0 mmol/L/hour
- Reduce capillary blood glucose by 3.0 mmol/L/hour
- Maintain potassium between 4.0 and 5.5 mmol/L

Prognosis

Has improved with better clinical care and mortality now stands at 0.67%.

Hyperglycaemic Hyperosmolar State (HHS) (formerly HONK)

Specific diagnostic criteria for HSS do not exist; however, commonly recognised features are:

- Hypovolaemia
- Hyperglycaemia (usually >30 mmol/L)
- No hyperketonaemia (<3 mmol/L) or acidosis (pH >7.3, bicarbonate >15 mmol/l)
- Osmolality usually >320 mosmol/kg

A mixed HSS and DKA can occur.

Epidemiology

Incidence estimated at less than 1 case per 1,000 person-years. Typical patient is elderly with multiple co-morbidities.

Aetiology

The causes of HHS include:

- Infection
- Poor diabetes control
- Myocardial infarction
- Stroke
- Pancreatitis
- Drugs (eg sympathomimetics, beta-blockers, corticosteroids or diuretics)

Pathophysiology

Hyperglycaemia occurs due to relative insulin deficiency or insulin resistance. There is still sufficient insulin to prevent cellular metabolism switching to fatty acid catabolism therefore preventing

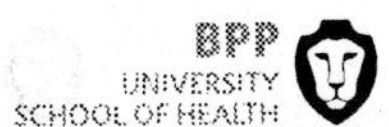

ketoacidosis. Uncontrolled hyperglycaemia leads to osmotic diuresis and serum hyperosmolarity leading to profound dehydration and altered neurological states. Relative hyper-viscosity due to dehydration increases the risk of venous thromboembolism. Untreated or poorly managed HHS can lead to DIC.

History

- Symptoms often develop over multiple days and are more insidious than those of DKA; however, due to the progression over numerous days the metabolic disturbances and severity of dehydration is usually greater
- Drowsiness, confusion, generalised weakness
- Visual impairment
- Leg cramps
- Nausea and vomiting – less common than in DKA
- Symptoms relating to precipitating factors such as fever, productive cough and dysuria
- Current hypoglycaemic therapy and compliance and any recent changes to medication

Examination

- Tachycardia
- Hypotension (or postural hypotension)
- Seizures
- Reduced level of consciousness – despite the previous title, hyperosmolar non-ketotic osmotic coma, coma is relatively rare and represents severe disease
- Raised temperature (if septic) or hypothermia
- Signs of source of infection eg pneumonia, meningitis
- Signs of dehydration: reduced skin turgor, dry mucous membranes and reduced urine output
- Neurological examination – focal neurological signs can occur such as one sided weakness and these can easily be misidentified as a stroke

Investigations

Blood tests:

- FBC
- CRP
- U&Es: usually hypernatremia but beware severe hyperglycaemia can cause pseudo-hyponatremia
- Serum osmolality: usually >320 mmol/Kg
- Capillary + lab glucose measurements
- ABG: possible mild metabolic acidosis but pH typically >7.3
- Consider checking cardiac enzymes to rule out silent MI

Microbiology:

- Blood cultures

Imaging:

- CXR: may show evidence of consolidation

Others:

- ECG: may show ischaemic changes.
- Urinalysis: glucose and possibly minimal ketones. May also show leucocytes and nitrites which may indicate UTI. If so, send urine sample for microscopy, culture and sensitivity.

Management

(Guidelines based on joint British diabetes societies inpatient care group 2012)

General measures:

- A to E assessment.
- Consider antibiotics if evidence of infection.
- Urinary catheter to monitor fluid balance.
- Keep nil by mouth if vomiting or reduced GCS; an NG tube may be required.
- Consider ITU review if haemodynamically compromised or significantly reduced level of consciousness. The guidelines have criteria which indicate severe HSS.
- Treat the underlying cause.
- Close monitoring (initially hourly) with regular clinical review, careful monitoring of glucose, electrolytes, fluid status and osmolality. The patient should be monitored for complications of electrolyte shifts eg cerebral oedema and central pontine myelonylisis.
- DVT prophylaxis: significantly greater risk of thrombosis compared to DKA. Guidelines recommend prophylactic LMWH.
- All patients should be assumed to be at high risk of foot ulceration. The heels must be appropriately protected and daily foot checks undertaken.
- Diabetes specialist nurse/diabetologist referral.

Specific therapies:

Fluid replacement:

- Patients are usually profoundly dehydrated.
- 0.9% saline is the fluid of choice. Only switch to 0.45% saline if the osmolality is not declining despite adequate fluid balance on assessment.
- Replacement should be less vigorous than with DKA.

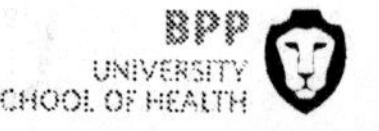

- If blood glucose falls below 14 mmol/l commence 10% glucose (125ml/hr) alongside the 0.9% saline.
- The aim is to achieve a positive balance of 3–6 litres by 12 hours. Then replace the remainder of the estimated fluid losses over the next 12 hours.
- As long as it is safe to do so the patient can drink fluids; it is essential that an accurate fluid balance chart is maintained.
- Fluid balance is especially important if the patient is elderly or has co-morbidities such as congestive cardiac failure.
- Potassium replacement as above for DKA.

Insulin replacement

- Recommended when the blood glucose is no longer falling with IV fluids alone. However, it should be started immediately alongside fluids when there is significant ketonaemia (1 mmol/L or urine ketones >2+).
- Insulin should be given as a fixed rate intravenous insulin infusion (FRIII) at 0.05 units/kg/hour.

Prognosis

Mortality is at 15–20% even with effective treatment. Prognosis is worse in the elderly.

Hypoglycaemia

Although the exact definition is highly debated, clinically on the wards it is often taken as being a plasma glucose of <4 mmol/L.

Epidemiology

Most commonly occurs in patients being treated for diabetes mellitus with insulin or oral hypoglycaemics.

Aetiology

Causes of hypoglycaemia include:

- Overtreatment with insulin or oral hypoglycaemics (including deliberate overdose)
- Excess alcohol
- Hepatic, renal or cardiac failure
- Sepsis
- Post-gastric bypass
- Adrenal insufficiency
- Insulinoma
- Insulin autoimmune hypoglycaemia (rare)

Pathophysiology

- Adrenergic symptoms typically start to appear when glucose concentrations fall below 3.0 mmol/L. They are due to increased secretion of glucagon, adrenaline, cortisol and growth hormone as the body tries to increase the plasma sugar levels. These may include sweating, anxiety, palpitations, nausea, hunger, and tremor.
- Neuroglycopenic symptoms are a result of cerebral hypoglycaemia. These include blurred vision, dizziness, confusion, lethargy and drowsiness. Focal neurological symptoms may be seen and in severe cases there may be seizures, coma and cardiac arrest.

History/examination

- History of diabetes
- Treatment of diabetes including doses and what medications have actually been taken
- Medication history
- Time since last meal and nature of meal
- Awareness of 'hypo'
- Response of hypo symptoms to carbohydrate intake
- Adrenergic symptoms as above
- Neuroglycopenic symptoms as above
- Alcohol history

Investigations

Blood tests:

- FBC
- U&Es and CRP
- LFTs
- Drug screen
- Both capillary and laboratory glucose
- HbA1c: shows whether recent control has been too tight
- C-peptide and proinsulin: if insulinoma suspected

Specialist tests: exist for the rare conditions.

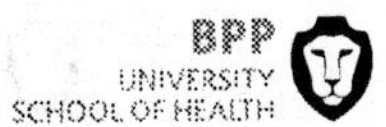

Management

Alert and orientated	Confused or drowsy BUT intact swallow reflex	Unconscious OR unsafe swallow
Rapid acting oral glucose: 15 g eg 1.5 tubes Glucogel, 4 GlucoTabs or Lucozade	Buccal glucose eg Hypostop/glucogel	IV access: 100 ml 20% glucose or 150 ml 10% glucose
Followed by long acting carbohydrate eg sandwich	Consider requirement for IV access	Check at 15 mins
Recheck BG at 15 mins if still <4 mmol/L repeat above	If consciousness regained give long acting carbohydrate	If no IV access give 1 mg IM Glucagon (takes approx. 15 mins to work)
	Check BG at 15 mins	Check BG at 15 mins

Table 3.64: Management of hypoglycaemia

Cushing's disease/syndrome

Cushing's syndrome results from prolonged exposure to excess glucocorticoids (endogenous or exogenous).

Cushing's disease results from a pituitary adenoma causing an ACTH dependent glucocorticoid excess.

Epidemiology

Incidence thought to be 10–15 per million.

Aetiology

Cushing's syndrome can be ACTH dependent or non-ACTH dependent:

ACTH dependent	ACTH independent
• Pituitary adenoma (80%) • Ectopic ACTH secretion (particularly lung cancer)	• Exogenous glucocorticoid administration (most common) • Benign adrenal adenoma • Adrenal carcinoma • Nodular adrenal hyperplasia

Table 3.65: Aetiology of Cushing's syndrome

Pathophysiology

Glucocorticoid (cortisol) release from the adrenal cortex is stimulated from ACTH from the pituitary gland, which in turn is secreted in response to CRH from the pituitary. The hypothalamus-pituitary-adrenal axis is controlled physiologically with negative feedback. Pathologies affecting this axis can cause excess cortisol release.

History/examination

There is a large spectrum of clinical manifestations from subclinical to severe symptoms.

- Drug history
- Skin manifestations: easy bruising, purple striae, skin atrophy, poor wound healing, hirsutism, acne, pigmentation (with ACTH dependent cases)
- Psychiatric disturbances: typically, depression or psychosis
- Recurrent infections
- Diabetes
- Moon facies and facial plethora
- Buffalo hump
- Obesity (particularly truncal obesity and supraclavicular fat pads)
- Hypertension
- Oligo/amenorrhoea
- Reduced libido
- Osteopenia, osteoporosis and unexplained fractures
- Proximal myopathy

Investigations

Usually multiple tests are needed to make a diagnosis and are best co-ordinated by a specialist. Before any testing occurs exogenous glucocorticoid use must be excluded.

The diagnosis of Cushing's syndrome is established when at least two of the different first line tests are abnormal.

The diagnosis is in two stages:

1. Confirm the diagnosis:
   i) Four possible tests can be used:
      - Low-dose dexamethasone suppression test
      - 24-hour urinary free cortisol. This should be done 3 times. Need at least 2 out of 3 to be 3 times the laboratory upper limit of normal

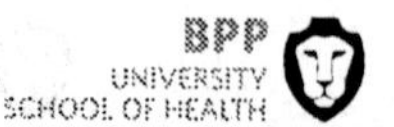

- Midnight plasma cortisol: due to the loss of the normal circadian rhythm of cortisol levels, a midnight level of greater than 50 mmol/l is indicative
- Late night salivary cortisol (two measurements are usually required)

Beware of Pseudo-Cushing's syndrome which can have the clinical features and biochemical evidence of raised cortisol; however, is not caused by problems with the pituitary-adrenal axis. Common causes include depression, severe obesity and chronic alcoholism.

2. Localise the lesion and determine the cause:
   i) ACTH levels will distinguish ACTH and non-ACTH dependent causes:
      - Low ACTH levels indicate an ACTH-independent cause
      - Raised ACTH levels indicate an ACTH-dependent cause

Blood tests:

- U&Es: can show hypokalaemia
- Glucose: high
- Corticotrophin releasing hormone level

Imaging:

This will depend on the results of the diagnostic tests:

- CXR: to exclude lung cancer
- MRI: of pituitary
- CT: of abdomen to visualise the adrenals

Others:

- Inferior petrosal sinus sampling

Management

- Cushing's disease: surgery, ie trans-sphenoidal microsurgery is the main-stay of treatment. Radiotherapy (usually as an adjunct to surgery). Bilateral adrenalectomy may rarely be necessary.
- Adrenal disease: adrenalectomy unilateral or bilateral.
- Ectopic ACTH secretion: excision of source.
- Exogenous glucocorticoid therapy: reduce dose or stop drug.

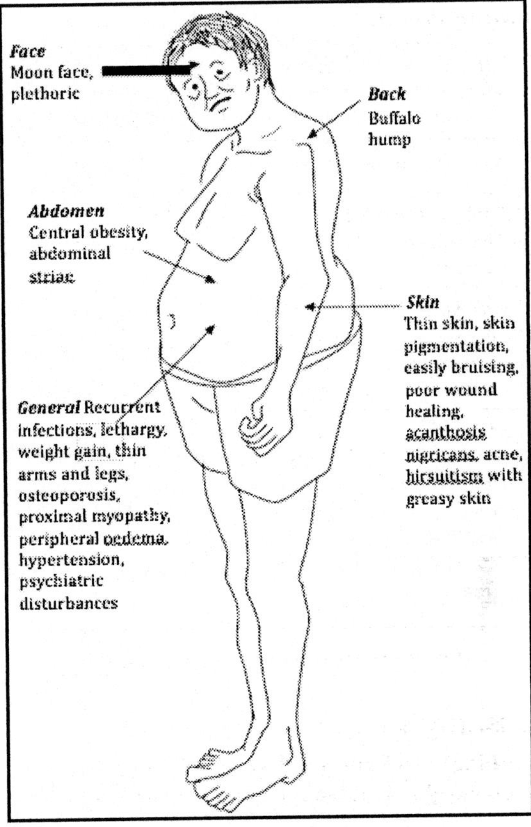

Figure 3.29: Signs and symptoms of Cushing's syndrome

- There are numerous pharmacological agents that can be used individually, in combination and alongside the above treatment options. These include cabergoline, pasreotide mifepristone, mitotane, ketoconazole, metyrapone and etomidate. The specific agent and dosing is decided by the specialist.

Prognosis

Untreated has a high mortality (50% in 5 years).

Primary adrenal insufficiency (Addison's disease)

Adrenal insufficiency is when the adrenal glands do not produce one or more of the three classes of hormones normally produced. These are the glucocorticoids, mineralocorticoids and androgens. This is despite a normal or raised ACTH level.

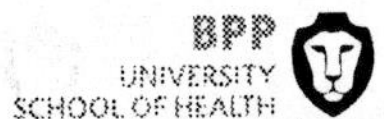

Epidemiology

Incidence is estimated to be 35–120/1,000,000 per year and females are predominantly affected. It may present with insidious onset or acutely with an adrenal crisis.

Aetiology and pathophysiology

- Autoimmune (85–90% cases in the west): can also be seen as part of the polyglandular syndromes
- TB (7–20% in the west)
- Metastases: predominantly lung, breast and lymphoma
- Drugs: ketoconazole, fluconazole, rifampin, phenytoin
- Haemorrhagic infarction (eg antiphospholipid syndrome)
- Fungal infection in immunocompromised individuals
- Congenital: congenital adrenal hypoplasia, enzyme deficiencies

History/examination

- Described as the 'master of non-specificity' due to its highly non-specific symptoms
- Weight loss and anorexia
- Fatigue
- Myalgia and weakness
- Abdominal pain, diarrhoea and vomiting
- Reduced libido
- Depression
- Salt craving
- Past medical or family history of autoimmune diseases, especially type 1 diabetes
- Look for signs of dehydration (including postural hypotension)
- Hyperpigmentation particularly on the face, neck, buccal mucosa and palmar creases

Investigations

Blood tests:

- U&Es: hyponatremia and hyperkalaemia, with raised urea in dehydration
- Low calcium
- Glucose: hypoglycaemia
- TFTs
- Random cortisol: will be low (usually taken at 0900)
- ACTH: will be high in primary adrenal insufficiency

Confirm the diagnosis:

- Short synacthen test: 250 microgram synacthen (a synthetic ACTH) is given IM at 0900 and serum cortisol measured at 0, 30 and 60 minutes. A normal response is for the cortisol to rise to more than 450 nmol/L or an incremental rise of at least 150 nmol/L.
- Adrenal autoantibodies.

Other:

- Chest X-ray: looking for TB
- CT: of the abdomen may reveal metastases or a primary tumour

Management

- Patient education and information
- Medic alert bracelet
- Provide written information and include information about the Addison's Disease self-help group

Hormone replacement:

- Different steroids can be used but typically:
  - Hydrocortisone three times daily with a higher dose in the morning
  - Fludrocortisone titrated to symptoms and clinical findings
  - Ensure additional glucocorticoid is given during acute illness: patient taught to increase home steroids if mild disease, if admitted to hospital may need to be converted to IV hydrocortisone

Adrenal crisis:

A potentially life-threatening complication of Addison's disease and manifests with the typical symptoms but at a more extreme level.

Triggers include:

- Infection
- Trauma
- Surgery
- Stopping steroid treatment

If an adrenal crisis is encountered, management includes:

- IV hydrocortisone

- Aggressive fluid replacement
- Correction of hypoglycaemia and any other electrolyte imbalances
- Septic screen

Prognosis

With careful adherence to replacement therapy a normal life expectancy is seen.

Conn's syndrome

Epidemiology

Conn's syndrome accounts for approximately 33% cases of primary hyperaldosteronism. It is more common in women. Other causes of primary hyperaldosteronism include adrenal hyperplasia, familial hyperaldosteronism and adrenal carcinoma.

Aetiology

Conn's syndrome is a form of primary hyperaldosteronism resulting from a unilateral aldosterone-secreting adrenal adenoma.

Pathophysiology

Mineralocorticoid secretion from the Zona Glomerulosa of the adrenal cortex is governed by the renin-angiotensin system. Excess secretion, independent of the RAS, can be due to a number of pathologies, one of these being Conn's syndrome. The extra aldosterone acts at the distal renal tubule where it promotes sodium and water uptake leading to hypertension. It also leads to potassium loss and subsequent hypokalaemia.

History/examination

- Features of hypokalaemia including cramps, weakness and palpitations from tachydysrhythmias
- Hypertension, especially younger onset (below age 50)
- Polyuria and polydipsia may be reported

Investigations

Blood tests:

- U&Es: classically hypernatremia and hypokalaemia, but up to 50% of Conn's are normokalaemic
- Aldosterone – should be raised
- Renin: a high/normal renin, in the absence of diuretic therapy, excludes the diagnosis. Renin is expected to be low in Conn's
- ABG: shows metabolic alkalosis

Imaging:

- Adrenal CT/MRI

Others:

- Saline infusion test
- Selective adrenal venous sampling

Management

- Laparoscopic adrenalectomy with pre-operative spironolactone
- In non-surgical candidates, ongoing treatment with amiloride or spironolactone

Prognosis

If remains untreated, the patient faces all the risks induced by ongoing hypertension and in addition the risk of cardiac arrhythmias from hypokalaemia.

Phaeochromocytoma

Epidemiology

A rare condition which affects less than 0.2% of hypertensive patients. Prevalence is equal in males and females. There is a peak incidence between 40 and 50 years old.

Aetiology

The majority of phaeochromocytomas are tumours affecting chromaffin cells of the adrenal medulla. A small number will be extra-adrenal and affect the paraganglion cells in the ANS. Most tumours are sporadic; however, there may be familial predisposition and approximately 30% are thought to be hereditary. Hereditary tumours are associated with a number of other conditions:

- MEN type 2
- Neurofibromatosis type 1
- Von Hippel-Lindau syndrome

There is a 10% rule which describes the fact that 10% of phaeochromocytomas will be:

- Familial
- Bilateral
- Malignant
- Extra-adrenal

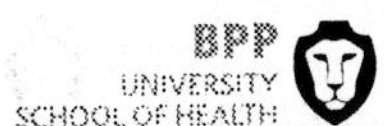

Pathophysiology

- Phaeochromocytomas cause hyper-secretion of catecholamines (adrenaline, noradrenaline and rarely dopamine) and hence symptoms are related to increased stimulation of alpha and/or beta adrenergic receptors.
- Malignant tumours are histologically similar to benign tumours; however, they either metastasise or have local invasion. Common sites of metastases are:
  - Liver
  - Lymph nodes
  - Bone

History/examination

- Symptoms are present in 50% and are typically paroxysmal
- Episodic headache, sweating and tachycardia (palpitations) make up a classic triad
- Paroxysmal/persistent hypertension
- History of diabetes mellitus
- Familial history of phaeochromocytoma and endocrine disorders
- Panic attacks
- Pallor
- Tremor
- Occasionally an abdominal mass may be palpable
- Neurofibromas + café au lait spots

Investigations

Diagnosis is through 24-hour urine collection and measurement of urinary catecholamines, vanillylamdelic acid and metanephrines **or** plasma fractionated metanehprines.

Blood tests:

- U&Es: renal impairment/failure may be present
- Glucose: impaired glucose tolerance may occur due to high levels of catecholamines
- Bone profile: hypercalcaemia may be present in patients with primary hyperparathyroidism related to MEN 2 syndrome
- TFTs: elevated in MEN 2

Imaging:

- Abdominal CT can detect adrenal phaeochromocytomas of 0.5 cm and extra-adrenal phaeochromocytomas of 1 cm diameter
- MRI to localise tumour
- MIBG scintigraphy scan + FDG-PET scan

Genetic testing: if meets certain criteria

Management

- Control of hypertension with alpha blockers then adding beta-blockers is achieved pre-operatively to prevent precipitating a hypertensive crisis.

Prognosis

Benign phaeochromocytoma

- Normal life expectancy if surgery successful
- 95% 5-year survival rate
- Recurrence more likely in hereditary disease

Malignant

- Untreated 50% 5-year survival rate
- Unpredictable: factors improving survival include early diagnosis and excision of primary tumour

Hyperthyroidism

Hyperthyroidism is an excessive quantity of thyroid hormones in the circulation.

Epidemiology and aetiology

Hyperthyroidism can be primary, when the abnormality relates to the thyroid gland itself, or secondary when it is secondary to excess TSH in the circulation. It can also be iatrogenic eg exogenous thyroid hormones intake of caused by drugs that increase thyroid levels such as: levodopa and iodine containing IV contrast agents.

Common causes as below:

Primary causes	Secondary causes (very rare)
Graves' disease (75%), Women > men (10:1), typically 20-40 years of age. Autoimmune basis.	Pituitary adenoma (TSH secreting)
Toxic multinodular goitre. Commonest cause in the elderly.	Thyroid hormone resistance syndrome
Thyroid adenoma (toxic)	
Thyroiditis (10%) – post partum thyroiditis, De Quervains thyroiditis	

Table 3.66: Causes of hyperthyroidism

History/examination

History	Examination
Family history	Thin patient
High iodine intake	Fine tremor of hands
Eye pain – 'grittiness', changes in visual acuity or colour vision	Palmar erythema
Childbirth	Onycholysis
Recent infections	Thyroid acropachy
Weight loss despite a normal or increased appetite	Lid lag
Sweating and heat intolerance	Thin hair
Irritability, hyperactivity and insomnia	Goitre
Nervousness and psychosis	Brisk tendon reflexes
Oligomenorrhoea +/- infertility	Muscle weakness, proximal myopathy
Decreased libido	Pruritus + urticaria
Diarrhoea	Gynaecomastia
Fatigue	
Palpitations, tachycardia and AF	
Cardiac failure, particularly in the elderly	

Table 3.67: History and examination findings of hyperthyroidism

Graves' disease

Examination:

- Usually a painless diffuse goitre (may have a bruit on auscultation)
- Ophthalmopathy:
  - Eye signs in approximately 30%, which are more severe in smokers.
  - Lymphocytic infiltration of the muscles and fatty tissues of the eye with oedema and later fibrosis, causing forward displacement of the eye leading to proptosis (exophthalmos). Examination will reveal prominent white sclera below the cornea as the patient looks straight ahead. Can be asymmetrical. It frequently causes corneal damage and keratitis as the patient is unable to close the eyelids fully. In severe cases there may be chemosis (oedema of the conjunctiva), an increase in the intraocular pressure, and papilloedema.
  - Complex ophthalmoplegia: may occur because of weakness in the extra-ocular muscles.
- Pretibial myxoedema
  - Affects 2% of Graves' disease sufferers
  - Painless thickening of the skin and subcutaneous tissue over the shin
- Thyroid acropachy
  - Rare (<1%)
  - Almost all have ophthalmopathy and pretibial myxoedema
  - A similar appearance to finger clubbing
  - X-rays may reveal some subperiosteal bone formation

Investigations

Blood tests:

- FBC: must be performed prior to commencing anti-thyroid drugs as they may cause agranulocytosis.
- Thyroid function tests: in primary hyperthyroidism: raised T3 and T4 and low TSH levels. In secondary hyperthyroidism: may be an increased TSH if the cause is hypothalamus-pituitary dysfunction.
- Serum antibodies against thyroglobulin, thyroid peroxidase and thyrotropin-receptor antibodies in Graves' disease.
- In subacute thyroiditis CRP and ESR are often raised.

Imaging:

- Ultrasound thyroid.
- Isotope scans aid in the differentiation between Grave's and toxic adenomas. Increased uptake in graves, decreased in thyroiditis.

Others:

- ECG: to diagnose any rhythm abnormalities especially atrial fibrillation
- FNA: to differentiate between malignant and benign nodules

Management

Medication:

Anti-thyroid drug therapy is first-line for all patients:

- Carbimazole/Methimazole and Propylthiouracil:
  - Reduces production of thyroid hormone
  - Titrate according to TFTs or use the 'block-replace' regimen where levothyroxine is given alongside these medicines when the patient is made hypothyroid
  - Patients must be warned regarding the risk of agranulocytosis with Carbimazole (<0.1% of patients) and advised to seek medical attention if they develop fever or a sore throat

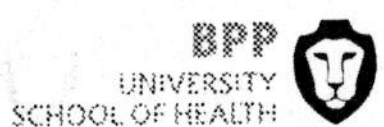

- Propylthiouracil known to cause severe liver failure especially in children and is reserved for pregnancy and thyroid storm
- In Grave's disease remission is usually achieved at 18–24 months after which attempts may be made to stop antithyroid drugs

Propranolol is useful in early stages of treatment and is effective in controlling symptoms such as palpitations and tremor. If B-blockers are contraindicated, calcium channels blockers can be used.

Radioactive iodine therapy:

- Increasingly first-line treatment in teenagers. Also in relapsed Grave's and those with toxic nodular hyperthyroidism.
- Can take three to four months to take effect.
- Can't be given to pregnant or breast feeding females and must avoid pregnancy for six months after.
- Can worsen thyroid eye disease.
- Regular TFTs are mandatory and treatment with levothyroxine may be required.

Surgery:

- Partial thyroidectomy is the most common procedure performed with the aim of normalising the patient's thyroid function.
- Useful in patients with large or retrosternal goitres, a solitary toxic adenoma, those who cannot tolerate drug therapy or who have relapsed post-therapy.
- Potassium iodide is used by some surgeons prior to surgery in order to reduce the vascularity of the gland and minimise the risks of haemorrhage.
- Specific complications include hypothyroidism, left recurrent laryngeal nerve damage, parathyroid gland damage, and haemorrhage into the neck with laryngeal oedema.

Prognosis

- A treatable disease
- Graves' ophthalmopathy may not completely resolve on treatment
- There is increased mortality due to cardio- and cerebrovascular disease if left untreated

Thyrotoxic crisis (thyroid storm)

Epidemiology

This is an uncommon but life-threatening medical emergency with a mortality around 20–30%. It can occur in both known hyperthyroidism and in previously undiagnosed cases.

Aetiology

Precipitating factors are:

- Acute inter-current illness, particularly severe sepsis but also myocardial infarction, surgery and trauma
- Other causes include: radioiodine, iodine-based contrast media and withdrawal of anti-thyroid drugs

History/examination

Patients present with features of severe thyrotoxicosis and hyperpyrexia. In addition: seizures, psychosis, coma and signs of heart failure may be present. GI symptoms may be mistaken for acute surgical abdomen.

Management

Treatment should be initiated promptly:

- Resuscitate the patient with oxygen, IV fluids and place an NG tube if required.
- Prescribe a loading dose of propylthiouracil.
- Potassium iodide (Lugol's solution) given four hours later.
- Intravenous beta-blockers effectively reduce the symptoms of tachycardia and anxiety. Diltiazem can be used if propranolol contraindicated.
- Steroids (hydrocortisone) IV should be given.
- Any specific treatments of precipitating causes
- Patients who fail medical therapy should be treated with therapeutic plasma exchange or thyroidectomy.

Prognosis

Prognosis is poor unless there is quick recognition and management of symptoms. Even with early diagnosis and appropriate treatment, the mortality rate ranges from 10–30%. This increases to 50–90% if left untreated.

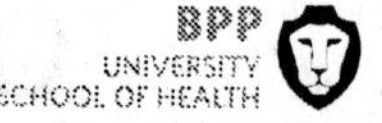

Hypothyroidism

Hypothyroidism results from a deficiency of thyroid hormones.

Epidemiology and aetiology

The prevalence of overt hypothyroidism is 0.1–2%; however, subclinical hypothyroidism is more common at 4–10% adults. Hypothyroidism is 5–8 times more common in women than men. It can affect individuals of any age but is most common in middle age or older patients.

Like hyperthyroidism, hypothyroidism can be primary or secondary. There are also iatrogenic causes including amiodarone, lithium and the treatment of hyperthyroidism (accounts for one-third of cases in developed countries).

Primary causes (95%)	Secondary causes (very rare)
Iodine deficiency (commonest cause worldwide)	Hypopituitarism – reduced TSH
Autoimmune disease (commonest cause in developed world): atrophic thyroiditis, Hashimoto's thyroiditis	Hypothalamic dysfunction – reduced TRH
Infiltrative diseases: amyloidosis, sarcoidosis	
Congenital: thyroid agenesis	

Table 3.68: Causes of hypothyroidism

History/examination

Many symptoms are non-specific and tend to be present for many months/years prior to the development of signs of the disease.

History	Examination
Tiredness	Large body habitus
Weight gain despite decreased appetite	Hoarse voice
Cold intolerance/cold peripheries	Dry skin and hair
Cognitive impairment	Loss of hair in outer third eyebrows
Depression	Myxoedema – soft tissue swelling typically peri-orbitally and on the dorsum of the hands
Constipation	Carpal tunnel syndrome
Oligomenorrhoea or amenorrhoea	Goitre/thyroidectomy scar
	Bradycardia
	Slow relaxing reflexes
	Ataxia
	Proximal myopathy
	Heart failure

Table 3.69: History and examination findings in hypothyroidism

Investigations

Blood tests:

- FBC: may show anaemia. Typically, macrocytic or normocytic patterns
- TFTs: confirm the diagnosis of primary hypothyroidism by revealing a low T4/T3 level with a raised TSH level
- Anti-thyroid antibodies (thyroglobulin or thyroid peroxidise): are strongly positive in Hashimoto's thyroiditis
- Lipid profile: raised cholesterol + triglycerides

Imaging:

- Chest X-ray: to identify any pericardial or pleural effusions
- USS: if asymmetric goitre

Others:

- ECG: sinus bradycardia with low voltage QRS complexes
- A biopsy may reveal lymphocytic infiltration, which is a typical feature

Management

Primary disease is managed with levothyroxine:

- Titrated to normalise TSH.
- Take care in patients with ischaemic heart disease and the elderly. Start with a low dose and titrate slowly.
- T4 has a long half-life (one week) so full clinical response and changes in TSH levels may take up to six weeks.

Subclinical' hypothyroidism (normal T4 but TSH <10 mU/l) does not need pharmacological treatment, but TFTs should be monitored every 6 months.

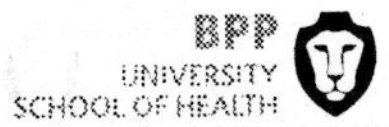

If secondary hypothyroidism is suspected:

- Important not to start levothyroxine
- Hypopituitary disease must be excluded as if there is a reduced reserve of ACTH, treatment with thyroxine replacement alone may cause an acute Addisonian crisis

Prognosis

Life expectancy is normal unless there is the presence of accelerated ischaemic heart disease.

Myxoedema coma

Epidemiology

This is a rare medical emergency, mostly affecting elderly individuals. 90% of patients are female.

Aetiology

It is precipitated by exposure to cold weather, infections, sedative treatment and anything which impairs the respiratory system. It can occur in patients which known hypothyroidism or as a new diagnosis.

History/examination

The principal presenting signs are hypothermia, features of hypothyroidism and reduced level of consciousness. Despite the name, coma is not seen in everyone. Seizures can occur. Other features include hypotension, hypoventilation, bradycardia, hypoglycaemia and hyponatremia.

Management

- Thyroxine replacement is required, IV levothyroxine is the first choice.
- IV hydrocortisone should be administered as the adrenal glands are thought to function poorly in severe hypothyroidism.
- General supportive measures including IV fluids, slow re-warming, treatment of underlying infection and correction of electrolyte disturbances and hypoglycaemia.

Prognosis

Associated with a poor prognosis especially in elderly individuals. The mortality rate is between 20% and 50%.

Acromegaly

Acromegaly is a chronic, progressive disease caused by excessive secretion of growth hormone (GH), usually from a pituitary adenoma.

Epidemiology

The prevalence is around 1:140,000–250,000 individuals. Males and females tend to be affected equally with an even distribution amongst all ethnic groups. Mostly diagnosed in individuals aged between 40 and 50 years, although the clinical features are often evident from the mid 20s.

Aetiology

Results from a growth hormone-producing pituitary tumour in the majority of cases (>98%). This may be seen as part of the MEN-1 syndrome. Excess growth hormone releasing hormone (GHRH) and ectopic production of GH are very rare causes.

Pathophysiology

The chronic excessive circulating GH on the peripheral tissues via the stimulation of insulin-like growth factor 1 (IGF-1) production cause the clinical features.

History/examination

History:

- Often an insidious onset and symptoms precede diagnosis by years
- Change in facial appearance – ask if there are any old photos to compare
- Changes in size of hands/feet – changes in glove or shoe size. Or rings no longer fit
- Increase in hat size (if known)
- Headache and visual disturbances (presenting feature in 25% of patients); bitemporal hemianopia
- Carpal tunnel syndrome
- Oligomenorrhea and galactorrhoea in females
- Reduced libido/impotence in males
- Deepening voice
- Breathlessness and peripheral oedema indicative of heart failure
- Arthropathy
- Excessive sweating
- Past history of diabetes/impaired glucose tolerance, hypertension and obstructive sleep apnoea. Ask specifically about colonic polyps or cancer

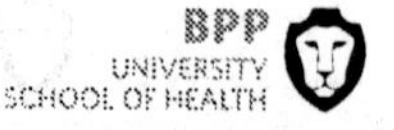

Examination:

- Hands: large and moist from sweating (only in active disease). Classically described as 'spade-like' with a 'doughy' feel to the handshake
- Axillae: skin tags and acanthosis nigricans
- Face: prominent supraorbital ridges, enlarged nose, lips and tongue (macroglossia). Thickened greasy skin
- Mouth: interdental separation and prognathism (protruded lower jaw) with malocclusion
- Eyes: test visual fields
- Neck: palpate for goitre
- Chest: gynaecomastia and galactorrhoea. Check for displaced apex beat +/- signs of heart failure

Investigations

Blood tests:

- GH release occurs as 'pulses' with low levels between pulses. Hence measurement is not always a useful test; however, if levels are persistently low the diagnosis of acromegaly is very unlikely
- Insulin-like growth factor 1 (IGF-1) levels: will be raised
- OGTT: considered the best diagnostic test. An OGTT should suppress GH; however, in acromegaly will typically fail to suppress
- Other tests of pituitary function: prolactin, TFT, cortisol and LH/FSH

Imaging:

- MRI: of the pituitary gland is very sensitive for revealing the pituitary adenoma
- Chest X-ray or CT chest and abdomen: may be required in the rare cases of ectopic GH production to locate the source
- Total body scintigraphy with radiolabelled somatostatin – localises tumour

Other:

- ECG
- Formal visual field perimetry
- Colorectal cancer screening including regular colonoscopy starting at 40 years old. The frequency of checks depends on the colonoscopy findings and disease severity

Management

Treatment should be considered in all individuals diagnosed with acromegaly due to the increased mortality and morbidity seen with the disease. The disease is best managed in specialist centres with close collaboration between an endocrinologist, a pituitary surgeon and possibly a radiotherapist. Response to therapy is measured by assessing the growth hormone levels as well as serial IGF-1 measurements.

Surgical management:

- First-line treatment is trans-sphenoidal surgery
- Results in clinical remission in around 90% of patients with micro-adenoma; however, only around 50% with a macro-adenoma
- Pituitary tissue is preserved as much as is possible
- Complications include infection (meningitis 2%), diabetes insipidus (2%), cerebrospinal fluid rhinorrhoea (2%) and hypopituitarism (10%)

Medical management:

- Octreotide/Lanreotide/Pasreotide:
  - Synthetic analogues of somatostatin
  - First-line medical therapy, used if surgery unsuccessful or not possible
  - Significantly reduces the level of GH and IGF-1, with a response in around 60% of patients
  - Side effects: increased frequency of gallstones, nausea, abdominal discomfort and loose stools
- Dopamine agonists:
  - Used if surgery unsuccessful or impossible
  - Also have a use in tumour reduction prior to therapy such as surgery
  - Achieves biochemical cure in relatively few patients (around 30%)
  - Cabergoline or bromocriptine are the most commonly used. Risk of cardiac fibrosis so echo is required beforehand
- Pegvisomant:
  - A highly selective GH receptor antagonist. Normalises IGF-1 in 90–100% of patients but GH levels increased during treatment and no decrease in tumour size is seen

Radiotherapy:

- Usually used following unsuccessful pituitary surgery and medical therapy
- Can also be used in conjunction with Octreotide or a dopamine agonist as the biochemical response to radiotherapy is very slow and may take up to ten years or even more
- Drawbacks are the length of time to achieve biochemical remission and the side effect of hypopituitarism

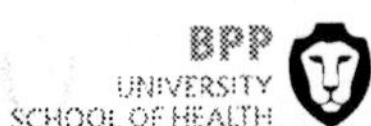

Prognosis

If left untreated, acromegaly leads to much reduced life expectancy with the majority of deaths occurring from heart failure, coronary artery disease, and secondary to hypertension.

Aggressive management of both the primary adenoma and its sequela such as hypertension, sleep apnoea and diabetes is improving both morbidity and mortality.

Electrolyte disturbances

Hypernatraemia

Defined as serum sodium > 145 mmol/L.

Epidemiology

Precise incidence unknown.

Aetiology

Almost always due to water loss or impaired ability to drink. Common causes in the hospital include infection, persistent vomiting, reduced oral intake in the unwell elderly patient and HHS. Rarer causes are diabetes insipidus and Mineralocorticoid excess eg in Conn's syndrome.

Pathophysiology

This depends on the aetiology.

History/examination

- Any symptoms of infection
- Vomiting/diarrhoea
- Past history of diabetes
- Mobility (in the elderly)
- Assessment of hydration status shows:
  - Hypotension (or postural hypotension)
  - Skin turgor
  - Dry mucous membranes

Investigations

Blood tests:

- FBC
- U&Es
- Inflammatory markers: CRP
- Glucose

Management

Rehydration: The oral route is preferable and the aim should be to reduce the concentration by a rate of no more than 0.5 mmol/L per hour.

Prognosis

A full recovery is usual with careful fluid balance monitoring.

Hyponatraemia

Serum sodium (Na) of <135 mmol/L.

Epidemiology

Precise incidence unknown, but thought to occur in up to 15% of inpatients.

Aetiology

Hyponatraemia may be divided into three forms.

Pathophysiology

The serum and total body sodium levels are inextricably linked to water balance and hyponatraemia can be caused by a relative lack of sodium or excess of water. The average 70 kg man has 42 L water (60% of body weight), made up in the following compartments:

- 28 L intracellular fluid
- 4 L extracellular fluid (of which 10.5 L is interstitial fluid and 3.5 L is intravascular fluid)

Usual Osmolality:
2 x [Na+ + K+] + urea + Glucose = 280mOsm/kg

Water balance is controlled by ADH which increases water resorption by stimulating the insertion of aquaporins, ie water channels, in the distal nephron and collecting duct. This is regulated by hypothalamic osmoreceptors and atrial baroreceptors. Sodium balance is controlled by the actions of ANP (reduces Na reabsorption) and aldosterone (increases Na reabsorption) on the kidneys.

SIADH is seen only in euvolaemic states when diuretic use, Addison's disease and hypothyroidism

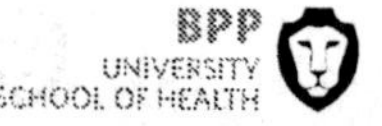

Type	Diseases
Hyper-osmolar	Hyperglycaemia
Iso-osmolar	Pseudohyponatraemia (serum lipaemia or excess immunoglobins). Beware the sample taken from a 'drip arm' may also be pseudohyponatraemic
Hypo-osmolar	**Hypervolaemic** • Renal failure • CCF • Cirrhosis • Nephrotic syndrome **Euvolaemic** • Syndrome of inappropriate ADH secretion (SIADH) • Hypothyroidism • Psychogenic polydipsia **Hypovolaemic** • Diarrhoea (also high output stoma) • Vomiting • Sweating • Burns • Trauma • Diuretics • Salt-losing nephropathy • Addison's Disease

Table 3.70: Three forms of hyponatraemia

have been excluded. Tests will reveal hyponatraemia with a plasma osmolality < 270 mOsm/kg but an inappropriately concentrated urine with urine sodium > 20 mmol/L and urine osmolality > 300 mOsm/kg.

Causes of SIADH include:

- Chest infection
- Malignancy: pancreas, gastric, lung
- Intracranial pathology, classically subdural haematoma but also meningitis, abscess and MS as well as post-neurosurgical intervention
- Drugs eg SSRI antidepressants

History/examination

- Ultimately, depends on underlying aetiology
- Acute hyponatraemia:
  - Acute history of headache
  - Vomiting
  - Confusion
  - Seizures
  - Coma
- Chronic hyponatraemia:
  - Insidious history of anorexia
  - Headache
  - Muscle cramps
  - Deteriorating cognitive function
- Assessment of fluid volume status may show fluid overload or fluid deficiency:
  - Fluid overload: raised JVP, dependent oedema and signs of pulmonary oedema
  - Fluid deficiency, dry mucous membranes, delayed capillary refill and postural or absolute hypotension

Further examination will be directed to help establish the underlying cause.

Investigations

Blood tests:

- FBC: get baseline values
- LFTs: get baseline values
- Bone profile: get baseline values
- Glucose: get baseline values
- TFTs: get baseline values
- Plasma osmolality: get baseline values
- U&Es

Imaging:

- CXR
- CT brain: if subdural haemorrhage is suspected as a cause of SIADH

Others:

- Echocardiography
- Urinalysis: urine osmolality and sodium concentration
- ECG: if there is congestive cardiac failure
- Other tests will be governed by the clinical scenario and probable underlying cause

Management

- Establish underlying cause and direct treatment accordingly.
- In the elderly there may be a number of contributory causes.
- In chronic hyponatraemia beware of correcting serum sodium too quickly as there is a risk of central pontine myelinolysis: aim for an increase of no more than 0.5 mmol/L/hour.

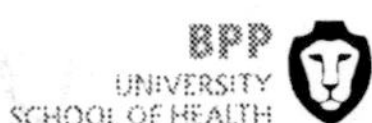

- Frequent monitoring of sodium levels and an accurate fluid-balance record should be maintained.
- Any contributory drugs (especially diuretics or Citalopram) should be stopped or changed.

Acutely unwell and significantly symptomatic:

- A to E assessment and resuscitation
- IV NaCl. May require hypertonic saline with caution
- Add IV Furosemide, especially if at risk of fluid overload

Hypervolaemic hyponatraemia:

- Water restriction
- Diuretic use

Hypovolaemic hyponatraemia:

- IV normal saline

Euvolaemic hyponatraemia:

- Addison's: steroids
- Hypothyroidism: levothyroxine
- Psychogenic polydipsia: fluid restriction

SIADH:

- Fluid restriction
- If this does not work: Demeclocycline

Prognosis

A full recovery is usual if the underlying cause can be found and treated.

Hyperkalaemia

Defined as serum potassium >5.5 mmol/L with severe serum potassium >6.5 mmol/L.

Epidemiology

Precise incidence unknown.

Aetiology

The major causes of hyperkalaemia are:

- Renal failure
- Drugs: Angiotensin converting enzyme inhibitors, potassium sparing diuretics
- Significant tissue breakdown eg rhabdomyolysis, tumour lysis, burns
- Metabolic acidosis, causing a movement from the intracellular to the extracellular space
- Addison's disease

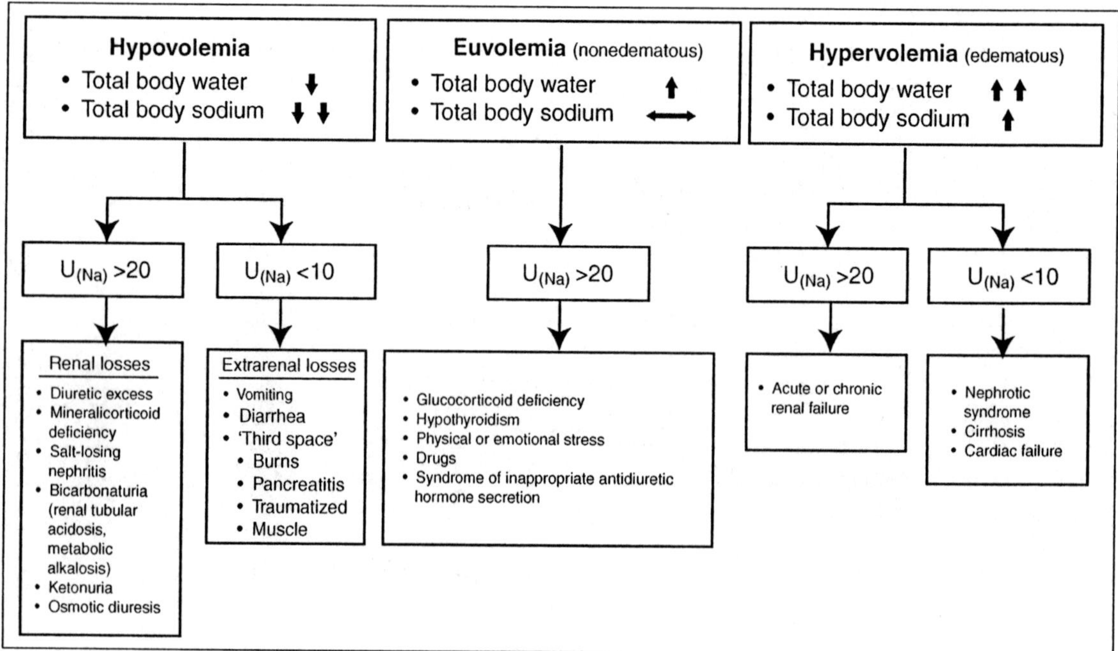

Figure 3.30: A diagnostic algorithm for the causes of hyponatraemia

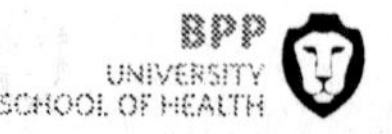

- Iatrogenic potassium overload
- Pseudohyperkalaemia: haemolysis of the blood sample

Pathophysiology

Potassium is one of the major cations in the body which is approximately 98% intracellular. The body's levels are predominantly regulated by the balance between GI absorption and renal excretion. Hyperkalaemia is a classic cause of cardiac arrhythmias.

History/examination

- Often asymptomatic, ie an incidental finding
- Symptoms often vague: fatigue, lethargy and generalised weakness
- Palpitations
- Trauma
- Drug history
- Risk factors for renal impairment eg history of hypertension and diabetes
- May be unremarkable
- Irregular pulse caused by ectopic beats

Investigations

Blood tests:

- U&Es: potassium level and evidence of renal impairment
- ABG: acid-base status
- Digoxin levels if taking Digoxin (hyperkalaemia increases Digoxin toxicity)

Others:

- ECG: shows changes that are progressive with increasing serum potassium, ie heart blocks, flattening of P waves, tenting of T waves, widening of QRS, ventricular tachycardia.

Management

Based on Resuscitation Council (UK) guidelines. It depends on degree of hyperkalaemia and hence the potassium levels should be carefully monitored. Patient with a mild to moderate hyperkalaemia should be on a cardiac monitor until the hyperkalaemia is resolved.

Mild (5.5–6.0 mmol/L):

- Stop drugs predisposing to hyperkalaemia
- Ensure adequate hydration
- Consider calcium resonium
- Consider furosemide

Moderate (6.0–6.5 mmol/L):

- Insulin/dextrose: typically 15 units actrapid in 50 ml 50% glucose over 15 minutes

Severe (>6.5 mmol/L):

- Calcium chloride 10 ml 10% IV
- Salbutamol nebuliser
- Consider sodium bicarbonate
- Consider haemodialysis

In cardiac arrest:

- Calcium chloride 10 ml 10% IV
- Sodium bicarbonate 50 ml 8.4% IV
- Insulin/dextrose. Typically 15 units actrapid in 50 ml 50% glucose

Prognosis

The higher the potassium level, the greater the risk of VT and cardiac arrest; however, with prompt and effective treatment a full recovery should be expected.

Hypokalaemia

Defined as serum potassium < 3.5 mmol/L. However, moderate serum potassium levels are 2.5 to 3.0 mmol/L while severe serum potassium levels are less than 2.5 mmol/L.

Epidemiology

Precise incidence unknown.

Aetiology

Commonly due to urinary or GI loss of potassium. Clinical symptoms rarely occur unless serum potassium is less than 3.0 mmol/L. The main causes are:

- Decreased potassium intake
- Increased potassium entry into cells
- Increased potassium excretion
- Dialysis/plasmapheresis

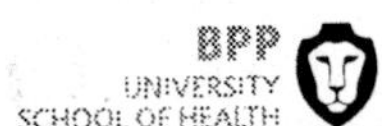

Pathophysiology

Mechanism	Features
Decreased potassium intake	• Rare • Associated with very restricted diets • Anorexia nervosa • Increased potassium entry into cells eg alkalosis, catecholamine signaling, salbutamol, insulin • Hypokalaemic periodic paralysis • Increases in blood cell production (eg after administration of folic acid or B12 in megaloblastic anaemia or granulocyte-macrophage colony-stimulating factor in neutropenia)
Increased loss from GI tract	• Vomiting • Diarrhoea • Ileus • Villous adenoma
Increased loss in urine	• Diuretics • Mineralocorticoid excess • Salt-wasting nephropathies eg Bartter's or Gitelman's syndromes, tubulo-interstitial disease, hypomagnesaemia, metabolic acidosis or polyuria
Increased loss through sweating	• Hot climate • Cystic fibrosis • Burns
Chronic alcoholism	

Table 3.71: Pathophysiology of hypokalaemia

History/examination

- Usually asymptomatic
- Presence of a likely cause – vomiting, diarrhoea, alcoholism
- Drug history, especially diuretic use
- Muscle weakness can sometimes be a feature of acute hypokalaemia
- With decreasing potassium, fatigue and cramps are a feature
- Most likely unremarkable

Investigations

Blood tests:

- U&Es
- TSH: hyperthyroidism is associated with hypokalaemic periodic paralysis
- ABG: in particular to measure the pH

Others:

- Urine potassium
- ECG: classical changes are ST depression, T wave flattening and U waves. AF or other arrhythmias may be seen

Management

- Potassium replacement. Bearing in mind that since most of the body's potassium is intracellular, a reduction in serum potassium may reflect a significant total body deficit.
  - Mild/moderate hypokalaemia: oral tablets (each contains around 12 mmol potassium).
  - Moderate/severe hypokalaemia: IV replacement at around 10 mmol/hour, or 20 mmol/hour via a central line with close cardiac monitoring.
  - Cardiac arrest or peri-arrest: The Resuscitation Council's guidelines are 20 mmol/min over 10 minutes followed by a further 10 mmol over the next 10 minutes.

Case Study: Making the best of things...

Emily Brown was nearing 30. She had a high powered job in the city and had steadily been working her way up the career ladder for the last decade – a feat all the more remarkable because she had also been battling bulimia throughout those years. It had all started when she was 18, overwhelmed, not so much by the academic pressures, but the aesthetic demands placed on a young woman by modern society. Gradually, anorexia progressed to bulimia, and as the number of business lunches increased, Emily sought ever more extreme methods to keep her ultra-slim figure – and, so she imagined, her job. The first time she went to see the GP, Emily weighed 8 stone, was regularly taking handfuls of laxatives and was barely managing to get through the day because she felt so tired and unwell. Her potassium level was 2.1, but her ECG was normal. The GP started some oral replacement and tried to address the underlying cause of Emily's eating disorder. However, nothing worked and the GP decided to settle for trying to keep her safe, continuing the oral potassium and performing regular potassium checks and ECGs and gradually Emily began to feel a little bit better and gradually was able to use some psychological support to battle her way through her tunnel of darkness.

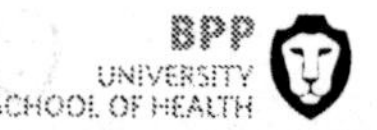

- During replacement regular monitoring of potassium levels are necessary.
- Stop any causative drugs.
- Replacement of magnesium if also low.

Prognosis

Prompt and effective treatment is essential as hypokalaemia may progress to cause cardiac arrest.

Hypercalcaemia

Defined as calcium more than 2.6 mmol/L.

Epidemiology

It is a common, often incidental finding. 5% of hospitalised patients have hypercalcaemia.

Aetiology

Most cases are due to hyperparathyroidism (usually primary but can be due to secondary and tertiary) and malignancy. Most common malignancies are breast, lung, prostate, ovary, kidney and myeloma. Parathyroid hormone related peptide, osteolysis, vitamin D dependent (lymphoma) and ectopic PTH release are all involved in malignancies leading to hypercalcaemia. Other causes (10% of hypercalcaemia cases):

- Sarcoidosis
- Tuberculosis
- Drugs: thiazide diuretics, calcium/vitamin D, lithium
- Endocrine: thyrotoxicosis, acromegaly
- Prolonged immobilisation
- Rhabdomyolysis (calcium low in the acute phase)
- Familial hypocalciuric hypercalcaemia

Pathophysiology

Depends on the aetiology.

History/examination

- Asymptomatic (50%)
- Symptoms usually imply severe hypercalcaemia (>3.5 mmol/L)
- The classical symptoms:
  - 'Bones': bone pain/fractures
  - 'Groans': nausea/vomiting, constipation
  - 'Stones' (renal): polyuria/polydipsia; loin pain
  - 'Psychic moans' (psychiatric): depression/confusion
- Past or family history of cancer
- Cough, smoking history
- None (if mild)
- Dehydration
- Look for signs of underlying malignancy eg clubbing secondary to lung carcinoma, breast lump
- Erythema nodosum (sarcoid or TB)
- Reduced level of consciousness
- Seizures

Investigations

Blood tests:

- FBC
- U&Es: look for evidence of dehydration and renal impairment
- LFTs
- Glucose
- Mg2+
- Inflammatory markers
- Bone profile
- PTH
- Consider myeloma screen (paired serum and urine protein electrophoresis for Bence-Jones protein) and PSA

Imaging:

- CXR
- AXR: may show renal stones
- Plain X-ray of any areas of bony pain
- Consider bone scan

Others:

- ECG: may show bradycardia and atrio-ventricular (AV) block

Management

- IV fluid rehydration
- Furosemide will help calcium excretion but only once fully rehydrated
- Stop any calcium tablets and thiazide diuretics
- May need IV bisphosphonate (Pamidronate 60–90 mg) especially if refractory and painful
- After IV bisphosphonate it takes at least 72 hours before the calcium levels fall and the effects last around three weeks. Beware re-treating too early as inevitably hypocalcaemia will be the consequence)
- Haemodialysis as a last resort

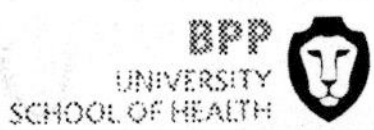

- Monitor calcium levels and ensure decreasing
- Treat the underlying cause (eg parathyroidectomy, steroids for sarcoidosis)

Prognosis

Very dependent on cause, but in the case of malignancy with bony metastases it will be poor.

Hypocalcaemia

Defined as calcium less than 2.1 mmol/L.

Epidemiology

Precise incidence unknown. It is present in 88% of critically ill patients admitted to ICUs.

Aetiology

Decreased levels of calcium in circulation can be due to:

- Vitamin D deficiency
- Chronic renal failure
- Hypoparathyroidism: iatrogenic, HIV-related, pseudohypoparathyroidism, idiopathic, autoimmune

Increased loss of circulating calcium can be due to:

- Rhabdomyolysis
- Acute pancreatitis

Drugs can also induce hypocalcaemia. Critical illnesses such as sepsis, burns and having multiple transfusions are known to cause hypocalcaemia as well as hypomagnesaemia.

Pathophysiology

Calcium levels are primarily controlled by PTH and Vitamin D. PTH is released from the parathyroid gland in response to low calcium and causes increased resorption from bone and increased 1-a hydroxylation of vitamin D. 1,25(OH)2-Vitamin D increases calcium resorption from the intestine and kidney.

Hypocalcaemia is mainly secondary to imbalance in calcium absorption, excretion and distribution.

History/examination

- Lack of access to sunlight eg elderly people staying indoors, religious dress
- Medical history: thyroid/parathyroid surgery
- Paraesthesia: classically peri-oral but also fingertips and toes
- A range of behavioural changes and neuropsychiatric symptoms may be reported: cognitive impairment, depression, lethargy, irritability, anxiety and parkinsonism
- Non-specific symptoms of fatigue and muscle weakness
- Abdominal pain: if pancreatitis suspected
- Chronic hypocalcaemia may be asymptomatic
- Trousseau's sign: carpal spasm in response to ischaemia secondary to vascular occlusion with a BP cuff for three minutes
- Chvostek's sign: tapping over cranial nerve VII by the ear gives brief contraction/twitching of ipislateral peri-oral muscle resulting in contraction of a corner of the mouth
- Carpo-pedal spasm

Features of chronic hypocalcaemia:

- Cataracts
- Extra-pyramidal symptoms eg parkinsonism
- Skin and hair changes:
  - Dermatitis
  - Eczema
  - Hyperpigmentation
  - Psoriasis
  - Brittle hair with patchy alopecia
  - Brittle nails with transverse groove
  - Dementia may be present in which case a Mini Mental Status Examination must be performed

Investigations

Blood tests:

- U&Es
- Bone profile
- LFTs: albumin level
- Mg^{2+}
- More advanced tests such as PTH and Vitamin D levels if required

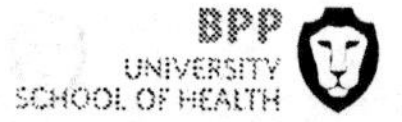

Others:

- ECG: may show prolonged QT interval, T wave inversion, heart block
- USS: of the kidneys is necessary if CRF is found

Management

- Calcium gluconate (or chloride) 10 ml of 10% IV over 10 to 20 minutes. Repeated if necessary
- Treat any concurrent hypomagnesaemia
- Oral calcium and vitamin D supplements

Prognosis

- Good prognosis if treated promptly
- Must be treated as it can result in cardiac arrest

Hypomagnesaemia

Defined as serum magnesium <0.6 mmol/L.

Epidemiology

Incidence is unknown.

Aetiology

The control of magnesium homeostasis is the balance between gastrointestinal absorption and renal excretion. Unlike other ions there is no direct hormonal control over this, although PTH does increase GI absorption. Causes of hypomagnesaemia include:

- Malnutrition
- Alcohol dependence
- Refeeding syndrome
- Diarrhoea and vomiting (including high output stomas)
- Chronic diuretic use
- Bartter syndrome
- TPN
- Acute pancreatitis

Pathophysiology

The pathophysiology is dependent on the aetiology.

History/examination

- Weakness
- Tremor
- Seizures
- Paraesthesia
- Nystagmus
- Tetany

Investigations

Blood tests:

- Mg2+
- U&Es: hypomagnesaemia has many shared causes with hypokalaemia
- Calcium: hypomagnesaemia impairs PTH secretion causing hypocalcaemia

Others:

- ECG: may show T wave changes, U waves and prolonged QT interval, ventricular ectopics, and Torsades de pointes

Management

Magnesium replacement – orally if asymptomatic or IV if severe/symptomatic

- Replacement of potassium and calcium if necessary

Prognosis

Good if detected and treated.

Further reading and references

1. Addison's Disease Self-Help Group, www.addisons.org.uk.
2. Drivers Medical Group. (2009) *For Medical Practitioners: At a glance guide to the current medical standards of fitness to drive.* Swansea, DVLA.
3. Resuscitation Council (UK). (2008) *Advanced Life Support.* 5th Edition. London, Resuscitation Council.

Palpitations

Differential diagnosis

Type	Diseases
Arrhythmias	Tachycardias Long QT syndrome Bradycardias Atrial fibrillation (AF) Extrasystoles

Table 3.72: Differential diagnosis of palpitations

Palpitations are an abnormal awareness of the heartbeat. It is a very common presentation in all medical settings.

Tachycardia

Tachycardia is defined as a rate greater than 100 bpm. There are two main categories:

- Supraventricular/narrow complex (where the focus of rhythm is generated at or above the atrioventricular (AV) node)
- Ventricular/broad complex (focus is below AV node)

Narrow complex arrhythmias (QRS duration less than 120 ms/3 small squares):

- Sinus tachycardia
- AF with fast ventricular response
- Atrial flutter
- Atrial tachycardia
- AVNRT
- AVRT

Ventricular tachycardias (QRS duration more than 120 ms/3 small squares):

- Monomorphic
- Polymorphic (eg Torsades de Pointes)

Epidemiology

Tachycardias are very common, especially sinus tachycardia and AF.

Aetiology and pathophysiology

There are many causes of tachycardia dependent on the specific type of tachycardia:

Sinus tachycardia:

A physiological response to a stressor. This is managed by treating the underlying cause eg:

- Hypovolaemia
- Drugs eg caffeine, alcohol, amphetamines
- Endocrine abnormalities eg hypoglycaemia, hyperthyroidism, phaeochromocytoma
- Anxiety and panic disorder
- Anaemia
- Sepsis
- Pregnancy
- After exercise

Atrial tachycardia:

- An abnormal pattern of electrical activity that originates in the atria but not the SA node
- Can be sustained
- Usually seen in structural heart disease
- Can be focal or a re-entrant circuit
- Sometimes multifocal, giving P waves of differing morphology
- Management involves breaking the abnormal circuit and/or ablating the initiating focus

Atrial flutter:

- A macro re-entrant circuit in the atria, usually around the tricuspid valve, generating a very fast atrial response (typically 300 bpm).
- The AV node filters this, classically giving a 2:1 block and a ventricular response of 150 bpm.
- ECG shows a 'saw-tooth' baseline, best seen in leads II, III, aVF and V1.
- 60% are precipitated by an acute intercurrent illness eg sepsis.

AVNRT:

- The most common form of SVT.
- The AV node has two conduction pathways; a fast and a slow conducting. The fast usually dominates and has a longer refractory period.

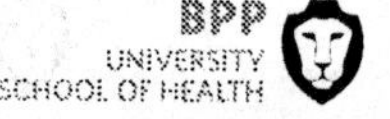

- If a premature beat hits the AV node when the slow pathway is active but the fast pathway is still refractory, the slow pathway conducts the impulse to the ventricles but in addition the impulse is turned around within the AV node and is conducted back to the atria by the fast pathway (which is no longer refractory), initiating the SVT. This results in a retrograde P wave that may be visible on an ECG.

AVRT:

- An accessory pathway outside of the AV node is capable of conduction between the atria and ventricles.
- Orthodromic: the impulse travels via the AV node then back to the atria via the accessory pathway.
- Antidromic: the initial conduction from the atria to the ventricles is via the accessory pathway, resulting in a broad QRS complex.

Wolff-Parkinson-White (WPW):

- Conduction from the atria to the ventricles via an accessory pathway generates a degree of ventricular pre-excitation.
- This is seen on the ECG as a shortened PR interval and a delta wave.
- Increased risk in AF: The usual filter to the ventricular response, the AV node, is bypassed by the accessory pathway giving a very rapid (250–300 bpm) 'pre-excited' AF.
- At high risk of degenerating into ventricular fibrillation (VF).

Ventricular tachycardia:

- Always a very worrying sign!
- Always get senior help.
- High risk of degenerating into pulseless VT.

Polymorphic VT:

- Torsades de Pointes is usually non-sustained but risks degenerating into VF
- There is a characteristic ECG where the QRS complexes appear to twist around the axis
- Associated with a long QT interval
- Other associations are with hypomagnesaemia and hypokalaemia, hence frequently seen in alcoholics

History/examination

- Onset and progression:
  - When and how often do palpitations occur?
  - How long do they last?
  - Do they occur occasionally or as sustained episodes?
- Are they fast or slow?
- Regular or irregular? It is often helpful to ask the patient to tap out the rhythm of the palpitations.
- Any associated symptoms – chest pain, dizziness or shortness of breath, collapse or loss of consciousness?
- Personal/family history of abnormal heart rhythms, pacemakers, sudden deaths or any endocrine/metabolic abnormalities eg thyroid disease
- Drug history: prescribed, non-prescribed, illicit drug use, alcohol and caffeine intake
- Assess tachycardic patients using the standard A to E approach
- Full cardiovascular examination
- Look for signs of sepsis and dehydration
- Examine the thyroid gland (and the drug chart)

Investigations

The key investigation is a 12 lead ECG. It is important to note whether the patient is experiencing palpitations or chest pain at the time the ECG is taken.

If no abnormalities are found on the 12 lead ECG, the patient may have a paroxysmal arrhythmia which may be detected on 24 hour ambulatory ECG monitoring or, if the palpitations do not occur frequently, an event monitor or implantable loop recorder.

ECG:

- 12 lead ECG
- 24 hour ambulatory ECG monitoring (24 hour tape)

Blood tests:

- FBC
- Renal function
- TFT
- Magnesium
- Glucose
- Cardiac enzymes

Others:

- Echocardiogram
- (Event monitor or implantable loop recorder)

There are three questions you need to consider when attempting to interpret the ECG of someone who presents with tachycardia:

1. Are the QRS complexes narrow or broad?
2. Are there P waves?
3. Is it regular or irregular?

Management

- The management of tachycardia is summarised in the tachycardia algorithm from the Resuscitation Council.
- Look for the adverse signs early and seek senior help immediately if they are present (or you feel you need support).
- All patients should be constantly monitored and reassessed so that any deterioration in cardiac output may be recognised early.
- If DC cardioversion is required, an anaesthetist will be needed to sedate or intubate the patient whilst this is happening.
- The precise number of joules required varies depending on the defibrillator used, so local policies should be known. The shock should be synchronised to avoid precipitating VF, but this is not unknown even with a synchronised shock.

Regular broad complex tachycardia (without compromise):

If a decision needs to be made as to whether it is VT or SVT with aberrant conduction (eg SVT with LBBB), it may be possible to see a previous ECG to help, or certain features on the ECG may imply VT (concordance, fusion and capture beats).

If in doubt it should be treated as VT and the usual management would be with amiodarone.

Irregular broad complex tachycardia (without compromise):

More complicated and it is important to get help if this is seen. Again a recent ECG will be invaluable to guide treatment.

AF with bundle branch block should be treated as pre-excited AF, caused by WPW syndrome. It is important to diagnose, as treating this with drugs that slow AV node conduction may precipitate VT/VF. The best treatments are with amiodarone, flecainide or DC cardioversion. Drugs to be avoided include Digoxin, Diltiazem, Verapamil and Adenosine.

Torsades de Pointes should be treated by stopping any medications which prolong the QT interval and correcting any electrolyte imbalances.

Regular narrow complex tachycardia:

Treated with vagal manoeuvres (blowing into a syringe is perhaps the easiest).

If unsuccessful then adenosine (6 mg, 12 mg, 12 mg – warn the patient that it will make them feel truly awful – almost as if they are about to die – but that this will pass within a few seconds).

Record a rhythm strip (using the printer on the defibrillator is usually the most convenient) whilst giving these treatments.

	Narrow or broad	P waves	Regular or irregular
Sinus tachycardia	Narrow	Yes	Regular
Atrial tachycardia	Narrow	Yes but may be abnormal morphology	Regular
Atrial fibrillation	Narrow	No	Irregularly irregular
Atrial flutter	Narrow	May see sawtooth flutter waves	Regular (75, 100 or 150 bpm depending on level of block). Can be irregular if variable block
AVNRT/AVRT	Narrow	May be seen after QRS complex due to retrograde conduction	Regular
Monomorphic VT	Broad – same amplitude	Can occasionally be seen, though no fixed relation to QRS	Regular
Polymorphic VT	Broad – varying amplitude	Can occasionally be seen, though no fixed relation to QRS	Regular

Table 3.73: ECG features of tachycardia

This has a good chance of cardioverting an SVT, and if the underlying rhythm is atrial flutter this will be unmasked and the diagnosis made.

Irregular narrow complex tachycardia:

The commonest is AF and the treatment is outlined in the AF section.

All rhythms:

Following successful treatment for the tachycardia it is important to record the 12 lead ECG. This will show any underlying arrhythmia (eg Wolff- Parkinson-White syndrome, Brugada syndrome or long Q-T syndrome) which could predispose to future tachyarrhythmia.

The patient will need referral to a cardiologist for ongoing medical management, consideration of electrophysiological studies and radiofrequency ablation to identify and break any aberrant conduction pathways. Any episodes of VT will need referral for consideration of an implantable defibrillator.

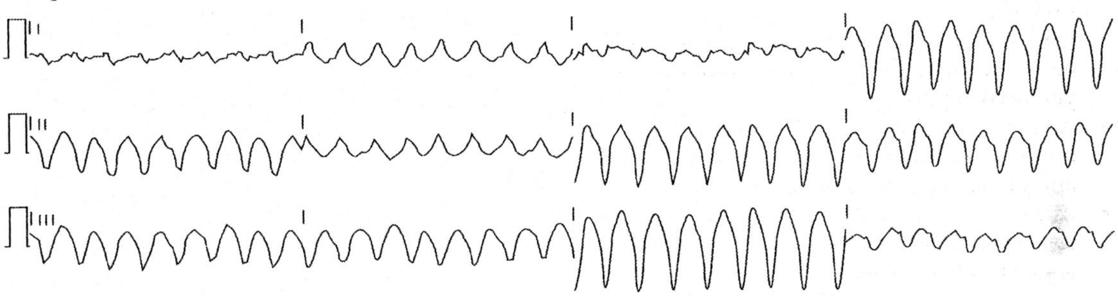

Figure 3.31: Ventricular tachycardia

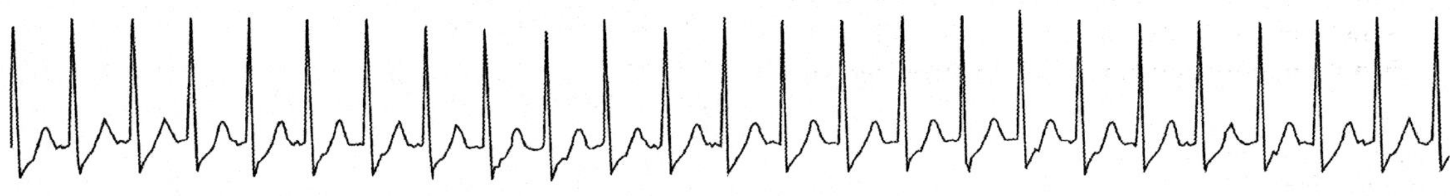

Figure 3.32: SVT in lead II

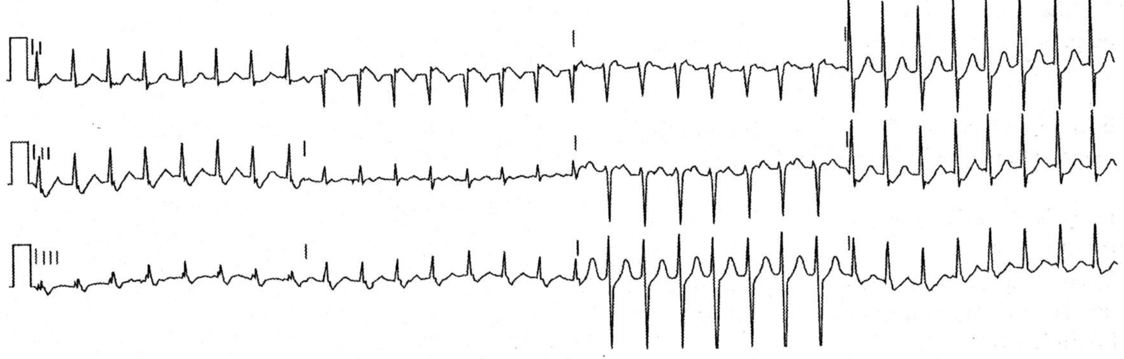

Figure 3.33: AVNRT

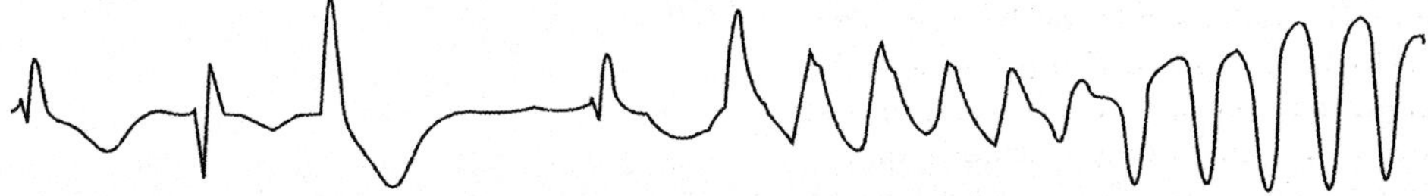

Figure 3.34: Torsades de Pointes

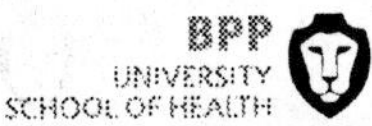

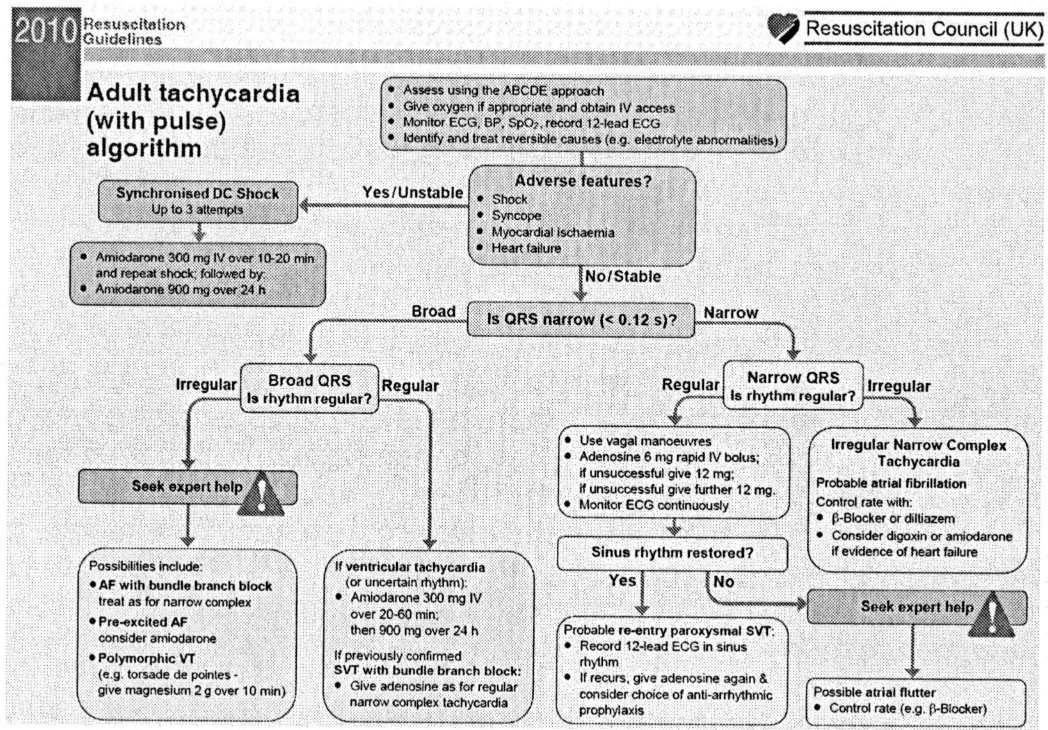

Figure 3.35: Adult tachycardia (with pulse) algorithm. (Reproduced with permission from Resuscitation Council UK)

Long QT syndrome

Epidemiology

Estimated prevalence of 20/100,000.

Aetiology

1. Congenital causes
   i) Romano-Ward syndrome (autosomal dominant)
   ii) Jervell, Lange-Nielsen syndrome (autosomal recessive, associated with deafness)
   iii) At least 12 genes associated with LQTS have been discovered so far, and hundreds of mutations within these genes have been identified. Mutations in 3 of these genes account for about 75% of long QT syndrome:
      - LQT1 – KCNQ1
      - LQT2 – HERG
      - LQT3 – SCN5A
2. Acquired causes include:
   i) Electrolyte imbalances (hypokalaemia, hypomagnesaemia and hypocalcaemia)
   ii) Drugs (Amiodarone, Sotalol, antihistamines)

Pathophysiology

LQTS causes malfunction of cardiac ion channels. This tends to prolong the duration of the ventricular action potential (APD), which extends repolarisation, thus lengthening the QT interval. This abnormal repolarisation causes differences in myocyte refractory periods, meaning some parts of the myocardium might be refractory to subsequent depolarisation while others are ready.

EADs – occurring more commonly in LQTS can be propagated to neighbouring myocytes due to differences in the refractory periods, leading to re-entrant polymorphic ventricular arrhythmias – Torsades de Pointes.

This may either revert spontaneously back to sinus rhythm causing syncope or degenerate to ventricular fibrillation causing sudden death.

EADs are caused by excessive prolongation of the action potential resulting in re-opening of certain L-type calcium channels during the plateau phase of the cardiac action potential.

In addition, sympathetic activity can increase the activity of the L-type calcium channels which increases the frequency of EADs. This provides a rationale for why the risk of sudden death in individuals with LQTS is higher during increased adrenergic states such as exercise or excitement.

History/examination

- Palpitations, syncope, seizures (sudden death) in the first three decades.
- This is secondary to cardiac dysrhythmias, in particular VT and VF. These can be provoked by an external trigger eg a loud noise but commonly occur during sleep.
- As per 'palpitations' history/examination.

Investigations

ECG:

- 12 lead ECG: A resting ECG does not always demonstrate a prolonged QT interval, making diagnosis difficult.
- 24 hour holter monitor.

On the ECG the QT interval will vary with heart rate, so the corrected QT interval must be calculated (QTc). Normally this will be automatically done by the ECG machine, but it can be calculated using the Bazett formula: QTc = QT / square root of RR interval. In adults a prolonged QTc is defined as >0.45 secs.

Blood tests:

- Genetic testing is available via specialist clinics.

Cardiac stress test:

- May unmask the LQTS.

Management

- Advice on lifestyle (avoid contact sports) and avoidance of drugs which prolong the QT interval.
- A beta-blocker can be used to shorten the QT interval.
- High risk cases can be fitted with an implantable defibrillator.

Prognosis

- Mortality can be as high as 70% over 10 years in untreated patients.

Top tip:
Quit while you can...

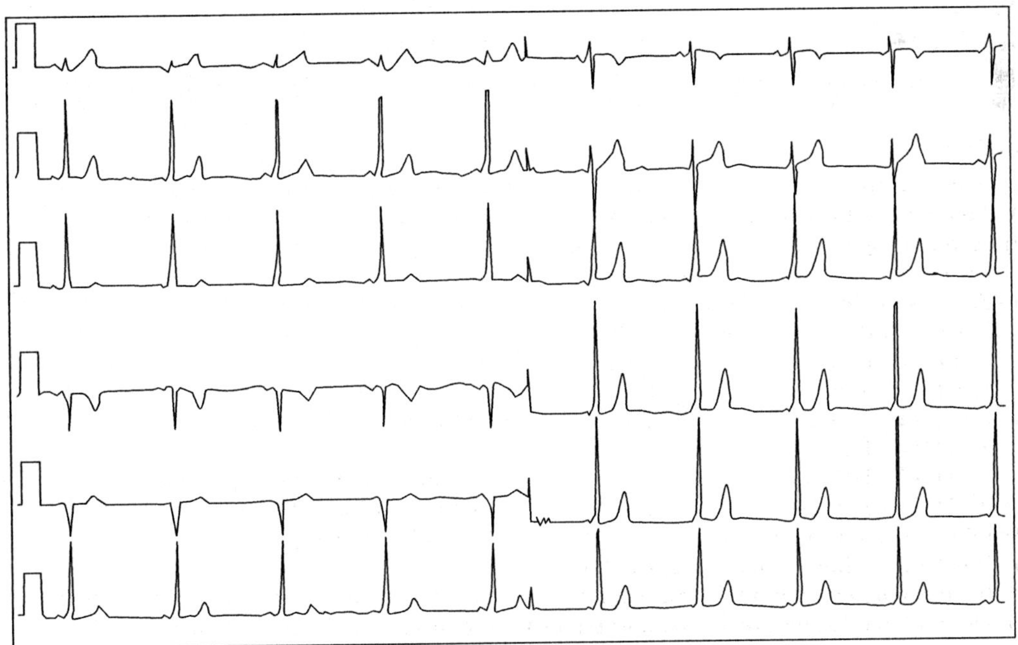

Figure 3.36: WPW

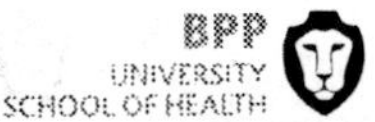

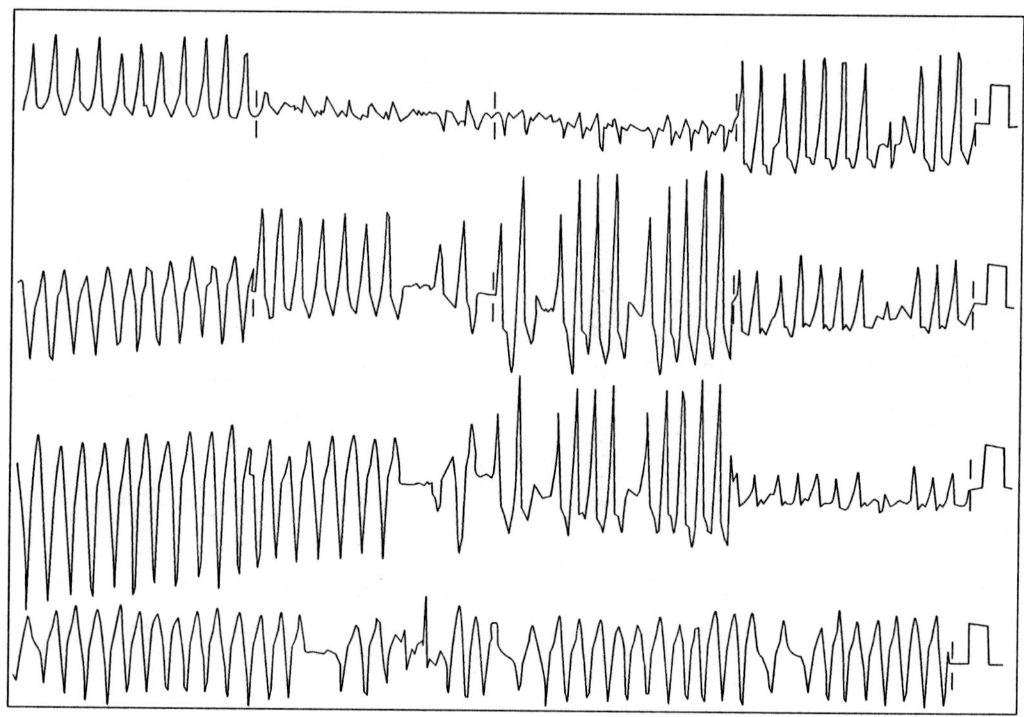

Figure 3.37: WPW with AF (pre-excited AF)

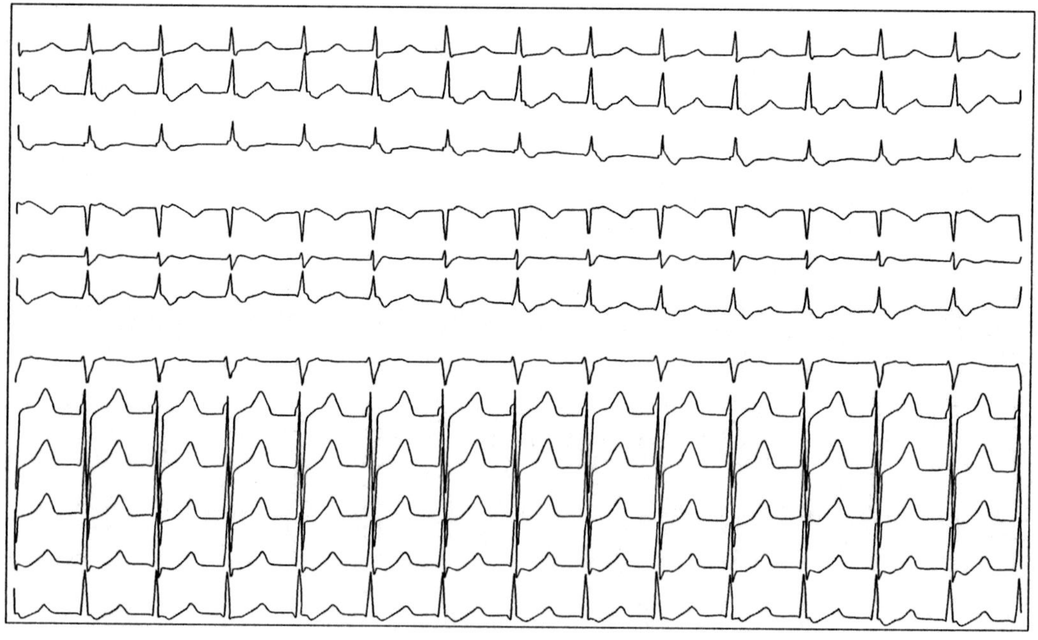

Figure 3.38: AVNRT

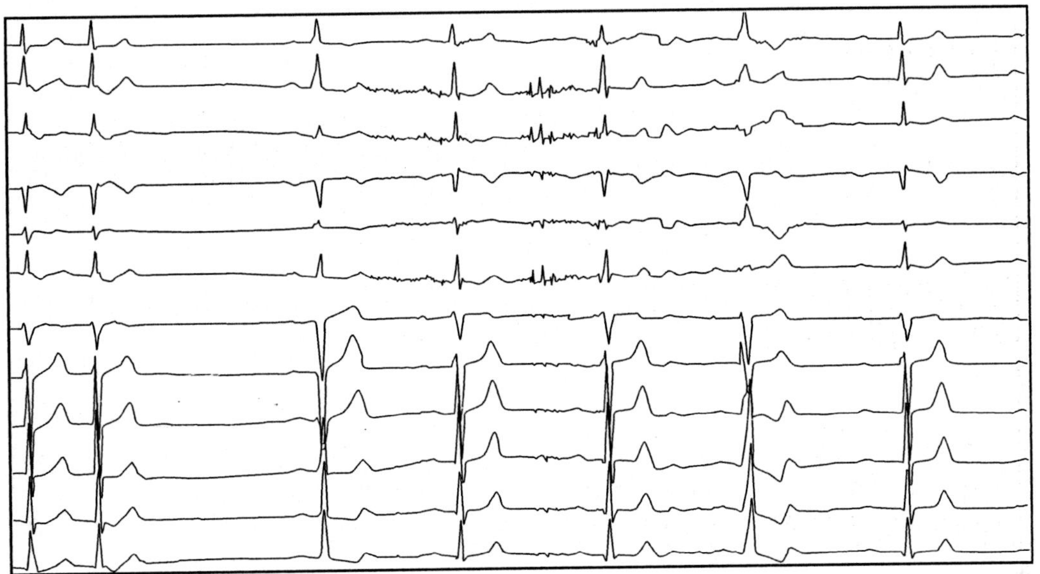

Figure 3.39: AVNRT terminating during adenosine IV push

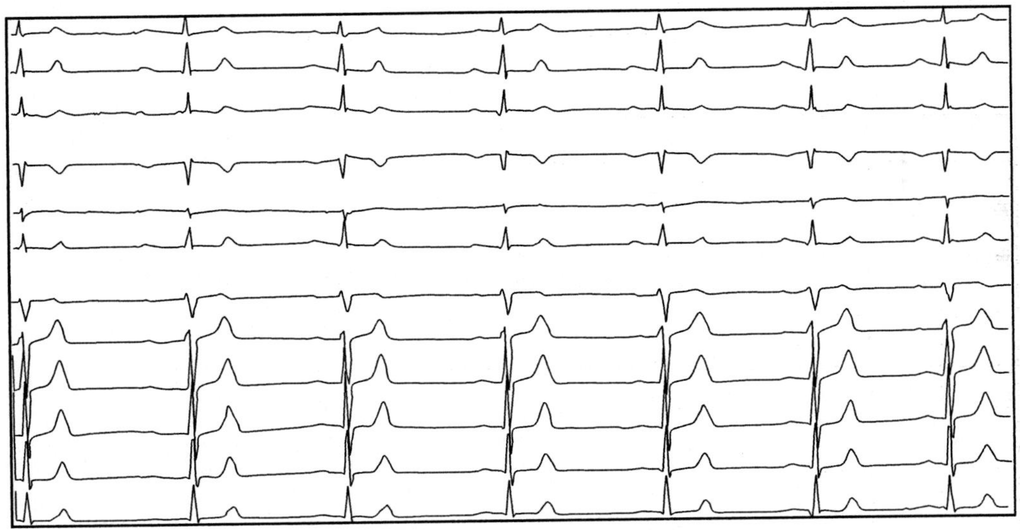

Figure 3.40: Sinus rhythm post-adenosine

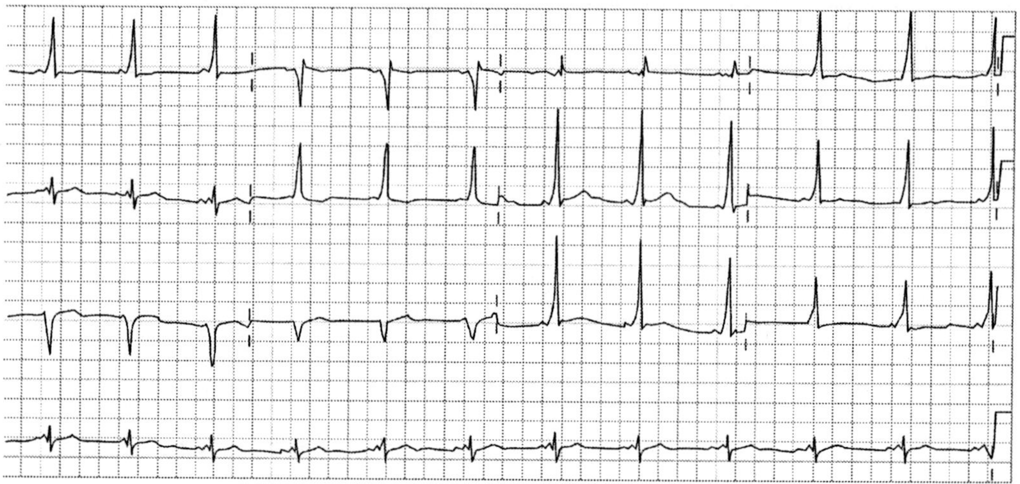

Figure 3.41: ECG of Wolff-Parkinson-White syndrome. Note the short PR interval and upsloping delta wave in the QRS complex

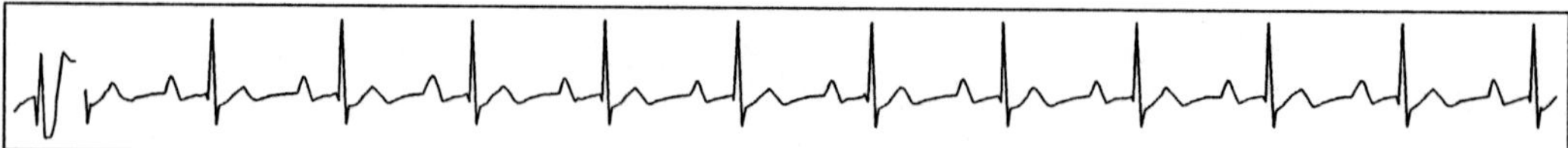

Figure 3.42: First degree heart block

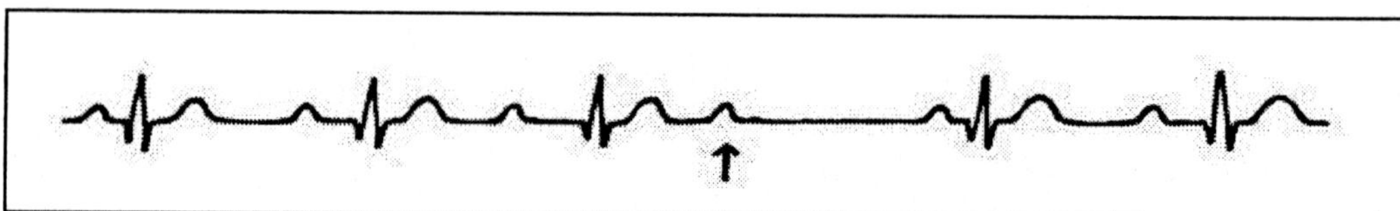

Figure 3.43: Mobitz type I heart block

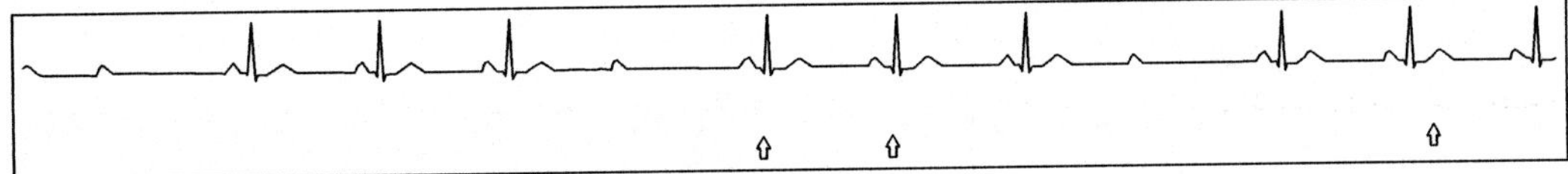

Figure 3.44: Mobitz type II heart block

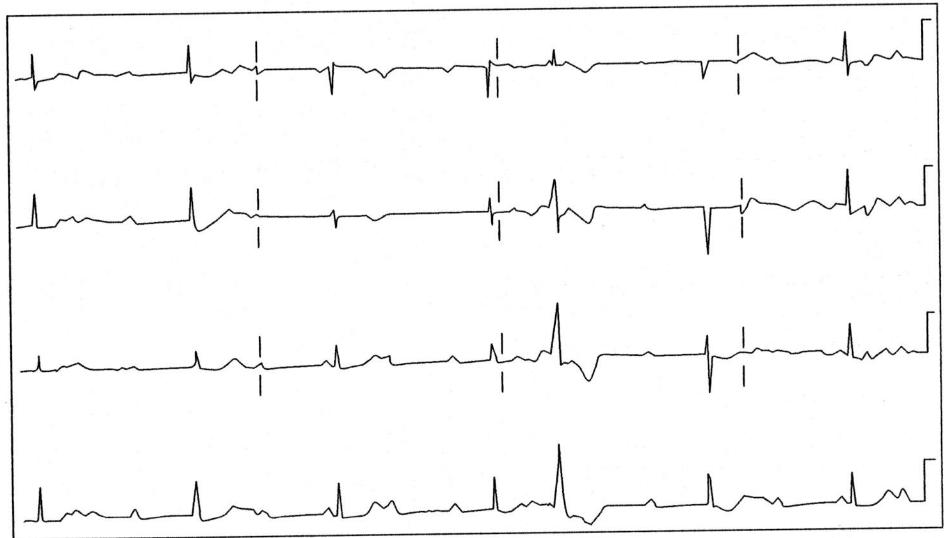

Figure 3.45: Complete heart block

Bradycardia

Bradycardia is defined as a rate less than 60 bpm, with extreme bradycardia less than 40 bpm. Palpitations with bradycardia may be caused by a sinus bradycardia or a degree of 'block' in the normal conducting system of the heart. However, the more usual presentation of bradycardias is with syncope or presyncope.

Aetiology

Causes of bradycardia and heart block include:

- Idiopathic: resulting from fibrosis of the conduction pathways
- Myocardial ischaemia (especially inferior MI)
- Drugs which slow or block electrical conduction in the heart (eg beta-blockers, Digoxin and calcium channel blockers)
- Electrolyte disturbance (eg hyperkalaemia)
- Infective: Endocarditis with aortic root abscess, Lyme disease
- Infiltrative diseases: Sarcoidosis and amyloidosis
- Post-cardiac surgery especially aortic valve replacement
- Physiological, especially in athletes

Pathophysiology

Heart block:

Heart block is a disturbance in the electrical conduction system below the level of the SA node that causes transient or permanent impairment of conduction of the normal electrical impulses. There are three degrees of heart block:

First degree: A prolonged PR interval (>200 msec or >5 small squares) but all atrial impulses are conducted through to the ventricles. See Figure 3.42.

Second degree Mobitz type I (Wenckebach): The PR interval increases with each beat until the P wave fails to conduct to the ventricles leading to a dropped beat. The cycle then repeats itself. See Figure 3.43.

Second degree Mobitz type II: the PR interval is constant but only a proportion of P waves are successfully conducted to the ventricles. See Figure 3.44.

Third degree or complete heart block: complete electrical dissociation between the atria and the ventricles. Although regular P waves and QRS

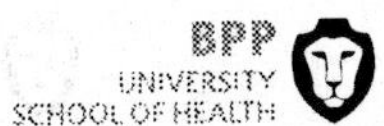

complexes are seen, there is no association between them. The ventricular rate is typically 30–50 bpm. See Figure 3.45.

First degree and Wenckebach are relatively benign arrhythmias and may be found in fit young athletes. The level of the block is at the AV node, and consequently the QRS complexes are all narrow complex. No specific treatment is required unless it is drug-induced.

Mobitz type II and complete heart block are at risk of degenerating into a higher degree block or asystole. They are never physiological and should always be investigated and referred to a cardiologist. The level of block is below the AV node in the His-Purkinjie system. The precise level will determine the QRS morphology – if the block is in the bundle of His (25% cases) the QRS duration will be normal but the lower down the system the block, the wider the QRS and the greater the likelihood of degeneration. In third degree block there is no conduction and an alternative ventricular pacemaker generates the pulse, hence the QRS may be wide.

Sick sinus syndrome (or SA node disease or tachy-brady syndrome) can cause both palpitations and syncope/presyncope. Usually idiopathic in origin, it can also be caused by ischaemic heart disease, cardiomyopathy and amyloidosis. It can be problematic to treat, as controlling the tachycardic element can worsen the bradycardic element. Sometimes a pacemaker is required to allow the tachycardia to be treated successfully with antiarrhythmic drugs.

Investigations

ECG:

- 12 lead ECG
- 24 hour ambulatory ECG monitoring

Blood tests:

- FBC
- U&Es: checking for electrolyte abnormalities, in particular hypokalaemia
- Cardiac enzymes

Echocardiogram:

Others:

- Event monitor or implantable loop recorder (Reveal device)

Top tip:

Don't rush. Whereas some of you may be absolutely passionate about your chosen speciality and have secured your dream job, you're definitely in the minority. Taking a year out was the best decision I made – I've had an amazing year, got a master's degree, done some research, had time to take a break and go on holiday, made a decision about specialties, and am now looking forward to starting training again. Some of my friends are even taking two or three years out and are having a fantastic time. Medicine can feel like a treadmill at times, with pressure to always get to the next stage, but taking time out can give you a new perspective – and can be a lot of fun!

Management

- The management of bradycardia is outlined in the adjacent algorithm from the Resuscitation Council.
- Assess the patient using the standard A to E approach advocated by the Resuscitation Council.
- Look for the adverse signs and commence treatment with atropine.
- If the patient can be stabilised they should be reviewed by a Cardiologist to consider pacemaker insertion.
- If the patient cannot be stabilised then either a temporary pacing wire should be inserted or transcutaneous pacing commenced until a definitive pacemaker can be inserted.
- The decision to insert a permanent pacemaker is ultimately made by a cardiologist in conjunction with the patient. Indications include a documented asystole of greater than three seconds or Mobitz type II/complete heart block.

Atrial fibrillation

Epidemiology

Atrial fibrillation affects about 1% of the population, but the prevalence dramatically rises with age, reaching 10% in those aged over 80.

Aetiology

- Hypertension
- Ischaemic heart disease

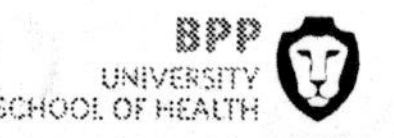

2010 Resuscitation Guidelines

Resuscitation Council (UK)

Adult bradycardia algorithm

- Assess using the ABCDE approach
- Give oxygen if appropriate and obtain IV access
- Monitor ECG, BP, SpO_2, record 12-lead ECG
- Identify and treat reversible causes (e.g. electrolyte abnormalities)

Adverse features?

- Shock
- Syncope
- Myocardial ischaemia
- Heart failure

YES → **Atropine** 500 mcg IV

NO → Risk of asystole?

Satisfactory response?

YES → Risk of asystole?

NO → Interim measures

Interim measures:

- Atropine 500 mcg IV repeat to maximum of 3 mg
- Isoprenaline 5 mcg min^{-1} IV
- Adrenaline 2-10 mcg min^{-1} IV
- Alternative drugs *

OR

- Transcutaneous pacing

→ **Seek expert help**
Arrange transvenous pacing

Risk of asystole?

- Recent asystole
- Mobitz II AV block
- Complete heart block with broad QRS
- Ventricular pause > 3 s

YES → Interim measures

NO → **Observe**

***Alternatives include:**

- Aminophylline
- Dopamine
- Glucagon (if beta-blocker or calcium channel blocker overdose)
- Glycopyrrolate can be used instead of atropine

October 2010

5th Floor, Tavistock House North, Tavistock Square, London WC1H 9HR
Telephone (020) 7388-4678 • Fax (020) 7383-0773 • Email enquiries@resus.org.uk
www.resus.org.uk • Registered Charity No. 286360

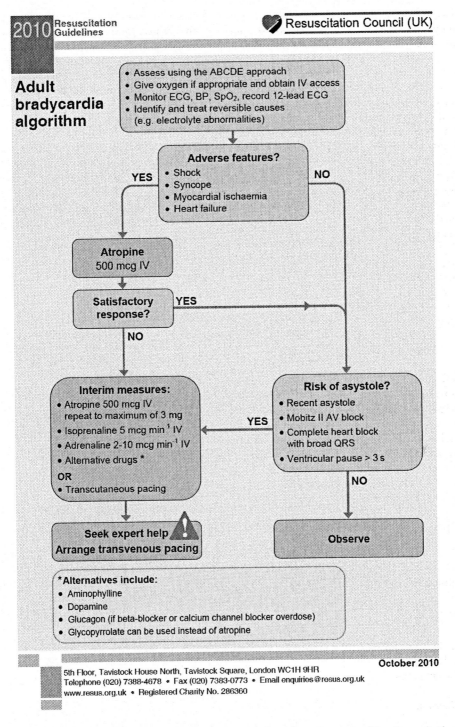

Figure 3.46: Resuscitation Council Bradycardia Management Algorithm. Courtesy of the Resuscitation Council UK. Reproduced with permission

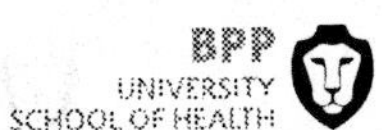

- Alcohol
- Hyperthyroidism
- Mitral valve disease (stenosis or regurgitation)
- Heart failure
- Sepsis
- Postoperative
- Electrolyte disturbance (hypokalaemia, hypocalcaemia and hypomagnesaemia)
- Cardiac tumours (eg atrial myxoma)
- 'Lone' AF (patients under 60 in whom no other cause is identified)

Pathophysiology

Atrial fibrillation is characterised by chaotic electrical activity within the atria which prevent their normal co-ordinated contraction. The commonest site for the initiation of AF is around the pulmonary veins. The electrical activity in the atria is conducted to the ventricles in an unpredictable way leading to irregularly irregular ventricular systole.

If atrial fibrillation persists, electrophysiological remodelling occurs within the atria which favours continued fibrillation, making it harder for the heart to be cardioverted to sinus rhythm.

As the atria do not effectively contract, ventricular filling depends almost entirely on passive filling during ventricular diastole which reduces cardiac output by 10–20%. In situations where passive filling of the LV is impaired (eg in diastolic heart failure or restrictive cardiomyopathy), the onset of AF can prevent adequate cardiac output thus leading to decompensated heart failure.

In addition to the effects of atrial fibrillation on cardiac output, the lack of effective atrial contraction during the cardiac cycle results in stasis of blood, predisposing to thrombus formation. This may result in systemic thromboembolism including TIA or stroke, mesenteric ischaemia or acute limb ischaemia. The risk of thromboembolism is greatest during the transition from AF to sinus rhythm and vice versa.

Classification

Atrial fibrillation may be classified according to its duration and persistence. Management depends on whether the AF is of new onset (which may favour rhythm control) or prolonged and resistant to cardioversion (which may favour rate control and anticoagulation).

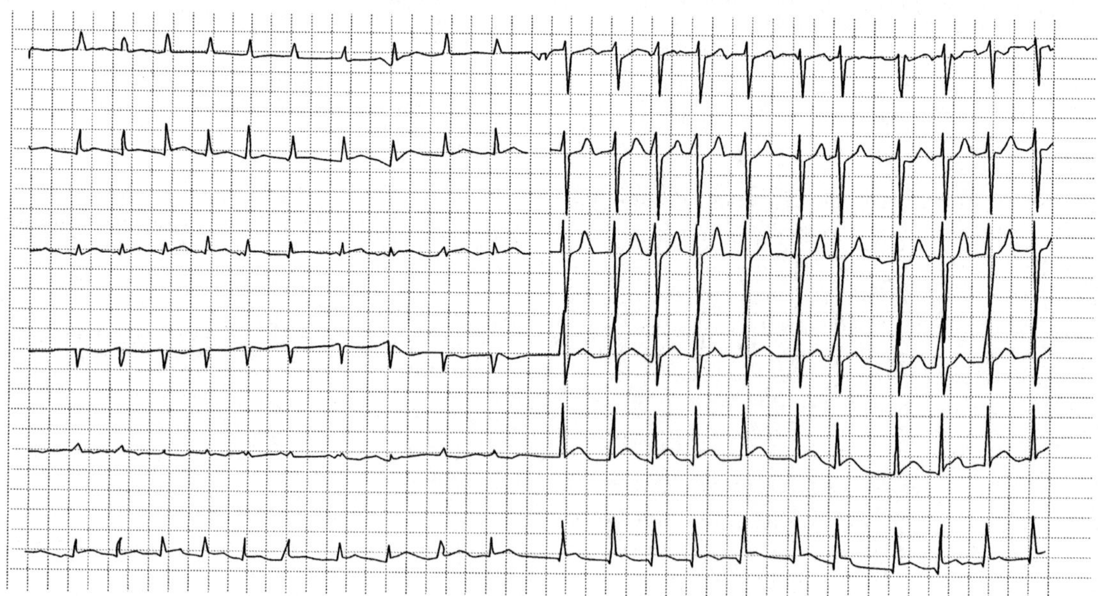

Figure 3.47: AF with fast ventricular response

1. Paroxysmal: <7 days in duration and terminates spontaneously
2. Persistent: >7 days in duration and would potentially last indefinitely if not cardioverted
3. Permanent: >7 days in duration but not possible to successfully revert to sinus rhythm

History/examination

- As per 'palpitations' history/examination

Investigations

Blood tests:

- U&Es: hypokalaemia
- Mg: hypomagnesaemia
- Bone profile: hypocalaemia
- TFTs

ECG:

Irregularly irregular R-R interval and absence of P waves (an irregular baseline is seen in between the QRS complexes). If uncertain, compare the R-R interval between different QRS complexes with a piece of paper to see if they are the same or vary.

Others:

Echocardiography: to establish systolic and diastolic heart function, look for any structural heart disease and measure left atrial size. An enlarged left atrium may make it more difficult to maintain sinus rhythm.

Management

There are two main aspects which need to be considered in managing patients with AF:

1. Optimising cardiac output – either by rhythm control or rate control
2. Anticoagulation to prevent the risk of thromboembolism

NICE CG180: Atrial Fibrillation 2014 (rate vs rhythm control)

Offer rate control as the first-line strategy to people with atrial fibrillation, except in those:

- Whose AF has a reversible cause
- Who have heart failure primarily caused by AF
- With new-onset AF
- With atrial flutter whose condition is suitable for an ablation strategy to restore sinus rhythm
- For whom a rhythm control strategy would be more suitable based on clinical judgement.

1. Offer a standard beta-blocker or a rate-limiting calcium-channel blocker as initial monotherapy
2. If monotherapy does not control symptoms add: beta-blocker, diltiazem or digoxin
3. Consider digoxin monotheraoy for non-paroxysmal AF in sedentary patients
4. Do not offer amiodarone for long-term rate control.

Consider pharmacological and/or electrical rhythm control for people with AF whose symptoms continue after controlling heart rate or when a rate-control strategy has not been successful.

1. **Cardioversion**
    a. If AF >48 hrs: electrical rather than pharmacological cardioversion
    b. Amiodarone therapy 4 weeks prior – 12 months post electrical cardioversion to maintain sinus rhythm
2. **Pharmacological**
    a. Standard beta-blocker – unless contraindicated
    b. Dronedarone after successful cardioversion in paroxysmal/persistant AF (in particular cases)
    c. Amiodarone in those with LV impairment or heart failure
    d. No class 1c antiarrythmic drugs to those with ischaemic/structural heart disease
    e. 'Pill-in-the-pocket' strategy to those with infrequent/paroxysmal/precipitant-induced symptoms (if suitable for individual patient)

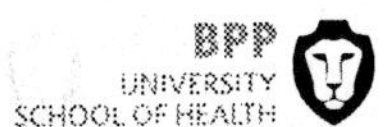

Rate vs rhythm control:

The choice between rate and rhythm control of atrial fibrillation depends on whether it is paroxysmal, persistent or permanent, and on whether the atrial fibrillation is causing significant symptoms (eg palpitations or worsening heart failure). It should also be noted that some studies (eg AFFIRM) have demonstrated that in elderly asymptomatic patients there is no advantage of rhythm control over rate control in reducing mortality and may, in fact, increase morbidity owing to side effects from antiarrhythmic drugs. In all cases a clear underlying reversible cause should be sought and treated.

Anticoagulation in AF:

Long-term anticoagulation should be considered in all patients with AF. It is important to calculate the relative risks of thromboembolic events and bleeding.

Risk of thromboembolic events:

Use the CHA2DS2-VASc stroke risk score to assess risk in people with any of the following:

- Symptomatic or asymptomatic paroxysmal, persistent or permanent atrial fibrillation
- Atrial flutter
- A continuing risk of arrhythmia recurrence after cardioversion back to sinus rhythm

	0	1	2
Age	<65	65-74	>75
Sex	Male	Female	
CHF history	No	Yes	
Hypertension	No	Yes	
Stroke/TIA/ thromboembolism	No		Yes
Vascular disease	No	Yes	
Diabetes	No	Yes	

Table 3.74: CHA2DS2-VASc stroke risk score

Scores:
0 – low risk (0% rate thromboembolic events at 1 year)
1 – intermediate risk (0.6% rate at 1 year)
>1 – high risk (3% rate at 1 year)

Bleeding risk:

Use the HAS-BLED score to assess the risk of bleeding in people who are starting or have started anticoagulation. Offer modification and monitoring of:

- Uncontrolled hypertension
- Labile INR
- Concurrent medication eg aspirin or NSAIDs
- Harmful alcohol consumption

For most people the benefit of anticoagulation outweighs the bleeding risk but for those at high bleeding risk close monitoring may be required. Do not withhold anticoagulation simply because the individual is at risk of having a fall.

HAS-BLED – estimates the risk of major bleeding for those with AF on anticoagulation:

1. **Hypertension** (+1)
   (Uncontrolled, >160 mmHg systolic)
2. **Renal Disease** (+1)
   (Dialysis, transplant, Cr >2.26 mg/dL or >200 µmol/L)
3. **Liver Disease** (+1)
   (Cirrhosis or Bilirubin >2x Normal or AST/ALT/AP >3x Normal)
4. **Stroke** (+1)
5. **Prior Major Bleeding or Predisposition to Bleeding** (+1)
6. **Labile INR** (+1)
   (Time in Therapeutic Range <60%)
7. **Age > 65** (+1)
8. **Medication Usage Predisposing to Bleeding** (+1)
   (Antiplatelet agents, NSAIDs)
9. **Alcohol or Drug Usage History ≥8 drinks/week** (+1)

Interventions to prevent thromboembolic events:

Do not offer stroke prevention therapy to people aged under 65 with AF and a CHA2DS2-VASc score of 0 for men and 1 for women. Offer anticoagulation to people with a score of 2 or above, taking bleeding risk into account.

Anticoagulation:

Anticoagulation may be with apixaban, dabigatran etexilate, rivaroxaban or a vitamin K antagonist. Antiplatelets should not be offered solely for stroke prevention monotherapy in AF.

1. **Apixaban**
   Recommended in nonvalvular AF for those with:
   i) Prior stroke or TIA
   ii) An age of 75 or older
   iii) Hypertension
   iv) Diabetes mellitus
   v) Symptomatic heart failure
2. **Dabigatran etexilate**
   Recommended in non-valvular AF for those with:
   i) Previous stroke, TIA or systemic embolism
   ii) LV ejection fraction <40%
   iii) Symptomatic heart failure – NYHA class 2 or above
   iv) An age of 75 or older
   v) 65 or older with one of: diabetes mellitus, coronary artery disease or hypertension
3. **Rivaroxaban**
   Recommended in non-valvular AF for those with:
   i) Congestive heart failure
   ii) Prior stroke or TIA
   iii) An age of 75 or older
   iv) Hypertension
   v) Diabetes mellitus
4. **Vitamin K antagonists**
   May be offered as an alternative anticoagulation option to those with AF but requires careful self-monitoring and monitoring of the time in therapeutic range (TTR) by the prescribing practitioner. Should be regularly reviewed and alternatives considered if suitable.

Cardiomyopathies

Differential diagnosis

Type	Disease
Cardiomyopathy	**Hypertrophic cardiomyopathy (HCM)** **Dilated cardiomyopathy (DCM)** **Restrictive cardiomyopathy (RCM)** Arrythmogenic right ventricular cardiomyopathy (ARVC) Left ventricular non-compaction cardiomyopathy Takotsubo cardiomyopathy (TCM)

Table 3.75: Differential diagnosis of cardiomyopathy

Hypertrophic cardiomyopathy (HCM)

The presence of increased ventricular wall thickness or mass in the absence of loading conditions (eg hypertension, aortic valve stenosis) sufficient to cause the observed abnormality.

Epidemiology

HCM is a clinically heterogeneous but relatively common autosomal dominant genetic heart disease. The prevalence is approximately 1:500 to 1:2,000 and is probably the most frequently occurring cardiomyopathy.

HCM is the commonest cause of sudden cardiac death in the young, including trained athletes, and is an important substrate for heart failure disability at any age.

Morphologic evidence of disease is found by echocardiography in approximately 25% of first-degree relatives of patients with HCM.

Aetiology

According to the presence or absence of LV outflow tract obstruction, HCM can be defined as obstructive or non-obstructive.

1. Hypertrophic obstructive cardiomyopathy (HOCM)
2. Apical hypertrophic cardiomyopathy (non-obstructive variant of HCM)

Genetic:

Familial HCM occurs as an autosomal dominant Mendelian-inherited disease in approximately 50% of cases. There are defects in several of the genes encoding the sarcomeric proteins, such as myosin heavy chain, actin and tropomyosin, resulting in abnormal myocardial calcium kinetics and calcium fluxes.

In the young, HCM is often associated with congenital syndromes. Unlike the adult form of the disease, various patterns of inheritance are seen eg Noonan and Leopard syndrome (autosomal dominant) and Friedreich's ataxia (autosomal recessive).

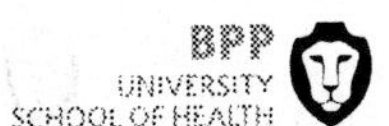

Along with wide genetic variation, there is also heterogeneity in phenotypic expression, resulting in a huge range of clinical symptoms. Phenotypic variability is related to the differences in genotype, with specific mutations associated with particular symptoms, the degree of hypertrophy and prognosis.

Other contributing factors:

- Abnormal sympathetic stimulation
- Abnormally thickened intramural coronary arteries
- Subendocardial ischaemia and increased diastolic stiffness
- Cardiac structural abnormalities resulting in disrupted cardiac mechanics

Pathophysiology

The most salient feature of HOCM is an abnormal dynamic pressure gradient across the LV outflow tract. This is related to narrowing of an already small outflow tract (due to marked asymmetric septal hypertrophy and possibly an abnormal location of the mitral valve) by the systolic anterior motion of the mitral valve against the hypertrophied septum. The likely cause of this is a Venturi effect resulting from increased ejection velocity produced by the abnormal LV outflow tract orientation and geometry.

In addition, most patients have an abnormal diastolic function, which impairs ventricular filling and increases filling pressures, despite a normal or small ventricular cavity.

History/examination

- Dyspnoea – the most common presenting symptom, occurring in as many as 90% of symptomatic patients
- Angina
- Palpitations
- Orthopnea and paroxysmal nocturnal dyspnoea – early signs of congestive heart failure
- Peripheral oedema
- Dizziness (often exacerbated by medications such as GTN, diuretics and vasodilating antihypertensives)
- Pre-syncope and syncope
- Sudden cardiac death – highest incidence in pre-adolescent and adolescents (up to 6% pa) though approximately 1.5% overall)
- Precordial palpation: double/triple apical impulse resulting from a forceful left atrial contractile against a non-compliant left ventricle
- Heart sounds: split second heart sound; S3 gallop in children and indicating decompensated heart failure in adults; fourth heart sound (atrial systole against non-compliant LV); ejection systolic murmur; pansystolic murmur of mitral regurgitation; early diastolic murmur of aortic regurgitation in 10%
- Biferiens pulse (collapse followed by secondary rise due to increased velocity through LV tract in early systole, whch declines as the gradient develops and then rises again in late systole)
- JVP – prominent 'a' wave caused by diminished right ventricular compliance
- Pulmonary oedema in severe HCM

Investigations

Blood tests:

- Genetic testing is becoming increasingly available, which can be used to identify asymptomatic family members.

ECG:

- LV hypertrophy and ST-T wave abnormalities
- Axis deviation (right or left)
- Conduction abnormalities (P-R prolongation, bundle-branch block)
- Sinus bradycardia with ectopic atrial rhythm
- Atrial enlargement
- Uncommon findings: abnormal and prominent Q wave in the anterior precordial and lateral limb leads, short P-R interval and AF (poor prognostic sign)

Imaging:

- CXR: Cardiac size may range from normal to significantly increased with left atrial enlargement frequently giving a 'double-density' appearance.
- Echocardiography:
  - Abnormal systolic anterior leaflet motion of the mitral valve
  - LV hypertrophy
  - Small ventricular size
  - Septal hypertrophy
  - Left atrial enlargement
  - Mitral valve prolapse and regurgitation
  - Decreased mid aortic flow
  - Partial systolic closure of the aortic valve in mid systole

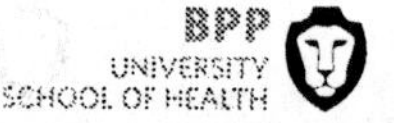

- Myocardial perfusion imaging: may show reversible defects
- Cardiac MRI: similar features as echocardiography but also combines perfusion imaging

Cardiac catheterisation:

- Determines the degree of outflow obstruction, cardiac haemodynamics, diastolic characteristics of the LV, LV anatomy and, importantly, the coronary anatomy.

Electrophysiology studies:

- May identify conduction abnormalities, sinus node dysfunction and the potential for inducible arrhythmias.

Management

Patients should be advised to avoid strenuous activity such as intense sporting activities. This is particularly important for athletes.

Multidisciplinary involvement is a vital element of effective management.

1. **Risk stratification:**
   In all patients with hypertrophic cardiomyopathy it is essential to risk stratify in order to identify which patients are at risk of sudden cardiac death.
   i) Tests: history, ECG, exercise test, Holter monitor, Echocardiogram
   ii) Major risk factors:
      - Prior cardiac arrest
      - Spontaneous sustained ventricular tachycardia
      - Family history of premature sudden cardiac death
      - Unexplained syncope
      - LV thickness >30 mm
      - Abnormal BP response to exercise
      - VT on Holter or exercise
   iii) If there is evidence of sustained or symptomatic VT or VF: ICD with or without amiodarone is offered
   iv) If there is no evidence of sustained VT or VF, patients can be risk stratified:
      - 0 risk factors: Reassure adults and reassess children
      - 1 risk factor: Individualise decision-making based on presence of other factors
      - 2 risk factors: ICD with or without amiodarone

2. **Symptomatic management:**
   Aim to alleviate symptoms of dyspnoea, chest pain and syncope by decreasing the left ventricular outflow tract gradient.

   This may be achieved by reducing ventricular contractility, increasing ventricular volume, increasing ventricular compliance and outflow tract dimension.

   i) If no symptoms: no treatment
   ii) If mild symptoms are present: beta-blockers, calcium channel antagonists
   iii) If moderate to severe symptoms are present in non-obstructive HCM:
      - Beta-blocker or Verapamil
      - Diuretics (use cautiously) in obstructive HCM
      - Beta-blocker or Verapamil
      - Add Disopyramide to beta-blocker if symptoms and gradient persist
      - Invasive therapies – surgical septal myectomy, alcohol septal ablation, pacemaker, mitral valve replacement
      - Cardiac transplantation in refractory cases

Dilated cardiomyopathy (DCM)

DCM is the presence of left ventricular dilatation and systolic dysfunction in the absence of abnormal loading conditions or coronary artery disease sufficient to cause global systolic impairment. Right ventricular dilatation and dysfunction may be present but are not necessary for the diagnosis.

Epidemiology

The prevalence is approximately 1 in 5,000 in the UK. It can affect both children and adults, but is most common in middle-aged men. Familial disease is present in 25% of patients in Western populations with a predominant autosomal dominant inheritance.

Aetiology

Inherited:

Familial DCM has incomplete and age-dependent penetrance and is linked to more than 20 loci and genes. Like HCM, it is genetically heterogeneous. Autosomal dominant mutations in cytoskeletal, Z-band, nuclear membrane and intercalated disc protein genes as well as the contractile sarcomeric proteins are responsible for many cases.

Other inheritance patterns are less frequent.

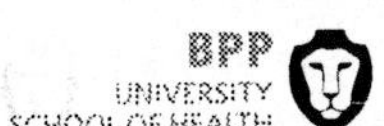

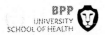

Non-inherited:

There is a broad range of primary and secondary causes of DCM:

- Chronic excessive alcohol consumption
- Infections (eg viral endocarditis/myocarditis, parasites, protozoa, Chagas disease)
- Drugs (eg anthracyclines, cocaine, metamphetamine, heavy metals)
- High-output states (eg anaemia, thyrotoxicosis, tachycardias)
- Collagen vascular disease
- Glycogen storage disease, type IV
- Thiamine, zinc and phosphate deficiency
- Amyloidosis
- Phaeochromocytoma
- Kawasaki disease
- Eosinophilic (Churg-Strauss syndrome)
- Pregnancy

Pathophysiology

DCM may result from any conditions that promote cardiomyocyte injury or loss. It is characterised by ventricular chamber enlargement and systolic dysfunction with normal LV wall thickness. Ventricular enlargement and dysfunction generally leads to progressive heart failure with further decline in LV contractile function.

Sequelae include ventricular and supraventricular arrhythmias, conduction system abnormalities, thromboembolism, and sudden or heart failure-related death. Compensatory mechanisms associated with low cardiac output induce reflex upregulation of sympathetic tone and the renin-angiotensin axis, causing increased release of vasopressin, aldosterone, and atrial natriuretic peptide. Stimulation of these hormonal tracts results in volume expansion, which induces vasoconstriction. Vasoconstriction increases afterload that, in turn, decreases stroke volume. As cardiac output depends on stroke volume and heart rate, vasoconstriction ultimately contributes to decreased cardiac output.

History/examination

It is important to determine the severity of disease, possible causes, and symptomatology. Symptoms are a good indicator of severity.

- Past medical history – risk factors
- Prior history/family history of MI/heart failure/cardiomyopathy or sudden cardiac death
- Drug history
- Social history (alcohol/tobacco/illicit drugs)
- Fatigue and dyspnoea
- Palpitations
- Orthopnoea/PND
- Peripheral oedema/increased abdominal girth (later sign of congestive heart failure due to elevated right heart pressures)
- Dizziness
- Pre-syncope/syncope
- Precordial palpation: laterally/inferiorly displaced apical impulse para-sternal heave
- Heart sounds: AF, S3 gallop (decompensated cardiac heart failure), pansystolic murmur (mitral regurgitation)
- Elevated JVP with large 'a', 'c' and 'v' waves due to increased right heart pressures and tricuspid regurgitation
- Goitre
- Pulmonary oedema/pleural effusion
- Hepatomegaly
- Ascites (portal hypertension)
- Cyanosis
- Clubbing
- Muscle wasting (inherited dystrophies)

Investigations

Blood tests:

- FBC: to investigate any cause of anaemia and treat iron deficiency anaemia
- LFTs: can be elevated, which may suggest alcoholic disease, haemochromatosis, hepatic congestion and/or hepatic infarction
- TFTs
- U&Es: an elevated creatinine, hyponatraemia (RAS activation and associated with worse prognosis)
- Cardiac biomarkers: the precise role of cardiac biomarkers is still being defined. However, there is evidence that patients who present with elevated markers experience more severe failure and higher mortality:
  - Cardiac enzymes - acute or recent myocardial injury
  - BNP is sensitive and specific in diagnosing heart failure and changes can reflect response to treatment
- Magnesium levels should be closely followed because low levels may cause chronic hypokalaemia and predispose to arrhythmia such as AF

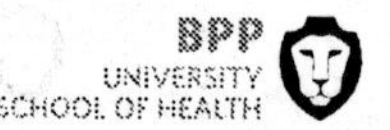

ECG:

- Identifying LV enlargement and estimating other chamber sizes
- Non-specific ST-T and Q wave changes
- AF or premature ventricular complexes are common (increases the likelihood of heart failure)
- Conduction delay, particularly LBBB

Imaging:

- CXR – cardiomegaly, signs of pulmonary oedema and venous congestion.
- Echocardiography – in acute decompensated heart failure to establish cause; to differentiate DCM from HCM or restrictive cardiomyopathies. Dilated chambers, thin walls and co-existent valvular disease are most common.
- Cardiac MRI – more accurate for left ventricular thrombus, gold standard for assessing biventricular systolic function and allows tissue characterisation.

Others:

- Urine pregnancy test
- Urine toxicology screen
- Histology: endomyocardial biopsy may be helpful in diagnosing myocarditis, connective tissue disorders, and amyloidosis

Management

Risk stratification:

Risk stratification of patients with DCM in the era of device implantation is not well described.

In DCM, mid-wall fibrosis determined by CMR is a predictor of the combined end point of all-cause mortality and cardiovascular hospitalisation. In addition, mid-wall fibrosis by CMR predicts sudden cardiac death/VT. CMR may therefore help in the risk stratification of patients with DCM, which may have value in determining the need for ICD therapy as primary prophylaxis for ventricular tachyarrhythmias (VT/VF).

The presence of severe left ventricular systolic dysfunction (LVEF) < 30% may be sufficient to warrant ICD therapy as primary prophylaxis for ventricular tachyarrhythmias (VT/VF).

Medical management:

Goals include: symptom relief, improved cardiac output, shortened hospital stay, fewer hospital admissions, reversal of injury process, and decreased mortality.

- ACEI or ARII receptor antagonists
- Aldosterone antagonists eg spironolactone
- Loop or thiazide diuretics
- Digoxin: A positive inotropic effect and ventricular rate control in AF
- Cardioselective beta-blockers, eg Bisoprolol or Carvedilol
- Vasodilators: Hydralazine, IV GTN, ISDN and Nesiritide (recombinant DNA form of human BNP that dilates veins and arteries. Used temporarily in the management of decompensated heart failure)
- Anticoagulants: restrict to patients in AF, with artificial valves, and with known mural thrombus

Cardiac resynchronisation therapy (biventricular pacing):

Improves overall efficiency of cardiac function, if there is evidence of electrical dyssynchrony on ECG (broad LBBB with QRS duration >120 ms) and/or mechanical dyssynchrony on echocardiography (inter- and intra-ventricular dyssynchrony).

Results in cardiac haemodynamic improvements, symptomatic benefits and reduced mortality and hospitalisation rates compared to those achieved with optimal medical therapy.

Lead positioning – right atrial lead, right ventricular lead, coronary sinus lead to pace the LV. Resynchronisation pacing generators have defibrillation capabilities (biventricular ICD).

Current indications for cardiac resynchronisation therapy:

- The presence of severe left ventricular systolic impairment
- NYHA Class III or IV symptoms despite optimal medical therapy with ACE inhibitors, beta-blockers, and/or other appropriate pharmacologic measures
- Evidence of significant inter- or intra-ventricular conduction delay

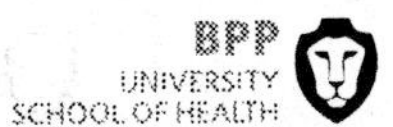

Surgical management:

- Left ventricular assist devices – a bridge to transplantation and are being evaluated as permanent implants in those who are not candidates for heart therapy
- Partial left ventriculectomy (Batista procedure) – reduces the LV diameter, which is thought to improve ventricular function
- Heart transplantation: if all other management options fail to control symptoms

Prognosis:

The severity of disease on initial diagnosis has been shown to be inversely proportional to the long-term survival.

In general for DC, the 60-day mortality rate following hospital admission due to an exacerbation of CHF is 8–20% depending on the population studied.

Restrictive cardiomyopathy

A myocardial disease characterised by restrictive filling and reduced diastolic volume of either or both ventricles with normal or near-normal systolic function and wall thickness. Increased interstitial fibrosis may be present.

Epidemiology

The least common type of cardiomyopathy accounting for approximately 5% of all cases of primary heart muscle disease.

Aetiology

- Idiopathic
- Familial:
  - Often autosomal dominant – may be related to mutations in troponin I or desmin
  - Rarely autosomal recessive inheritance – haemochromatosis associated with HFE gene mutation or glycogen storage disease
  - X-linked – Anderson-Fabry disease
- Infiltrative
  - Amyloidosis
  - Glycogen storage disease
  - Sarcoidosis
  - Systemic sclerosis
- Endocardial pathology:
  - Endomyocardial disease with hypereosinophilia (Loeffler endomyocarditis)
  - Diurectics in obstructive HCM (use cautiously)
- Malignancy:
  - Carcinoid heart disease
  - Metastatic myo- and endocardial infiltration
- Anthracycline toxicity
- Post-cardiac transplantation or mediastinal irradiation

Pathophysiology

RCM results in increased myocardial stiffness which causes ventricular pressure to rise with only small increases in volume. This reduced compliance leads to diastolic heart failure. The LV cannot fill adequately at normal diastolic pressures, leading to a reduction in cardiac output due to reduced left ventricular filling volume.

In the early stage of disease, systolic function usually remains normal. Ventricular wall thickness is increased secondary to myocardial infiltration with amyloidosis, though not as pronounced as in HCM. As the disease progresses, systolic function may begin to deteriorate. Reduced left ventricular filling volume leads to reduced stroke volume and low cardiac output symptoms (eg fatigue, lethargy), whereas increased filling pressures cause pulmonary and systemic congestion.

RCM can therefore result in left or right heart failure or complete heart block due to fibrosis at the SA or AV nodes.

History/examination

- Past medical history: radiation or chemotherapy, cardiac transplantation, systemic disease
- Drug history: Methysergide
- Family history: Cardiomyopathy or sudden cardiac death
- Fatigue and dyspnoea
- Palpitations
- Angina
- Orthopnoea and PND
- Peripheral oedema and increased abdominal girth
- Thromboembolism
- Pre-syncope and syncope
- Sudden cardiac death
- Precordial palpation: Parasternal (right ventricular) heave
- Heart sounds: AF, S3 gallop, pansystolic murmurs of mitral and tricuspid regurgitation
- Weight loss/cardiac cachexia

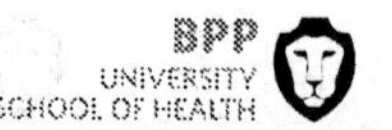

- Decreased pulse volume due to low cardiac output
- Elevated JVP with rapid 'x' and 'y' descents. May rise during inspiration (Kussmaul sign)
- Pleural effusions
- Hepatomegaly
- Ascites or gross peripheral oedema

Investigations

Blood tests:

- FBC with peripheral smear to identify eosinophilia
- Renal function
- LFTs
- Haematinics: to screen for haemochromatosis
- Serum BNP level

ECG:

- Findings depend on the stage of the disease and the specific diagnosis.
- May be normal or just show some non-specific ST-T wave changes.
- Rhythm disorders, particularly AF.
- Conduction abnormalities are uncommon in amyloidosis.
- Myocardial infiltration and/or small vessel induced ischaemia or infarction may give rise to a pseudo-infarct pattern.
- Low QRS voltage is common in amyloidosis.

Imaging:

- CXR: Cardiomegaly and often bilateral pleural effusions may also be identified.
- Echocardiography:
  - Ventricular size may be normal or reduced with normal wall thickness.
  - Diffuse ventricular hypertrophy is common with amyloidosis and other infiltrative diseases.
  - Both atria will be dilated.
  - Mural thrombus and cavity obliteration are seen in obliterative RCM.
  - Abnormal myocardial texture seen as 'speckling' is characteristic of amyloidosis.
  - Transmitral flow patterns and tissue Doppler imaging identify diastolic dysfunction.
- Cardiac MRI: Detailed assessment of pericardial thickness and abnormal myocardial interstitium.
- CT: Similar to MRI in its ability to assess pericardial thickness. CT is better able to detect pericardial calcification as occurs in constrictive pericarditis.

Cardiac catheterisation:

- Accentuated filling occurs in early diastole, which terminates abruptly at the end of the rapid filling phase. When pressure tracings are taken at this point, they show a characteristic diastolic dip and a plateau or a square-root sign.

Others:

- Cardiac biopsy: useful if non-invasive studies have failed to establish a clear diagnosis.
- Fine needle aspiration of abdominal fat may demonstrate amyloidosis and is safer than cardiac biopsy.
- Liver biopsy is performed for the diagnosis of haemochromatosis.

Management

Treatment goal is to reduce symptoms by lowering elevated filling pressures without significantly reducing cardiac output.

Current agents are not very effective in treating disorders of myocardial relaxation, therefore treatment is limited to:

- Low dose thiazide or loop diuretics to reduce cardiac preload
- Long-acting nitrates to reduce preload – eg isosorbide mononitrate or GTN patch
- Digoxin – use with caution in amyloidosis as potentially arrhythmogenic
- Anticoagulation for patients with a history of thromboembolism or atrial fibrillation
- Amiodarone – maintenance of sinus rhythm is important to preserve the atrial contribution to ventricular filling

Targeted therapies:

- Melphalan (anti-plasma cell therapy) may slow the progress of AL amyloidosis by stopping production of the paraprotein responsible for the amyloid formation.
- In the early phase of Loeffler endocarditis, corticosteroids, cytotoxic agents (eg hydroxyurea) and interferon may be used to suppress the intense eosinophilic infiltration of the myocardium alongside conventional heart failure medication, which improves symptoms and survival.
- In haemochromatosis, chelation therapy or venesection is effective to decrease the iron overload.

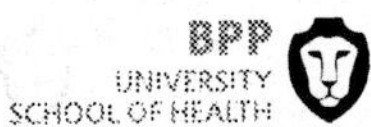

Prognosis

Disease course varies depending on the pathology and treatment but is often unsatisfactory.

The prognosis of patients with primary systemic amyloidosis remains poor, with a median survival of approximately two years despite intervention with alkylating-based chemotherapy in selected cases.

The importance of an accurate diagnosis of RCM is to distinguish it from constrictive pericarditis, which also presents with restrictive physiology but is frequently curable by surgical intervention (pericardiectomy).

Further reading and references

1. Assomull, R.G., Lyne, J., Prasad, S.K., et al. (2006) Cardiovascular Magnetic Resonance, Fibrosis, and Prognosis in Dilated Cardiomyopathy. *J Am Coll Cardiol* 2006; 48: 1977–1985.
2. Baker, D.W. and Wright, R.F. (1994) Management of heart failure. IV. Anticoagulation for patients with heart failure due to left ventricular systolic dysfunction. *JAMA* 1994; 23–30; 272(20): 1614–8.
3. Dimarco, J.P., Ellenbogen, K.A., Epstein, A.E., et al. (2008) ACC/AHA/HRS 2008 guidelines for Device-Based Therapy of Cardiac Rhythm Abnormalities: executive summary. *Heart Rhythm* 2008; 5(6): 934–55.
4. Andersson, B., Arbustini, E., Elliott, P., et al. (2008) Classification of the cardiomyopathies: a position statement from the European society of cardiology working group on myocardial and pericardial diseases. *European Heart Journal* 2008; 29(2): 270–276
5. Gage, B.F., Shannon, W., Waterman, A.D., et al. (2001) Validation of clinical classification schemes for predicting stroke: Results from the national registry of atrial fibrillation. *JAMA* 2001; 285(22), 2864–2870.
6. National Institute for Health and Clinical Excellence. (2014) *Atrial Fibrillation* (CG180). [Online]. Available from: www.nice.org.uk/guidance/cg180?unlid=2021544602016101584650 [Accessed 7 November 2016].
7. Sudden arrhythmic death syndrome, www.sads.org.uk/drugs_to_avoid.htm – website detailing drugs to avoid.
8. Maron, B.J., Thiene, G., Towbin, J.A., et al. (2006) American Heart Association; Council on Clinical Cardiology, Heart Failure and Transplantation Committee; Quality of Care and Outcomes Research and Functional Genomics and Translational Biology Interdisciplinary Working Groups; Council on Epidemiology and Prevention. Contemporary definitions and classification of the cardiomyopathies: an American Heart Association Scientific Statement from the Council on Clinical Cardiology, Heart Failure and Transplantation Committee; Quality of Care and Outcomes Research and Functional Genomics and Translational Biology Interdisciplinary Working Groups; and Council on Epidemiology and Prevention. *Circulation* 2006; 113: 1807–1816.
9. The Atrial Fibrillation Follow-up Investigation of Rhythm Management (AFFIRM) Investigators. (2002) A Comparison of Rate Control and Rhythm Control in Patients with Atrial Fibrillation. *NEJM* 2002; 347: 1825–33.
10. UK Resuscitation Council. (2016) *Advanced Life Support*. 5th Edition. London: Resuscitation Council.
11. Ko, D.T., Woo, A., You, J.J., et al. (2007) Life expectancy gains and cost-effectiveness of implantable cardioverter/defibrillators for the primary prevention of sudden cardiac death in patients with hypertrophic cardiomyopathy. *Am Heart J* 2007; 154(5): 899–907.

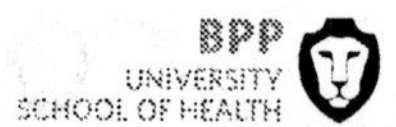

Poisoning

Common poisons

Type of drug use	Poisons
Medicinal	**Paracetamol** **Salicylates** **Opiates** **Benzodiazepines** **Tricyclic antidepressants (TCA)**
Recreational	Cannabis Heroin **Cocaine** **Ecstasy** Gamma-hydroxybutyrate (GHB) Amphetamines Lysergic acid diethylamide (LSD) Ketamine

Table 3.76: Common medicinal and recreational poisons

Poisoning in general

Epidemiology

Poisoning accounts for 10% of UK hospital admissions, about one-third of which are due to Paracetamol. Although poisoning is a major cause of death in the under-50 year olds, less than 1% of those admitted to hospital die. Major causes of death are recreational drugs, antidepressants, Paracetamol and carbon monoxide.

Aetiology

Poisoning may be accidental, which is often the case in young children, or deliberate. Deliberate poisoning can either be as part of a completed suicide or an act of DSH. On occasions poisoning can also be an act of terrorism or due to occupational, recreational, environmental and iatrogenic reasons. Deliberate poisoning often involves more than one drug, with alcohol being the commonest second agent. Poisoned patients will often admit to what they have taken, but the admitting doctor should keep an open mind, especially in patients with a reduced GCS, and consider poisoning in the differential diagnosis.

Pathophysiology

The pathophysiology is dependent on the poison ingested.

History/examination

- Causative agent: the signs and symptoms depend on the nature of substance(s), amount and time taken. Look for any supporting evidence of the causative agent, eg packets of pills brought in by the patient, family and friends or the ambulance service.
- Past medical, drug and psychiatric history: depression, previous episodes of DSH and medications which could produce toxicity.
- Indicators of suicidal intent – the details surrounding the incident eg was it planned, was the patient hoping to be found, was there a suicide note?
- Environment: the nature of the work/activity the patient was involved in, chemicals that were used in the processes, any Hazchem information.

Investigations

Blood tests:

- FBC
- U&Es
- LFTs
- Calcium
- Glucose
- Clotting
- Specific drug levels: Paracetamol and Salicylate should always be taken in the unconscious patient and any in whom there is doubt about the medication that may have been taken. Digoxin and iron are also readily available if indicated. Other tests can be requested but take some time to obtain the results, eg Carbamazepine
- ABG: acidosis is very common in acute poisoning

Imaging:

- CXR: especially if concurrent aspiration is suspected

Others:

- Toxicology screen: may be required, but is not universally available
- Dipstix tests: can be used to test for recreational drug use. These are expensive and not widely available in clinical areas
- ECG: findings vary depending on the toxin

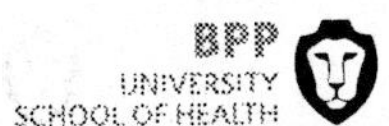

Management

This is dependent on the cause; however, there is a general management to follow for all poisons.

1. **Structured assessment:**
   i) A to E approach.
   ii) Focus on the effects of the causative agent eg looking for signs of hypotension, assessing the GCS and checking the ECG for QT prolongation in TCA overdose.
2. **Supportive therapy:**
   i) Protect the airway, potentially intubating the patient until the patient is capable of protecting their own airway.
   ii) Treat and manage hypoxia.
   iii) Correct hypotension with fluid replacement and vasopressors if required.
   iv) Control seizures and correct electrolyte imbalances.
   v) Warm the patient if necessary.
3. **Specific measures:**
   i) Reducing absorption: activated charcoal can be used for a wide range of toxic agents, but is only beneficial if used within the first hour post-ingestion. Gastric lavage, emesis and cathartics have no evidence to support an improvement in outcomes and may cause morbidity.
   ii) Increasing elimination: urine alkalinisation can be beneficial in the treatment of salicylate poisoning.
   iii) Antidotes: See Table 3.77 for more detail.

Poison	Antidote
Benzodiazepines	Flumanezil*
Beta-blockers	Glucagon
Calcium channel blockers	Calcium chloride
Cyanide	Hydroxocobalamin, dicolbalt edentate, sodium nitirite, sodium thiosulphate
Digoxin	Digibind
Heparin	Protamine sulphate
Iron	Desferrioxamine
Methanol, ethylene glycol	Ethanol
Nerve agents	Atropine, pralidoxime
Opioids	Naloxone
Paracetamol	N-acetylcysteine (NAC), methionine
Warfarin	Vitamin K

Table 3.77: Antidotes for common poisons. (*) antidote used only for the reversal of iatrogenic over-sedation

4. **Psychiatric assessment:**
   Psychiatric assessment is necessary prior to discharge. Although not always intended as a suicide attempt, an act of DSH increases the likelihood not only of further episodes, but also of future completed suicide.
   Certain characteristics of the act may point to suicidal intent:

   i) Evidence of premeditation
   ii) Suicide note
   iii) Precautions/timing to avoid discovery
   iv) Not seeking help during or afterwards
   v) Admission of suicidal intent
   vi) Older age
   vii) Male

   The patient should be sympathetically nursed in a bed which is easily observed and referred to psychiatric services as per local protocols.

The British Association of Emergency Medicine produced a list of antidotes that should be stored in all EDs in 2006. In the EDs or EAU you will have access to the following resources:

- Toxbase
- National Poisons Information Service
- UK Medicines Information Service
- BNF

Paracetamol

Epidemiology

Paracetamol poisoning is the commonest method of self-poisoning accounting for 50% of all cases.

Aetiology

Both deliberate self-harm (including attempted suicide) and accidental overdose are seen.

Pathophysiology

Paracetamol is conjugated in the liver to Paracetamol glucuronide and sulphate. 5–10% is oxidised by the cytochrome P450 enzymes into NAPQI, which is highly toxic. This is normally detoxified by conjugation with glutathione. However, in overdose, the conjugation pathways are saturated resulting in large quantities of NAPQI and this depletes the glutathione stores leading to hepatocyte damage.

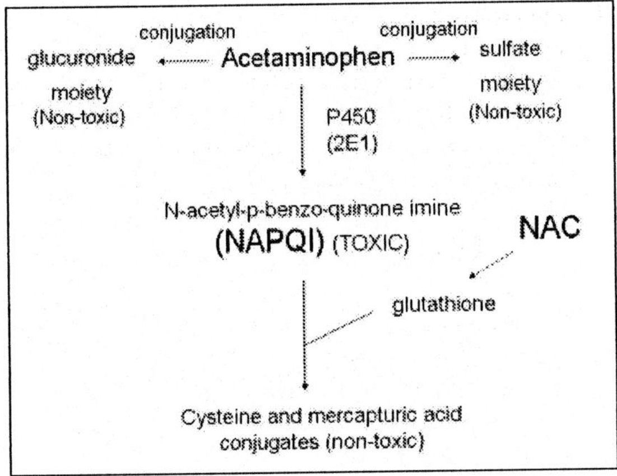

Figure 3.48: Metabolism of paracetamol and method of action of N-acetylcysteine

History/examination

- The amount ingested
- The time since ingestion and if doses were staggered
- Any other drugs taken, especially alcohol
- Risk factors for additional toxicity, eg liver disease, high alcohol consumption, eating disorders
- May report nausea, vomiting and anorexia
- In large overdoses there may be reduced level of consciousness and metabolic acidosis
- In late presentation there may be signs of liver failure

Investigations

Blood tests:

- Paracetamol and salicylate levels: taken at least four hours post-ingestion
- LFTs
- Coagulation screen
- ABG: checking for metabolic acidosis

Management

Plasma Paracetamol levels should govern treatment. These should be taken at least four hours post-ingestion and, using the normogram available in the BNF, administer the treatment.

In the event of a large overdose, ie at least 12 g of Paracetamol in total or 150 mg/Kg, the treatment should begin immediately without waiting for blood levels.

If there is doubt about the time that the overdose was taken, take bloods and commence NAC infusion.

Dose of NAC administered should be:

- 150 mg/kg over 1 hour
- 50 mg/kg over 4 hours
- 100 mg/kg over 16 hours

Treatment with NAC has been associated with mild elevation of the INR. Patients who have a marginally elevated INR, ie 1.3 or less, but normal transaminase levels (ALT or AST) after all three doses, do not require further monitoring or treatment with NAC. If both the INR and transaminases are still elevated, then repeat another bag of 100 mg/Kg over 16 hours.

Approximately 5% of patients show symptoms of allergy to NAC with rash and wheeze. In this case the infusion should be stopped, chlorpheniramine given, and the infusion resumed at a slower rate.

The King's College criteria were developed to provide a prognostic indicator in acute liver failure. If the patient fulfils these criteria, they should be referred to the local tertiary liver transplant unit as soon as possible.

1. Acute liver failure secondary to paracetamol overdose:
   i) pH <7.30 or
   ii) INR >6.5 and serum creatinine >300 in patients with grade 3 or 4 hepatic encephalopathy
2. Acute liver failure (not secondary to paracetamol overdose)
   i) INR >6.5 or any three of:
   ii) Age <10 or >40
   iii) Duration of jaundice before hepatic encephalopathy >7 days
   iv) Aetiology
   v) INR >3.5
   vi) Serum bilirubin >300

Timeline for treatment following presentation in ED

0–4 hours:

- If jaundice/hepatic tenderness and ingestion >36 hours previously, start NAC immediately.
- NAC treatment may also be considered immediately if more than 150 mg/Kg (or 12 g in an adult) or the ingestion timing was staggered.
- Consider activated charcoal if more than 12 g of Paracetamol has been ingested within the last hour.
- At four hours from ingestion, measure the plasma Paracetamol concentration.

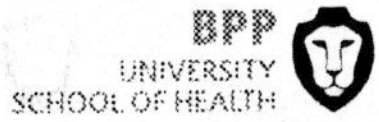

4-8 hours:

- Measure plasma Paracetamol concentration.
- NAC treatment may be considered if more than 150 mg/Kg of Paracetamol has been ingested whilst awaiting the four-hour sample results.
- Assess treatment needs using the standard normogram and commence NAC if appropriate.
- If the ingestion was >15 hours ago or the last intake of a staggered ingestion was >24 hours ago and paracetamol levels are still detectable then NAC treatment should be commenced.
- Treatment should be started within 8 hours for maximal benefit. If it is commenced within this time frame, the risks of renal and hepatic toxicity are minimal.
- After NAC administration, INR and hepatic enzyme levels have normalised, the patient can be discharged with advice to return if vomiting/ jaundice develop (providing the mental health team have reviewed the patient and provided appropriate input).

Prognosis

- Liver transplant may be required for a few patients and they must be identified as early as possible, preferably by the second day.
- An arterial pH <7.30 on the second or subsequent day after overdose is found in about 70% of cases with a poor prognosis.
- A combination of INR >6.7, plasma creatinine concentration greater than 300 micromol/L and grade 3 or 4 hepatic encephalopathy is associated with a 17% survival rate.
- An increase in prothrombin time/INR between the third and fourth days after overdose also indicates a poor prognosis.
- Liver transplantation is probably contra-indicated in patients with severe hypotension, severe cerebral oedema and serious infection.

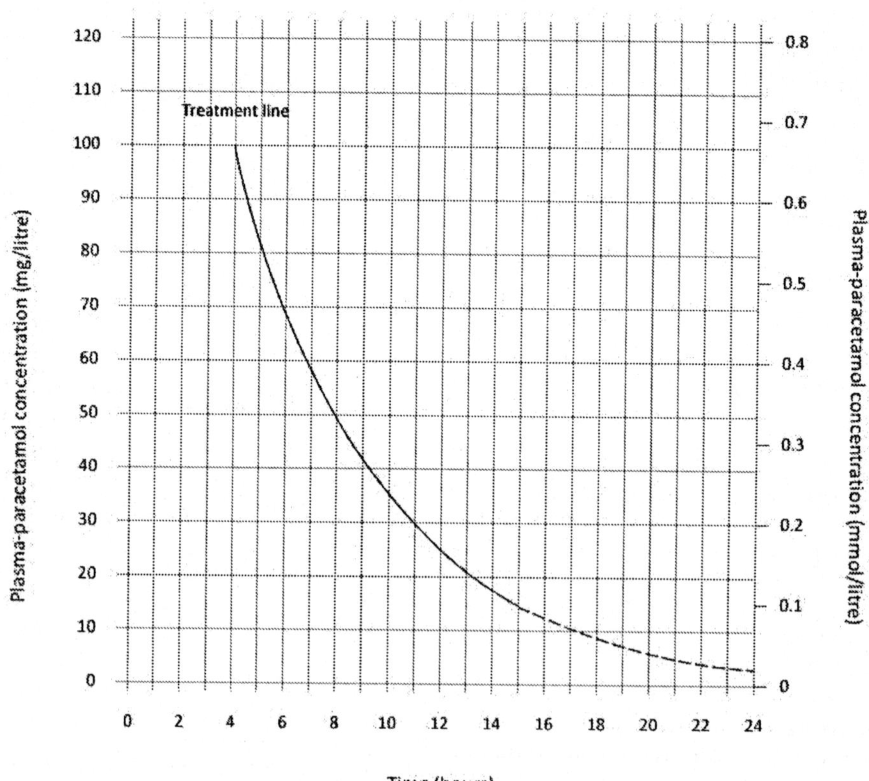

Figure 3.49: MHRA treatment normogram for Paracetamol overdose

Salicylates

Epidemiology

There were over 3,000 hospital admissions in England during 2007–2008 for salicylate poisoning.

Aetiology

Salicylate poisoning is usually due to aspirin overdose but it can be caused by the ingestion of oil of wintergreen.

Pathophysiology

A toxic dose of salicylate is >150 mg/Kg and severe toxicity is between 330 and 500 mg/Kg. Doses of over 500 mg/kg are potentially lethal. The respiratory centre is stimulated to give tachypnoea with the resultant respiratory alkalosis. The acidic nature of salicylate gives a metabolic acidosis. There is also an uncoupling of the normal intracellular oxidative phosphorylation resulting in hyperpyrexia.

History/examination

- How much aspirin and when was it taken
- Any other toxins ingested
- Nausea and vomiting
- Abdominal pain
- Lethargy
- Tinnitus
- Dizziness
- Hyperthermia
- Tachypnoea
- Respiratory alkalosis
- Metabolic acidosis
- Hypoglycaemia
- Confusion
- Seizures
- Coma
- Examine for non-cardiogenic pulmonary oedema which has an increased risk in the elderly and smokers with underlying chronic lung disease

Investigations

Blood tests:

- Salicylate levels
- Baseline blood tests are required
- U&Es: may be raised if dehydrated from vomiting and hyperventilation
- Glucose
- ABG

Others:

CXR – pulmonary oedema

Management

- Activated charcoal
- After initial levels, repeat blood tests should be taken at three hour intervals until the serum salicylate level starts to decrease
- IV fluids to correct hypotension
- Urine alkalisation may be required, especially with severe acidosis, using IV sodium bicarbonate
- Severe toxicity requires haemofiltration
- Mental health team referral as per ED protocol

Opiates

Epidemiology

Opioid poisoning is an increasing problem. Morphine and diamorphine, as well as heroin, are all drugs of abuse and accidental recreational overdoses are common. Deliberate poisoning is less common and iatrogenic overdose should always be considered in the deteriorating patient who has been prescribed opiates.

Aetiology

Opioids are common drugs of abuse in the forms of heroin, morphine and diamorphine but opioids are also commonly used analgesics in hospital patients.

Pathophysiology

Opioids act on the opioid receptors. Individuals have varying responses to opioids and hence doses that may be fine in one individual may cause an overdose in a sensitive individual. There are a number of common opioids, with significant variation in half-life.

Opiate	Half-life (hours)
Morphine	3
Diamorphine	3
Codeine	3.5
Dihydrocodeine	4
Tramadol	6
Methadone	12–18

Table 3.78: Common opiates and their half-life

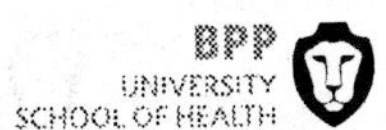

Morphine is metabolised to morphine-6-glucuronide in the liver, which is excreted by the kidneys. Renal impairment can prolong the half-life and increase the possibility of toxicity. The effects in overdose will also be potentiated by simultaneous ingestion of alcohol and other centrally acting drugs.

History/examination

- Which opioid(s), when and by what route
- Any other toxins ingested
- Reduced respiratory rate
- Hypotension
- Bradycardia
- Pin-point pupils
- Reduced level of consciousness
- Vomiting and delayed gastric motility
- Needle and track mark in IV users – exclude any abscesses
- Hallucinations
- Rhabdomyolysis in patients have been immobile for long periods

Investigations

Blood tests:

- FBC
- U&Es – impaired renal function will affect opioid half-life
- LFTs

Others:

- ECG
- Respiratory rate and saturations

Management

Conscious patient:

- A to E assessment.
- Activated charcoal is a possibility if the overdose definitely occurred in the previous hour.
- If the patient has clinical signs then observe them until fully awake.
- Consider giving Naloxone. The patient will then need observing for at least six hours.
- If the patient has no clinical signs then observe for at least four hours after ingestion of a standard release preparation or at least eight hours after a modified (slow) release preparation.

Unconscious patient:

- A to E assessment.
- Activated charcoal is a possibility if the overdose definitely occurred in the previous hour.
- Administer 0.4–2 mg IV Naloxone and repeat the dose if there is no response within 2 minutes.
- Large doses (4 mg) may be required in a seriously poisoned patient. Intramuscular (IM) Naloxone is possible if necessary.
- Failure of a definite opioid overdose to response to large doses of Naloxone suggests that another CNS depressant drug or brain damage is present.
- Beware of an aggressive response from an opioid addict because their 'fix' is ruined when giving Naloxone.
- Naloxone has a short serum half-life (30–80 minutes) in comparison to the opiates it reverses so repeat doses or an IV infusion may be necessary.
- Observe the patient carefully for at least six hours after the last dose of Naloxone because further administration may be required.

Benzodiazepines

Epidemiology

Not as common as a drug of abuse, but very commonly used for sedative purposes in hospital. Often prescribed to patients with anxiety related disorders including depression.

Aetiology

The cause of benzodiazepine poisoning is usually iatrogenic.

Pathophysiology

There are a number of common benzodiazepines and they all have significant variation in half-life. However, their duration of action is less than the half-life. Benzodiazepines are positive allosteric modulators of GABA-A receptors and therefore potentiate the inhibitory effects within the CNS.

Benzodiazepines are very rarely fatal unless co-ingested with other CNS depressants.

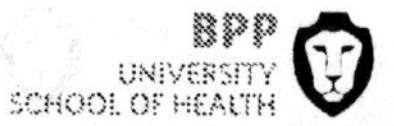

Drug	Half-life (including active metabolites) (hours)
Flumazenil	1
Midazolam	1.8
Nitrazepam	10
Temazepam	20
Diazepam	36
Chlordiazepoxide	36

Table 3.79: Common benzodiazepines and their half-life

History/examination

- Which benzodiazepine(s), when and by what route
- Any other toxins
- Drowsiness
- Respiratory depression
- Impaired balance
- Slurred speech
- Diplopia and nystagmus
- Bradycardia
- Hypotension
- Hypothermia
- Amnesia
- Ataxia
- Coma

Investigations

No specific investigations are required.

Blood tests:

- Baseline blood tests
- Paracetamol, salicylate and alcohol levels
- ABG if significant respiratory depression

Management

- Supportive management is the mainstay.
- Flumazenil (200 micrograms) is the antidote for benzodiazepines (GABA-A antagonist) but its use in overdose is controversial. It can be used with caution in the management of iatrogenic overdose but it is not licensed for the management of deliberate overdose of benzodiazepines. This is due to the risk of inducing uncontrollable seizures.

Tricyclic antidepressants

Epidemiology

The incidence of TCA overdose is decreasing with the reduction in prescription numbers and a move towards safer classes of antidepressants.

Aetiology

The most common cause of TCA overdose is due to suicide attempts.

Pathophysiology

TCAs have multiple effects which include blocking of MAO reuptake, anticholinergic action and blockade of ion channels, in particular sodium ion channels. There are cardiovascular effects as a result of adrenoceptor blockade.

History/examination

- Which TCA(s) were taken and when
- Any other toxins
- Reduced level of consciousness
- Seizures
- Anticholinergic features such as dry mouth, blurred vision, urinary retention and constipation
- Dilated pupils
- Tachycardia
- Upgoing plantars
- Brisk reflexes
- Hypoxia
- Bradypnoea and respiratory acidosis
- Metabolic acidosis
- Hypokalaemia
- Hypotension
- Cardiac conduction abnormalities: prolonged QT interval and atrio-ventricular (AV) nodal conduction delays

Investigations

Blood tests:

- Baseline blood tests
- ABG

Others:

- ECG

Management

- Activated charcoal if presenting <1 hour
- IV fluid therapy to treat hypotension
- Inotropes may be necessary
- Monitor for respiratory depression – intubation may be necessary
- Cardiac monitoring
- Control seizures
- Sodium bicarbonate can be used in severe poisoning and may help control dysrhythmias
- If GCS <8 will require ICU referral and intubation to protect the airway

Recreational drugs

It is likely that you will encounter patients admitted to hospital who are suffering from adverse reactions to the recreational use of drugs of abuse. It is useful to be familiar with some of the street terms that people may use to describe these drugs and the treatment required.

Recreational drug	Street name
Cannabis	Skunk, grass, dope, hash, gange
Heroin	H, horse, smack, junk, brown, gear, china white, skag
Cocaine	Coke, Charlie, snow, white
3,4-methylenedioxy-methamphetamine (MDMA)	Ecstasy, E, pills, doves, XTC, disco biscuits, Bruce Lees, echoes, hug drug, burgers, Smarties, magic beans, Mitsubishis, Rolexes, dolphins, snow ball, callies, eccies, little fellas, dids and yokes
Gamma-hydroxybutyrate	Liquid E, liquid X
Ampetamines	Speed, whizz, billy, uppers
Lysergic acid diethylamide (LSD)	Acid, sugar, trips, tabs, sid, Bart Simpsons, blotter, micro dots, liquid, Lucy, stars, lightening flash, paper mushrooms, rainbows, flash and hawk
Ketamine	Special K, K, ket, super k, vitamin K, green, Mr Soft and techno smack

Table 3.80: Common recreational drugs and their street names

Drug	Pathophysiology	Symptoms	Investigations	Treatment
Cocaine	CNS stimulant Cerebral artery vasospasm	Chest pain Hallucinations/agitation Pupil dilatation Tachycardia Dysrhythmia Hypertension Hyperpyrexia Seizures	Baseline bloods Cardiac enzymes ECG AXR (abdominal packing) CT chest (aortic dissection)	Supportive Benzodiazepines Cooling ACS protocol
Ecstasy	Release and reuptake inhibition of presynaptic dopamine, serotonin and noradrenaline Release of cortisol, prolactin, ACTH and ADH	Hyperthermia Dehydration Hyponatraemia Serotonin syndrome Teeth grinding Nystagmus Urinary retention Pupil dilatation Tachycardia	ECG Baseline bloods	Supportive Catheterisation IVI and careful fluid resuscitation ICU support
Ketamine	NMDA receptor antagonist Acts on opioid and monoamine receptors	Hallucinations/agitation Tachy/bradycardia Hyper/hypotension Vomiting Seizures Diplopia Nystagmus Respiratory depression LUTS – culminating in ketamine-induced vesicopathy	Baseline bloods ECG Bladder scan	Supportive Catheterisation ICU support anticholinergics and specialist urology support

Table 3.81: Summary of commonly abused drugs

Further reading and references

1. Bateman, D.N. and Vale, A. (2007) *Poisoning*. Oxford: Medicine Publishing, pp10–12.
2. Joint Formulary Committee. (2016) *British National Formulary*. 71st Edition. London: Pharmaceutical Press.
3. Flatley, J. and Hoare, J. (2008) *Drugs Misuse Declared: Findings from 2006/2007 British Crime Survey. Home Office National Statistical Bulletin*. London: Home Office.
4. National Poisons Information Service, www.npis.org.
5. Alexander, G.J., Hayllar, K.M., O'Grady, J.G., et al. (1989) Early Indicators of prognosis in fulminant hepatic failure. *Gastroenterology* 1989; 97 (2): 439–45.
6. Royal College of Emergency Medicine. (2013) *Guidelines for Paracetamol Overdose*. [Online]. Available from: www.rcem.ac.uk/RCEM/Quality_Policy/RCEM/Quality-Policy/Quality-Policy.aspx [Accessed 7 November 2016].
7. Toxbase, www.toxbase.org.

Rash

Differential diagnosis

System/Organism	Disease
CNS	Meningococcal septicaemia/ meningitis
Infection	Viral or fungal infection
Atopy/allergen-related	**Dermatitis and eczema**
Autoimmune	**Psoriasis**
Hormonal	**Acne vulgaris**
Fungal	**Tinea (ringworm)**
Others	**Lichen planus** Scabies Molluscum contagiosum Leprosy Erysipelas **Bullous disease:** **Dermatitis herpetiformis** **Pemphigoid** **Pemphigus vulgaris** Measles
Yeast	**Pityriasis rosacea** **Pityriasis versicolor**
Systemic	Skin manifestations of systemic disease **Erythema nodosum** **Herpes simplex** **Drug-related rashes:** **Erythema Multiforme**

Table 3.82: Differential diagnosis of rash

The most important differential to consider in medicine is meningococcal septicaemia or meningitis (see section on fever). The more chronic skin conditions are generally managed in General Practice and thus may be encountered by an F2 doctor doing a GP placement. However, many hospital inpatients will also have co-existing skin complaints, which can significantly impact on their quality of life, so a basic understanding of their management is important for all doctors.

Dermatitis and eczema

Epidemiology

Affects around 3% of the population, and 10% of children aged under 5 years. It is a relapsing condition that often starts in infancy and continues into adulthood.

Aetiology

A mixture of polygenic inheritance and environmental influences. If one parent is atopic the risk for children developing the condition is 30% but this increases to 50% if both parents are affected. Strong detergents, chemicals, animal fur, house mites and woollen clothes can exacerbate the condition in particular individuals and dairy products may precipitate the rash in some children.

Pathophysiology

An inflammatory response within the skin to an exogenous agent, heightened by an endogenous sensitivity in some individuals to react to environmental allergens. There is often a familial tendency towards atopy, with family members having an induced incidence of co-existing asthma, hay fever, conjunctivitis, or eczema.

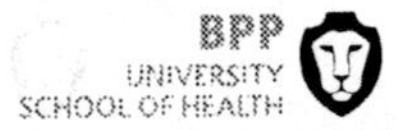

There are three types of dermatitis:

1. Contact dermatitis, resulting from a response to irritants or an allergic reaction
2. Seborrhoeic dermatitis
3. Atopic dermatitis

History/examination

- A diffuse rash with patchy, irritating and occasionally painful lesions. It is associated with erythema, oedema, dry and flaky skin.
- There may be vesicles and bullae, which can burst and leave areas which are raw and weepy.
- The most commonly affected regions are 'flexor areas, but extensor surfaces may also be involved in those with pigmented skin.
- Pruritus is common.
- Secondary bacterial infection (usually Staphylococcal) may occur, causing surrounding cellulitis.
- Around chronic lesions the skin may become thickened and scaly (lichenification).
- Histological findings reveal an initial epidermal oedema, which subsequently results in vesicle formation (more numerous on soles and palms).
- Pitting and ridging of the nail-bed is a common associated feature.

1a. Contact dermatitis (irritant):

- Results from continuous exposure to physical or chemical irritants.
- The history may be consistent with occupational exposure precipitating the rash.
- Occupations such as hairdressing, engineering and nursing are associated with an increased risk.

1b. Contact dermatitis (allergic):

- Previous allergen exposure and sensitisation is required.
- The rash will only be present where there has been allergen exposure.
- A thorough history followed by a patch test should help identify the allergen.
- Common allergens include: chromates, nickel, dyes, perfumes, plants and some preservatives found in cosmetics and creams.

2. Seborrhoeic dermatitis:

- An erythematous, pruritic, and scaly rash which involves the greasy areas of the skin such as the scalp, eyebrows, nasal and ear creases and around the head. The axillae, inframammary and perineal regions may also be involved.

3. Atopic dermatitis:

- Characterised by reaction to an environmental allergen.
- Features include asthma, rhinitis, conjunctivitis, and dermatitis.
- It affects up to 25% of individuals in the UK.
- Mainly presents in infancy and is accompanied by other atopic features.
- A positive family history is very common.
- The rash tends to affect the flexor areas and is pruritic and erythematous. Constant scratching especially in childhood can result in lichenification.

Investigations

Blood tests:

- FBC – possible eosinophilia
- Serum IgE: levels are characteristically raised

Others:

- Skin prick test: performed using common environmental allergens and usually yields positive results
- Skin swabs for microbiology MC&S may be necessary to confirm secondary infection of skin lesions

Management

- The mainstay of management is to remove or reduce exposure to the responsible agents
- Avoidance of wool clothing
- Dietary changes such as a lactose-free diet may be helpful
- Gentle soap substitutes or washing with just water
- Bath oils eg oilatum or balneum may be soothing
- Topical steroids will provide symptomatic relief.
- Aqueous or emollient cream application is often helpful eg hydromol
- Non-sedating oral anti-histamines may relieve pruritus
- Topical Tacrolimus has recently been used for mild to moderate disease
- For severe disease, systemic therapy with steroids or other immunosuppressants such as Ciclosporin or Azathioprine can be used
- Secondary infection of skin lesions may require oral antibiotics eg Flucloxacillin +/- Benzylpenicillin are commonly used

Psoriasis

Epidemiology

1–2% of individuals in the UK are affected. Usually affects ages 16–22 or 55–60. It can range from a mild form where it is not clinically obvious to a chronic and severe form where it may cause the patient to be incapacitated with severe aesthetic deformity. Occasionally it has an acute, life-threatening presentation.

Aetiology

Psoriasis is an autoimmune disease that is often associated with a positive family history. Inheritance is polygenic and influenced by environmental factors, which include:

- Infection, eg group A *Streptococcus*
- Drugs, eg Lithium
- Ultraviolet light
- Alcohol intake/smoking status

Pathophysiology

A skin biopsy illustrates an increase in skin turnover. The granular layer is usually absent and the upper epidermis consists of polymorphonuclear abscesses. There will be dermal capillary dilatation. There are several different types of psoriasis:

1. **Chronic plaque psoriasis**
   i) The most common type.
   ii) It characteristically involves pink/red scaly plaques on the extensor skin surfaces, in particular the knees and elbows, and may also involve the ears, scalp and lower back region.
   iii) New psoriatic plaque lesions tend to form at sites of skin trauma which is known as Köbner's phenomenon.
   iv) Lesions may be associated with pruritis or pain.
2. **Flexural psoriasis**
   i) Usually presents at a later age.
   ii) Well-defined, erythematous, shiny plaque lesions mainly in the flexor areas such as the groin, underneath the breasts, and in the natal cleft. However, it is not associated with scaling.
3. **Guttate psoriasis**
   i) Mostly seen in children and young adults.
   ii) Characteristically described as 'raindrop' type lesions, small circular or oval shaped plaque lesions appear around two weeks after a Streptococcal sore throat.
   iii) It has a tendency to resolve spontaneously over a two month period even if no treatment is given.
4. **Palmoplantar pustular psoriasis**
   i) Pustules confined to the hands and feet.

Erythrodermic and pustular psoriasis are the most severe forms, with diffuse and severe skin inflammation. Both forms may occur together in what is known as 'Von Zumbusch' psoriasis. These are potentially life-threatening in nature. The associated features include malaise, pyrexia, and circulatory disturbance. The pustules contain a sterile collection of inflammatory cells.

History/examination

Acute presentation:

- Multiple small skin lesions over the body, limbs, scalp, natal cleft and umbilicus.
- Lesions are round, silver and scaly in nature with an erythematous base and can be removed leaving small areas of bleeding (Auspitz sign).
- There is usually resolution over a two to four month period but a small number of patients will develop chronic lesions.
- Köbner's phenomenon may be seen.

Chronic presentation:

- Lesions (as described above) which mainly affect the extensor surfaces of the skin, in particular the back, elbows, knees and scalp, characteristically symmetrical
- Coarse pitting of the nail bed as well as onycholysis
- If the flexor regions are involved the lesions are smooth and form confluent areas which are erythematous and pruritic
- Psoriatic arthropathy affects around 5–10% of individuals with psoriasis, and may predate the skin disease. Patterns of arthropathy vary and include:
  - Asymmetrical involvement of the hands and feet
  - Symmetrical involvement, mimicking rheumatoid arthritis
  - Sacroiliitis
  - Arthritis mutilans

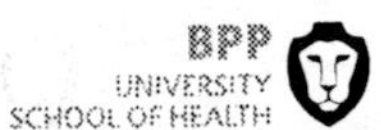

Investigations

This is a clinical diagnosis based on the appearance of the skin. There are no specific blood tests or diagnostic procedures.

Histology:

- Skin biopsy: May be performed in order to exclude other diagnoses. It will show clubbed Rete pegs if positive for the presence of psoriasis.

Management

For all patients, a thorough understanding of the disease and its chronic nature is essential. It is particularly important for individual patients to learn to identify and avoid potential relapse triggers.

A multidisciplinary approach is often required, involving secondary care level dermatological support and appropriate input to manage complications such as increased cardiovascular risk and depression.

Topical therapy:

- Salicylic acid lotion or ointment. It helps reduce hyperkeratotic and scaly lesions and it can be used as an adjunct with coal tar or dithranol.
- Coal tar paste is not commonly used because although it is an effective therapy, it causes staining of the clothes and has an offensive odour. It is available in shampoo form and is effective for scalp lesions. Baths in coal tar are very effective when there are extensive skin lesions.
- Dithranol is a skin preparation which is usually left on lesions for up to two hours. However, it can cause irritation and a low strength preparation is used initially. Again there may be staining of the skin, hair and clothes.
- Calcipotriol is a vitamin D analogue which is effective in mild to moderate psoriatic lesions.

Systemic therapy:

- PUVA is an effective treatment in clearing lesions and delaying the recurrence of the disease in chronic cases. However, it has been associated with an increased risk of skin cancer.
- Retinoids are vitamin A derivatives. Retinoid use is limited to severe cases which are resistant to other treatments. It can cause dry skin and lips associated with cracking and bleeding. Hair loss is also common. Other side effects include generalised myalgia, hepatic dysfunction and hyperlipidaemia. Retinoids are also potentially teratogenic and therefore pregnancy must be avoided for two years after taking acitretin.

Prognosis

Psoriasis is a chronic condition, where periods of stability will be interspersed with disease flares. The disease course is variable in each individual. Early onset and familial history are negative prognostic features. Increased mortality rates generally result from cardiovascular or psychological complications or the side effects of medication.

Acne vulgaris

Epidemiology

Acne vulgaris mostly affects individuals during puberty but the onset of the condition can occur up to the age of 40 years. It affects 85% people at some point during adolescence.

Aetiology

Acne vulgaris is typified by an increased size and activity of the sebaceous glands. The underlying aetiology of this is multifactorial. It is made more likely by environmental factors such as trauma, cosmetics and some medications (including topical corticosteroids). There is a postulated polygenic genetic influence, with high concordance seen in twin studies. Other influences are endocrine (hyperandrogenism), hence it is associated with polycystic ovaries in females (90%).

Pathophysiology

The rate of sebum production directly correlates with the severity of acne. Keratin can block the hair follicles and cause a build-up of sebum which results in the characteristic blackheads known as 'comedones'. An inflammatory reaction is seen at the hair follicles, which is increased by colonisation with the bacterium *Propionibacterium acnes.*

Secondary bacterial infection of these blackheads can commonly occur.

History/examination

- Acne vulgaris causes:
  - Seborrhoea
  - Comedones
  - Papules

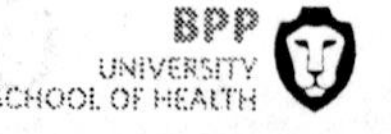

  - Pustules
  - Nodules
  - Cysts
  - Scars
- Common areas of distribution:
  - Face
  - Upper thorax
  - Shoulders
- The skin is greasy and the lesion may result in scarring which persists into adulthood.

Investigations

This is mostly a clinical diagnosis based on the findings of history and examination. There are no formal investigations for the diagnosis of acne.

Management

No treatment is required for the majority of adolescent sufferers. Keeping the face and other affected areas clean may help, but excessive washing is of no benefit.

Control of hormone secretion with the combined OCP is effective in females.

Topical treatment with Benzoyl peroxide cream, antibiotics such as Erythromycin, topical retinoids or other topical keratolytics such as salicylic acid help with the skin lesions.

Oral antibiotics such as Oxytetracycline or Erythromycin are given for at least six months and are effective in moderate disease.

After failure of the above treatment, oral Isotretinoin, a vitamin A analogue, is useful for severe disease. However, it is associated with side effects such as dry skin, myalgia, hyperlipidaemia, and hepatic dysfunction. Due to its teratogenic potential, it cannot be used in pregnancy.

Tinea (ringworm)

Epidemiology

A common condition, particularly amongst children. It is heavily contagious and commonly transmitted via skin-to-skin contact or contaminated areas such as the shower or pool. Cats are known to be carriers.

Aetiology

Fungal organisms which are present within the skin's keratin layer are mostly responsible. These incluce *Trichophyton, Microsporum* and *Epidermophyton.* The fungus grows and multiplies over the skin, nails and scalp. Depending on the body site affected, tinae pedis, tinae cruris and tinae capitis can be diagnosed.

Pathophysiology

Fungal infection of the skin.

History/examination

1. ***Tinea pedis:***
   i) The most common form and involves the inter-digital skin, especially between the fourth and fifth metatarsals
   ii) Possible nail involvement
   iii) White, fissured and pruritic lesions
   iv) Secondary streptococcal can develop, which are often recurrent
   v) May resemble atopic dermatitis
2. ***Tinea cruris:***
   i) Infection in the groin and upper, inner thigh region
   ii) Raised, discrete lesions with a scaly extending margin
   iii) Pruritic
3. ***Tinea capitis:***
   i) Localised hair loss with underlying scaling of the skin
   ii) Mostly affects pre-pubertal children – spread by close contact
   iii) Circular patches of pustular lesions
   iv) Secondary infection is common

Investigations

Others:

- Wood's light examination: can be used to illustrate fluorescence of the lesions which is characteristic in tinea capitis.

Management

- For a localised problem, topical treatment with anti-fungals such as Imidazole, Clotrimazole, Miconazole, or Terbinafine is effective.
- For a widespread problem, systemic treatment may be necessary especially if there is hair or nail involvement. For example, oral Terbinafine

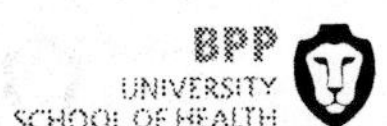

or Itraconazole tends to be effective but they are only initiated following laboratory confirmation of the diagnosis.

Pityriasis rosea

Epidemiology

Young adults are mostly affected between the ages of 10 and 30 years. The incidence is estimated at between 0.1% and 3%. However, individuals of all ages as well as both males and females are thought to be susceptible. It is an acute condition which tends to be self-limiting.

Aetiology

Tends to occur in clusters amongst close contacts. Most cases are in the spring and autumn seasons with a relatively low rate of recurrence. It is thought that although no specific bacteria, fungus or virus has been implicated, human herpes virus 6 and 7 are thought to have a role.

Pathophysiology

The exact mechanisms which result in the initiation of the disease process are poorly understood.

History/examination

- A 'herald patch' characteristically appears prior to the development of the rash. This is a distinct red brown oval shaped lesion with a scaly appearance which tends to appear over the abdomen or scapula.
- A pruritic macular rash develops at one to two weeks and tends to last up until six weeks.
  - It involves the trunk and the upper regions of the limbs (characteristically known as the 'christmas tree' distribution)
  - Lesions are oval shaped with a scaly border
  - Usually appear at natural skin creases
- Often occurs in clusters within families or in schools.
- Other accompanying features include headache, fever, nausea and fatigue.

Investigations

There are no specific investigations for diagnosis which is predominantly clinical in nature.

Management

Usually, self-resolving within six weeks and therefore requires no specific treatment.

Occasionally mild sedatives may be required to provide symptomatic relief as well as topical steroid preparations.

Lichen planus

Epidemiology

Lichen planus is not commonly encountered but it mostly affects middle-aged individuals. It tends to affect women more than men with a 3:2 ratio.

Aetiology

Cause is unknown but viral or autoimmune nature is suspected. Several drugs including anti-malarial drugs, gold, and anti-tuberculous drugs can produce similar lesions. Only half of the lesions resolve by around nine months.

Pathophysiology

The exact mechanisms which result in the initiation of the disease process are poorly understood.

Key features in the history/examination

- Pruritic and irritating rash involving the flexor surfaces of the forearm, wrist, trunk and ankles.
- Nail involvement in up to 10% of patients.
- Distinct shiny papules, which are usually purplish and polygonal in shape.
- Wickham's striae are fine white lines which pass through the lesions.
- Lesions tend to form at areas of skin excoriation or injury (Köbner's phenomenon).
- There may be widespread lesions or a few and confined to one area.
- Other areas such as the oral mucosa or nails may be involved. Characteristically, a 'lace-like' appearance in the mouth may be the only sign of the disease.
- Lesions usually resolve within six months; however, recurrence is common.

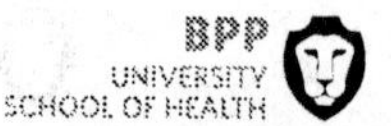

Investigations

Histology:

- Skin biopsy: lymphoid infiltration of the epidermal basal cells, with a saw-toothed appearance at the dermis-epidermis junction.

Management

Topical treatment with steroids may provide symptomatic relief until the lesions subside.

If lesions are extensive, they tend to be associated with severe pruritis which responds to systemic steroid therapy.

Rosacea

Epidemiology

Rosacea is 3 times more common in females with a peak incidence between the ages of 30 and 60.

Aetiology

It is precipitated by factors such as hot drinks, sunlight exposure, alcohol, and occasionally the use of topical steroids.

Pathophysiology

Pathological mechanisms are unclear. A number of hypotheses exist, including vascular abnormalities, degeneration of the dermal matrix and certain environmental factors, as well as microorganisms such as *Helicobacter pylori*. High levels of an abnormal form of the antimicrobial protein called cathelicidin have been reported in patients with rosacea. Studies are still ongoing to determine the role of this protein.

History/examination

- Characteristic rash over cheeks, nose, chin and forehead.
- The skin is red with papules and pustules as well as telangiectasia.

Investigations

The majority of patients with rosacea have very mild symptoms and therefore are not formally diagnosed or treated. It can mostly be diagnosed from clinical examination or with a trial of treatment in order to confirm the diagnosis when it is suspected.

Management

Long-term oxytetracycline may be effective in suppressing the rash. It is usually given for two months followed by a rest period of two months prior to re-starting therapy.

Pityriasis versicolor

Epidemiology

A common skin infection affecting around 2% to 8% of the population at some stage. It mostly affects adolescents and young adults, especially where there is a warm and humid environment.

Aetiology

Pityriasis versicolor is a yeast infection usually due to *Pityrosporum orbiculare*. This is commonly found on the skin surface and growth is encouraged by a warm and humid environment.

Pathophysiology

The exact mechanisms which result in the initiation of the disease process are poorly understood.

History/examination

- Characteristic truncal reddish-brown, scaly lesions which vary in size and can form a confluent rash.
- It can result in depigmentation despite effective treatment – may give the appearance of vitiligo.

Investigations

Histology:

- Skin scrapings: confirm the diagnosis.

Others:

- Wood's light examination: may also aid in diagnosis as it causes yellow fluorescence.

Management

- Selenium sulphide (2.5%), a topical anti-fungal, is the mainstay of treatment.
- Topical treatment with Imidazole may be required for long periods if the rash is severe.

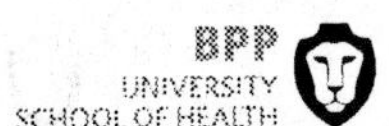

Drug-related rashes

Epidemiology

Drug-related rashes affect 1–2% of hospitalised patients.

Aetiology

Any drug can potentially cause a skin reaction, ranging from the trivial to life-threatening. The patient's medications must be considered as a cause in any patient presenting with a rash.

The most common causes are:

- Antibiotics, in particular the penicillins, which usually appears at around 10–12 days
- Penicillamine, Angiotensin converting enzyme (ACE) inhibitors, Allopurinol and Thiazides

Pathophysiology

Different individuals may react in different ways to the same drug but the features of these rashes include:

- Maculopapular (morbilliform)
- Eczematous
- Urticarial
- Purpuric

Key features in the history/examination

1. **Maculopapular rash:**
   i) The most common presentation of a drug-related reaction, with Penicillin often the causative agent.
   ii) Flat coloured lesions less than 1 cm in diameter combined with palpable lesions of less than 5 mm in diameter.
2. **Urticarial rash:**
   i) Usually caused by penicillins and aspirin.
   ii) Up to 2% of all patients receiving treatment with penicillin have a reaction.
   iii) There is a cross-reaction in one in ten penicillin-allergic patients who are treated with a cephalosporin.
   iv) It results from mast cell degranulation with histamine release as well as other vasoactive agents which cause erythema and oedema.
   v) Characteristically causes formation of pruritic erythematous wheals but widespread angio-oedema can also result.
   vi) Reactions tend to be more common in adults, who will have had a previous exposure to the drug.
   vii) Rarely, some patients have a serious anaphylactic reaction within minutes of drug exposure including hypotension, wheeze and arthralgia.
   viii) Other drugs which may potentially cause an urticarial rash include:
   - ACE inhibitors
   - Barbiturates
   - Salicylates and NSAIDs
   - Streptomycin
   - Sulphonamides
   - Tetracyclines
   - Phenothiazines
   - Chloramphenicol
3. **Purpura:**
   i) A rash resulting from capillary damage.
   ii) Usually indicative of a severe drug reaction.
   iii) Drugs which cause bone marrow suppression (including gold and carbimazole) result in thrombocytopaenic purpura.

Investigations

- Investigations guided by the patients' clinical presentation.
- Essential to take a thorough history including a full drug history as well as any previous allergies.
- A careful clinical examination will indicate any investigations which may be required.

Management

All likely drug precipitants should be stopped if at all possible.

Symptoms of pruritus respond well to oral antihistamines and mild topical steroids.

When patients have acute anaphylactic reactions (fortunately this is rare) they should be treated according to the Resuscitation Council (UK) guidelines. This involves IV fluid resuscitation and 0.5 mg Adrenaline IM injection (strength 1:1,000) as well as Chlorpheniramine and systemic steroids.

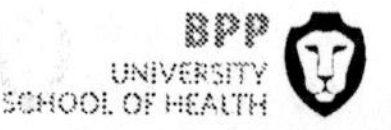

Erythema nodosum (systemic illness)

Epidemiology

Erythema nodosum is usually found in those aged 20 to 50 years and the male to female ratio is 1:5.

Aetiology

Erythema nodosum most commonly results from sarcoidosis (around one-third of cases) but it may accompany Streptococcal infection such as in rheumatic fever. It is also a feature of tuberculosis, UC and Crohn's disease. It can result from drug use such as the sulphonamides, penicillins and salicylates. Often it is idiopathic. It is commonly recurrent in nature.

Pathophysiology

A panniculitis due to an immunological reaction to a variety of different causes.

History/examination

- Characteristically there will be tender, erythematous, raised lesions on the shin which occasionally involves the thighs and upper limbs.
- The lesions change colour progressively to that similar to a bruise.
- Almost half of patients will also have arthropathy of the lower limbs.

Investigations

Blood tests:

- If sarcoidosis suspected, check calcium and serum ACE levels.

Imaging:

- CXR: bilateral lymphadenopathy if sarcoid suspected

Management

Treatment is directed towards the specific underlying cause of the disease.

Mostly symptomatic management including bed rest, elevation of the legs and using compression bandages and wet dressings, as well as non-steroidal anti-inflammatory drugs.

Where the cause is unknown, potassium iodide has been shown to be effective for persistent lesions.

Corticosteroids are used in severe cases which are unresponsive to the standard treatment.

Herpes zoster/shingles (systemic disease)

Epidemiology

Worldwide, the incidence is between 1 and 3 cases per 1,000 per year, and 4 to 12 cases per 1,000 per year in those aged over 65 years.

Aetiology

Shingles is caused by the reactivation of the varicella zoster virus.

Pathophysiology

Shingles is often precipitated by immunosuppression, which is increasingly likely in older age.

History/examination

- Cluster of blistering lesions with an erythematous base. They can become filled with pus and subsequently crust over.
- They occur within the distribution of a nerve root and tend to cause pain and tingling prior to the appearance of the lesions (can be more than one dermatome).
- The pain can be severe and intolerable.
- Prior infection with varicella zoster virus is necessary for the development of shingles as it remains latent within the dorsal root ganglia until reactivation occurs due to a reduced resistance in the host, for example, as a result of immunosuppression.
- The main complication is post-herpetic neuralgia where there is severe and persistent pain in the distribution of lesions. Eye symptoms may also arise if the ophthalmic nerve is involved.

Investigations

Diagnosis is primarily made after visual inspection of the lesions.

Blood tests:

- VZV specific IgM antibody: this is only present during chicken pox or herpes zoster and not when the virus is dormant.

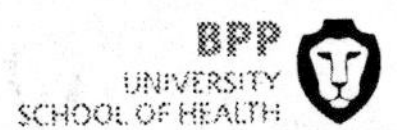

Management

- Patients require isolation from susceptible individuals at least until the lesions are crusted over in order to minimise the risk of spread.
- Oral Acyclovir should be used to hasten healing of the lesions.
- Immunosuppressed individuals must be treated with IV Acyclovir.
- Analgesia is key in symptom relief.
- Antibiotics may be required if there is secondary bacterial infection.

Post-herpetic neuralgia:

- Symptoms of neuralgia are confined to the area of skin affected by the herpes zoster rash.
- The onset of pain tends to follow the healing and crusting over of lesions.
- Gabapentin, Amitriptyline and carbamezepine are most effective for neuralgic pain.

Dermatitis herpetiformis (bullous disease)

Epidemiology

Primarily a disease with onset in the second and third decades of life.

Aetiology

Dermatitis herpetiformis is seen in patients with gluten sensitivity. Up to 80% of individuals are positive for HLA B8.

Pathophysiology

IgA is deposited in the dermal papillae. Untreated, the severity varies according to the amount of gluten ingested.

History/examination

- Intensely pruritic vesicular rash.
- The buttocks are usually affected but the extensor aspects of the elbows and knees, the interscapular region and scalp can also be affected.
- Initially there are clusters of small urticarial blistering lesions which tend to be symmetrical in nature.

Investigations

Blood tests:

- IgA antibodies: Presence of IgA antibodies will be detected.

Histology:

- Skin biopsy: This will reveal the IgA deposits.

Management

- A gluten-free diet.
- Oral Dapsone is usually used.
- Sulphonamides can also be used for the skin lesions.
- Secondary infection with bacteria is common.

Pemphigoid (bullous disease)

Epidemiology

The incidence is approximately 5/100,000 per year and the elderly population is mostly affected. It is slightly more common in women than in men.

Aetiology

An autoimmune skin disease when bullae form as a result of an immune reaction where there is formation of autoantibodies targeting the type XVII collagen portion of hemidesmosomes. It will rarely involve the mucous membranes. There is infiltration of neutrophils, lymphocytes and eosinophils.

Pathophysiology

Lesions form at the basement membrane in between the dermis and epidermis (deeper than in pemphigus vulgaris). There is deposition of IgG in the basement membrane.

History/examination

- The limbs, trunk and rarely mucous membranes are affected.
- There may be a preceding pruritis prior to the onset of lesions.
- Tense bullae (up to 3 cm), although these may be absent with signs of excoriation.
- Lesions may form in areas of skin trauma, but it does not break as easily as in pemphigus vulgaris.
- Nikolsky's sign will be negative.

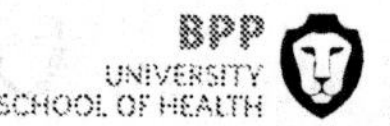

Investigations

Blood tests:

- Antibodies: Test for any antibodies against bullous pemphigoid antigens 1 and 2 (BPAG1/2).

Management

- A referral to the dermatologist.
- Oral Prednisolone is usually sufficient for control of lesions and it may be used long term in small doses.

Pemphigus vulgaris (bullous disease)

Epidemiology

A very rare condition nowadays with an incidence of less than 1/100,000 per year. It usually occurs in late-middle aged individuals.

Aetiology

An autoimmune disease where antibodies form against desmoglein which is responsible for the attachment of adjacent epidermal cells via attachment points known as desmosomes. Autoantibodies attack the desmogleins and cause separation of the cells, and hence the epidermis becomes unglued causing acantholysis. Blisters form which slough off and result in sores forming.

Pathophysiology

The epidermis is split above the basal layer and the epidermal cells degenerate. The tissue will be positive for IgG.

Key features in the history/examination

- Large, lax, superficial lesions.
- Most patients tend to present with extensive erosions of the skin with only a few progressing to form bullae.
- These lesions occur over the limbs and trunk regions.
- Oral lesions are common and may be the sole presenting feature.
- Nikolsky's sign: the superficial skin layer can be moved over the deeper skin layers causing the layers to break down and hence increasing susceptibility to infection.
- The break in the epithelium predisposes to infection.
- Lesions tend to occur where there has been a breach in the skin surface.
- Pain is often very severe.
- The patient may also present with systemic features of fever and feeling generally unwell.

Investigations

Histology:

- Skin biopsy: characteristic epidermal features

Management

- Referral to a dermatologist.
- High doses of steroids are required to control the lesions.
- Occasionally, Azathioprine and IV immunoglobulin therapy is indicated.

Erythema multiforme

Epidemiology

A common condition, with a peak incidence between 20 and 30 years.

Aetiology

The rash may be associated with drug therapy such as with Penicillin, Sulphonamides, Salicylates and Barbiturates. Infection with the herpes simplex virus for example can also result in characteristic lesions.

Pathophysiology

IgM immune complex deposition in the superficial microvasculature of the epidermis and mucous membranes.

History/examination

- Either a skin disorder alone or with systemic features such as fever, sore throat, headache, arthralgia, diarrhoea and vomiting.
- The skin rash, if present, usually follows the symptoms. It is erythematous, of varying morphology that may become bullous.
- Usually the limbs are involved first and the rash then spreads to the trunk and eventually may involve the entire body, including the buccal mucosa.
- Characteristic 'target' lesions usually occur late, which are erythematous concentric rings.

- Stevens-Johnson syndrome is a severe form of the disease where there are systemic features of the condition with multiple lesions in the oral cavity, conjunctiva, anal and genital regions.

Investigations

Diagnosis is clinical and based on the appearance of the skin lesions associated with the specific risk factors or associated pre-disposing conditions.

Histology:

- Skin biopsy: Microscopic examination of the tissue can also aid diagnosis when it is uncertain.

Management

- Usually resolves spontaneously within five to six weeks but recurrence is common.
- All drug treatment should be withdrawn as far as possible.
- Mild topical steroids are effective in reducing symptoms of pruritus.
- Those with suspected Stevens-Johnson syndrome will require systemic steroids to suppress and control the lesions.

Top tip:

1. Don't panic. 2. Listen. 3. Enjoy yourself – all branches of medicine offer the most wonderfully rewarding, varied and endlessly fascinating career. This is the dramatic side, more practically: Keep a bottle of water in the office of the ward you're on most.

Further reading and references

1. DermNet New Zealand, www.dermnetnz.org.
2. National Institute for Health and Clinical Excellence. (2004) *Frequency of application of topical corticosteroids for atopic eczema* (TA81). [Online]. Available from: www.nice.org.uk/guidance/ta81 [Accessed 7 November 2016].
3. National Institute for Health and Clinical Excellence. (2004) *Tacrolimus and pimecrolimus* (TA82). [Online]. Available from: www.nice.org.uk/guidance/ta82 [Accessed 7 November 2016].
4. National Institute for Health and Clinical Excellence. (2007) *Atopic eczema in children* (CG057). [Online]. Available from: www.nice.org.uk/guidance/cg57 [Accessed 7 November 2016].
5. National Institute for Health and Clinical Excellence. (2007) *Adalimumab for the treatment of psoriatic arthritis* (TA125). [Online]. Available from: www.nice.org.uk/guidance/ta125 [Accessed 7 November 2016].
6. National Institute for Health and Clinical Excellence. (2008) *Infliximab for the treatment of adults with psoriasis* (TA134). [Online]. Available from: www.nice.org.uk/guidance/ta134 [Accessed 7 November 2016].
7. Resuscitation Council (UK). (2008) *Advanced Life Support*. 5th Edition. London: Resuscitation Council.

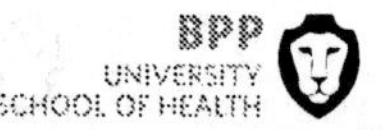

Seizures

Differential diagnosis

System/Organ	Disease
Neurological	Epilepsy Structural brain lesion eg post-stroke, space occupying lesion (SOL) and tumour
Cardiovascular	Seizure-type activity during syncope SAH Intracerebral haemorrhage
Infective	Meningitis Encephalitis Abscess
Drugs/Toxins	Alcohol
Metabolic	Disorders of glucose, calcium, sodium Hypoxia

Table 3.83: Differential diagnosis of seizures

Seizures consist of abnormal sudden synchronous discharge of neurons in the cerebral cortex.

Epilepsy

A chronic condition characterised by recurrent, ie two or more, unprovoked seizures. There is more than one type of epilepsy and they all have differences in clinical features and the way they are managed. Diagnosis is usually made by a neurologist and the history plays a major part in this.

Epidemiology

Prevalence varies around the world but it is thought to be about 10/1,000 in the UK with about 600,000 people in the UK having epilepsy. The overall incidence is 50/100,000 per year with bionodal peaks in younger and older age groups. However, alcohol can precipitate epilepsy at any age.

Aetiology

Primary idiopathic epilepsy is likely to have a polygenic underlying cause, but this is not well understood. Chromosomal causes, such as trisomy 21 and single gene inheritance as in tuberous sclerosis (on chromosomes 9 and 16) and neurofibromatosis (on chromosomes 17 and 22), also exist.

Cerebrovascular disease is the commonest cause of adult-onset epilepsy, with a greater seizure risk seen with SAH and intracerebral haemorrhage than ischaemia. Perinatal insults such as hypoxia and cerebral infections (CMV, *Toxoplasmosis gondii,* bacterial meningitis, HIV, malaria or cystercicosis) can all result in epilepsy.

Other causes include:

- Trauma
- Benign or malignant intracerebral tumours
- Neurodegenerative diseases
- Metabolic or toxic causes eg alcohol or hypoglycaemia

Pathophysiology

The first fit:

A single fit does not make a diagnosis of epilepsy, but does warrant careful investigation. Making the diagnosis can be difficult, and a careful history and examination needs to be conducted. Unless the fit has happened in front of you and therefore you have observed the prodrome, the seizure and the aftermath, then the key will be a witness account. You must try hard to find and contact any witnesses, and if referring on to a neurology or 'first fit' clinic, stress the importance of taking the witness along.

If the examination, blood tests and ECG are normal it is safe to discharge the patient and perform the rest of the investigations and consider management as an outpatient in the first fit clinic. However, some red flags necessitate admission:

- More than one seizure in 24 hours
- Failure to make a full recovery
- Focal neurological signs
- Pregnancy/post-partum seizures, which carry a risk of being the presentation of eclampsia or cerebral venous thrombosis
- Evidence suggestive of intracerebral sepsis

Classification:

Epilepsy can be classified into partial and generalised. Generalised seizures involve synchronised electrical discharge in both hemispheres and these seizures always involve impairment of consciousness. Partial seizures refer to focal electrical abnormalities within

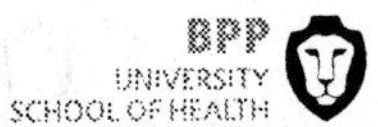

a part of the brain. However, partial seizures can progress to become secondarily generalised. It is important to make a specific diagnosis as treatments and prognosis differ between different subtypes.

Type of epilepsy	Subtypes
Partial Seizures	**Simple Partial:** No loss of consciousness. Flushing and sweating. Feelings of fear, panic, sadness, happiness, or feeling detached from what's going on around you. Experiencing smells and tastes. Flashbacks. 'Deja vu' and 'jamais vu'.
	Complex Partial: Impairment of consciousness. Automatisms such as chewing, swallowing and lip-smacking. Staggering around and wandering off.
	Generalised: Temporal lobe epilepsy – may be simple, partial, complex partial (if bilateral) or become secondarily generalised.
Generalised Epilepsy	**Absence Seizures:** Sudden loss of awareness, lasting only a few seconds, sometimes many times daily. Staring, eyelid flickering is seen. Formally called 'petit mal seizures'.
	Tonic: Rhythmical shaking of limbs and head. This may be a focal or generalised epilepsy.
	Clonic: Stiffness and extension of limbs and neck. This may be a focal epilepsy with focal signs or generalised.
	Tonic-clonic: The 'classical' seizure whereby there is an initial clonic phase followed by a tonic phase.
	Atonic: Synonymous with 'drop attacks'.

Table 3.84: The different subtypes of partial and generalised seizures

History/examination

Prodrome:

- What was the patient doing at the time
- Standing/sitting/lying
- Unusual behaviour
- Unusual movements
- Other symptoms eg pallor/palpitations

Fit:

- Injuries: lateral tongue bite
- Urinary incontinence
- Loss of consciousness
- Witness description of seizure

Afterwards:

- What do you remember next?
- Duration of confusion
- Any focal neurology

Important to check:

- Past history (problems with birth, cerebral infections, stroke)
- Family history
- Drug history

The examination will most likely be normal between seizures, but a full neurological examination is mandatory.

Investigations

Blood tests:

- FBC
- U&Es
- LFTs
- Glucose, magnesium and calcium levels: are important to exclude a cause for the seizure
- CK levels: usually raised post-ictally
- Prolactin: not a reliable indicator

Imaging:

- CT brain: to exclude underlying structural abnormality.
- MRI brain: more sensitive to exclude an underlying structural abnormality. The NICE considers this to be the neuroimaging modality of choice.

Others:

- ECG: any underlying cardiac arrhythmia.
- EEG: The inter-ictal EEG may be normal but it may show characteristic abnormalities such as the three per second spike and wave pattern seen in primary generalised epilepsy. It should be used as a tool to support the diagnosis where there is clinical suspicion and to help define the subtype of epilepsy.

Management

- Multidisciplinary management involving a Nurse Specialist, Consultant Neurologist and General Practitioner (GP).
- Information and education to patients and their relatives in verbal and written form.

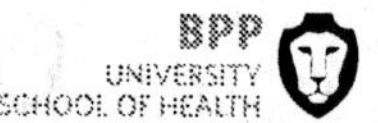

- Patients should be empowered and involved in treatment decisions, and a management plan agreed.
- Information should be given about the possible side effects of medications and the importance to withdraw them only under medical supervision.
- There are many online resources eg Epilepsy Action that patients may find useful.
- Advice needs to be given about driving. The patient needs to be informed that it is their responsibility to inform the DVLA and refrain from driving. This is best done in front of a witness and must be clearly documented in the medical notes.
- For an 'incidental' seizure on the ward in a known epileptic, it may be normal for them but it is important to ensure safety and privacy during the fit. Only intervene if the seizure is prolonged or unusual for them. This emphasises the importance of taking a good history, even if seizures are not the presenting complaint.

Pharmacological treatments:

Drug treatments should almost always be initiated and monitored by a specialist. Different medications are preferred in different subtypes of epilepsy and, once interactions and side-effect profiles are taken into consideration, the precise management will be tailored to the individual. This has been shown in recent trials such as the 'Study of Standard and New Anti-Epileptic Drugs (SANAD), 2007'. Some examples of the current practice are:

1. Partial seizures: Carbamazepine, Lamotrigine, Valproate
2. Absence seizures: Lamotrigine, Valproate
3. Tonic-clonic: valproate, lamotrigine, carbamazepine, levetiracetam, phenytoin

Side effects of pharmacological treatments:

All AEDs cause side effects that range from trivial to serious. Patients should be made aware of these during discussions about management options.

- Common, non-specific: nausea and vomiting, diarrhoea and rash as well as ataxia and nystagmus in toxicity
- Induction of the cytochrome P450 enzymes with Phenytoin, Carbamazapine and Phenobarbital (especially important in patients taking Warfarin, Theophylline and the OCP)
- Carbamazapine: diplopia in toxicity
- Lamotrigine: Stevens-Johnson syndrome
- Phenytoin: gum hypertrophy
- Vigabatrin: visual field defects

Withdrawal of pharmacological treatments:

- This should always be done under the supervision of a specialist team.
- Should be done slowly and one drug at a time.
- Risk of recurrence of seizures is greatest in the first six months and in the presence of a structural brain lesion.
- Again patients must be warned about stopping driving and referred to the DVLA guidelines.

Status epilepticus:

Classically defined as a seizure lasting longer than 30 minutes, or a series of seizures without regaining consciousness. However, since most seizures last less than two minutes there has recently been a move to define a seizure lasting longer than five minutes as impending status and treat. Status epilepticus is a medical emergency which, without prompt, effective treatment, carries a significant mortality. The longer the seizure is allowed to continue, the more refractory to treatment they become and the higher the risk of morbidity. Management involves:

- A to E assessment, ensuring patent airway and IV access
- Local policies differ, but a typical sequence of medications might be:
  - IV lorazepam
  - Phenytoin infusion
  - Paraldehyde IM
  - General anaesthetic
- IV glucose if hypoglycaemic
- Thiamine IV if alcohol thought to be contributory
- AED levels and ABG
- Urine toxicology if appropriate

Pregnancy and epilepsy:

- Women of childbearing age should be given information in advance of commencing AED treatment.
- Many AEDs are enzyme-inducers and reduce the efficacy of oral contraceptive agents, in particular the progesterone only pill, so contraception failure is more likely.
- The risk of seizure-associated mortality is increased during pregnancy and there is a 50% infant and 30% maternal mortality with status epilepticus.

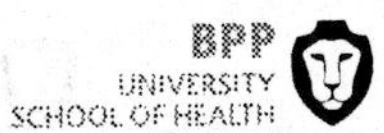

AEDs should therefore be continued during pregnancy.

- Pregnancy is related to an increase in seizure frequency. This is in part due to the fall in the levels of some AED during the second and third trimesters. This is particularly important with Lamotrigine.
- AEDs are linked to congenital malformations eg neural tube defects with Valproate use and a reduced IQ in childhood, again especially with Valproate.
- Give folic acid supplementation.
- Give vitamin K during the last four weeks of pregnancy.
- Encourage registration with the UK Epilepsy
- and Pregnancy Register which aims to collate information about the frequency of major malformations in children whose mothers take AEDs.
- If status epilepticus occurs during pregnancy or delivery, an emergency C-section should be performed.
- The AED dose may need reducing post-partum if it has been increased during pregnancy.
- AEDs are found in breast milk but this should not be seen as a contraindication during breast-feeding.

Prognosis

Epilepsy is a chronic condition which requires sensitive multidisciplinary management in view of the social implications, multiple medication side-effects and issues around pregnancy.

It is associated with a raised SMR, especially in the under-40s and those with severe epilepsy. This is thought to be due to:

- SUDEP
  - The mechanism is not understood.
  - Male sex and poor medication concordance increase the risk but it is not seen in idiopathic epilepsy in childhood.
- Accidental death eg trauma and drowning
- Suicide, especially in severe and temporal lobe epilepsy

Further reading and references

1. Drivers Medical Group. (2009) *For Medical Practitioners: At a glance guide to the current medical standards of fitness to drive.* Swansea, DVLA.
2. UK Epilepsy and Pregnancy Register, www.epilepsyandpregnancy.co.uk.
3. Epilepsy Action, www.epilepsy.org.uk.
4. National Institute for Health and Clinical Excellence. (2004) *The epilepsies: diagnosis and management of the epilepsies in adults in primary and secondary care* (CG020). [Online]. Available from: www.nice.org.uk/guidance/cg20 [Accessed 7 November 2016].
5. Al-Kharusi, A.M., Alwaidh, M., Marson, A.G., et al. (2007) The SANAD study of effectiveness of valproate, lamotrigine, or topiramate for generalised and unclassifiable epilepsy: an unblinded randomised controlled trial. Lancet 2007; 369: 1000–1015.

Top tip:

I'd say strive for perfection but don't beat yourself up if it's not always possible. No wait, better, buy nurses chocolates and make friends with the ones who can do bloods.

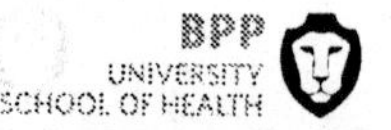

Weakness and paralysis

Differential diagnosis

System/Organ	Disease
Common	**Stroke/Transient Ischaemic Attack** **Multiple Sclerosis** **Guillain-Barré syndrome** **Motor Neurone Disease** **Myasthenia gravis** **Spinal cord compression/Trauma**
Other	Vitamin deficiency Hyponatraemia Hypocalcaemia

Table 3.85: Differential diagnosis of weakness and paralysis

Stroke/transient ischaemic attack

The World Health Organization defines stroke as 'a clinical syndrome consisting of rapidly developing clinical signs of focal (or global in case of coma) disturbance of cerebral function lasting more than 24 hours or leading to death with no apparent cause other than a vascular origin'.

TIA has been traditionally defined as a focal neurological impairment lasting less than 24 hours; however, it has been increasingly recognised that a cut-off of 1 hour is more appropriate.

Epidemiology

150,000 people per year have a stroke in the UK (approximately 1 every 5 minutes). It is the third highest cause of mortality in the UK, and the most common cause of disability.

In England, the estimated annual incidence of TIA is 150–200 per 100,000 per year; however, this is likely to be an underestimate as a number will go either unnoticed or unreported.

Stroke and TIA predominantly affects those over 65 but 1,000 people under the age of 30 suffer a stroke per year. One in four women and one in five men will have a stroke if they live to be 85.

Aetiology

There are two types of stroke:

	Ischaemic (85–90%)	Haemorrhagic (10–15%)
Modifiable risk factors	Smoking Hypertension Diabetes mellitus Hyperlipidaemia Atrial fibrillation Valvular heart disease Coagulopathy (eg antiphospholipid syndrome, Systemic Lupus Erythematosus (SLE)	Smoking Hypertension Diabetes mellitus Alcohol excess Drug treatments – ie anticoagulants
Unmodifiable risk factors	Increasing age Race – African, Asian, Afro-Caribbean Previous history of stroke/TIA Increasing age	Amyloid angiopathy Race – African, Asian, Afro-Caribbean Berry aneurysms Arterio-venous malformation

Table 3.86: Ischaemic and haemorrhagic stroke types

Pathophysiology

Acute ischaemic stroke is caused by a thrombosis, either from rupture of atherosclerotic plaque or from an embolus (eg caused by atrial fibrillation or carotid artery plaque). Both of these lead to an occlusion in an intracranial artery (most commonly the middle cerebral artery) causing ischaemia. An ischaemic stroke may also occur at a 'watershed' area between the distribution of two cerebral arteries (typically the middle and posterior) following a period of hypotension causing hypoperfusion of these areas. Haemorrhagic stroke is caused by vascular rupture leading to bleeding into either the subarachnoid space or an intra-paranchymal haemorrhage. An infarct may show 'haemorrhagic transformation' whereby the initial infarct triggers a secondary haemorrhage.

TIA shares a common aetiology and pathophysiology with ischaemic stroke.

History/examination

- Time and date of onset of symptoms
- Duration of symptoms
- Risk factors for cerebrovascular disease
- Contraindications to thrombolysis

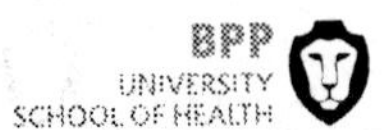

- Premorbid level of social functioning, eg walking, washing and dressing, existing care package
- Left or right handedness
- General examination: pulse rate and rhythm, neck bruits, fundoscopy, gait
- MMSE
- Examine using National Institute of Health Stroke Scale (NIHSS) or ABCD2 score for TIA
- Full, detailed neurological examination
- Examination will need to be repeated to document any recovery
- Strokes are commonly classified clinically using the Bamford/Oxford Community Stroke Project Classification

Item	Score range
Level of consciousness (LOC) 1a.LOC questions 1b.LOC commands	0–3 0–2 0–2
Best gaze	0–2
Visual fields	0–3
Facial weakness	0–3
Motor arm	0–4 (right and left)
Motor leg	0–4 (right and left)
Limb ataxia	0–2
Sensory loss	0–2
Body language	0–3
Dysarthria	0–2
Extinction and inattention	0–2

Table 3.87: NIHSS

A	Age	> 59	1 point
B	BP on presentation	Systolic >139 mmHg or Diastolic >89 mmHg	1 point
C	Clinical Features	Unilateral weakness Speech disturbance without weakness Other	2 points 1 point 0 point
D	Duration	>59 minutes 10–59 minutes <10 minutes	2 points 1 point 0 point
D	Diabetes	Presence	1 point

Table 3.88: ABCD score for TIA

OCSP	Clinical features	Vascular basis
Total Anterior Circulation Syndrome 20% of strokes	Higher cortical dysfunction (visual neglect or dysphasia) and Hemiparesis in at least two of face/arm/leg and Homonymous hemianopia	Usually proximal middle cerebral artery or internal carotid artery
Partial Anterior Circulation Syndrome 35% of strokes	Isolated higher cortical dysfunction or two out of: higher cortical dysfunction, hemiparesis, homonymous hemianopia	Usually branch middle cerebral artery occlusion
Posterior Circulation Syndrome 25% of strokes	Isolated homonymous hemianopia or Brain stem (cranial nerve palsies). May have contralateral motor/sensory deficit Bilateral motor/sensory deficit or Cerebellar signs	Occlusion of vertebral, basilar, cerebellar or posterior cerebral artery
Lacunar Syndrome 20% of strokes	Pure motor stroke or Pure sensory stroke or Sensorimotor stroke or Ataxic hemiparesis May be 'silent' and asymptomatic	Usually thrombosis occluding a smaller, deeper artery

Table 3.89: The Bamford/Oxford Stroke Classification

Sensorimotor signs:

- Unilateral upper and lower limb weakness and facial drooping are indicative of stroke
- Pronator drift
- Unilateral sensory impairment in upper and lower limb or face

Speech signs:

- Aphasia
- Dysphasia (expressive or receptive)
- Dysarthria

Opthalmic signs:

- Eye movements
- Visual neglect
- Partial visual field loss

Cerebellar signs:

- Ataxia
- Nystagmus
- Past-pointing
- Dysdiadochokinesis

Investigations

Blood tests:

- FBC
- ESR
- U&Es
- LFTs
- Bone profile
- TFT
- Glucose: to exclude hypoglycaemia as cause of symptoms
- Lipid profile
- If no clear cause for the stroke, especially in the younger age group, check thrombophilia screen, vasculitis and antiphospholipid screen and haemoglobin electrophoresis for sickle cell anaemia. Consider HIV testing with appropriate consenting

Imaging:

- CXR
- CT brain: to identify aetiology of stroke. An acute infarct may not be clearly visible
- MRI brain may be required in cases of diagnostic doubt and especially in cases of brainstem stroke
- Carotid dopplers

Others:

- ECG – to check for dysrhythmia such as atrial fibrillation
- Echocardiography – this may be a 'bubble ECHO' to exclude a patent Foramen Ovale, especially if no risk factors found for stroke
- 24 hour tape if paroxysmal arrhythmia suspected

Management

Acute management of ischaemic stroke:

- A to E assessment.
- Oxygen therapy if saturations are less than 94%.
- Thrombolysis using alteplase following local policy – if onset of symptoms within three hours and no contraindications for thrombolysis. This may involve transport to a tertiary thrombolysis centre.

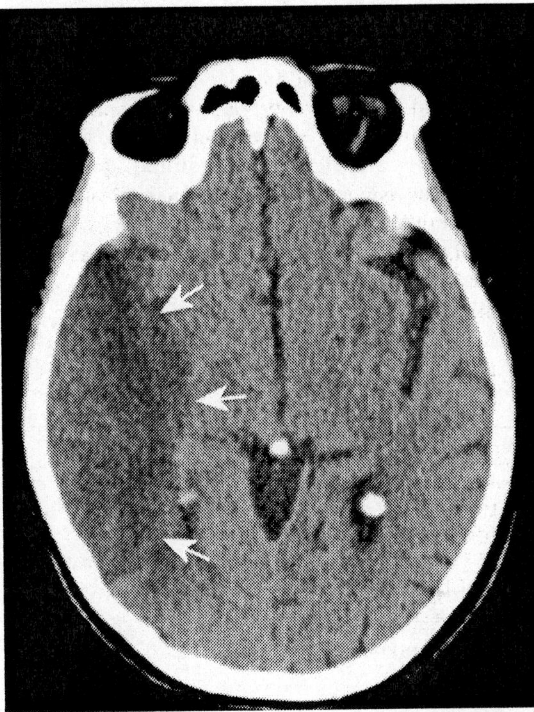

Figure 3.50: Non-contrast CT head showing a large area of hypo density in the right temporo-parietal lobe (arrows) in keeping with an acute ischaemic infarct in the middle cerebral artery territory

Acute management of haemorrhagic stroke:

- A to E assessment
- Oxygen therapy if saturations are less than 94%
- Discuss with neurosurgeons as surgery may be required

Acute management of TIA:

- There will be a local protocol for the precise pathway to follow in the Emergency Department.
- Broadly:
  - If ABCD2 score 3 or less, refer as outpatient to TIA clinic for investigation
  - If ABCD2 score 4 or more, admit for urgent investigations (eg carotid Doppler)

All patients with stroke are best managed on a multidisciplinary stroke unit, which has proven to result in reduced death and disability. Interventions should include:

- Swallow assessment – if suspicious of a swallowing deficit, this should be initially assessed during the initial clerking procedure, and onward referral

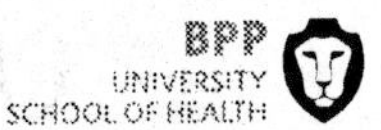

made to Speech and Language Therapy (SLT) if required
- Early mobilisation
- Early involvement of physiotherapy
- Early nutritional assessment and consideration of naso-gastric feeding if required
- Early detection and correction of physiological derangements – ie pyrexia
- Early discharge planning in a multidisciplinary setting

A stroke can be a traumatic and upsetting experience for the patient and family, therefore appropriate psychological support is essential:

- Verbal and written information should be given about the diagnosis.
- The patient and family should be involved as much as possible in treatment, goal-setting and discharge planning.
- Details of the stroke association and other national and local support groups should be given.

Secondary prevention – stroke and TIA:

- Lifestyle changes including smoking cessation, exercise and weight loss
- Antiplatelet treatment: aspirin 300 mg for the first 14 days followed by clopidogrel 75 mg after both stroke or TIA unless contraindicated
- Aim for tight blood pressure control
- Lower cholesterol
- Consider anticoagulation with rivaroxaban or warfarin if atrial fibrillation cause of ischaemic stroke
- Carotid Doppler followed by carotid endarterectomy if indicated

Prognosis

TIA – overall risk of progression to full stroke within 3 months is 11% but is dependent on the ABCD2 score

ABCD2 Score	7 day mortality	3 month mortality
0–3	1%	3%
4–5	6%	10%
6–7	12%	18%

Table 3.90: 7 day and 3 month mortality according to ABCD2 score

Stroke – varies according to the clinical stroke syndrome as well as co-morbidities

	TACS		PACS		LACS		POCS	
	30 day	1 year	30 day	1 year	30 day	1 year	30 day	1 year
Death	40	60	5	15	5	10	5	20
Dependent	55	35	40	30	40	30	30	20
Independent	5	5	55	55	65	60	65	60

Table 3.91: Percentage mortality and morbidity post-stroke, from the Bamford classification

Haemorrhagic – significantly higher mortality and morbidity than ischaemic stroke

Multiple sclerosis (MS)

Epidemiology

MS is predominantly a disease of young adults with a mean age of onset 29–33 years old. It affects more women than men with a male:female ratio of 3:2. There is a prevalence of 110 per 100,000 in the UK and it is more common in Caucasians. 67% of patients present with relapsing remitting illness, 5–10% have benign disease course with infrequent relapses and 11% of patients have a gradual disease progression from outset.

Aetiology

MS is an autoimmune disease affecting the white matter in the CNS thought to be triggered by genetic and environmental factors. It is 20–40% more common in first degree relatives. Genes in Human Leucocyte Antigen and Interleukin region are thought to be involved.

Environmental factors implicated:

- Toxins
- Viral exposure – although none have been found to be causative
- Sunlight exposure

A diagnosis of MS is not made on the first presentation of focal demyelination. The first episode is considered a clinically isolated syndrome; a diagnosis of MS requires subsequent relapses involving different parts of the CNS. The exception is where radiological imaging demonstrates temporal and anatomical dispersal of demyelination.

Relapses may be triggered by infections, post-partum changes, surgical procedures, trauma and stress.

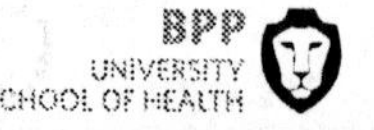

Three clinical patterns of MS are recognised:

- Relapsing and remitting (80%)
- Secondary progressive
- Primary progressive

Pathophysiology

Relapsing-remitting MS is believed to be an autoimmune disease mediated by T-cells against the myelin sheath although it appears that B-cells also play a part.

CD4 T cells are thought to become activated in the peripheral blood system and migrate across the blood-brain barrier where they react with the myelin sheath. This causes the release of cytokines which activate macrophages and B-cells that cause inflammation and leads to the destruction of oligodendrocytes with demyelination of the axons.

Destruction of the myelin sheath leads to slowing in nerve conduction which leads to symptoms of relapse. Inflammation eventually subsides and sheaths remyelinate. However, over time the axons die, leaving progressive neurological deficits (secondary progressive disease).

History/examination

There are a wide range of signs and symptoms dependent on the site of inflammation in the brain or spinal cord and residual physical dysfunction following previous relapses:

- Fatigue
- Weakness
- Clumsiness
- Visual disturbances
- Dizziness
- Poorly defined paraesthesiae
- Weakness or numbness in one or more limb
- 25% present with optic neuritis
- L'hermitte phenomenon – electric shock sensations in spine, arms or legs following flexion of neck
- Internuclear ophthalmoplegia may be present
- Optic atropy – optic disc pallor, decreased visual acuity, decreased colour vision, relative afferent papillary defect and central scotoma
- Diplopia
- Spasticity

Investigations

Blood tests:

- Baseline FBC, U&Es, LFTs
- ESR and CRP
- ANA, ANCA, Rheumatoid Factor, ENA and Anti-dsDNA
- TFTs
- B_{12}
- Antiphospholipid and anticardiolipin antibodies

Imaging:

MRI brain and spinal cord: are the most important diagnostic test. Multiple hyperdense regions are seen, usually in the periventricular white matter, especially on the FLAIR sequences.

Others:

- Lumbar Puncture: determine CSF cell count, protein and oligoclonal IgG (present in 98% of patients with MS)
- EEG: delayed visual evoked potentials in 80–90% of patients

Clinical presentation	Additional data needed
2+ relapses and evidence of 2+ objective lesions on MRI	None
1 relapse and evidence of 1 objective lesion on MRI	Positive CSF and 2+ lesions demonstrated on MRI or a further relapse
Insidious neurological progression suggestive of MS	Positive CSF and MRI evidence of: 9+ lesions in brain or 2+ lesions in spinal cord or 4–8 lesions in brain and 1 lesion in spinal cord

Table 3.92: Modified McDonald Criteria

Management

- Patient education, empowerment and participation in the decision-making process
- Support for patient, family and carers
- Provide information about support groups for instance the Multiple Sclerosis Society
- Multidisciplinary involvement:
  - Neurologist
  - GP
  - Occupational therapist
  - Specialist pain service
  - Physiotherapist

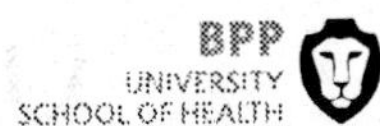

  - Psychologist
  - Acute exacerbations: corticosteroids
- Treatment of symptoms:
  - Depression: antidepressants (SSRIs etc as appropriate)
  - Pain: Gabapentin, Pregabalin, Amitriptyline
  - Spasticity: Baclofen, Dantrolene, Diazepam, Tizanidine, Botulinum toxin, physiotherapy
  - Bladder disturbance: Oxybutanin, Tolterodine, catherisation
  - Tremor: Clonazepam, Primidone
  - Erectile dysfunction: Sildenafil
- Disease modification treatment:
  - NICE guidelines recommend Nataluzimab for rapidly evolving and severe relapsing-remitting MS
  - Dimethyl fumarate, Teriflunomide or fingolimod are recommended for active, but not rapidly progressing relapsing-remitting disease
  - Alemtuzumab is an option for relapsing-remitting disease
  - NICE guidelines do not recommend the uses of interferon-beta and glatiramer acetate.
  - In aggressive diseases that do not respond to Nataluzimab other immunosuppressants may be used such as Cyclo-phosphamide.

Prognosis

The prognosis is improving with aggressive treatment of relapses, but it is still the case that 10 years after diagnosis, 10% of patients are wheelchair-bound and around half are unable to maintain employment.

Guillain-Barré (acute inflammatory demyelinating polyradiculopathy or AIDP)

Epidemiology

This is the most common neuromuscular cause of paralysis. There is a prevalence 1–2/100,000 per year with males being affected more than females. There are bimodal age peaks at 15–35 and 50–75.

Aetiology

Two-thirds of patients have a history of recent gastro-intestinal or respiratory infection in the preceding one to three weeks. Infections include:

- *Camplyobacter jejuni*
- Heptatis B
- Cytalomegavirus
- *Mycoplasma pneumoniae*
- Epstein-barr virus
- Varicella-zoster
- HIV

Other risk factors include post-partum and malignancies such as lymphoma and vaccinations.

Pathophysiology

Cellular and humoral immune mechanisms are implicated. It is proposed that the preceding infection leads to a production of antibodies to specific gangliosides and glycolipids. Antibodies react with myelin to cause demyelination.

History/examination

- A rapidly progressive ascending weakness
- Weakness reported in 60% of cases in 1–3 weeks following infection reaching its peak at around 4 weeks after onset
- Back or leg pain
- Sensory loss starting in lower limb
- Paralysis starting in lower limbs
- Dyspnoea
- Shortness of breath
- Ascending and symmetrical weakness varying in severity from minimal, to tetraplegia with respiratory paralysis
- Hypotonia
- Absent or reduced reflexes
- Facial weakness

Autonomic changes can include the following:

- Tachy/bradycardia
- Facial flushing
- Paroxysmal hypertension
- Orthostatic hypotension
- Anhidrosis and/or diaphoresis

40% of patients present with respiratory or pharyngeal weakness:

- Dyspnoea
- Shortness of breath
- Slurred speech
- Dysphagia

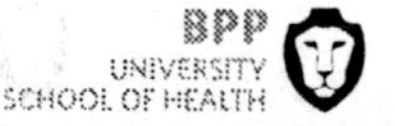

Investigations

Blood tests:

- FBC
- U&Es
- Inflammatory markers – CRP and ESR
- Anti-GQ1b if Miller-Fisher variant suspected

Microbiology:

- If any evidence of ongoing infection, send relevant samples

Imaging:

- MRI (usually if diagnostic doubt)

Other:

- ECG: variety of arrhythmias
- Lumbar puncture: CSF will show elevated protein (may be absent in first week of disease)
- Nerve conduction studies
- Spirometry: vital capacity measurements govern the need for ventilation

Management

- Intubation and assisted ventilation in patients with respiratory weakness and paralysis necessary in around 30% of patients
- Plasma exchange
- Immunoglobulin infusion
- IV Methylprednisolone (although studies have shown no benefit)
- Recognition, treatment and prevention of complications are as important as any treatment:
  - Monitor forced vital capacity 4 hourly (<15 ml/ Kg indication for ventilation)
  - DVT prophylaxis
  - Physiotherapy
  - Occupational therapist
  - Speech and language therapy swallow assessment
  - Pain – non-steroidal antiflammatory drugs, amitryptiline, carbamazepine, gabapentin, opiates

Prognosis

Mortality of 5%

Motor neurone disease

Epidemiology

This is a relatively rare disease with approximately 5,000 cases in the UK at any one time. There is increased risk with age and the incidence is highest between the ages 55 to 75. Motor neurone disease (MND) is 50% more common in males than females.

Aetiology

The cause and pathology behind MND is not very well understood. It is thought to be due to interplay between genetics and exogenous factors. Familial MND tends to have an earlier onset and about 20% of cases have mutations in the copper/zinc superoxide dismutase gene. Other genetic variants have been found but only in very small numbers.

Potential environmental factors:

- Physical activity
- Smoking
- Mechanical and electrical injury
- Exposure to neurotoxins
- Occupations – farmer, military service, professional football

The symptoms of MND are caused by degeneration of Betz cells, pyramidal tracts, cranial nerve nuclei and anterior horn cells.

Pathophysiology

Pathophysiology is dependent on the aetiology.

History/examination

Lower limb onset:

- Difficulty in walking
- Unsteadiness
- Foot drop
- Tendency to stumble
- Heaviness
- Stiffness in one or more limbs

Upper limb onset:

- Loss of functional hand dexterity
- Poor grip
- Proximal arm weakness
- Muscle wasting particularly in the hands
- Fascilations especially of the large proximal limbs

Bulbar onset:

- Dysarthria
- Dysphonia with nasal, hoarse or tight voice
- Dysphagia

Respiratory onset:

- Breathlessness
- Orthopnea
- Hypercapnic features from overnight hypoventilation fatigue, reduced exercise tolerance, hypersomnolence and morning headaches

On examination concurrent upper motor neurone and lower motor neurone signs in the absence of sensory impairment or pain are suggestive of MND. However, any combination of motor neurone signs may be elicited.

Upper motor neurone signs:

- Hypotonia
- Brisk reflexes
- Extensor plantar responses

Lower motor neurone signs:

- Muscle wasting
- Fasciculations
- Reduced/absent reflexes

Typically examination findings include:

- Wasting of tibialis anterior
- Wasting of small muscles of hands particularly first dorsal interosseous and thenar eminence
- Claw-like hand due to weakness of finer and wrist extensors
- Foot drop due to weak ankle dorsiflexion
- No sensory signs are found

Investigations

Blood tests:

- CK: often up to four times normal level
- TFTs: hypo- and hyperparathyroidism can mimic MND
- Serology: both HIV and Lyme disease can mimic MND

Imaging:

- MRI: for upper motor neurone signs

Other:

- Lumbar puncture: in atypical presentation to exclude inflammatory or infiltrative disease
- Electromyography (EMG): can demonstrate the extent of the disease

Management

- Patient education, empowerment and participation in the decision-making process
- Information about support groups eg the Motor Neurone Disease Association
- Multidisciplinary approach with input from:
  - Nurse specialists
  - Physiotherapist
  - Occupational therapist
  - Speech and language therapist
  - Respiratory physicians
  - Gastroenterologists
  - Palliative care team

Respiratory support:

- Early intervention with non-invasive ventilation to support and prevent hypoventilation.
- Signs indicative of requirement are nocturnal desaturation, hypercapnia and forced vital capacity less than 50%.

Nutritional support:

Signs suggestive of need for intervention:

- Aspiration
- Continued weight loss
- Choking episodes
- Tiring whilst eating

An early gastrostomy is the intervention of choice, ideally performed when forced vital capacity is greater than 50%.

Pharmacological intervention:

- Riluzole
  - NICE recommends for ALS form; however, it is often given to all forms
  - Prolongs survival by at least three months

Symptom relief:

- **Paroxysmal choking/laryngospasm:** sublingual lorazepam and positioning
- **Dyspnoea:** oral or nebulised morphine, sublingual lorazepam in conjunction with NIV

- **Difficulty coughing and clearing secretions:** nebulised saline, carbocysteine. Ensure adequate fluid intake. Suction and cough assist devices
- **Spasticity:** baclofen, dantrolene, tizanidine
- **Cramps and fasciculations:** quinine, carbemazepine, diazepam and physiotherapy
- **Drooling:** hyoscine patch, amitriptyline, atropine, botulinum toxin to salivary glands
- **Constipation:** lactulose, docusate, movicol. Ensure adequate fibre and fluid
- **Emotional lability:** amitriptyline, SSRI

Prognosis

- Variable from a number of months to ten years
- Majority of patients survive two to three years from diagnosis
- Poor prognosis is linked to age at onset and respiratory or bulbar presentation

Type	Features
Amyotrophic lateral sclerosis (ALS)	75% of cases 50% progress to bulbar Mixed upper and lower motor neurone clinical features starting in limbs
Progressive bulbar palsy (PBP)	20% of cases Most common in older women Poor prognosis
Progressive muscular atrophy (PMA)	5% of cases Lower motor neurone signs at onset More significantly common in men than women Over 50 years at onset Possible slower disease progress
Primary lateral sclerosis (PLS)	0.5% of cases Upper motor neurone signs at onset, often starting in lower limbs 50% convert to ALS Survival over 10 years is common
Flail arm syndrome	Rare Proximal lower motor neurone weakness of arms
Flail leg syndrome	Rare Lower motor neurone weakness of legs

Table 3.93: The different types of MND

Myasthenia gravis

Epidemiology

The incidence of Myasthenia gravis is approximately 10/100,000 per year. There is a bimodal distribution for age with a peak in the 20s (early onset) and a peak in the 60s (late onset). The early onset is more common in females whereas the late onset is more common in men.

Aetiology

Myasthenia gravis possibly has a genetic link. 75% of patients have some form of thymus abnormality and 50% of thymoma patients have Myasthenia gravis. Interestingly, Penicillin may induce or aggravate the disease.

There is a link to diabetes mellitus, thyrotoxicosis, rheumatoid arthritis and SLE. However, most cases are idiopathic.

Pathophysiology

The majority of patients have auto-antibodies against the acetylcholine nicotinic post synaptic receptor (AChR). These actions reduce the number of receptors and block the sodium ion channel which leads to a reduction in neurotransmission and therefore fatiguable muscle weakness. Patients become symptomatic once acetylcholine receptors are reduced to 30%. It is thought that the thymus is the site of generation of auto-antibodies but it is not known what stimulates production.

History/examination

- Generalised weakness
- Reduced exercise tolerance that improves with rest
- Initially symptoms may be intermittent occurring after repeated use of the muscle
- Full and accurate medication history – many medications may provoke exacerbations
- On examination 85% of patients have ptosis and diplopia (caused by a complex opthalmoplegia)
- The key element is the fatigueability: ask the patient to look upwards at your outstretched finger. The patient's eyelids will slowly droop over a few minutes as the muscles fatigue
- May have facial muscle involvement: mild cases – weakness of eye or lip closure; severe cases – may have expressionless face with slack muscles
- Neck muscle weakness may be present

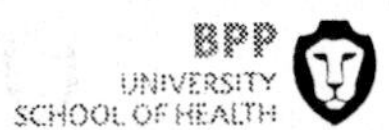

- Limbs may have proximal rather than distal weakness
- Severe presentations may have bulbar and respiratory involvement
- Severe exacerbations:
  - Lack of tone in whole body
  - Unable to lift head from chest
  - Nasal quality to voice
  - Slack, expressionless face
  - Absence of gag reflex
  - Lack of cough and presence of pneumonia

Antibiotics	Macrolides Fluroquinolones Aminoglycaside Tetracycline Chloroquine
Anti-arrhythmic	Beta-blockers Calcium channel blockers Quinidine Lignocaine Procainamide Trimethaphan
Other	Lithium Chlorpromazine Muscle relaxants Levothyroxine Adrenocorticotropic hormone (ACTH) Corticosteroids

Table 3.94: Medications reported to exacerbate Myasthenia gravis

Investigations

Blood tests:

- Serology: antibodies to AChR present in 50% of ocular patients, 85% of general patients

Imaging:

- CT: to check for thymus abnormality

Others:

- Electrophysiology: testing the reduction in evoked action potential following repetitive nerve stimulation to assist in the diagnosis. Increased 'jitter' seen in single fibre studies
- Tensilon test (rarely performed)

Management

- Acetylcholinesterase inhibitors eg pyridostigmine
- Prednisolone: commencing may exacerbate symptoms so treatment should be started as an inpatient if bulbar or respiratory symptoms present
- May require other immunosuppression/steroid sparing agents eg azathioprine
- Thymectomy

Spinal cord compression

Epidemiology

Worldwide, trauma is the most common cause of spinal chord compression. There are 4,000 cases of metastatic spinal cord compression per year in the UK. 85% of spinal cord tumours are metastatic. Spinal epidural abscess is found in 2.8 cases per 10,000 admissions which is increasing due to increased IV drug use. Osteoporosis is the commonest cause of vertebral fractures leading to spinal cord compression.

Aetiology

Can occur as a result of:

- Spinal cord trauma
- Disc herniation
- Vertebral compression fracture
- Spinal tumour – either primary or metastatic
- Infection

Commonest causes of vertebral compression fractures	Common tumours metastasising to bone	Infections
Osteoporosis Osteomyelitis Pathological fractures Corticosteroid therapy (secondary osteoporosis) Spinal subluxation Osteomalacia	Breast Bronchus Prostate Renal	Discitis Pott's disease (Tuberculosis of spine) Epidural abscess

Table 3.95: Common causes of spinal compression

Pathophysiology

Compression of the spinal cord is caused by either stretching (ie spinal cord subluxation) or pressure (ie tumour, disc herniation). Both lead to damage to the myelinated tracts and cell bodies in the spinal cord. The subsequent damage leads to reduction or cessation of sensation and motor functions.

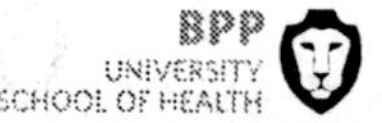

History/examination

- Acute onset suggestive of trauma or disc herniation
- Chronic onset suggestive of malignancy or osteoporosis
- History of:
  - Primary tumour that metastasises to bone
  - Bone metastases
  - IV drug use
- Numbness
- Parathesias – may be mild in early chronic forms
- Bladder and bowel dysfunction
- Signs of neurogenic shock may be present on examination in acute presentations:
  - Hypotension
  - Bradycardia
  - Warm, dry extremities
  - Peripheral vasodilation
  - Poikilothermia
  - Decreased cardiac output
- Loss of motor function and sensation distal to the spinal level
- May have local deformity of spine
- Spinal tenderness may be present
- Hyper-reflexia

Investigations

Blood tests:

- FBC: to check for signs of infection
- ESR and CRP
- Bone profile

Microbiology:

- Blood cultures if infection is suspected
- Lumbar puncture if infection is suspected

Imaging:

- CXR: to rule out lung primary
- Spinal X-ray: to check for vertebral fracture
- CT spine
- MRI spine

Management

Stabilisation and supportive treatment

Acute traumatic spinal cord injury:

- Immobilisation
- Decompression and stabilisation
- Corticosteroids – usually dexamethasone
- Prevention of complications (DVT prophylaxis, peptic ulcer prevention, physiotherapy etc)

Malignancy related options:

- Surgery to decompress
- Radiotherapy to shrink tumour
- Corticosteroids – usually dexamethasone
- Prevention of complications – as above

Infection related:

- Antibiotics based on sensitivity of organism. Most effective if continued to 12 weeks
- Surgery
- Prevention of complications – as above

Prognosis

Malignancy related recurrence rate of 7–9% with multiple metastases increasing the risk.

Infection related: there is no reported risk of recurrence.

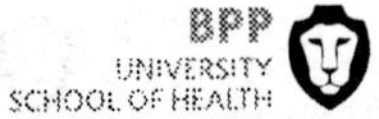

Further reading and references

1. Bamford, J., Dennis, M., Sandercock, P., et al. (1991) Classification and natural history of clinically identifiable subtypes of cerebral infarction. *Lancet* 1991; 337: 1521–6.
2. British Thoracic Society and Society of Cardiothoracic Surgeons of Great Britain and Ireland Working Party. (2001) Guidelines on the selection of patients with lung cancer for surgery. *Thorax* 2001; 56: 89–108.
3. Johnson, S.C., Nguyen-Huynh, M.N., Rothwell, P.M., et al. (2007) Validation and refinement of scores to predict very early stroke risk after transient ischaemic attack. *Lancet* 2007; 369: 283–92.
4. Motor Neurone Disease Association, www.mndassociation.org.
5. MS Society, www.mssociety.org.uk.
6. National Institute for Health and Clinical Excellence. (2002) *Multiple sclerosis – beta interferon and glatiramer acetate: guidance* (TA32). [Online] Available from: www.nice.org.uk/guidance/TA32 [Accessed 7 November 2016].
7. National Institute for Health and Clinical Excellence. (2003) *Multiple Sclerosis* (CG08). [Online] Available from: www.nice.org.uk/guidance/CG8 [Accessed 7 November 2016].
8. National Institute for Health and Clinical Excellence. (2007) *Alteplase for the treatment of acute ischaemic stroke* (TA122). [Online] Available from: www.nice.org.uk/guidance/ta122 [Accessed 7 November 2016].
9. National Institute for Health and Clinical Excellence. (2007) *Multiple sclerosis – natalizumab* (TA127). [Online]. Available from: www.nice.org.uk/guidance/ta127 [Accessed 7 November 2016].
10. National Institute for Health and Clinical Excellence. (2001) *Guidance on the use of Riluzole (Rilutek) for the treatment of Motor Neurone Disease* (TA20). [Online]. Available from: www.nice.org.uk/guidance/ta20 [Accessed 7 November 2016].
11. The Royal College of Physicians. (2008) *National clinical guideline for stroke*. 3rd Edition. London: RCP.
12. Stroke Association, www.stroke.org.uk.
13. World Health Organization. (1978) *Cerebrovascular Disorders*. Geneva: Offset Publications.

Top tip:

I wish somebody had told me this...it has literally saved at least one life, and the lack of knowledge has cost one. If an elderly patient is brought in 'not quite right' or 'just a bit more confused' etc, admit them! They ARE septic. They will not mount a temperature because their hypothalami are not functioning. They will not mount a white cell response because their marrow is screwed. Take cultures, dip the urine, check the CRP, get a chest film and an ECG. If they don't tank now, they will soon.

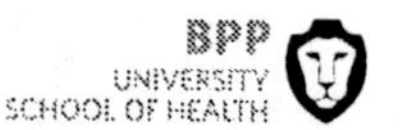

Chapter 4
Core clinical cases in surgery

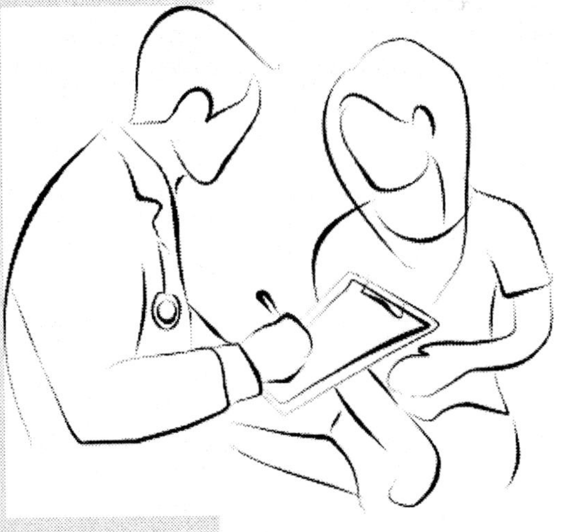

Chapter 4

Core clinical cases in surgery

Acute abdominal pain

Differential diagnosis

System	Disease
Gastrointestinal	**Peptic ulcer disease** **Acute intestinal obstruction** **Diverticulitis** Colon cancer **Acute appendicitis** **Meckel's diverticulum** Mesenteric infarction **Ischaemic colitis** Ulcerative colitis Crohn's disease Volvulus
Hepato-biliary	**Biliary colic** **Acute cholecystitis** **Ascending cholangitis**
Pancreas	**Acute pancreatitis**
Spleen	**Splenic rupture**
Gynaecological	**Ectopic pregnancy** **Ovarian torsion** Pelvic inflammatory disease
Urinary tract	**Renal and ureteric calculi** Urinary tract infection (UTI) including pyelonephritis Urinary retention Testicular torsion
Vascular	**Ruptured abdominal aortic aneurysm (AAA)** **Aortic dissection** **Mesenteric infarction**
Others	Haemorrhagic cyst Rectus sheath haematoma Retroperitoneal haemorrhage Psoas abscess

Table 4.1: Differential diagnosis of acute abdominal pain

Top tip:
Answer your bleep promptly and answer it with a smile!

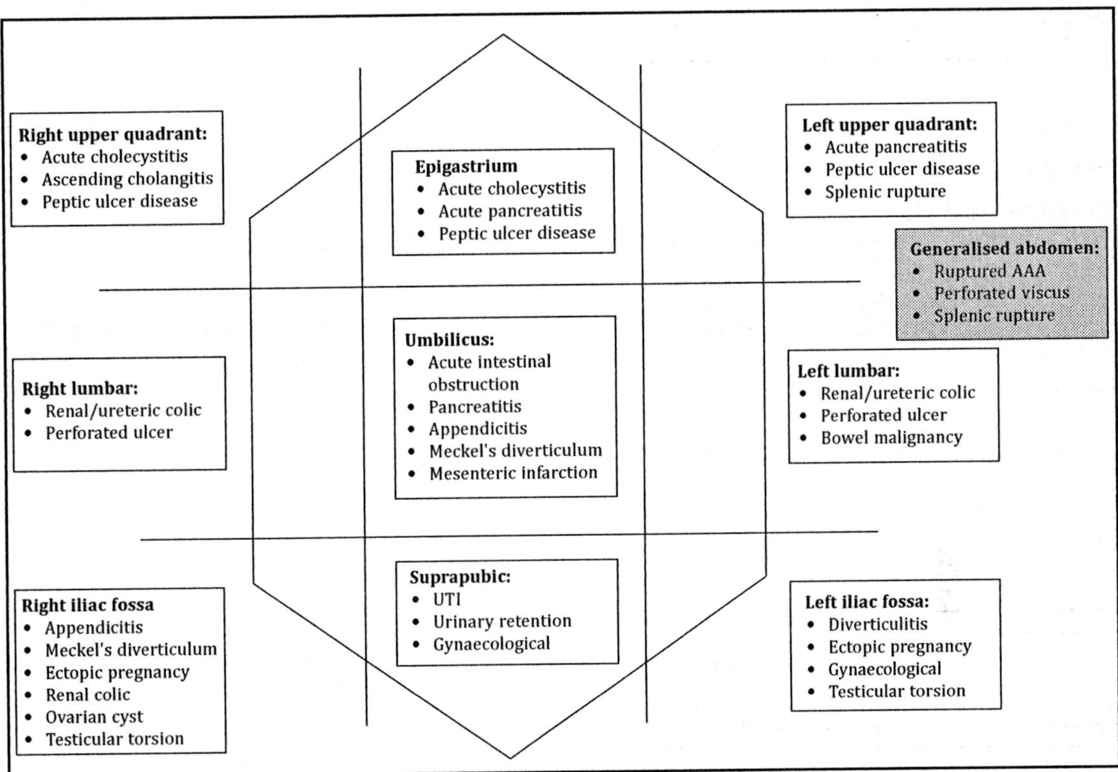

Figure 4.1: Potential diagnoses of pain in each area of the abdomen

Top tip:

Try to find some joy in what you do, every day! There are always going to be some days where you feel either underappreciated, underpaid, overworked, overqualified for boring tasks, or underqualified for challenging situations. However, I believe you should still strive to find a little joy; the patient's family you were able to reassure, that unusual diagnosis you were able to spot, the timeliness you were able to steer the ward round in, the new procedure you learnt. Whatever it is for you, and even if it's hard sometimes, find the joy of this really fantastic profession!

Gastrointestinal structures

Peptic ulcer disease

Epidemiology

Common sites of peptic ulcers include the duodenum and the stomach. Duodenal ulcers (70–80%) are more common than gastric ulcers, and usually occur in men between the ages of 35 and 55. Gastric ulcers occur later in life typically between 55 and 65 years.

Aetiology

Infection with *Helicobacter pylori* is the main cause of duodenal ulcers. It is present in approximately 80% of cases. *H. pylori* is a spiral shaped Gram negative bacillus, with potent urease activity. It releases cytotoxins which damage mucosal membranes degrading the stomach's defensive barrier and allowing further damage of the mucosa by gastric acid.

NSAIDs are a risk factor for the development of peptic ulceration, by reducing the mucosal defences against gastric substances. They inhibit the production of prostaglandins G_2 (PGG_2) and prostaglandin E_2 (PGE_2), which are involved in stimulating mucus secretion and encouraging blood flow to the gastric mucosa.

Other risk factors include steroids, smoking and states of extreme physiological stress eg burns or major trauma.

Pathophysiology

Duodenal ulcers usually occur in the first part of the duodenum. Anterior duodenal ulcers are prone to perforate while posterior duodenal ulcers tend to bleed. Malignancy in the duodenal region is rare.

Gastric ulcers tend to be larger than duodenal ulcers. Chronic ulcers are commonly found on the lesser curve of the stomach and can erode posteriorly into retroperitoneal structures such as the pancreas and surrounding vasculature.

History/examination

- Gastric and duodenal ulcers cannot be differentiated on symptoms alone.
- Attacks of epigastric abdominal pain, lasting for days to weeks with intermittent periods of complete relief. The pain can also radiate to the back.
- Onset of pain can occur immediately after a meal but typically occurs two hours after eating food. It is aggravated by spicy foods and relieved by milk.
- Nausea, vomiting and heartburn.
- If there is chronic bleeding symptoms of anaemia can arise. However, in acute presentations haematemesis and malaena may also be seen.
- Tenderness in the epigastric region.
- A perforation presents with signs of localised or generalised peritonitis.

Investigations

Blood tests:

- FBC – anaemia secondary to bleeding.
- Serological testing: will identify the presence of antibodies to *H. pylori*. However, it can remain positive for 6–12 months after eradication. In such cases the urea breath test can be used.

Endoscopy:

- OGD: direct visualization of the oesophagus, stomach and duodenum. Very sensitive and biopsies can be taken to differentiate benign and malignant disease and identify the presence of *H. pylori*.

Imaging:

- Double contrast barium meal: is performed rarely, if endoscopy is not possible. This is useful to identify most ulcers and a hiatus hernia.
- Ultrasound may exclude other causes of epigastric pain (gallstones).

Others:

- Urease CLO test: involves the biopsy sample and a solution of urea being placed together with a pH indicator.
- Urea breath test: involves the patient ingesting a solution containing non-radioactive labelled urea. High levels of CO_2 in the patient's breath before and after ingestion of the solution confirms the diagnosis.

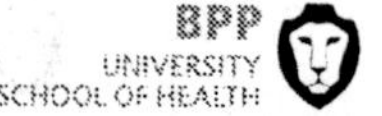

Management

General advice for patients is to avoid alcohol, smoking, stress, and the ingestion of NSAIDS (eg aspirin).

The majority of management is medical with surgical management usually reserved for complications, the most common being bleeding or perforation.

Medical management:

1. ***H. pylori* eradication:**

   A seven day course of antibiotics and anti-acid drugs such as PPI. A typical regime: Amoxicillin, Clraithromycin and Omeprazole eradicates *H. pylori* in approximately 90% of patients.

2. **Acid reduction:**
   - i) Reducing acid alone results in ulcer healing within one to two months of treatment but ulcers will recur if *H. pylori* is not eradicated.
   - ii) PPIs such as Omeprazole inhibit hydrogen ion release from gastric parietal cells. Peptic ulcers will usually heal within two weeks and patients generally experience symptom relief within a few days.
   - iii) H2 receptor antagonists block stimulation of gastric acid secretion.
   - iv) Barrier drugs (Sucralfate, Bismuth compounds): enhance mucosal defence mechanism by providing a protective layer on the epithelial surface.

Surgical management for duodenal ulcers:

- Elective surgery for peptic ulcers is now rare, but the primary procedure is a truncal vagotomy and pyloroplasty.

Surgical management for gastric ulcers:

The principle of surgical treatment is to remove the ulcer and the gastrin secreting zone.

- Billroth I gastrectomy:
  - The distal part of the stomach is removed and a gastroduodenal anastomosis is performed.
  - Approximately 90% of gastric ulcers are treated this way.
- Billroth II gastrectomy or Polya gastrectomy:
  - Performed if Billroth I too technically difficult.
  - The antrum and the distal body of the stomach are removed, followed by closure of the duodenal stump. The remaining stomach is anastomosed to a small bowel loop (jejunum).
- Vagotomy and ulcer excision

Surgical management for perforated ulcers:

There are three surgical options:

- Abdominal washout and repair of the defect by approximation of ulcer edges or use of omental patch (most common)
- Excision of the ulcer
- Gastrectomy

NICE guidance for dyspepsia/peptic ulcer disease

- Offer lifestyle advice: avoidance of smoking, alcohol, coffee, fatty foods and weight loss
- Review medications: NSAIDS, steroids, bisphosphonates, nitrates
- First-line treatment: PPI with H2 receptor antagonist if inadequate response
- Offer *H. pylori* testing to all – carbon-13 urea breath test/stool antigen test/laboratory serology
- First-line treatment for *H. pylori*: 7 days of omeprazole, amoxicillin and clarithromycin or metronidazole
- Treat confirmed ulcers with 8 weeks of PPI +/- *H. pylori* eradication
- For unhealed ulcers consider: non-adherence, malignancy, failure to detect *H. pylori*, inadvertent NSAID use and Zollinger-Ellison/Crohn's disease

(NICE guideline CG184 – 2014)

Acute intestinal obstruction

Epidemiology and aetiology

Intestinal obstruction can be divided into small and large bowel obstruction. Small bowel obstruction accounts for 5% of all acute surgical hospital admissions. The commonest causes of small bowel presentations are: adhesions (60%), malignancy (5%) and strangulated hernia (10%). Large bowel obstruction commonly arises due to colorectal malignancy and accounts for 15% of all cases.

Location of obstruction	Causes
Obstruction in the lumen	Faecal impaction, food bolus, tumour, gallstone ileus, foreign body.
Obstruction in the wall	Tumours, diverticulae, Crohn's disease, congenital atresia.
Obstruction outside the wall	Volvulus, strangulated hernia, adhesions, intussusceptions.
Obstruction in neonates and infants	Stenosis, imperforate anus, meconium ileus, Hirschsprung's disease, strangulated hernia.

Table 4.2: The classification of intestinal obstruction according to location and the causes of each type

Pathophysiology

When a bowel lumen becomes obstructed, the bowel distal to the obstruction empties and the bowel proximal to the obstruction dilates usually with gas and fluid from the intestinal walls. Intestinal peristalsis increases in an attempt to overcome the obstruction. This results in intestinal colic felt as crampy abdominal pain.

Simple intestinal obstruction occurs when the bowel is obstructed without the blood supply to the bowel being compromised. Strangulated obstruction occurs when the blood supply to the affected segment of the bowel is acutely impaired.

Increasing bowel distension can result in perforation due to increased pressure. If strangulated, the blood supply is acutely impaired and ischaemia rapidly develops. This weakens the mucosal layer of the bowel leading to early perforation – bacteria and associated toxins leak into the peritoneal cavity, often leading to peritonitis.

History/examination

- There are four classic features of acute intestinal obstruction: **pain, vomiting, distension** and **constipation.**
- Sudden onset of severe colicky abdominal pain.
- Central abdominal pain indicates small bowel obstruction. Lower abdominal pain suggests large bowel obstruction.
- Vomiting is usually an early feature of small bowel obstruction but occurs late in large bowel obstruction, when it may become faeculant.
- Distension is dependent on the site of the obstruction. Often, there is typically more distension the more distal the obstruction.
- Absolute constipation ie passing no faeces or flatus. This is a sign of complete intestinal obstruction and it is an early feature of large bowel obstruction.
- Relative constipation is defined as the passing of flatus but not faeces.
- Signs may include pyrexia, dehydration, localised tenderness on palpation and visible peristalsis.
- Abdominal scars from a previous operation should lead to suspicion of adhesional intestinal obstruction.
- Bowel sounds are increased and 'tinkling' in nature.
- Rectal examination may identify an obstructing mass or faecal impaction.
- A collapsed rectum on the rectal exam suggests a mechanical obstruction, whilst a gas-filled rectum suggests pseudo-obstruction.
- There are specific features associated with strangulating obstruction:
  - Pyrexia and tachycardia
  - Colicky abdominal pain becoming constant
  - Abdominal tenderness and rigidity
  - Reduced or absent bowel sounds
  - Raised WCC with bowel infarction

Investigations

Blood test:

- FBC: may reveal a raised white cell count
- U&Es: deranged as a result of dehydration
- ABG: high lactate and metabolic acidosis are signs of bowel strangulation

Imaging:

- CXR: to exclude perforation.
- AXR: loops of distended bowel are seen and a fluid level may be visible on an erect film. The dilated loops (>3.5 cm diameter) of small bowel obstruction are usually centrally placed with striation passing across the total bowel width known as valvulae conniventes. The dilated loops of large bowel obstruction (5 cm diameter) usually lie peripherally with haustra – indentations that do not cross the total width of the bowel.
- Barium/contrast (gastrografin) follow through/ enema. Contrast is used with a series of X-rays to identify the level of intestinal obstruction. This is not indicated if perforation is clinically suspected.
- CT: This will identify the specific site and cause of the bowel obstruction, and may provide evidence of bowel perforation.

Management

Immediate management:

- In simple obstruction, first-line management is often conservative. This will include:
  - A to E assessment and resuscitation (large amounts of fluid sequestered in the gut, with losses from vomiting, means that a significant amount of fluid is required).
  - Insertion of a nasogastric tube (NG) allows decompression of the bowel. Gastric contents are also emptied reducing the risk of aspiration.

This combination of therapy is often referred to as 'drip and suck'.

Additional steps:

- Insert a urinary catheter to accurately monitor fluid balance
- Broad spectrum IV antibiotics in all cases of strangulation
- Analgesia
- Nil by mouth
- Insertion of rectal catheter/flatus tube for cases of volvulus

In cases where perforation is not felt to be imminent these conservative measures can be trialled for up to 72 hours. If there is no improvement following these, the next step is surgical management. This is most effective in adhesional obstruction.

Surgical management is first line for cases of suspected or impending perforation and strangulation, as well as for causes which are unlikely to settle spontaneously eg malignant obstruction, or where the patient is acutely unstable. Malignancy may be radiologically/ endoscopically stented as a bridge to definitive surgery or as a palliative measure.

Surgical management:

- The surgical procedure of choice is an open midline laparotomy.
- The affected bowel is inspected carefully, to identify any non-viable areas (loss of peristalsis, loss of the normal sheen, green or black discolouration, loss of pulsation of the blood vessels within the mesentery). If non-viable bowel is identified, a resection is required.
- Small bowel obstruction: non-viable section completely resected and a primary anastomosis performed. This is usually a very successful procedure due to the good blood supply.
- Large bowel obstruction: if the obstruction is proximal to the splenic flexure, it is resected with a primary ileo-colic anastomosis. Left sided lesions are resected and the remaining bowel is brought out to the abdominal surface as a colostomy. The rectal stump can be oversewn as in a Hartmann's procedure or brought to the surface as a mucous fistula. A reversal procedure with anastomosis can be performed at a later date.
- In the event of bowel perforation and intra-abdominal contamination the risk of anastomotic breakdown is significantly higher. A stoma may be performed as a diversion, either instead of a bowel anastomosis or to protect one that was created and again can be reversed later.

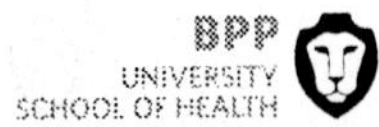

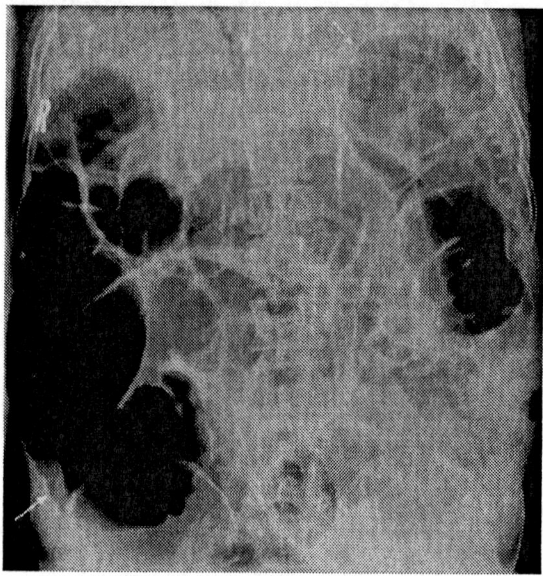

Figure 4.2: AXR of an 80-year-old woman who presented with abdominal distension and constipation. Note dilated peripheral loops of bowel (arrows) with a lack of complete haustral markings in keeping with large bowel obstruction

Diverticulitis

Epidemiology and aetiology

Diverticula are protrusions of the mucosa and submucosa through the muscle layers of the bowel wall. They occur as a result of bowel wall weakness or increased intraluminal pressure. Low dietary fibre intake and constipation cause a rise in intraluminal pressure, colonic wall muscle hypertrophy and increased segmentation.

Diverticulosis is often seen after the age of 50, with colonic diverticula more common in western countries. They are usually found on the left colon (90% involving the sigmoid colon) but can affect the entire colon. Approximately 15% of patients with diverticulosis (diverticula in the colon) develop acute diverticulitis (inflammation of these diverticulae due to infection). Other complications of diverticulosis include diverticular bleeding, stricturing and obstruction and fistulation with surrounding structures.

History/examination

- Acute onset of lower abdominal pain, commonly on the left
- The pain becomes generalised and increases in severity with diverticula perforation
- Malaise, vomiting, diarrhoea or constipation
- Bleeding or mucus per rectum and symptoms of anaemia may be present
- Pyrexia
- Lower abdominal and left iliac fossa tenderness with guarding
- A possible mass, representing the sigmoid colon, which is tender and thickened
- A tender mass may be palpated on digital rectal examination if the sigmoid has looped into the pelvis
- A perforated diverticulum produces signs of localised or generalised peritonitis

Investigations

Blood tests:

- FBC: may reveal a raised white cell count
- Inflammatory markers: check for elevated CRP
- U&Es

Imaging:

- CT: the investigation of choice in the acute phase.
- The Hinchey classification describes the severity of diverticulitis, whilst excluding other causes of abdominal pain.
- Double-contrast barium enema: can be used to view the whole of the large bowel and demonstrate stenosis, fistulas, and peri-colic abscesses. It is less invasive than endoscopy but small polyps or carcinoma may be missed.

Endoscopy:

- Flexible sigmoidoscopy/colonoscopy: allows visualisation of the sigmoid colon/the whole large bowel. In acute attacks the procedure may be painful and the mucosa will be inflamed increasing the risk of iatrogenic perforation. It is commonly used once the acute attack has passed (six to eight weeks). These investigations allow confirmation of the diagnosis and can rule out contemporaneous pathology eg malignancy under direct vision.

Initial management

1. **Conservative management:**
   Most acute attacks of diverticulitis settle with conservative management.

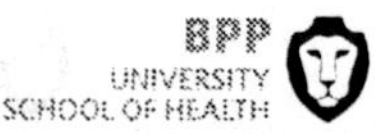

2. If not improving or systemically unwell patient:
   i) A to E assessment
   ii) IV access and resuscitation of the patient if necessary
   iii) IV fluids
   iv) Broad spectrum IV antibiotics (Penicillin and Metronidazole)
   v) Appropriate analgesia eg IV opioid and an anti-emetic
   vi) Outpatient large bowel endoscopy once acute phase settled

Surgical management:

A perforated diverticulum resulting in generalised peritonitis requires the patient to undergo an emergency laparotomy whereas a small localised perforation can be managed conservatively with IV antibiotics +/- CT guided drainage of a local collection.

A further 10% of patients with recurrent attacks will also need elective surgical management where the affected segment of the bowel is removed and an end-to-end anastomosis is performed.

If obstruction develops, a Hartmann's procedure and resection of the affected area may be required. This involves closing the rectum and bringing the left colon out to the abdomen, forming a colostomy. This may later be reversed or may be permanent.

Perforation: can be managed with a number of different procedures:

- Laparotomy with an abdominal wash out and omental patch repair
- Primary resection and Hartmann's procedure
- Primary resection and anastomosis

Hinchey classification of diverticulitis	
Stage 1	Diverticulitis with pericolic/ mesenteric abscess
Stage 2	Diverticulitis with walled off pelvic abscess
Stage 3	Diverticulitis with generalised purulent peritonitis
Stage 4	Diverticulitis with faecal peritionitis

Table 4.3: Hinchey classification of diverticulitis

Acute appendicitis

Epidemiology

One of the most common surgical emergencies; lifetime prevalence of approximately 6–8%.

Pathophysiology

Acute appendicitis in some cases initially starts as infective/non-infective mucosal inflammation and lymphoid tissue hyperplasia, with a patent appendiceal lumen. Intraluminal pressure increases as a result of continuous mucus and inflammatory exudate secretion, causing obstruction of lymphatic drainage and resulting in mucosal oedema and ulceration. Spontaneous resolution may occur with IV antibiotics. However, with progression, the appendix becomes distended, with an ischaemic wall. This allows bacterial spread through the submucosa resulting in acute appendicitis. If left untreated, this can lead to perforation and subsequent peritonitis.

History/examination

- Central abdominal colicky pain (visceral), which moves to the right iliac fossa, due to peritoneal inflammation (somatic)
- Pain is usually aggravated by movement and relieved by lying still
- With perforation symptoms may temporarily resolve, due to relief of tension; however, they then increase and present as generalised peritonitis
- Anorexia and vomiting
- Constipation (and sometimes diarrhoea)
- Pyrexia, tachycardia, right iliac fossa guarding, percussion tenderness and rebound tenderness (difficult to illicit if guarding is present)
- Painful digital rectal examination due to a pelvic appendix or pus in the pouch of Douglas
- With generalised peritonitis, the abdomen is rigid, bowel sounds are absent, and the patient has signs of sepsis

Symptom	Early feature	Late feature
Pain	Peri-umbilical Pain	Moves to the right iliac fossa
Temperature	Apyrexial	Slight or high pyrexia
Pulse rate	Normal pulse rate	Raised as a response to temperature
Vomiting	Usually follows onset of pain	–
Anorexia	Constant	Constant

Table 4.4: The early and late features of acute appendicitis

Specific signs associated with acute appendicitis:

- McBurney's point tenderness: tenderness at two-thirds from the umbilicus to the anterior superior iliac spine.
- Rovsing's sign: right iliac fossa pain on left iliac fossa palpation. Psoas sign: if the appendix is positioned on the psoas muscle, the patient will lie with the right hip flexed with aggravation of pain on hip extension.
- Obturator sign: when the hip is flexed and rotated, this results in spasm of the obturator muscle. If the appendix is inflamed and in contact with the obturator the patient will experience pain in the hypogastrium.

Investigations

The diagnosis of acute appendicitis is usually clinical; however, routine investigations are performed.

Blood test:

- FBC: may reveal a raised white cell count
- U&Es: important particularly in the elderly patient with other co-morbidities

Urinalysis:

- Urine dipstick: may show blood and leucocytes as a result of ureteric irritation and inflammation.
- Beta-human chorionic gonadotropin to rule out pregnancy (particularly ectopic) in all women of reproductive age.

Imaging:

- Erect CXR and AXR: used to exclude perforation or ureteric colic. Both of these are not indicated in young patients with good clinical signs of appendicitis.
- Abdomino-pelvic USS: commonly performed in young women to exclude ovarian pathology ie ruptured cyst or ovarian torsion. USS cannot accurately identify the appendix unless it is markedly enlarged but it can highlight the presence of free fluid within the abdomen, which collaborates with a diagnosis of appendicitis.
- CT: this is 98% sensitive at diagnosing appendicitis, but is reserved for older patients where malignancy is suspected. Patients are exposed to a dose of high radiation, and so this is not a routinely used investigation. It may also demonstrate an appendiceal mass/abscess common in cases that present >1 week after the onset of pain.

Management

- Immediate management: A to E assessment and resuscitation
- Monitoring of blood pressure, heart rate, oxygen saturations, and urine output (via urinary catheter in seriously ill patients
- IV fluids
- IV Paracetamol + additional analgesia, eg IV opioid and an anti-emetic
- Keep NBM
- Pre-operative IV antibiotics to reduce infective complications

Surgical management:

- Definitive treatment is to perform an open or laparoscopic appendicectomy – increasingly laparoscopic is the favoured approach.

Laparoscopic appendicectomy:

- Incision at umbilicus to expose peritoneum. Blunt trocar inserted. CO_2 insufflation
- Camera inserted, at least two further ports inserted under direct vision. Diagnostic laparoscopy – abdominal contents visualised, notably: appendix inflammation or gynaecological pathology in women
- Patient in head down position
- Appendix identified, mesoappendix dissected and mesoappendicular artery clipped and divided
- Appendix base divided (commonly Endoloops then scissors)
- Appendix removed in Endobag and extracted via periumbilical inscision
- Ports removed under direct vision. Scan abdominal cavity to ensure haemostasis

- Wounds closed with sutures +/- skin glue. Local anaesthetic infiltrated

Post-operatively: appropriate analgesia, encourage oral intake, early mobilisation, oral antibiotics and home as soon as possible.

Meckel's diverticulum

Aetiology and epidemiology

A Meckel's diverticulum is the remnant of the Vitello-intestinal duct, which usually disappears by the end of embryological development. The apex is adherent to the umbilicus or attached via a fibrous cord. It is found in approximately 2% of the population and inflammation is seen in 2% of these patients.

Pathophysiology

Located on the antimesenteric border, approximately 60 cm (2 feet) from the ileo-caecal valve, it has an average length of 2 inches. Therefore the rule of 2 (2%, 2 feet, 2 inches), helps with remembering here! They most commonly present in childhood (<2 years).

A Meckel's diverticulum is a true diverticulum encompassing all three layers of the intestinal wall, and possesses its own blood supply. It may contain ectopic mucosa, most commonly gastric or pancreatic. Such diverticulum are at risk of perforation, haemorrhage, and intussusception.

History/examination

- Asymptomatic/an incidental finding at operation.
- Acute inflammation gives signs and symptoms similar to those of appendicitis.
- Perforation presents with shock and an acute abdomen.
- Rectal bleeding may occur as a result of ulceration.
- They can present as a volvulus or intussusception with acute abdominal pain and signs of obstruction.

Investigations

Meckel's diverticulae are usually incidental operative findings. Certain investigations can aid the diagnosis.

Imaging:

Technetium-99 scan: radioactive technetium is injected and then absorbed by the gastric mucosa. The stomach will be outlined and in 90% of cases the site of the Meckel's diverticulum will be identified.

Barium follow through: will sometimes identify the diverticulum arising from the antimesenteric border.

Management

If the patient presents with an acute abdomen, an A to E assessment and resuscitation is required. A Meckel's diverticulectomy is the only choice for definitive management. If identified at operation (eg a diagnostic laparoscopy for possible appendicitis, these are often resected to prevent future complications.

Hepato-biliary structures

Biliary colic

Epidemiology

In western society 50% of women and 15% of men are diagnosed with gallstones. After approximately 5 years, 10% of these cases become symptomatic.

Aetiology

There are three types of gallstones if classified by composition.

1. Bile pigment stones (5%): seen in patients with excessive haemolysis eg due to sickle cell anaemia or thalassaemia. They are small, black, gritty and fragile. These stones are often found throughout the biliary tree, and in the ducts of patients with benign and malignant bile duct structures.
2. Cholesterol stones (20%): are more common in those who are older, female, and with increased weight. They are typically solitary and oval in shape.
3. Mixed stones (75%): are composed mainly of cholesterol with varying amounts of calcium phosphate, calcium carbonate, calcium palmitate and proteins.

A typical sufferer of gallstones is said to be a 'fat, fertile, female of 40'. However, gallstones can occur in men, usually in the older age group.

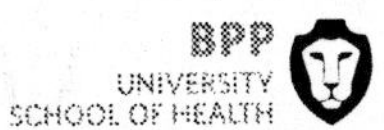

Pathophysiology

Biliary colic is the pain caused by muscle spasms of the gallbladder against a gallstone. This stone is usually lodged in the neck of the gallbladder (Hartmann's pouch) or the cystic duct.

History/examination

- Severe continuous pain in the epigastrium or right upper quadrant, which may radiate to costal areas, and the back or shoulders
- Nausea and vomiting
- Patient is unable to lie still
- Tachycardia
- Epigastric and right upper quadrant tenderness on palpation
- Examination may be unremarkable as most attacks only last for approximately six hours
- Attacks are particularly triggered following fatty meals

Investigations

Blood tests:

- FBC: may reveal a raised white cell count
- Liver function tests (LFTs): abnormal in cases of duct obstruction. In particular, high bilirubin and alkaline phosphatase (ALP)
- Amylase
- Renal function
- Glucose
- Clotting

Imaging:

- Erect CXR: to exclude perforation.
- USS: gallstones may be seen. The thickness of the gallbladder wall is a sign of inflammation (either acute or chronic).

Management

- Usually do not require inpatient management unless due to severe uncontrolled pain
- IV access should be gained
- Monitoring of blood pressure, heart rate and oxygen saturations
- IV fluids
- Analgesia, eg IV opioid and an anti-emetic
- A cholecystectomy can be arranged in a general surgical outpatient clinic once gallstones have been confirmed

The following are recommended by NICE:

- MRCP if ducts dilated +/- abnormal LFTs
- Laparoscopic cholecystectomy within 1 week for acute cholecystitis or after 4 weeks for elective surgery
- ERCP within 72 hours for those with CBD stones and jaundice and within 24 hours for CBD stones and cholangitis

Acute cholecystitis

Aetiology and epidemiology

Acute cholecystitis is inflammation of the gallbladder, commonly secondary to obstruction of the cystic duct by stones. It develops in 1–3% of patients with gallstones. Approximately 10% of cases are identified in adults over the age of 60, 5% of which will result in gallbladder perforation.

Pathophysiology

The inflammatory process of acute cholecystitis begins with obstruction of the cystic duct or gallbladder neck by a calculus. This obstruction results in the release of inflammatory mediators (eg prostaglandins), chemical irritation by bile acids, and a rise in intraluminal pressure.

A secondary bacterial infection may also occur. The most common organism found is *Esherichia coli;* others include Gram negative aerobic rods, anaerobes, and Enterocci.

Commonly, cystic duct patency is re-established within four to seven days. Recurrent attacks of acute cholecystitis lead to fibrotic thickening of the gallbladder wall – a characteristic feature of chronic cholecystitis. If the cystic duct remains obstructed there is increased inflammatory cell infiltration within the wall of the gallbladder. This can lead to haemorrhagic necrosis, gangrene, and perforation.

History/examination

- Right upper quadrant severe abdominal pain, lasting minutes to hours, which may radiate to the right side of the back and to the shoulder.
- Attacks of pain often start at night, waking the patient and may be ongoing for several weeks.
- With progressive infection the patient becomes systemically unwell.

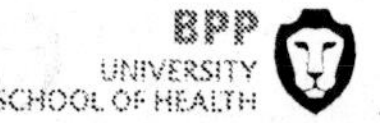

- Vomiting and symptoms of dyspepsia.
- Pyrexia and tachycardia.
- RUQ tenderness and guarding.
- Murphy's sign: during palpation of the right upper quadrant the patient is asked to take a deep breath in. The inspiration causes the gallbladder to descend onto the palpating fingers and if this elicits significant pain the sign is positive (due to inflammation). If repeated on the left, there should be no pain.
- Late features are:
  - A palpable mass (most likely the omental wall of the inflamed gallbladder or an empyema)
  - Rigid abdomen
  - Localised peritonitis or abscess formation, as a result of gallbladder perforation

Investigations

Blood tests:

- FBC: may reveal a raised white cell count
- LFTs: are abnormal in cases of duct obstruction. In particular, high bilirubin and ALP are seen
- Amylase
- U&Es
- Glucose
- Clotting

Imaging:

- Erect CXR to exclude perforation.
- USS: gallstones and a thickened gallbladder wall are seen. If the diameter of the common bile duct is >7 mm, it suggests the presence of stones within the duct.
- MRCP: the biliary tree is visualised and calculi may be detected.
- ERCP: more invasive than an MRCP with the added risk of precipitating pancreatitis. It involves endoscopic access of the bile duct, enabling visualisation of any calculi within the duct. If calculi are seen they can be removed at the same time, via a sphincterotomy.

Others:

- ECG: to rule out atypical presentation of ischaemic heart disease.

Management

Immediate management:

- A to E assessment
- IV access and resuscitation
- Monitoring of blood pressure, heart rate, oxygen saturations, and urine output (urinary catheter)
- IV fluids
- Analgesia, eg IV opioid and an anti-emetic
- NBM
- Broad spectrum IV antibiotics

Once there are signs of reducing inflammation (pyrexia and tachycardia settle), oral fluids and a fat free diet is recommended.

1. 80–90% of cases will settle with conservative treatment over 24–48 hours. These patients are readmitted 6–8 weeks later for an elective laparoscopic cholecystectomy.
2. The remaining 10% of cases will require urgent surgery. There is an increasing trend towards performing a cholecystectomy during the acute phase, as adhesions are yet to occur, making dissection easier.
3. When there is biochemical or imaging evidence of stones in the common bile duct an on-table cholangiogram could be performed to locate the stones. They can then be retrieved laparoscopically or with an ERCP.

Surgical management:

Laparoscopic cholecystectomy:

- A blunt trochar is inserted through the peritoneum and carbon dioxide inserted for abdominal insufflation.
- The laparoscope is inserted through the umbilical port and three further ports are sited under direct vision.
- The gallbladder is retracted upwards, lifting the liver and allowing full visualisation.
- The gallbladder neck is dissected off the liver.
- Calot's triangle (cystic duct, the common hepatic duct, and the inferior border of the liver edge) is identified to find the cystic artery.
- Cystic duct and artery clipped.
- The gallbladder is dissected off the liver and removed through the umbilical port.
- Irrigation and haemostasis.
- Skin closure, with a drain if concerns about bleeding.

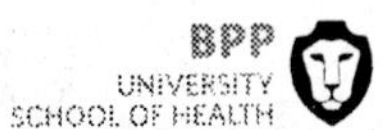

Note. Possible complications include those general to surgery: infection, bleeding, poor wound healing thromboembolic events and general anaesthesia.

And specifically: bile leak into the abdominal cavity.

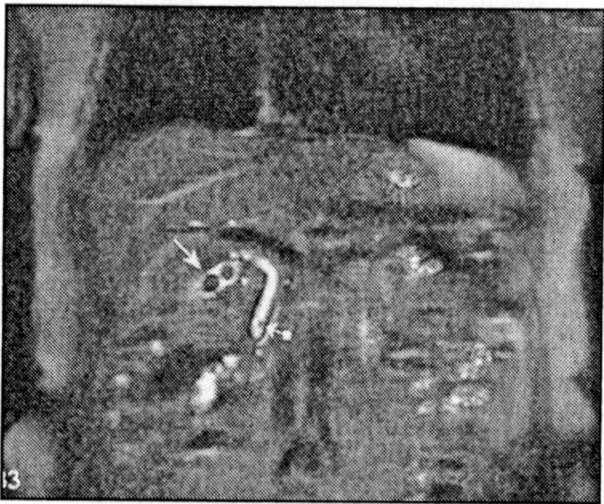

Figure 4.3: Magnetic resonance cholangiopancreatography showing gallstones within the gallbladder and common hepatic ducts (round-ended arrow)

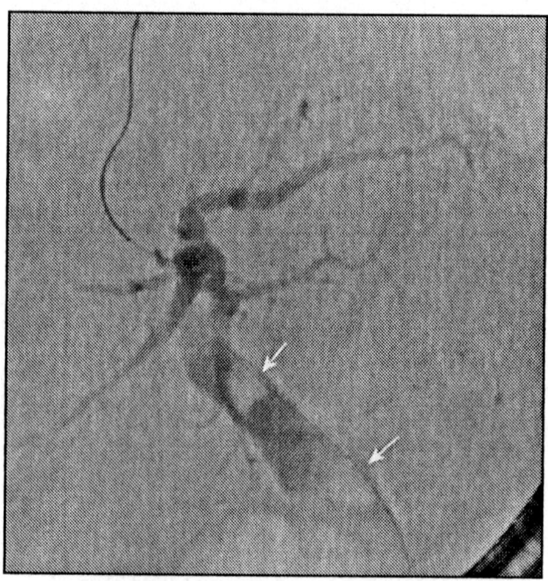

Figure 4.4: Endoscopic retrograde cholangiopancreatography showing dilated CBD with multiple filling defects suggestive of gallstones

Ascending cholangitis

Epidemiology

2–3% of patients with gallstones will present with severe complications of pancreatitis or ascending cholangitis.

Aetiology

The predisposing factors to cholangitis are: common bile duct stones, benign or malignant biliary strictures, and pancreatic or duodenal tumours. Cholangitis can occur following biliary reconstructive surgery and with bile duct instrumentation (eg ERCP).

Pathophysiology

Ascending cholangitis arises following bile duct obstruction causing biliary stasis and subsequent bacterial infection. Increased pressure following biliary obstruction causes increased pressure and thus an increased potential for stagnant contaminated bile to infect the bile duct and enter the blood stream causing septicaemia. This is a medical emergency, which can rapidly progress to SIRS leading to multi-organ failure.

History/examination

- Jaundice, rigors and abdominal pain (Charcot's Triad)
- Pyrexia and signs of sepsis may be present, eg tachycardia, sweating and low blood pressure.
- Clinical signs of jaundice (skin pigmentation and yellowing of the sclera)
- Tenderness in right upper quadrant with or without the presence of a positive Murphy's sign

Investigations

Blood tests:

- FBC
- LFTs: may be deranged with an obstructive picture (elevated bilirubin and ALP levels)
- CRP
- U&Es

Microbiology:

Blood cultures: should be sent when patients have a significant pyrexia or evidence of sepsis. The commonest bacteria associated with ascending cholangitis are the Gram negative bacilli (*E. coli*, Klebsiella and Enterobacter) and the gram positive *Enterococcus*.

Imaging:

USS: of the abdomen confirms dilated bile ducts and in some cases an MRCP is used to more accurately delineate the site of biliary obstruction.

Management

- A to E assessment
- Rehydration with IV fluids and IV antibiotics
- NBM
- Urgent biliary drainage: endoscopic of percutaneous transhepatic (ideally 24-48 hours after starting IV antibiotics but may need to be sooner if worsening, severe sepsis)

ERCP is preferred, as it enables: retrieval of bile duct stones, biopsy of sites of potential malignancy, and the deployment of plastic or metal stents in areas of narrowing. Where ERCP is not suitable (high proximal biliary obstruction or tight stricture) a percutaneous transhepatic cholangiography (PTC) is performed. This involves passing a tube for drainage from skin to bile duct under ultrasound guidance.

Pancreas

Acute pancreatitis

Epidemiology

Acute pancreatitis is relatively common, and accounts for approximately 3% of all cases of abdominal pain admitted to hospital in the UK. The disease has a mortality of 5–10%, with one-third of patients dying in the early acute phase from multi system organ failure.

Aetiology

The two common causes of acute pancreatitis include gallstones and alcohol, accounting for 60% and 20% respectively. A useful pneumonic, 'GET SMASHED', is used to identify the causes of acute pancreatitis:

- Gallstones
- Ethanol – commonest cause of recurrent pancreatitis
- Trauma
- Steroids
- Mumps (and other infections such as coxsackie B)
- Autoimmune diseases: vasculitis, SLE
- Scorpion venom: rare and not seen in the UK
- Hyperlipidaemia/hypothermia/hypercalcaemia
- ERCP
- Drugs: eg azathioprine and thiazides

Pathophysiology

In acute pancreatitis, pancreatic enzymes (trypsin, lipase, amylase) are released and activated resulting in auto-digestion of the pancreas. The process of pancreatitis occurs in a four stage process:

1. The patient presents with hypovolaemic shock as a result of oedema and abdominal fluid shift. The pancreas releases fluid and enzymes into the peritoneal cavity. This leads to the auto-digestion of fats and the subsequent development of necrosis.
2. The blood vessels are affected by the autodigestion, leading to haemorrhage into the retroperitoneal space. This tracking of blood-stained fluid may result in bruising at the abdominal flanks (Grey Turner's sign) or bruising at the umbilicus (Cullen's sign).
3. Ongoing inflammation progresses to necrosis of all or part of the pancreas and enzymes leak into the blood stream causing systemic effects.
4. The necrotic areas become infected resulting in a high mortality rate.

History/examination

- Rapid onset of constant, severe epigastric pain occurring over minutes and lasting for hours or even days. It may radiate to the back.
- Frequent vomiting is an associated symptom.
- On observation the patient may look well or extremely ill.
- Tachypnoea, tachycardia, and hypotension may be present.
- Mild jaundice as a result of common bile duct obstruction by the oedematous pancreatic head or gallstones.
- Tenderness on abdominal palpation, especially over the epigastric region, with or without guarding.
- Bluish discolouration at the flanks and umbilicus (Grey Turner's and Cullen's signs) is uncommon but it can develop over a few days.
- In 10–20% of cases a pleural effusion is present.
- Positive shifting dullness for the presence of ascites.

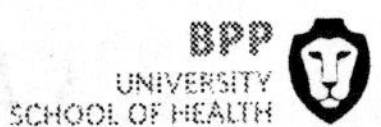

Investigations

Blood tests:

- FBC: may show a raised white cell count
- Amylase: will be grossly elevated in the acute phase
- Pancreatic lipase: is a more accurate marker than amylase as it has a longer half-life
- LFTs
- U&Es: to assess renal function
- Calcium: hypocalcaemia which can lead to tetany
- Inflammatory markers: CRP is a good marker of progress of acute pancreatitis
- Glucose: will be raised
- ABG: hypoxia can develop in severe cases

Imaging:

- CXR: may show a pleural effusion.
- AXR: a colon 'cut off' sign and a renal 'halo' sign may be seen.
- Abdominal USS: to assess for gallstones and possible dilatation of the common bile duct.
- CT: to assess disease severity, and identify any pseudocysts/fluid collection, which may require drainage. The visualisation of free fluid and air within pancreatic tissue indicates pancreatic necrosis. The Royal Society of Radiologists guidelines suggest CT is not indicated for the first 72 hours as these features present later.

Others:

- ECG: arrhythmia and absent T waves

Management

There are two common scoring systems used to assess the severity of the condition over the first 48 hours; Glasgow Imrie criteria and Ranson score.

Management for a mild attack: (Score <3)

- Conservative management on a general surgical ward is appropriate
- The patient is kept NBM
- IV fluids
- Frequent observation with repeated ABGs to assess acidotic state and lactate

Management for a severe attack: (Score ≥3)

- Aggressive management is required
- The patient is kept NBM with an NG tube sited
- High flow oxygen
- IV fluids as above
- IV analgesia: morphine titrated according to response
- Anti-emetic
- Strict fluid balance including a urinary catheter
- An identified biliary cause needs an urgent ERCP and sphincterotomy
- Support from and possible transfer to a HDU/ICU if necessary. May require inotropic support in severe sepsis
- Early enteral/parenteral nutritional support is important. Enteral feeding by naso-jejunal route has been shown to have lower complications but may require endoscopic placement
- Percutaneous drainage of pseudocysts may be required
- Surgery is avoided in the initial acute attack. However, it may be necessary for the patient to undergo debridement of the necrotic pancreas (necrosectomy) later in the disease particularly with infected necrosis
- If gallstones are identified on USS a laparoscopic cholecystectomy should be considered once the attack has settled

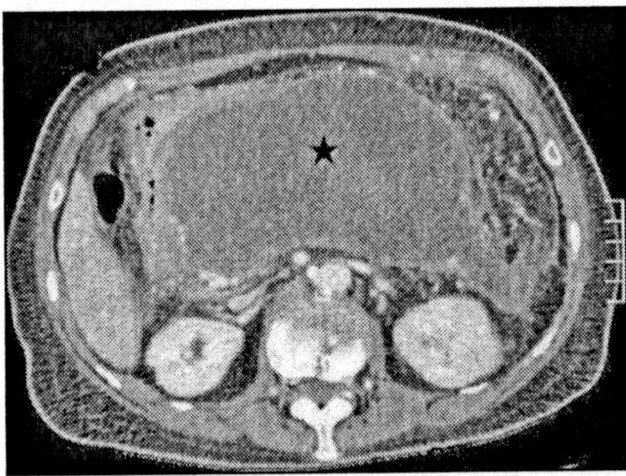

Figure 4.5: CT showing a large cystic collection in the anterior abdomen (star) with thick walls. This patient was recently discharged from the hospital after treatment for acute pancreatitis. Features are those of a large pancreatic pseudocyst

Glasgow Imrie criteria	Ranson score
1. Age >55 2. Blood glucose >11 mmol/L 3. Serum LDH >500 IU/L 4. AST >200 IU/I 5. White cell count >16 x 10^9/L 6. Blood urea >16 mmol/L 7. Serum calcium <2 mmol/L 8. Arterial pO_2 <8 kPa 9. Albumin <32 g/L	**On admission:** 1. Age >55 2. Blood glucose >11 mmol/L 3. Serum LDH >500 IU/L 4. AST >200 IU/L 5. White cell count >16 x 109/L **Within 48 hours:** 1. Blood urea >16 mmol/L 2. Serum calcium <2 mmol/L 3. Arterial pO_2 <8 kPa 4. Base deficit < –4 mmol/L 5. Haematocrit fall >10%

Table 4.5: The Glasgow Imrie criteria and Ranson score for assessing acute pancreatitis. One point is given for each criterion and if there is a score of three or more it indicates severe pancreatitis

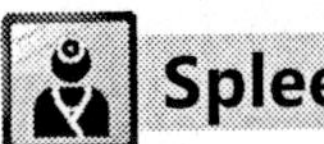

Spleen

Splenic rupture

Epidemiology

This is the commonest internal abdominal injury caused as a result of non-penetrating trauma.

Aetiology

Splenic rupture should be suspected after any trauma, especially injury to the left upper abdominal quadrant. If the overlying ribs are fractured this should increase clinical suspicion.

History/examination

Splenic rupture can have different presentations:

Haemorrhagic shock:

- Results from complete splenic rupture
- The spleen may have avulsed from its pedicle
- Death may occur rapidly
- Pallor
- Prolonged capillary refill time
- Drowsy and lethargic
- Tachycardic and hypotensive

Acute abdomen:

- Over hours, the patient may complain of abdominal pain (generalised or increased in the left flank)
- There is often referred left shoulder tip pain (Kehr's sign)
- Generalised or left sided abdominal tenderness on palpation
- Guarding and rigidity may be present
- Abdominal distension
- Bruising of the abdominal wall may be seen

Delayed rupture:

- Can occur hours to days after the injury
- Results from an enlarging splenic haematoma which suddenly ruptures
- Rare as haematoma generally identified by investigations early in presentation

Investigations

A diagnosis of a ruptured spleen is made clinically after a brief history and examination. If there is massive haemorrhage the surgeon may decide to proceed for an urgent laparotomy. If the patient is stable there may be time to perform a few specific investigations.

Imaging:

- CXR: rib fractures and a raised left hemi-diaphragm. Injury to the left lung (haemothorax or pneumothorax) may be apparent.
- AXR: the gastric bubble may be displaced to the right while the splenic outline and psoas shadow may not be seen. If there is a haematoma present in the spleen, the splenic flexure of the colon may be displaced downwards.

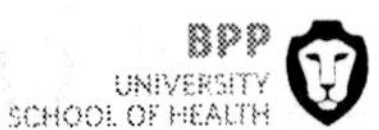

- Abdominal CT: will detect any splenic injury. Intra-abdominal fluid can be seen and damage to surrounding organs and structures can be identified.

Others:

- Urinalysis: the presence of haematuria may be suggestive of renal damage.

Management

Immediate management:

- A to E assessment and resuscitation as per ALS guidelines (will need IV fluids and blood products as soon as they are available)
- Appropriate analgesia (IV opioid and anti-emetic)
- Keep the patient NBM
- In a haemodynamically stable patient with a low grade splenic injury confirmed on CT, conservative management with close observation may be appropriate

Surgical management:

- If a patient requires resuscitation with blood products, an emergency splenectomy will be the next step, unless there is just a small laceration intra-operatively.

Post-splenectomy:

After a splenectomy has been performed patients are in an immunocompromised state.

- *Pneumoccal, Haemophilus* type B, and meningitis A and C vaccines should be given.
- Patients should receive annual flu vaccines.
- For patients at high risk from infection (age <16 or >50; poor response to pneumococcal vaccination; previous pneumococcal illness; underlying haematological malignancy): Penicillin V prophylaxis is recommended. The risk is highest in the first two years post-splenectomy.

Gynaecological structures

Ectopic pregnancy

Epidemiology

Ectopic pregnancies are defined as a fertilised ovum that has implanted outside the uterine cavity. It is becoming increasingly common, and in the UK alone it affects 1 in 60–100 pregnancies. Of these women approximately 10% will go on to have another ectopic pregnancy.

Aetiology

No specific cause has been identified. Any factor which damages the fallopian tubes can account for a tubal ectopic pregnancy. Other risk factors include assisted conception, pelvic and tubal surgery.

Pathophysiology

Ectopic pregnancies can occur at different sites. It affects <1% of pregnancies; however, there is an increase in risk with previous salpingitis and the use of intrauterine coil devices (IUDs).

The most common site is in the fallopian tube (95%). Other sites include the cervix, cornu, ovary, and abdominal cavity. With a tubal ectopic pregnancy the fallopian tube is unable to withstand the invasion of trophoblastic tissue. This results in bleeding into the lumen, which can result in rupture of the trophoblast. This leads to intra-peritoneal blood loss, which can be fatal. However, ectopic pregnancies can abort naturally without causing any symptoms.

History/examination

- Sudden onset of abdominal pain, which is initially colicky in nature and later becomes constant
- If a tubal ectopic pregnancy is present, the pain may be isolated to the right or left iliac fossa
- Abnormal dark vaginal bleeding
- Collapse
- Shoulder tip pain (suggesting intra-peritoneal blood loss)
- Tachycardia and hypotension (as a result of blood loss)
- Abdominal palpation may demonstrate guarding and rebound tenderness
- Vaginal examination: cervical excitation, tender adnexae, small uterus for expected gestational age and a closed cervical os

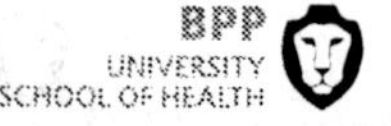

Investigations

Blood tests:

- FBC.
- Group and save and cross-match.
- Serum beta-hCG: more than 1,000 IU/L should show an intrauterine pregnancy on USS. In a viable pregnancy the serum beta-hCG rises by more than 66% in 48 hours. If the levels are rising slowly or falling, an ectopic or non-viable pregnancy may be present.

Urinalysis:

- Beta-hCG: should be performed in all women of reproductive age.

Imaging:

USS: may not visualise the ectopic pregnancy. It should identify an intrauterine pregnancy but if the uterus is empty the potential diagnosis is early gestation, a complete miscarriage or an ectopic pregnancy.

Management

Management of acute presentation:

- A to E assessment and resuscitation as appropriate as per ALS guidelines (IV fluids +/- blood products)
- Regular observations and strict fluid balance with a urinary catheter
- Analgesia eg IV opioid and an anti-emetic
- The patient is kept NBM
- Laparotomy and salpingectomy in haemodynamically unstable patients

Management of sub-acute presentation:

- A laparoscopic procedure is performed, either: salpingostomy (removal of the ectopic pregnancy) or salpingectomy (removal of the fallopian tube).
- If the ectopic pregnancy has not ruptured, is <35 mm in diameter, and serum beta-hCG is <5,000 IU/mL, a single dose of methotrexate can be given. Further doses may be required if unsuccessful. To ensure complete resolution, serial beta-hCG levels are performed every 48 hours until levels are low or undetectable.
- With small and unruptured ectopic pregnancies, and reducing beta-HhCG levels, no active treatment is required and the patient is managed conservatively.

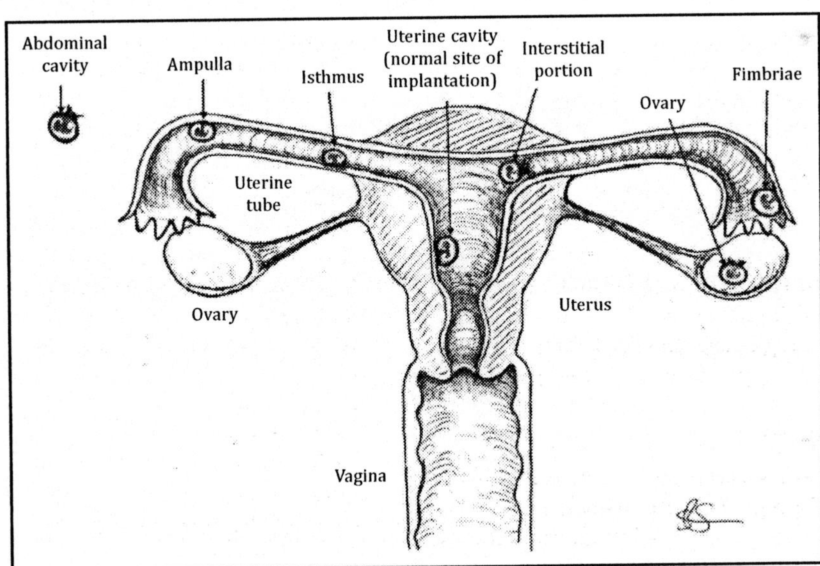

Figure 4.6: Sites of ectopic pregnancy

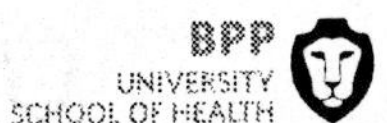

Ovarian torsion

Epidemiology

Ovarian torsion can occur at any age. However, approximately 70% of cases are seen in women less than 30. 17% of cases have been identified in those who are pre-menarchal or post-menopausal.

Aetiology

A number of factors have been identified as a cause of ovarian torsion. Torsion usually occurs as a result of an anatomical change or abnormality.

If it occurs in a young child the ovary is commonly normal, and the abnormality is usually a long fallopian tube or an absent mesosalpinx. During pregnancy an enlarged corpus luteum cyst predisposes to ovarian torsion. Women undergoing fertility treatment have an increased risk of ovarian torsion due to the increased number of luteal cysts, which increase the volume of the ovaries. Approximately 50–60% of cases involve an ovarian tumour.

Pathophysiology

Ovarian torsion typically occurs in an enlarged ovary and is usually unilateral. If there are ovarian masses involved in the case of torsion, they are commonly greater than 4–6 cm in size. Torsion can occur with masses of a smaller size.

History/examination

- Sudden onset of sharp, severe, unilateral abdominal pain, which increases in severity over time, can radiate to the back, pelvis or thigh and is exacerbated by exercise or movement
- Nausea, vomiting and fever
- Pyrexia and tachycardia are noted
- Abdominal palpation may identify a tender, unilateral, adnexal mass
- Signs of peritonitis are seen in late cases, as a result of ovarian necrosis

Investigations

Imaging:

- Pelvic USS: may show an ovarian enlargement that may be an ovarian mass or cyst.
- CT: can identify ovarian/pelvis masses or other causes of lower abdominal pain.

Management

- Involve seniors early!
- A to E assessment and resuscitation
- Analgesia eg NSAIDs or opioids
- Laparoscopy for diagnostic confirmation and treatment
- Possible oophoropexy (uncoiling the ovary and fixation to the pelvic wall)
- If on visualisation there is peritonitis or necrosis, the ovary and fallopian tube may be removed (salpingo-oophorectomy)

With early diagnosis and treatment there is excellent prognosis.

Urinary tract structures

Renal and ureteric calculi

Epidemiology

Renal tract calculi are common, with 50% of cases presenting between 30 and 50 years of age. It has a prevalence of 0.2% in the entire population.

Aetiology

Urinary tract calculi can occur without any explanation but there are three main predisposing factors:

1. Inadequate drainage (or stasis) of urine seen in cases of hydronephrosis or bladder diverticulum.
2. Increased amount of the normal constituents of urine, leading to supersaturated urine, which predisposes to calculi formation. This is seen in dehydration, hypercalcaemia eg hyperparathyroidism, gout or post-chemotherapy where there is increased uric acid production and in those with high oxalate levels.
3. The presence of abnormal urinary constituents, for example foreign bodies (stents, non-absorbable sutures, fragments of a urinary catheter). UTIs

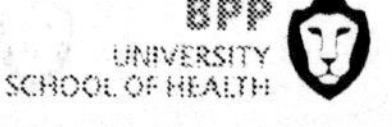

with obstruction may result in the production of epithelial slough and also tend to alter the urinary pH and precipitate stone formation (eg calcium phosphate stones). Cystine stone formation may occur as a result of an inborn error of amino acid metabolism.

Pathophysiology

There are three main constituents of urinary tract calculi; oxalate (60%), phosphate (30%), and urate (5%).

Oxalate stones have a hard, sharp surface that can damage the urinary epithelium. This results in bleeding from the tract causing the stones to appear black.

Phosphate stones are usually composed of calcium, ammonium, and magnesium phosphate. They are hard, chalky and white, are associated with a staghorn calculus and commonly found in patients with UTIs.

Urate stones are hard and brown with a smooth surface. Pure uric acid calculi are radiolucent.

The common sites for calculi impaction include the pelvi-ureteric junction, pelvic rim and vesico-ureteric junction.

History/examination

- Severe ureteric colic can occur if the stone impacts at the pelvic-ureteric junction, or moves down the ureter.
- The pain is generally a dull loin pain that radiates to the groin and is colicky in nature.
- Renal angle pain is noticed posteriorly, which is exacerbated by movement and palpation.
- If the pain radiates to the tip of the penis this can indicate a bladder stone.
- Some calculi may be asymptomatic.
- Nausea, vomiting, sweating and fever.
- The patient appears restless and cannot lie still.
- The lateral abdominal muscles are rigid.
- Percussion over the kidneys may illicit pain.

Investigations

Blood tests:

- FBC
- U&Es
- Calcium: raised serum calcium
- Phosphate levels
- Uric acid levels

Urinalysis:

- Visible or non-visible haematuria
- Nitrates and leucocytes suggest a possible UTI

Imaging:

- KUB: may show 90% of calculi.
- IVU: allows the anatomy of the renal tract to be visualised and identifies hydronephrosis and calculi. An IVU film must be compared to the plain KUB. Contraindications include contrast allergy, pregnancy, asthma, renal failure and patients taking metformin.
- A spiral, non-contrast CT scan: more sensitive in identifying renal calculi compared to an IVU. It can also diagnose and rule out other differential diagnoses, including ovarian cysts, and an aortic aneurysm.
- Dimercaptosuccinic acid (DMSA) scan: uses Technesium 99 and Dimercaptosuccinic acid to identify renal scarring, tumours and trauma.

Management

Conservative management:

- A to E assessment
- Analgesia eg morphine, pethidine, rectal diclofenac
- Encourage oral intake
- Ureteric stones less than 5 mm in size usually pass spontaneously

Long-term management:

- Ureteric stones: If the stone remains in the ureter and will not pass spontaneously intervention may be necessary.
- ESWL is used to shatter the stone. The smaller fragments can then be allowed to pass spontaneously.
- Ureteroscopy is the endoscopic removal of the stone. A dormia basket is used under direct visualisation. If the stone is too large for the basket the stones are fragmented using a laser.
- Open surgery, called ureterlithotomy, is used to gain access to the ureter, percutaneously to remove the ureteric stone.
- Renal stones: can also be managed with ESWL or a PCNL. Open surgery may be required to remove the stone, but this is very rare.
- In septic patients with an obstruction an emergency percutaneous nephrostomy tube is inserted and IV antibiotics are given.

- All patients should be encouraged to increase their oral intake to produce dilute urine.
- Indications for the removal of renal and ureteric calculi are: recurrent attacks of renal and ureteric colic, large/enlarging stones, bilateral renal obstruction/obstruction of a solitary kidney.

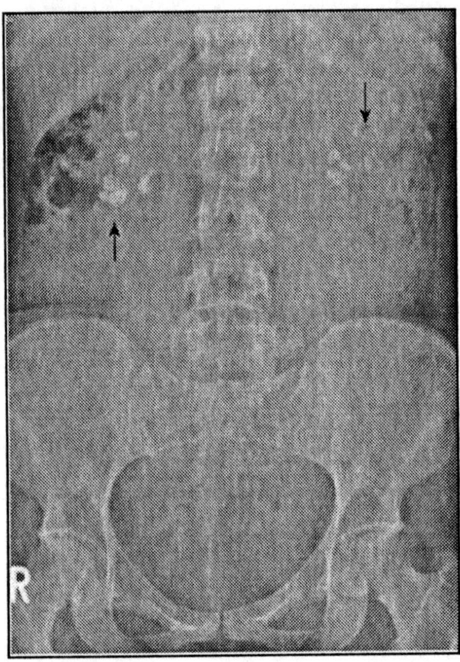

Figure 4.7: Plain X-ray of the abdomen showing bilateral multiple dense renal calculi (arrow)

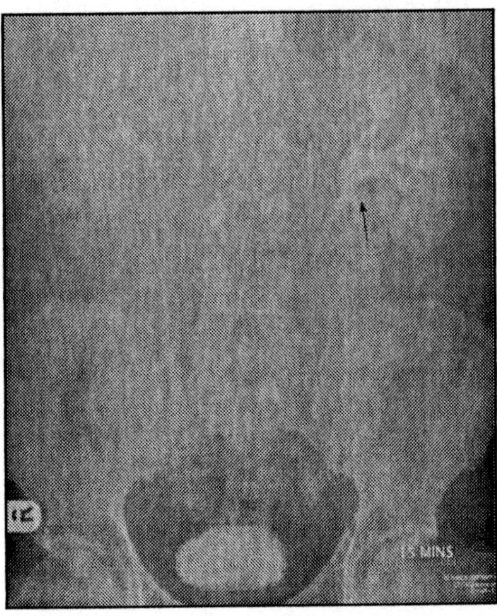

Figure 4.8: A 15 minute film from an IVU study showing delayed excretion of contrast from left kidney (arrow) with dilated pelvicalyceal system compared to the right side in keeping with mild hydronephrosis on the left

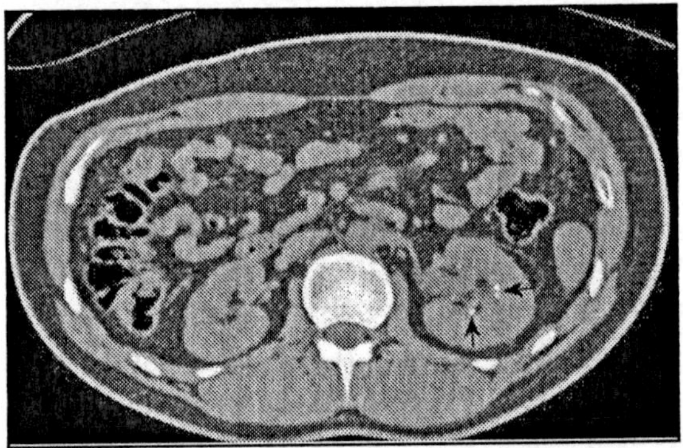

Figure 4.9: CT KUB examination showing three calculi in the left kidney (arrows). The right kidney is normal

Top tip:

Wash your hands and dry them before doing practical procedures – it allows you to more easily get gloves onto your hands which are likely to be sweaty and horrible on your first week in August!

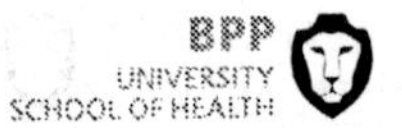

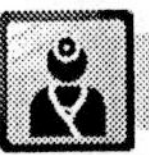

Vascular structures

Ruptured abdominal aortic aneurysm (AAA)

Epidemiology

An AAA is found in 2% of the population at autopsy. In 90% of cases they are found below the renal arteries (infra-renal). It has an incidence of 5% in patients with known coronary artery disease. AAAs can rupture anteriorly (20%) into the peritoneal cavity, and the remaining rupture posteriorly (80%) into the retroperitoneal space.

Aetiology

An AAA is defined as a greater than 50% increase in the normal aortic diameter (>3 cm in diameter). It is the commonest type of aortic aneurysm. Risk factors include: increasing age, smoking, atherosclerosis, hypertension, connective tissue disorders such as Marfan's syndrome and syphilis infection.

Pathophysiology

Elastin is a component of the connective tissue of the aorta which provides its tensile strength. In the normal human aorta there is gradual reduction in the amount of elastin in the distal portion of the aorta compared with the proximal segment. The walls in an AAA show elastin fragmentation and degeneration.

Risk factors for heart disease such as atherosclerotic plaques weaken artery walls, and disrupt the integrity of the tunica media. Smoking also causes arterial stiffness and thus predisposes vessels to damage.

Connective tissue disorders such as Marfan's syndrome and Ehlers-Danlos syndrome predispose patients to AAAs. Syphilis infection results in mycotic aneurysms but this is rarely seen today.

History/examination

- Severe, sudden onset generalised abdominal pain, particularly with radiation to the back and groin
- Associated symptoms include nausea, vomiting, cold legs and sweating
- Signs of shock (cold, clammy, tachycardia and hypotension)
- Altered levels of consciousness
- Absent femoral pulses in one or both groins
- A pulsatile mass on abdominal palpation
- A radio-radial delay is a well-known but rare sign of dissection involving the thoracic aorta

Investigations

Investigations should only be performed if the patient is haemodynamically stable, or if there is reasonable doubt about the diagnosis. Any delay in treatment may be fatal.

Blood tests:

- Crossmatch 6–8 units of blood
- FBC
- U&Es
- Glucose
- LFTs
- Clotting
- Venous or arterial blood gas: to check lactate and current state of tissue oxygenation

Imaging:

- AXR: an aneurysm may be difficult to palpate either due to hypotension, or the presence of a large retroperitoneal aneurysm. A plain film will show calcification in the wall of the aneurysm and loss of the 'psoas shadow'.
- CT abdomen: needed if the patient is known to have an aneurysm and presents with abdominal pain and is normotensive. A CT scan would be the most useful investigation to identify a leak. A CT scan can identify relevant anatomy such as the relationship of the aneurysm to the renal arteries and involvement of the common iliac vessels. It can provide information regarding the aortic angulation and dimensions, which are paramount if EVAR is to be considered. This investigation will not differentiate between an uncomplicated aneurysm and one that is about to rupture.
- CXR – widening of the aortic arch may indicate thoracic aortic aneurysm.

Others:

- ECG

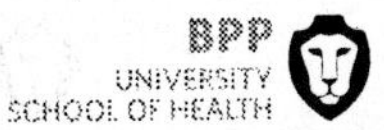

Management

Immediate management:

- 50% of patients with a ruptured AAA die prior to reaching hospital
- A-E assessment as per ALS guidelines
- Fluid resuscitation in accordance with principle of permissive hypotension ie not allowing SBP to rise above 90–100 mmHg as this may cause further bleeding
- IV analgesia and anti-emetic
- Accurate fluid balance – will require urinary catheter
- Preparation for emergency theatre: anaesthetic involvement, theatre staff and intensive care notification, consent

Surgical management:

- An open approach is traditionally employed.
- The neck of the aneurysm is clamped below the renal arteries and an artificial graft is sutured inside the aneurysm sac (may be straight or bifurcated).
- In specialist centres for non-ruptured aneurysms, EVAR repair may be considered. This decision is dependent on aneurysmal morphology, patient age, fitness for surgery and general expectations.
- Aneurysmal repair either traditionally or using EVAR confers significant mortality and morbidity, including acute renal failure, MI, and distal embolisation.

Aortic dissection

Epidemiology

Aortic dissection is a problem affecting adults mainly between the ages of 50 and 70. It is the most common emergency affecting the aorta.

Aetiology

The aortic wall is weakened by cystic medial degeneration and thus causing splitting of the wall to occur. Patients with atherosclerosis, hypertension and Marfan's syndrome are predisposed to aortic dissection.

Pathophysiology

Aortic dissection comprises of a tear in the aortic wall allowing blood to dissect between the middle and outer layers of the tunica media and adventitia, creating a false passage. This may rupture internally into the true lumen of the aorta creating a double lumen. If the aneurysm ruptures externally, it can result in cardiac tamponade and fatal haemorrhage. When the aortic layers separate, the lumen can become obstructed which leads to end-organ ischaemia.

Aortic dissections can be classified into Stanford type A and type B dissections. Type A occurs in two-thirds of all cases and affects the ascending aorta as well as the arch of the aorta. Type B occurs in one-third of all cases and affects the descending aorta only.

Top tip:

The hospital never sleeps. There will always be more to be done, and you can never finish everything. Hand over, go home, and don't worry about it until you're back in again. Otherwise you will go mad.

History/examination

- Sudden onset chest pain, which can radiate to the arms, neck or abdomen
- Typically a 'tearing interscapular pain'
- A new diastolic murmur (representing aortic regurgitation)
- Pulseless, cold legs from femoral artery occlusion
- Oliguria from renal artery occlusion
- Paraplegia or hemiplegia as a result of vertebral artery or carotid artery occlusion

Investigations

Imaging:

- CXR: widening of the mediastinum with the loss of aortic knob silhouette. A pleural effusion (haemothorax) may also be present.
- CT: identifies the origin and extent of the dissection.

Others:

- Echocardiogram: may demonstrate an intimal flap, a pericardial effusion and aortic regurgitation.
- ECG: inferior ECG changes from dissection of coronary orifices.

Management

Management of type A dissection:

- Surgery is recommended via a median sternotomy to initiate cardiopulmonary bypass, cross-clamp

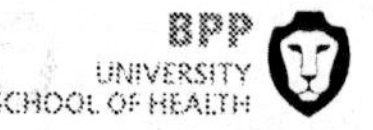

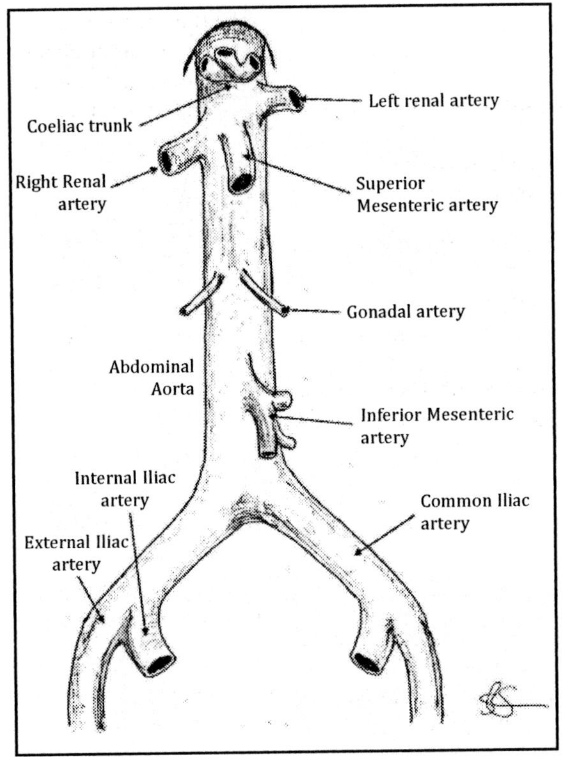

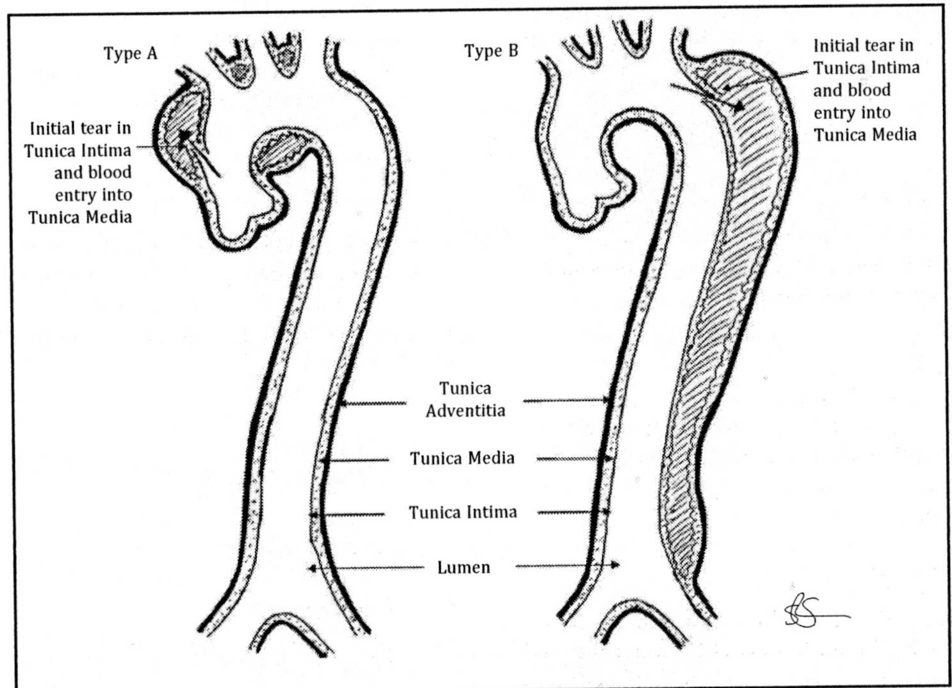

Figure 4.10: Type A and type B Aortic dissection

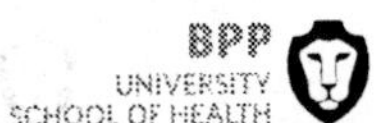

the aorta, resect the aneurysmal segment and insert a synthetic graft
- The aortic valve may need replacing and is often done using a composite graft consisting of a valve and tube

Management of type B dissection:

- Medical treatment is first-line: antihypertensive drugs are used to reduce the systolic blood pressure to prevent further dissection and thrombosis of the dissected segment may then occur.
- Surgery may be an option if: increasing pain indicated possible rupture, neurological symptoms develop or the aneurysm is increasing in size on serial CXRs.

Surgical complications include haemorrhage (20%), renal failure (20%), paraplegia (11%), MI (30%) and death (15%).

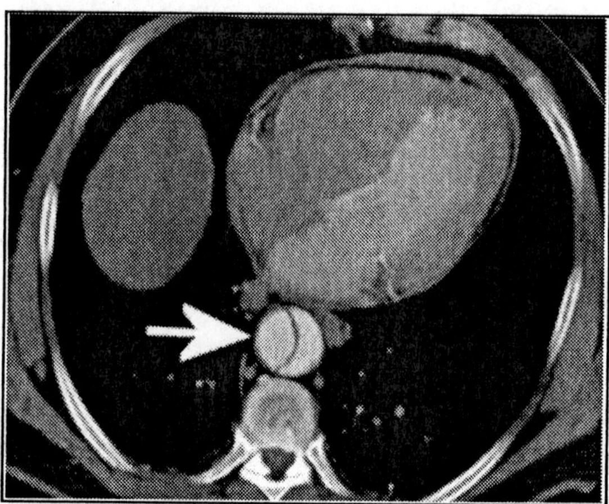

Figure 4.11: CT axial image of the chest showing a clear dissection flap in the descending thoracic aorta (arrow)

Prognosis

Two-thirds of surviving patients will die within seven years as a result of cardiac and cerebrovascular disease.

Mesenteric infarction

Epidemiology

Mesenteric ischaemia accounts for 1–2% of all gastrointestinal diseases. It is typically a disease of adults over the age of 50 and is a cause of 0.1% of all hospital admissions.

Aetiology

Acute intestinal ischaemia can occur as a result of arterial, venous, central, or peripheral vascular disease. The superior mesenteric vessels are the vessels most likely to be affected by emboli or thrombus.

Typically, emboli lodge at the branch of the middle colic artery (first large branch of the superior mesenteric artery). Mesenteric emboli can arise from the left atrium in AF, a mural thrombus after an MI, atheromatous plaque from an aortic aneurysm, and mitral valve vegetation. Mesenteric arterial thrombosis is usually secondary to atheroma but arterial occlusion can also be a result of post-aortic dissection.

Mesenteric venous thrombosis may occur as a result of pre-existing diseases including portal hypertension, sickle cell disease, women on the contraceptive pill, and thrombophillia.

Pathophysiology

The blood supply to the gut can be divided into three main parts. The foregut (stomach and duodenum) receives blood via the coeliac artery, the mid-gut (jejunum to distal transverse colon) receives blood via the SMA, and the hind-gut (remaining gut) receives blood via the inferior mesenteric artery.

Haemorrhagic infarction occurs with both arterial and venous occlusion but ischaemic infarction can occur with or without occlusion of the vessels. Thrombosis is commonly the cause of occlusion at the origin of the SMA.

The mucosal layer of the intestinal wall has little resistance to ischaemic injury, and therefore results in an oedematous intestine and mesentery. Bloodstained fluid then tracks into the bowel lumen and peritoneal cavity. Eventually gangrene and perforation of the ischaemic bowel occurs.

With small occlusions the patient may remain asymptomatic as a result of collateral circulation.

History/examination

- Sudden onset of colicky, central abdominal pain, which increases in severity over time
- Rectal bleeding, persistent vomiting and frequent defecation
- Evidence of recent MI, cardiac arrhythmia, and peripheral vascular disease should increase

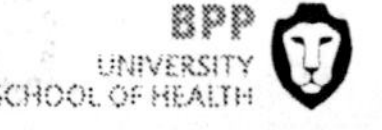

suspicion of mesenteric ischaemia
- Signs of hypovolaemic shock
- Mild abdominal tenderness in the early stages, with guarding and a rigid abdomen in the later stage
- Rarely a tender mass may be palpated, which represents the infarcted bowel
- Classically, the pain is disproportionate to the examination findings

Investigations

There are no specific laboratory investigations that are diagnostic of mesenteric ischaemia.

Blood tests:

- FBC: significantly raised white cell count
- Group and save, and cross-match
- ABG: metabolic acidosis and raised lactate may be present and are an indication of the patient's clinical condition

Imaging:

- Erect CXR: to exclude perforation
- AXR: thick intestinal walls may be seen
- CT: scan is not diagnostic but able to identify the site of bowel inflammation. It helps to exclude other differential diagnosis
- Mesenteric angiogram: can differentiate between embolic, thrombotic or non-occlusive ischaemia and also diagnose mesenteric vein thrombosis

Others:

- ECG: Acute MI or cardiac arrhythmias may be revealed.

Management

- A to E assessment in accordance with ALS guidelines and resuscitation as required.
- In early cases an SMA arteriotomy and embolectomy may be performed.
- Surgical management involves resecting the affected bowel. The viable bowel is then inspected the next day with a second look laparotomy.
- If the entire supply to the mesentery has been affected (the small intestine and right side of colon) the situation is usually fatal.
- Infarction of the large bowel alone is rare, but is managed with a transverse colectomy (if the ischaemia is confined to the transverse colon).
- Post-operative anticoagulation is required to prevent further emboli.

If successful it is important to address patient nutrition. Often patients will require permanent parenteral nutrition.

Further reading and references

1. Addiss, D.G., Fowler, B.S., Shaffer, N., et al. (1990) The epidemiology of appendicitis and appendectomy in the United States. *Am J Epidemiol* 1990; 132: 910–925.
2. Bulstrode, C.J.K., Russell, R.C.G. and Williams, N.S. (2000) *Bailey & Love's Short Practice of Surgery*. 23rd Edition. London: Arnold.
3. Calne, R., Ellis, H., and Whatson, C. (2002) *Lecture Notes on General Surgery*. 10th Edition. Oxford: Blackwell Publishing.
4. Goldberg, A. and Stansby, G. (2006) *Surgical Talk: Revision in Surgery*. 2nd Edition. London: Imperial College Press.
5. Gurusamy, K.S. and Samraj, K. (2009) *Early versus delayed laparoscopic cholecystectomy for acute cholecystitis (Review)*. The Cochrane Collaboration. John Wiley & Sons LT.
6. Department of Health UK. (2004) *Hospital appendicitis episode statistics: financial year 2004*. [Online]. Available from: www.hesonline.nhs.uk [Accessed 7 November 2016].
7. Humes, D.J. and Simpson, J. (2006) Clinical review: Acute appendicitis. BMJ 2006; 333.
8. Impey, L. (2004) *Obstetrics and Gynaecology*. 2nd Edition. Oxford: Blackwell Publishing.
9. Beckingham, I.J. and Indar, A.A. (2002) Clinical review: Acute cholecystitis. *BMJ* 2002; 325: 639–643.
10. Baillie, J. and Mergener, K. (1998) Fortnightly review: Acute pancreatitis. *BMJ* 1998; 316: 44–48.
11. Lingeman, J.E. and Miller, N.L. (2007) Clinical review: Management of kidney stones. *BMJ* 2007; 334: 468–472.
12. Katerndahl, D. and Munoz, A. (2000) Diagnosis and management of acute pancreatitis. *American Family Physician* 63.

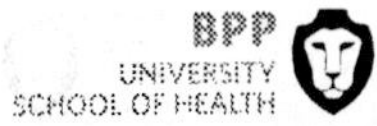

13. National Institute of Health and Care Excellence. (2015) *Gallstone Disease* (QS104). [Online]. Available from: www.nice.org.uk/guidance/qs104 [Accessed 7 November 2016].
14. National Institute of Health and Care Excellence. (2014) *Gallstone Disease – diagnosis and initial management* (CG188). [Online]. Available from: www.nice.org.uk/guidance/cg188 [Accessed 7 November 2016].
15. Stukel, T.A. and Urbach, D.R. (2005) Rate of elective cholecystectomy and the incidence of severe gallstone disease. *CMAJ* 172(8): 1015–9.
16. Weintraub, N.L. (2009) Understanding Abdominal Aortic Aneurysm. *NEJM* 361: 1114–1116.
17. Surgical Tutor, www.surgical-tutor.org.uk.
18. Yasuhara, H. (2005) Acute Mesenteric Ischemia: The challenge of Gastroenterology. *Surgery Today* 2005; Vol 3(3).

Rectal bleeding

Differential diagnosis

System	Disease
Upper gastrointestinal tract	Bleeding duodenal ulcer
Lower gastrointestinal tract	**Haemorrhoids**
	Anal fissure
	colorectal tumours
	Diverticular disease
	Ulcerative colitis (UC)
Others	Trauma
	Angiodysplasia

Table 4.6: Differential of rectal bleeding

Haemorrhoids

Epidemiology

This condition is extremely common and occurs in up to 50% of the adult population.

Aetiology

Haemorrhoids can be idiopathic but hereditary forms are seen too. Hereditary haemorrhoids are often seen in members of the same family. A theory of possible congenital weakness of the vein walls has been suggested. Leg varicose veins and haemorrhoids have been found to occur simultaneously.

The superior rectal veins lie within the connective tissue of the ano-rectum and drains into the inferior mesenteric vein. These veins engorge during increased abdominal pressure (commonly defecation).

Haemorrhoids are defined by their origin in relation to the dentate line which delineates the transition point from columnar epithelium above, to squamous below.

Predisposing factors can result in congestion of the superior rectal veins. These risk factors include:

- Straining due to constipation
- Pelvic tumour
- Pregnancy
- Use of purgatives
- Rectal carcinoma
- Enteritis and colitis (can exacerbate haemorrhoids)

Pathophysiology

Haemorrhoids are defined as 'vascular cushions containing a branch of the superior rectal artery and vein'.

They are external or internal in relation to the anus. External haemorrhoids are covered by skin and found below the dentate line, whereas internal haemorrhoids are covered by mucous membrane and found above the dentate line. Interio-external haemorrhoids is a term given to those internal haemorrhoids that prolapse.

Once the patient is placed into the lithotomy position major piles are located at the 3, 7, and 11 o'clock position. Each individual haemorrhoid can be divided into three parts:

1. The pedicle: found at the ano-rectal ring, and covered by a pale pink mucosa
2. The internal haemorrhoid: bright red or purple and originates from just above the dentate line
3. External associated haemorrhoid: covered by a layer of skin, with visible veins

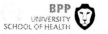

The complications of haemorrhoids include:

- Strangulation
- Thrombosis
- Ulceration and gangrene
- Fibrosis

Grade	Features
First degree	Do not prolapse but can bleed
Second degree	Prolapse on straining or defecation, but reduce spontaneously
Third degree	Prolapse and can only be manually replaced
Fourth degree	Prolapse and are irreducible

Table 4.7: The different grades of haemorrhoids

History/examination

- Bleeding is the most common symptom and it arises early in the disease. The blood is bright red and is seen around the motion not mixed in
- Mucous discharge is commonly associated with prolapsed haemorrhoids
- Pruritus
- Thrombosed, strangulated external haemorrhoids are swollen and very painful
- Prolapse occurs late in the disease and is seen in second to fourth degree haemorrhoids
- Rarely, symptoms of anaemia if profuse bleeding
- Exclude any palpable colonic masses and exacerbating factors such as a pregnant uterus, pelvic mass and enlarged liver
- Prolapsed piles are easily identified on rectal examination but internal haemorrhoids cannot be palpated

Investigations

Endoscopy:

- Proctoscopy: can show large prolapsed haemorrhoids encompassing tissue from above and below the dentate line.
- Sigmoidoscopy: to exclude any lesion further up the rectum eg polyp or tumour.
- Colonoscopy: performed if a further lesion is identified. A biopsy can be taken.

Management

Conservative treatment:

- Avoidance of straining when passing stool:
  - Encourage increased oral intake
  - Bulk laxatives
- Thrombosed, strangulated haemorrhoids can be treated with topical Lidocaine gel, ice packing, and analgesia.

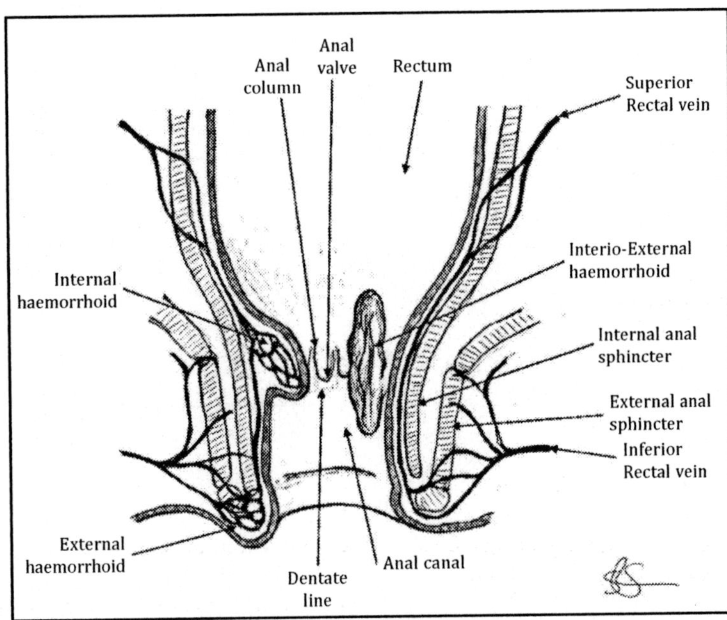

Figure 4.12: The different types of haemorrhoids

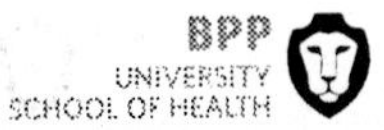

Sclerotherapy:

- Suitable for first and second degree haemorrhoids.
- 2–3 ml of 0.5% phenol in almond oil (sclerosing agent) is injected above each haemorrhoid.
- The injection is painless and further injections may be required at monthly intervals.

Haemorrhoid banding:

- Large first and second degree haemorrhoids are not suitable for injection therapy and are treated with banding.
- Tight elastic bands are placed at the base of the haemorrhoid pedicle, resulting in necrosis and spontaneous detachment. These are done above the dentate line, otherwise they can be very painful.

Haemorrhoidectomy (operative management):

- Performed for third or fourth degree haemorrhoids
- An alternative procedure is the minimally invasive Doppler-guided haemorrhoidal artery ligation of the terminal branches of the superior haemorrhoidal artery
- Early complications: pain, acute urinary retention and reactionary haemorrhage
- Late complications: secondary haemorrhage, anal stricture and an anal fissure
- Post-operative advice: regular analgesia, bulk laxatives, warm baths, dry and sterile dressings, outpatient review in four to six weeks

Anal fissures

Epidemiology

Anal fissure occurs predominantly in young to middle-aged adults and show no gender predominance.

Aetiology

Described as a longitudinal tear of the squamous epithelium lining the lower half of the anal canal from the anal verge to the dentate line. 90% of all fissures are found at the posterior site in the midline. It is not fully understood as to why this is the common site of occurrence; however, it is thought that during defecaetion this is where the majority of the pressure is applied.

Anterior anal fissures are more common in women, especially in those who are multi-parous. This is thought to be a result of damage to the pelvic floor following perineal tears during labour.

Anal fissures can be a complication of inflammatory bowel disease (normally Crohn's disease) or as a complication following haemorrhoid surgery.

After the initial formation of an anal fissure the pain experienced on defecation results in anal sphincter spasm, which extends the fissure line. This leads to the development of a spasm-fissure cycle.

Pathophysiology

Anal fissures can be acute or chronic. Acute anal fissures have a significant tear through the skin of the anal margin. The tear extends through the anal canal and there will be slight skin induration and oedema. There may also be spasms of the anal sphincter muscle.

In chronic anal fissures there is inflammation and induration of the fissure margins. The base of the fissure or lower border of the internal sphincter muscle may consist of scar tissue and, in long-term cases, fibrosis develops as well as continuous contraction of the sphincter muscles. In addition, there is an increased risk of infection, abscess, and fistula formation.

History/examination

- Pain on defecation that is sharp and stinging in character. It lasts one to two hours after the stool has been passed and as a result of anticipated pain the patient usually avoids passing stool.
- Pruritus.
- Bleeding is usually minimal and only noticed on wiping.
- A small amount of discharge.
- The anus should be examined but digital rectal examination may not be possible as a result of extreme pain.
- A sentinel pile may be identified in association with the fissure. This occurs because the base of the fissue becomes oedematous and hypertrophied.

Investigations

The diagnosis is clinical.

Management

Conservative management:

- Advice to avoid straining (use of bulk laxatives etc)
- Topical anaesthetic such as Xylocaine gels for analgesia

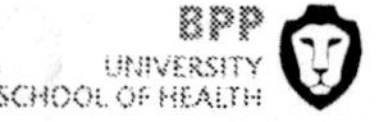

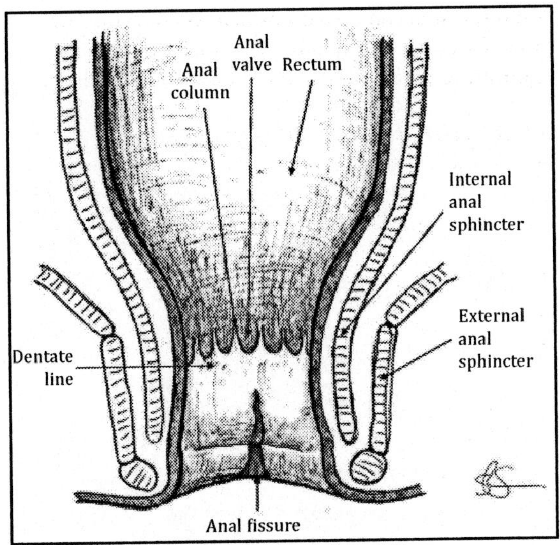

Figure 4.13: Anal fissure

- Topical nitrates (eg 0.2% glyceryl trinitrate paste) may cause relaxation of the internal sphincter
- Botulinum A toxin can be injected into the external anal sphincter to break the spasm-fissure cycle. This is less invasive and has a lower rate of faecal incontinence compared to sphincterotomy

Surgical management

Dilatation of the sphincter:

- Under general anaesthesia the index and middle finger are placed into the anus and it is dilated. It is important to not overstretch the anal sphincter as this can lead to incontinence (a major complication).

Anal sphincterectomy:

- The internal sphincter is divided and separated from the fissure.
- More suited for acute anal fissures.
- A small risk of incontinence following the procedure.

Further reading and references

1. Acheson, A.G. and Scholefield, J.H. (2008) Clinical review: Management of haemorrhoids. *BMJ* 2008; 336: 380–383.
2. Goldberg, A. and Stansby, G. (2006) *Surgical Talk: Revision in Surgery*. 2nd Edition. London: Imperial College Press.
3. Fox, T., Haas, G., and Haas, P. (1984) The Pathogenesis of haemorrhoids. *Disease of the Colon and Rectum* 1984; 27(7).
4. Nelson, R (2007). A Review of Operative Procedures for Anal Fissure. *Journal of Gastrointestinal Surgery* 2007; 6:284-289.

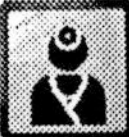

Haematuria

Differential diagnosis

Classification	Disease
Infections	Urinary tract infection (UTI) Tuberculosis
Cancers	**Renal tumours** **Bladder cancer**
Others	Urinary tract calculi **Polycystic disease** Bleeding disorder Glomerulonephritis **Trauma** Drugs

Table 4.8: Differential diagnosis of haematuria

Renal tumours

Epidemiology

Renal tumours are very uncommon and tend to present in adults over the age of 40. Male to female ratio is 2:1. Renal cell carcinoma or hypernephroma accounts for 2% of all adult malignancies. Wilms' tumour in children accounts for 8% of childhood cancers.

Aetiology

The aetiology is unknown but there are factors associated with the development of renal tumours. Carcinogens have been identified as a risk factor for transitional cell carcinoma. Those with chronic

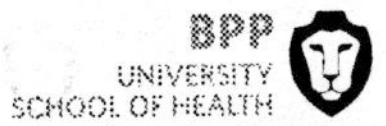

renal stones are at risk of developing squamous cell carcinoma (SSC). Renal cell carcinoma is associated with Von Hippel-Lindau disease and smoking is also a known risk factor.

Pathophysiology

Renal tumours can be benign (eg cysts) or malignant. Malignant tumours can be primary or secondary. While secondary tumours are rare, primary tumours can be classified as those arising from the pelvis and those from the kidney.

Tumours arising from the pelvis can either be transitional cell carcinomas, SSCs or papillomas. Transitional cell carcinomas are extremely malignant and occur where there is transitional cell epithelium present. SSCs commonly progress from squamous metaplasia.

History/examination

- Renal colic
- Hypertension
- A mass palpated in the loin
- Transitional cell carcinoma can be asymptomatic or present with painless haematuria
- Hypernephromas only occur in 11% of cases and generally patients only present in advanced disease. It may present with a classic triad of loin pain, loin mass and haematuria
- Varicocele is present in 1% of cases where the tumour has spread along the renal vein obstructing the testicular vein
- Anorexia and weight loss
- Pallor (anaemia)

Tumour	Features
Hypernephroma (Grawitz tumour)	• 80% of all renal tumours • Associations with Von Hippel-Lindau disease, and tuberous sclerosis • The tumour originates from the renal tubules and macroscopically looks like a large vascular mass
Nephroblastoma (Wilms' tumour)	• Childhood tumour usually affecting children below the age of 5 • Bilateral tumours in 5–10% of cases • The tumours are thought to originate from embryonic mesodermal tissue • There are known associations with congenital anomalies such as macroglossia, and aniridia • The tumours are large, pale and contain haemorrhagic areas

Table 4.9: Comparison of two main renal tumours

Investigations

Blood tests:

- FBC
- U&Es
- LFTs
- Calcium
- Clotting
- Group and save

Urinalysis:

- Urine dipstick: to demonstrate haematuria
- Cytology: for transitional cell carcinomas only

Imaging:

- CXR: to identify any metastasis
- IVU: will identify filling defects, hydronephrosis and any renal mass
- USS: may identify a mass and it can distinguish between solid and cystic tumours. The involvement of the inferior vena cava can be determined
- CT: for staging and assessment of the other kidney/ metastatic spread
- MRI: renal vein or caval thrombosis

Features of the kidney	Features of the spleen
• Ballotable • Moves down vertically on inspiration • Resonant to percussion as a result of overlying bowel	• Notched • Moves towards the right iliac fossa on inspiration • Dull to percussion as there is no overlying bowel

Table 4.10: Differentiating between the kidney and spleen

Management

- Nephroureterectomy is the surgical procedure of choice for transitional cell carcinomas. This involves removal of the entire renal tract on the affected side.

- Laparosopic or open radical nephrectomy is performed for large nephromas with a normal functioning kidney on the other side.
- A partial nephrectomy can be considered in small tumours of less than 4 cm and in those patients with a single functioning kidney. The local recurrence rate is <10%.
- In metastatic disease, palliative chemo- and radiotherapy is possible.

Prognosis

- Nephroblastomas have an 80% survival rate for the first 5 years in children less than 1. Recurrence commonly occurs within the first year but it is unlikely after 18 months.
- In operable hypernephromas there is a 70% survival after 3 years and 60% after 5 years. The 5-year survival with metastatic disease is 20%.

Bladder cancer

Epidemiology

Bladder cancer usually occurs in adults over the age of 65 years. It has an incidence of 1 in 5,000 in the UK, affecting 4 times as many men than women.

Aetiology

The aetiology remains unknown but there are a number of predisposing factors:

- Smoking
- Pelvic irradiation
- Industrial toxins from the dye industry such as beta-naphthylamine
- Chronic bladder irritation due to schistosomiasis, calculi or chronic infection
- Urachal remnants, eg embryological remnants between the umbilicus and the bladder

Schistosomiasis is associated with SSC with a peak age of incidence between the sixth and eight decades. The male to female ratio is 3:1.

Pathophysiology

90% of bladder cancers are transitional cell carcinomas. They can be solid, papillary, or both. SSC accounts for 7% and AC accounts for 2%. The tumour can spread directly to the rectum, vagina, prostate, and uterus. Renal failure can result due to obstruction of the ureters, leading to hydronephrosis. The liver and lung are the common sites for metastatic disease.

Stage	Level of spread
Ta	Confined to the mucosa
T1	Lamina propria is invaded
T2	The muscle is involved
T3	The perivesical fat is involved
T4	The tumour has invaded beyond the bladder to adjacent organs or to the pelvic wall

Table 4.11: Tumour, node and metastasis (TNM) staging

History/examination

- Commonly patients are asymptomatic
- Painless haematuria
- Dysuria, urgency and frequency
- Acute urinary retention (bladder neck obstruction)
- Suprapubic or pelvic pain
- Palpable mass
- Lymph nodes
- Hepatomegaly
- Shortness of breath if metastatic lung disease
- Signs of anaemia

Investigations

Blood tests:

- FBC
- U&Es
- LFTs
- Calcium
- Clotting
- Group and save

Urinalysis:

- Urine dipstick: to demonstrate haematuria
- Cytology: for transitional cell carcinomas only

Imaging:

- CXR: to identify metastases
- IVU: will identify filling defects, hydronephrosis and any renal masses
- USS: may identify a mass and distinguish between solid and cystic tumours. The involvement of the inferior vena cava can be determined

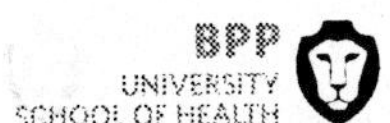

- CT: for staging and identification of metastatic spread
- MRI: renal vein or vena caval tumour thrombosis

Management

- All tumours are resected via TURBT.
- Stage Ta, T1, T2 and Grade G1, G2:
  - Intra-vesical chemotherapy with a repeat cystoscopy 8-10.
  - Intra-vesical immunotherapy using BCG is more effective than chemotherapy in treating recurrent disease. However, there are increased side effects.
  - All patients are followed up with regular cystoscopies at six month to one year intervals.
- Stage T3, T4 and Grade G3:
  - Radical radiotherapy
  - Cystectomy with the formation of an ileal conduit

Prognosis

Stage	Five-year survival rate
Ta/T1	70–80%
T2	40–50%
T3	25%
T4	Patients are dead with one year

Table 4.12: Five-year survival rates for bladder cancer

Polycystic disease

Epidemiology

Adult polycystic kidney disease usually presents in those aged between 30 and 60. It accounts for 8–10% of all end-stage renal disease (ESRD).

Aetiology

This is an autosomal dominant congenital condition. Polycystic kidney disease in children involves autosomal recessive inheritance and usually presents with renal failure. The aetiology of all renal cysts remains unknown.

Pathophysiology

Multiple cysts are present throughout the renal parenchyma. The cysts are different in size and can contain clear fluid, or coagulated blood.

Other associations include liver cysts (30%), cysts in the lungs, spleen and pancreas (10%) and intracranial berry aneurysms.

History/examination

- Abdominal mass: commonly bilateral
- Loin pain: is characteristically a dull, constant ache
- Severe pain may result if there is haemorrhage into the cysts
- Urinary retention and dysuria
- Uraemia: headache, anorexia and fatigue. There may also be drowsiness and vomiting
- Drowsy and lethargic
- Loin tenderness on palpation
- Irregular and knobbly kidney enlargement
- Hypertension (75%)
- Pyrexia and tachycardia with an infection

Investigations

Blood tests:

- U&Es: urea and creatinine are elevated in renal failure

Urinalysis:

- Urine dipstick: may reveal a UTI or haematuria

Imaging:

- USS: can identify cysts in adults. It is less useful in children as a result of the smaller sized renal cysts.
- IVU: the contrast will outline elongated and narrow calyces.

Management

- Medical treatment for renal failure and the associated hypertension (may include dialysis)
- Management of complications such as anaemia and infection – usually under the care of a nephrologist
- Nephrectomy if there is chronic loin pain, recurrent infections, haematuria and large kidneys
- A bilateral nephrectomy may be necessary to control severe hypertension

Trauma

Epidemiology

In the UK 90% of renal trauma is due to blunt trauma. Approximately 40% of these patients have associated intra-abdominal injuries.

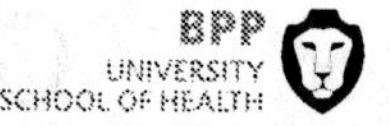

Aetiology

Injury to the kidney can result from a direct blow to the loin or a penetrating wound. Abdominal crush injury in road traffic accidents can also affect the kidneys.

Pathophysiology

The degree of damage can vary from mild bruising or a capsular haematoma to complete rupture. The kidney may also be partially or completely avulsed from its vascular pedicle.

History/examination

- Loin pain.
- Haematuria.
- Abdominal distension secondary to an ileus, as a result of a retroperitoneal haematoma.
- Examination may only reveal tenderness over the loin/renal angle on palpation.
- With blunt trauma, other organs are often involved, for example the liver and spleen. Signs and symptoms may arise as a result of damage to these organs.

Investigations

Urinalysis:

- Urine dipstick: visible (macroscopic) haematuria may develop a few hours post-injury.

Imaging:

- IVU: the contrast medium used may indicate rupture/damage to the renal calyces. A normal kidney will also be identified on the opposite side.
- USS: may identify a renal tear. Other injuries such as liver and spleen damage may also be detected.
- CT: used in all trauma patients to identify injuries.

Management

Immediate management:

- Manage as per ALERT guidelines with an A to E assessment
- Visible haematuria should result in bed rest, avoidance of physical activity and investigation to identify the cause
- Analgesia
- Antibiotics if infection suspected
- A three-way catheter may need to be placed if the patient goes into acute retention (likely clot retention) for bladder irrigation

Surgical management:

- 95% of cases are managed conservatively.
- Surgery may be required if there is progressive blood loss and an enlarging mass is identified in the loin.
- A nephrectomy is performed if there is life-threatening haemorrhage or severe post-trauma hypertension.
- Alternatively, renal embolisation can be performed to treat the haemorrhage.

Further reading and references

1. Feldman, A.S., Kaufman, D.S. and Shipley, W.U. (2009) Bladder Cancer. *Lancet* 2009; 374.
2. Parchment-Smith, C. (2006) *Essential Revision Notes for Intercollegiate MRCS: Bk.* 1. Knutsford: PasTest.
3. Parchment-Smith, C. (2006) *Essential Revision Notes for Intercollegiate MRCS: Bk.* 2. Knutsford: PasTest.
4. Elliott, M. and Kanani, M. (2003) *Applied Surgical Physiology Vivas.* Cambridge: Cambridge University Press.

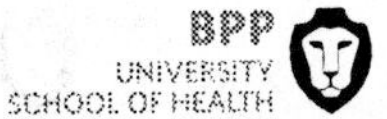

Urinary retention

Differential diagnosis

Sex	Disease
Both	**Acute urinary retention** **Urethral stricture** **Post-operative urinary retention** Renal tract cancer Urinary tract infection (UTI) Multiple sclerosis Drugs Constipation Prolapsed intervertebral disc
Male	**Benign prostatic hyperplasia (BPH)** Prostate cancer **Phimosis** **Paraphimosis**
Female	Retroverted gravid uterus

Table 4.13: Differential diagnosis of urinary retention

Acute urinary retention

Epidemiology

Acute urinary retention is very common. It is often seen post-operatively.

Aetiology

Urinary retention can be acute, chronic, or acute on chronic. The general causes are below:

No obstruction	Local causes
• Post-operative pain • Central nervous system conditions such as multiple sclerosis or a spinal tumour • Drugs eg tricyclic antidepressants and anticholinergics	• Urethral obstruction due to calculi or a blood clot • Abnormal wall pathologies eg stricture • Extrinsic compression eg prostatic enlargement, faecal impaction, pelvic tumour, or pregnant uterus

Table 4.14: The causes of acute urinary retention

History/examination

- Reduced or no passage of urine for several hours
- Lower abdominal pain, which can be severe in acute retention
- Signs of dehydration
- Pyrexia
- Suprapubic tenderness on palpation
- A palpable bladder that is dull to percussion
- Rectal examination may reveal an enlarged or hard prostate. Reduced anal tone and sacral sensation may be a sign of cauda equine syndrome – a surgical emergency!
- CNS/PNS examination to assess for neurological causes of urinary retention

Investigations

Blood tests:

- FBC: may show a raised white cell count.
- U&Es: renal function may be deranged.
- PSA level: determined before a rectal examination if assessing for prostate cancer. This will be falsely elevated in UTIs, acute prostatitis and following urethral instrumentation.

Urinalysis:

- UTI (after catheterisation)

Imaging:

- CXR: to identify metastatic disease.
- CTKUB: to check for urinary tract calculi.
- USS: to assess the residual volume in the bladder and look for any bladder abnormalities. Back pressure leading to hydronephrosis may be present with resultant dilated renal calyces and ureter.

Management

- Urethral catheterisation – measuring the residual volume and monitoring hourly output.
  - If unsuccessful, try a larger gauge catheter, if possible, which will be stiffer/coude tip catheter. After two unsuccessful attempts, consult a senior colleague who may attempt insertion of a urethral catheter or choose to site a suprapubic catheter.

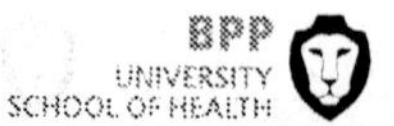

- Antibiotics to treat a UTI or to cover the infection risk of inserting a catheter.
- IV fluids and electrolyte correction if required.
- A TWOC should not be attempted within the first 24 hours after its insertion, due to the risk of relapse into retention.
- Some centres will organise urodynamics prior to TWOC if they have a residual greater than two litres.
- The underlying cause must be identified and treated.

Urethral stricture

Epidemiology

The true incidence of urethral strictures is unknown. However, there is an increase in the rate of stricture disease after the age of 55.

Aetiology

Urethral strictures may be congenital or acquired.

Type	Disease
Congenital	Meatal stenosis in hypospadias
Acquired	Trauma: mainly blunt trauma or instrumentation. Previous urethral or prostatic surgery Infection secondary to Chlamydia/ Gonococcal urethritis Perineal injury Pelvic fractures Balanitis xerotica obliterans (BXO)

Table 4.15: The causes of urethral strictures

Pathophysiology

The pathophysiology is dependent on the aetiology.

History/examination

- Hesitancy
- Poor stream or spraying of urine
- Post-micturition dribbling
- Painful ejaculation/micturition
- Urethral discharge if UTI/STI present

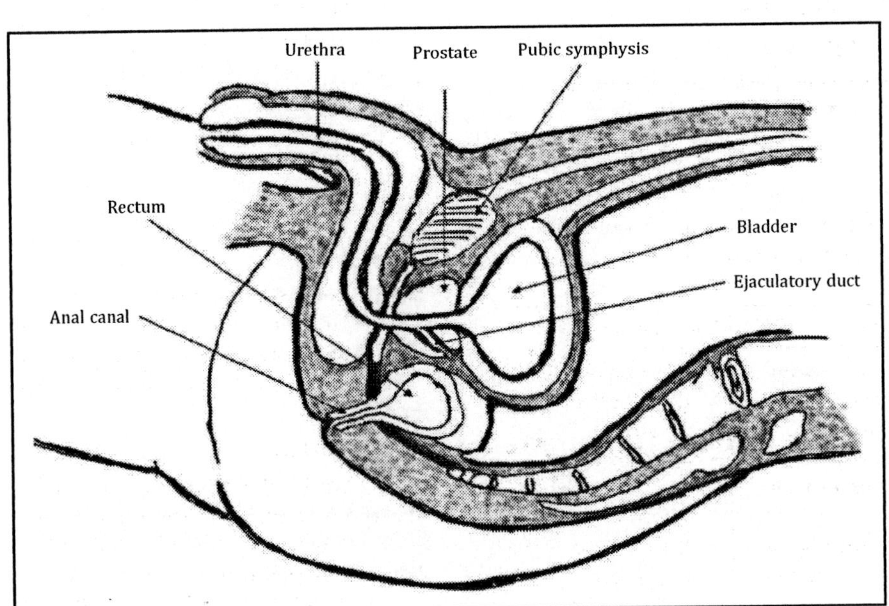

Figure 4.14: Anatomy of the male prostate

Investigations

Imaging:

- Urethrogram to identify site of stricture.
- Urethral USS: to assess the stricture and identify the presence of fibrosis. This can aid in determining the risk of recurrence.

Endoscopy:

- Cysto-urethroscopy: this can assist with treatment of the stricture, by performing dilatation of the stricture under direct vision. Dilatation can be carried out with metal dilators, gum-elastic bougies, or with self-dilators (eg catheters).

Others:

- Urodynamic investigations: the peak flow rate is reduced (peak flow less than 10 ml/sec) and there is a prolonged micturition time.

Management

- Intermittent dilatation
  - Symptomatic management and not a long-term cure, as there is a poor success rate with a high recurrence rate.
  - Complications include a false passage, infection and septicaemia.
- Optical urethrotomy:
  - The stricture is cut under direct vision, using a knife passed through the sheath of the urethroscope.
  - Suitable for short strictures.
  - There is a 50% recurrence rate; this can be reduced with post-operative intermittent dilatation.
- Urethroplasty:
  - Used for recurrent strictures
  - Stricture is excised with an end-end anastomosis

Post-operative urinary retention

Epidemiology

The incidence of post-operative urinary retention can range from approximately 10–55% depending on the type of procedure they have undergone.

Aetiology

It is common to see urinary retention after an operation involving the anal canal and perineal region. As a result, a urinary catheter is placed prior to the end of the procedure. Other common problems include:

- Difficulty passing urine whilst supine
- Embarrassment at using a bottle/bedpan
- Urinary retention may be missed in sedated patient
- Elderly male patients have a history of prostatic obstruction therefore had existing difficulties passing urine pre-operatively

History/examination

- Surgery under general anaesthesia in the previous 24–48 hours
- Lower abdominal pain and the inability to pass urine
- Suprapubic tenderness and a palpable bladder on abdominal palpation
- Dull percussive note overlying the bladder

Investigations

Diagnosis is usually clinical.

Imaging:

- Bladder scan to quantify the residual volume of urine within the bladder

Management

- Reassurance
- Running water/warm bath if possible
- Temporary urethral catheterisation

Benign prostatic hyperplasia

Epidemiology

This is a condition affecting men over the age of 50. Approximately 50% will have histological changes of BPH and 15% will complain of urinary symptoms.

Aetiology

The prostate consists of three lobes. It is the inner zone of the prostate that enlarges resulting in compression of the urethra. There are two known theories for BPH. The hormone theory suggests that the prostate gland enlarges as a result of reduced amounts of testosterone and increased amounts of oestrogen. The increased amount of oestrogen causes hyperplasia. The neoplastic theory suggests that the enlargement of the prostate occurs due to a benign neoplasm.

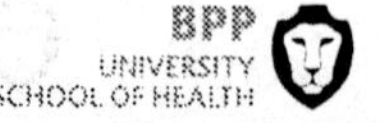

Pathophysiology

The prostate consists of glandular and stromal tissue. Through its lifetime it is influenced by hormonal change, which can result in enlargement of the gland. In addition, the prostate may be enlarged due to proliferation of epithelial and stromal tissue which then obstructs the urethra within the gland.

Enlargement of all of the three lobes of the prostate can lead to obstruction of the urethral lumen leading to urinary outflow obstruction.

Urinary outflow obstruction can result in:

- Bladder stones as a result of urinary stasis
- Bladder diverticula
- Bladder trabeculation as a result of bladder hypertrophy
- UTI
- Ureteric back pressure, leading to hydronephrosis and eventual renal failure

History/examination

- Obstructive urinary (voiding) symptoms include poor stream, straining, hesitancy, terminal dribbling and sudden onset of abdominal pain if there is acute urinary retention.
- Detrusor instability (storage) symptoms include frequency, urgency and nocturia.
- Symptoms of renal failure are headache, confusion and lethargy.
- Signs of uraemia are dry furry tongue, confusion and pallor.
- Abdominal palpation: large bladder that is dull to percussion and tenderness if there is acute urinary retention.
- Rectal examination: an enlarged smooth prostate. The lateral lobes are enlarged with a sulcus between the lobes. The examination should be performed after the bladder has been emptied because the gland is pushed down with a full bladder and therefore appears larger than it actually is.

Investigations

Blood tests:

- FBC: may show anaemia as a result of uraemia.
- U&Es: will be deranged in renal failure.
- PSA: is an indicator for prostate carcinoma. If levels are more than 4.0 ng/mL a TRUS can be performed. Multiple biopsies can be taken under TRUS guidance.

Urinalysis:

- Urine dipstick: to look for infection
- MSU: to look for infection

Imaging:

- CTKUB or USS: the upper urinary tract can be visualised to identify any complications such as hydronephrosis.

Others:

- Urodynamics: a urine flow test is performed in which the patient passes urine into a flow meter. A peak flow rate of less than 10 ml/sec suggests detrusor instability or obstructed urinary flow.

Management

Conservative management:

- May be appropriate if minimal symptoms present
- Limit evening fluid/caffeine/alcohol intake
- Simple bladder training where the patient holds urination mid-flow to reinstate control and gradually increases the amount of time they delay from the point where they would normally want to void
- Outpatient review in 6 months
- Approximately 65% will gradually suffer worsening symptoms

Pharmacological management:

The treatment of choice in those with moderate to severe symptoms (can combine treatments)

- α-adrenergic antagonist (eg Tamsulosin):
  - Cause bladder neck/prostatic smooth muscle relaxation
  - Faster acting than the 5α-reductase inhibitors
  - Postural hypotension is a significant side effect.
- 5α-reductase inhibitors (eg Finasteride):
  - Prevent conversion of testosterone to its active form, dihydro-testosterone, therefore reducing prostatic volume
  - Fewer side effects than α-adrenergic antagonists

Surgical management:

- Pre-operative counselling to inform patients of the complications:
  - Retrograde ejaculation occurs in 65%.
  - 5% will suffer with erectile impotence.
  - 15% will require a further procedure in 8–10 years.
  - Mortality rate is less than 0.5%.
  - Other complications include urethral stricture, sepsis, haematuria, urinary incontinence, UTI and TUR syndrome (hyponatraemia and confusion as a result of absorbing large volumes of irrigating fluid).
- Procedures include: TURP; open prostatectomy; laser prostatectomy and transurethral microwave thermotherapy.

Phimosis

Epidemiology

Phimosis is very common in young boys; however, it can present later in adult life. The true incidence of pathological phimosis in uncircumcised adult males is 1%.

Aetiology

The causes of phimosis include trauma, forceful retraction of the prepuce or recurrent balanitis. It can occur as a congenital lesion but this is rare.

Pathophysiology

Phimosis is the gross narrowing of the preputial orifice. In adult life it may present as a result of balanitis xerotica obliterans, in which the foreskin becomes thickened and will not retract. Patients may complain of painful intercourse, cracking or bleeding of the foreskin and infection.

History/examination

- Ballooning of the prepuce on micturition
- Urinary flow is a dribble
- Pain during sexual intercourse

Investigations

The diagnosis is clinical.

Management

- Antibiotics if infection is present
- Circumcision if indicated: (in adults) balanitis, splitting of a tight frenulum, and prior to treatment in penile carcinoma; (in children) phimosis and parental request

Paraphimosis

This is a condition where the foreskin has retracted beyond the glans, and cannot be replaced.

Epidemiology

Paraphimosis is common during infancy and adolescence. It has an incidence of approximately 1% in males over the age of 16 years.

Aetiology

Common causes include failure to replace the foreskin following urinary catheterisation insertion, masturbation, sexual intercourse, and occasionally during urination.

Pathophysiology

Venous and lymphatic drainage from the glans is obstructed, resulting in oedema and swelling. This may be followed by ischaemia of the glans.

Investigations

The diagnosis is clinical.

Management

- Manual reduction is first-line treatment after application of ice and aspiration of the glans. A dorsal block with local anaesthetic may be necessary.
- If manipulation fails a circumcision may be required.

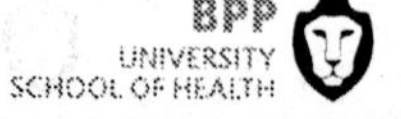

Further reading and references

1. Barry, M.J. and Roehrborn, C.G. (2001) Clinical Review: Extracts from 'Clinical Evidence' Benign Prostatic Hyperplasia. *BMJ* 2001; 323: 1042–1046.
2. Kanani, M. (2002) *Surgical Critical Care Vivas*. Cambridge: Cambridge University Press.
3. Bulstrode, C.J.K., Russell, R.C.G. and Williams, N.S. (2000) *Bailey & Love's Short Practice of Surgery*. 23rd Edition. London: Arnold.
4. Calne, R., Ellis, H. and Whatson, C. (2002) *Lecture Notes on General Surgery*. 10th Edition. Oxford: Blackwell Publishing.
5. Goldberg, A. and Stansby, G. (2006) *Surgical Talk: Revision in Surgery*. 2nd Edition. London: Imperial College Press.
6. Mundy, A.R. (2006) Review: Management of urethral strictures. Postgraduate *Medical Journal* 2006; 82: 489–493.

Limb pain

Differential diagnosis

Pathology	Disease
Venous	**Varicose veins** **Venous leg ulcers** Venous thrombosis
Arterial	**Arterial leg ulcers** **Acute limb ischaemia** Arterial stenosis Chronic limb ischaemia
Others	**Compartment syndrome** Small vessel disease

Table 4.16: Differential diagnosis of limb pain

Varicose veins

Epidemiology

Varicose veins are dilated superficial veins that affect 20% of the western population. 2% of these go on to develop associated skin changes, which can lead to ulcer formation.

Anatomy

There are two venous systems in the lower limbs. Both ensure blood from the skin and muscles of the legs is returned to the trunk.

Superficial venous system:

- The long (great) saphenous vein extends from just anterior to the medial malleolus along the medial aspect of the thigh and drains from the dorsum of the foot up to the sapheno-femoral junction in the groin.
- The short (small) saphenous vein is placed laterally and drains into the popliteal vein behind the knee. It is only involved in venous drainage of the skin and superficial tissue.

Deep venous system:

- This consists of a group of veins within the deep fascia, which surround the leg muscles.
- When the calf muscles contract, blood is pushed up towards the heart, with valves to prevent backflow and when the muscles relax blood flows from the superficial to deep systems like a pump.
- Smaller venous tributaries drain behind the knee into the popliteal vein, which ascends as the femoral vein and then the external iliac vein at the inguinal ligament.
- After this point venous return occurs through the common iliac vein, the inferior vena cava, finally entering the right atrium.

Perforators:

- These are veins that facilitate communication between the deep and superficial veins.
- They contain valves to prevent backflow from the deep to the superficial veins.

Aetiology

Varicose veins occur as a result of dysfunction of the valves in the leg veins. The exact mechanism is unknown but two theories have been proposed:

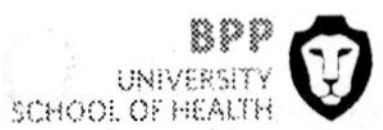

primary valve incompetence or structural weakness of the venous walls resulting in dilatation and valve disruption.

If both parents have been affected by varicose veins, offspring have an 80% chance of developing them as well. Environmental factors include standing all day, usually for occupational reasons. Oestrogen in pregnancy can cause varicose veins by inducing venous smooth muscle relaxation. Other environmental factors include previous DVT, abdominal or pelvic mass, ascites, obesity and constipation.

Pathophysiology

Varicose veins are thought to be a result of increased pressure within the superficial venous system. A patient at rest will have equal pressures in the superficial and deep venous systems. A patient carrying out any activity has increased pressure in the deep venous system. If the venous valves of the superficial system are incompetent, these veins will not be protected from the high pressures and varicosities will result.

History/examination

- Can be asymptomatic
- Leg discomfort or cramp-like pain
- Skin changes or ulceration
- Ankle swelling
- Pruritis
- Patients may complain for cosmetic reasons
- 'Long, tortuous and dilated' veins in the leg
- Small veins can have a diameter of 0.5 mm and appear purple/red in colour
- Larger veins are noted with a diameter of 1–3 mm and if the saphenous veins are affected the diameter can range from 5–15 mm
- Skin changes include pigmentation, eczema, ulceration, lipodermatosclerosis (wax like skin), and heamosiderin deposit (blue/purple discolouration caused by loss of red cells into the tissue due to increased venous pressure

Investigations

Clinical tests:

While modern imaging technologies have largely replaced clinical examinations, it is worth being aware of two tests to assess the site of incompetency:

1. **Trendelenburg's test:**

   i) Used to identify reflux of blood from the deep to superficial veins.
   ii) With the patient lying flat the superficial veins are emptied by elevating the leg.
   iii) A tourniquet is applied to the upper thigh (occlusion of superficial venous system at level of tourniquet).
   iv) The patient is then asked to stand.
   v) If the veins remain empty it can be safely assumed that the sapheno-femoral junction is incompetent and is the cause of the superficial venous reflux.
   vi) If the tourniquet does not control the varicose veins and allows the vein to fill with blood, the test can be repeated with the tourniquet placed lower down the leg until the point of control is reached.
   vii) This test can be repeated with application of a tourniquet to identify which set of veins have been affected.

2. **Tap test:**

   i) Fingers from one hand are placed over the sapheno-femoral junction.
   ii) A distal varicose vein is tapped.
   iii) A transmitted thrill may be felt over the sapheno-femoral junction if incompetent.
   iv) This occurs as there will be a column of blood in the vein due to the absence of vein valves.

Blood tests:

- FBC: baseline levels
- U&Es: baseline levels
- Clotting: baseline levels
- Group and save

Imaging:

- Doppler USS: Used to exclude arterial disease and detect venous reflux. The Doppler probe is placed over the sapheno-femoral junction and the venous flow in the common femoral vein is identified. The calf on the same side is gently squeezed to accelerate blood flow from the saphenous vein up the sapheno-femoral junction into the common femoral vein. A sound such as 'whoosh' is heard. When the calf is released a sound to illustrate reverse flow may be heard. An abnormal prolonged second 'whoosh' indicates valve incompetence as blood flows back unrestricted.

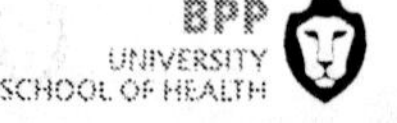

- Colour duplex scanning: This test outlines the veins of the legs. It can identify valve and perforator incompetence and it will confirm if the deep venous system is patent. This is essential before the patient is considered for any superficial venous avulsion.

Others:

- ECG prior to any operative procedure.
- Venography: A tourniquet is placed around the ankle and the superficial veins are occluded. Then a contrast medium is injected into the dorsum of the foot, where it will be passed through the deep venous system. Multiple X-rays are taken and any reflux through the deep and perforating veins can be seen.

Management

Conservative management:

- Management tends to be conservative unless the patient is particularly symptomatic.
- The underlying cause must be treated, eg weight loss or treatment for constipation.
- Compressive support stockings: provides symptomatic relief and the progression is reduced.
- Injection sclerotherapy: a sclerosing agent (sodium tetradecyl sulphate) is injected into the veins.
- Laser coagulation: can be used to treat small varicose veins.

Operative management:

- Operative treatment is usually offered to those with sapheno-femoral incompetence and/or major perforator incompetence.
- Trendelenburg procedure (high tie): the long saphenous vein is ligated at its entry point into the femoral vein and all its tributaries are ligated. This procedure has a high recurrence rate.
- Short saphenous vein ligation: the short saphenous vein is ligated deep in the popliteal fossa.
- Multiple avulsions: multiple stab incisions are performed to strip individual varicose veins.
- EVLA: thermal destruction of venous tissues. USS is used to map out the venous system and guide cannulation of the affected vein. The treatment is less invasive than the traditional high tie and has equal, if not lower, recurrence rates.

Site of incompetence	Distribution
Sapheno-femoral junction	Long saphenous distribution
Mid-thigh perforators	Short saphenous distribution
Sapheno-popliteal junction	Short saphenous and medial calf perforator distribution
Medial calf perforators	Mixed picture

Table 4.17: Distribution of varicose veins according to which perforators affected

Venous leg ulcers

Epidemiology

Venous leg ulcers are the most common type of leg ulcers, accounting for 80% of cases in the western community. Around 10% of leg ulcers are due to arterial disease, with 5–10% a result of mixed venous and arterial pathology.

Aetiology

Venous ulcers are thought to arise as a result of the constant high blood pressure within the veins of the lower legs due to venous insufficiency. Risk factors include increasing age, obesity, immobility, varicose veins, and a previous history of a DVT.

Pathophysiology

Venous ulcers can arise as a result of superficial or deep venous incompetence. This commonly is a result of valvular incompetence resulting in abnormal blood flow and venous congestion. These ulcers are seen proximal to the medial or lateral malleolus, typically along the medial gaiter region. There are often associated signs of long-standing venous disease, such as oedema, haemosiderin deposition, lipodermatosclerosis and varicose veins.

History/examination

- Pain, swelling and altered sensation.
- Varicose veins may be present.
- Peripheral pulses should be palpated and a complete peripheral vascular examination should be performed.
- Neoplastic changes along the edge of a long standing venous ulcer can occur (Marjolin ulcer).

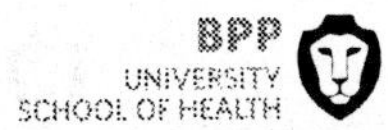

- Sensation may be altered in the limbs and ulcerated areas. Peripheral neuropathy is commonly seen with diabetic foot ulcers.
- Ankle-brachial blood pressures should be measured.

Investigations

Important for differentiating different types of ulcer.

Blood tests:

- FBC: baseline levels
- U&Es: baseline levels
- Clotting: baseline levels
- Group and save

Imaging:

- Duplex USS: required to assess the severity of arterial disease and collateral circulation
- Angiography: as above

Others:

- Ulcer biopsy: this can identify venous or arterial disease. Malignancy can also be detected.

Management

Conservative:

- Patients with deep venous incompetence and those who are unfit for surgery should be managed conservatively.
- Elevation to reduce venous pressure.
- Antibiotics for secondary infection.
- Multiple layer compression bandaging (usually by district nurses).
- Vascular stockings should be continued after healing to reduce risk of recurrence.

Surgical:

- In venous ulcers due to superficial venous incompetence, surgical removal of the associated varicose veins has been shown to promote healing.
- With large ulcers, skin grafting may be an option to encourage ulcer healing.

After an ulcer has healed the incompetent veins do not spontaneously resolve and therefore recurrence is common.

Arterial leg ulcers

Epidemiology

Approximately 10% of leg ulcers are due to arterial disease with 5–10% a result of mixed venous and arterial pathology.

Aetiology

Arterial ulcers result from an inadequate blood supply due to peripheral vascular disease, diabetes mellitus or trauma. Atherosclerosis is the major contributing factor to arterial ulcer formation. Other arterial vascular diseases that can cause ulcers include Raynaud's disease, Buerger's disease, scleroderma and rheumatoid vasculitis. Radiation and electrical burns can also result in arterial leg ulcers.

Pathophysiology

The initial ischaemia causes tissue necrosis which leads to the formation of arterial ulcers but then these ulcers fail to heal due to an inadequate blood supply. Arterial ulcers are often found at the most distal site of the circulation such as the tips of toes.

History/examination

- Intermittent claudication or rest pain of the lower limbs indicates the presence of peripheral vascular disease. Patients normally describe a cramp-like pain in the lower limbs on walking a particular distance which is relieved with rest.
- Arterial ulcers are usually very painful and pain may be leg position-dependent, ie aggravated by elevation.
- Surrounding skin is hairless and shiny.
- Nails are thickened due to fungal infection.
- Foot may appear pale, mottled or purple depending on the extent of ischaemia.
- Cool limb on palpation with delayed capillary refill.
- Distal foot pulses may be absent or weaker.

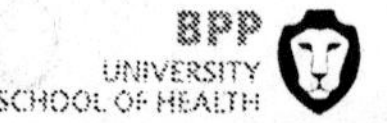

Arterial ulcer	Venous ulcer
Distribution on pressure areas of the foot. Common sites include heel, head of fifth metatarsal, tips of toes, ball of foot.	Distribution along the gaiter region (medial aspect of foot).
Painful.	Can be painless.
Punched out appearance with steep edges.	Superficial with gently sloping ragged edge.
Pale bloodless sloughy dry base.	Red velvety granulation tissue at the base and the ulcer margin has a slight blue rim.
Surrounding skin may be pale, shiny and hairless.	Surrounding skin shows evidence of venous insufficiency such as varicose veins, lipodermatosclerosis and haemosiderin deposition.

Table 4.18: Showing classical features of arterial and venous ulcers

Investigations

Blood tests:

- FBC: baseline levels
- U&Es: baseline levels
- Clotting: baseline levels
- Group and save

Imaging:

- Angiography: is required to assess the severity of arterial disease and it also provides a treatment option.
- Doppler USS and Duplex USS: indicate the degree of arterial flow. ABPI will demonstrate if there is a peripheral vascular disease component. The pressure at the ankle should be the same as the brachial artery pressure with the patient in the supine position.

ABPI	Severity
1	Normal
0.8–0.9	Some arterial insufficiency but not enough to cause symptoms
0.41–0.8	Correlates with claudication symptoms
<0.4	Rest pain

Table 4.19: The integrity of arterial blood flow as indicated by ABPI. Note diabetics can have heavily calcified vessels providing a falsely elevated ABPI reading

Others:

- Ulcer biopsy: This can identify venous or arterial disease. Malignancy can also be detected.

Management

Treatment for arterial ulcers is to improve the arterial circulation to the ulcer site thereby encouraging tissue healing.

Conservative and medical management:

This will reduce the chance of disease progression but alone is unlikely to achieve complete ulcer healing.

- Supervised exercise programmes
- Vasodilator therapy (eg naftidrofuryl oxalate)
- Smoking cessation
- Diet, weight management
- Anti-platelet drugs (Aspirin, Clopidogrel)
- Cholesterol reducing drugs
- Control of diabetes and blood pressure (if relevant)

Surgical management:

- The sites of stenosis must first be identified by an arteriogram with percutaneous angioplasty and stenting if applicable.
- Bypass grafting using synthetic material or autogenous vein is the standard surgical treatment. Aorto-iliac bypass, femoral-popliteal bypass, and distal bypasses are the main types of operations for arterial insufficiency.

Acute limb ischaemia

Acute limb ischaemia is a surgical emergency which can result in the patient losing a limb if they do not receive immediate treatment.

Epidemiology

There are approximately 5,000 cases per year in the UK.

Aetiology

The causes of an acutely ischaemic limb include thrombosis, embolism, trauma, aortic dissection, aneurysms and iatrogenic causes. Thrombus and emboli are the two most common causes.

Pathophysiology

Thrombosis accounts for 60% of cases. The main cause for this is plaque rupture within an already stenosed vessel. The three elements of Virchow's Triad – endothelial injury, hypercoagulability and blood stasis – determine thrombosis, thus predisposing factors include dehydration, malignancy, infection, immobility and thrombophilia.

An embolism accounts for 30% of cases. Defined as an abnormal mass of un-dissolved tissue that passes in the blood stream from one part of the circulation to another, a fluid or solid embolus can lodge within small diameter blood vessels. Predisposing factors include arrhythmias such as atrial fibrillation, atheromatous vascular disease, tumours, foreign body, air, cholesterol and a hypercoaguable state (eg protein C or S deficiency, polycythaemia, malignancy). Emboli commonly arise from a mural thrombus, mitral stenosis, and as a result of cardiac arrhythmias. They can lodge in any organ and cause ischaemia (eg limbs, brain, spleen, kidneys, lungs, and mesenteric vessels).

History/examination

- The six signs of an acutely ischaemic leg are:
  - Pain
  - Pallor
  - Perishingly cold
  - Paraesthesia
  - Paralysis
  - Pulselessness

The first three appear earlier and are therefore very important to detect.

Thrombus	Emboli
• History of intermittent claudication or rest pain • Onset occurs over hours • Signs of chronic vascular disease • The artery is hard to touch • No audible bruits	• History of recent MI and AF • No intermittent claudication • Onset occurs over seconds to minutes • No history of evidence of vascular disease • The artery is soft to touch • Audible bruit

Table 4.20: How to differentiate between a thrombus and emboli

Investigations

The diagnosis is clinical as without imminent treatment the patient may lose a limb.

Management

Immediate management:

- Early senior/vascular input
- Adequate analgesia
- IV access and fluids
- NBM
- IV heparin (5,000 units stat)
- Angiogram (only in patients with incomplete ischaemia)
- If acute limb ischaemia is due to thrombosis:
  - Thrombolysis eg TPA or streptokinase
  - Angioplasty and stenting
  - Emergency reconstruction with or without a fasciotomy
  - Amputation
- If acute limb ischaemia is due to an embolus:
  - Embolectomy with a Fogarty catheter
  - On table thrombolysis with unsuccessful embolectomy
  - Emergency reconstruction with or without fasciotomy
  - Amputation
- Post-operative management involves:
  - 48 hours of heparin infusion
  - Long-term anticoagulation with warfarin
  - Following acute management, investigations should be carried out to identify a possible embolic source eg echocardiography, 24 hour tape and USS of the aorta (to rule out an aneurysm)

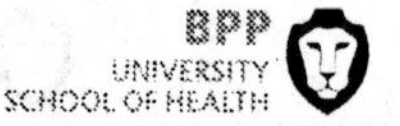

- Post-operative complications include:
  - Reperfusion injury – when oxygen is reintroduced, free radicals can damage vessel endothelium. This can result in compartment syndrome, acidosis, hyperkalaemia and shock
  - Compartment syndrome needs an urgent fasciotomy
  - Chronic pain

Compartment syndrome

Epidemiology

The incidence varies according to the aetiology.

Aetiology

- Fracture with subsequent haemorrhage (eg tibial or forearm fractures)
- Ischaemic reperfusion following injury
- Vascular puncture
- IV drug injection
- Tight fitting casts
- Prolonged limb compression
- Crush injuries
- Burns
- Vigorous exercise

Pathophysiology

Compartment syndrome is caused by increased tissue pressure in a fascial compartment impairing blood circulation to the muscles and nerves.

The normal mean interstitial tissue pressure is near 0 mmHg in non-contracting muscle. A pressure elevation of 30 mmHg or more results in compression of small vessels in the tissue, reducing nutrient blood flow and causing ischaemia and pain.

The commonest fascial compartments involved are the forearm and the leg. In the lower limbs, the anterior (extensors), posterior (flexors of the ankle), and peroneal (evertors) may be affected.

History/examination

- Pain: disproportionate to the injury sustained and aggravated by the passive stretching of the muscles in the compartment.
- Pale: the limb is pale, tense, swollen and shiny.
- Poikilothermia (cold): cool on palpation and there is a general tenderness to the affected compartment.
- Parasthesia: in the cutaneous nerve distribution of the affected limb.
- Paralysis: is normally a late finding when significant muscle ischaemia has occurred.
- Pulseless: this is a late finding and often indicates the time for limb salvage is passing.

Investigations

The diagnosis is made clinically.

Others:

Pressure gauge: the intra-compartmental pressure can be tested by using a pressure gauge cannulated into the affected tissue. Generally an intra-compartmental pressure of more than 30 mmHg indicates compartment syndrome and a fasciotomy will be required.

Management

- Removal of all skin coverings if present
- Surgical treatment with fasciotomy to decompress the affected limb

Prognosis

If compartment syndrome is left untreated it will eventually cause tissue hypoxia and necrosis. This will result in loss of the affected limb as well as rhabdomyolysis, causing acute renal failure.

Further reading and references

1. Hiatt, W.R. (2001) Medical treatment of peripheral arterial disease and claudication. *NEJM* 2001; 344: 1608–1621.
2. London, N. and Nash, R. (2000) Clinical review: ABC of arterial and venous disease – Varicose veins. *BMJ* 2000; 320: 1391–1394.
3. Parchment-Smith, C. (2002) *Surgical Short Cases for the MRCS Clinical Examination.* Knutsford: PasTest.

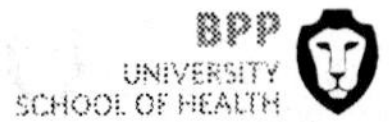

Lumps

Differential diagnosis

Structure	Disease
Skin	**Sebaceous cyst** **Benign naevi** **Lipoma** Neurofibroma Papilloma Kaposi's sarcoma Basal cell carcinoma (BCC) Bowen's disease Squamous cell carcinoma (SSC) Malignant melanoma
Neck	**Thyroglossal cyst** **Goitre** Thyroid cyst Primary thyroid tumour Solitary thyroid nodules Thyroid carcinoma **Branchial cyst** **Branchial sinus** **Dermoid cyst** Carotid body tumour **Pharyngeal pouch** **Salivary gland neoplasm** Acute parotitis Cystic hygroma
Breast	Breast cancer Fibroadenoma Lipoma Cyst abscess Haematoma
Groin and scrotum	**Incompletely descended testis** **Testicular torsion** **Hydrocele** **Varicocele** **Epididymal cyst** **Spermatocele** Testicular carcinoma **Epididymo-orchitis** Saphena varix Femoral artery aneurysm Haematoma Lipoma of the cord Inguinal lymph nodes
Hernias	Inguinal **Femoral** **Incisional** Umbilical Para-umbilical Epigastric Spigelian Obturator Lumbar Sciatic

Table 4.21: Differential diagnosis of a lump

Skin

Sebaceous cyst

Epidemiology

Sebaceous cysts are extremely common. They present between the ages of 20 and 30, and are twice as common in men as women.

Aetiology

Sebaceous cysts can arise due to blocked sebaceous glands, trauma or surgical disruption, swollen hair follicles and increased production of testosterone.

Infection with HPV and hereditary conditions such as Gardner's syndrome and basal cell naevus syndrome are also associated with sebaceous cyst formation.

Pathophysiology

Sebaceous cysts are sometimes referred to as epidermoid cysts. They occur following obstruction to the mouth of the sebaceous gland and can arise at any site where sebaceous glands are present. They are typically found on the scalp, face, scrotum and vulva. They do not occur on the soles of the feet or the palms of hands.

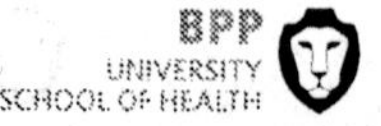

History/examination

- The cyst is a round, fluctuant, well-differentiated, smooth swelling attached to the skin.
- It moves freely with the skin over deeper lying structures.
- A central punctum is often present.
- The cyst usually contains offensive caseous material.
- Superimposed infection is common.
- Ulceration of the cyst can look like an SSC, which is known as 'Cock's peculiar tumour'.
- A sebaceous horn may form as a result of leakage and drying of the cyst contents.

Investigations

The diagnosis is largely clinical. In cases of possible malignancy, the lump should be excised and sent for histological analysis.

Management

- With uncomplicated sebaceous cysts surgical resection is the best option, including the surrounding capsule to limit recurrence. Currently in the UK this procedure requires a 'special funding' application to most CCG groups.
- The cyst should always be sent for histology for diagnostic confirmation.
- If there is infection and inflammation present an incision and drainage procedure is performed, but the capsule will need to be resected at a later date to prevent recurrence.

Benign naevi

Epidemiology

These are more common in fair-skinned individuals or those with hereditary predisposition.

Aetiology

Benign naevi can be congenital (as a result of embryological anomalies), and therefore are present from birth. Acquired benign naevi develop later in life and often occur as a result of sun exposure.

Pathophysiology

Melanocytes are clear cells found in the basal layer of the epidermis. Melanocytes arise from the embryonic neural crest and it is these cells which produce the brown pigment melanin. If these cells increase in number within the layers of the skin, they develop into benign pigmented naevi (moles).

Investigations

Benign naevi are diagnosed clinically. If malignant change is suspected a biopsy should be taken and sent for histological analysis.

Management

- Surgical excision may be considered for aesthetic indications or if the naevus is being irritated by clothing or shaving.
- All lesions excised are sent for histological analysis.

Type	Feature
Dermal naevi	• Also known as the common mole. • Appearances can vary as the naevus can be light or dark in colour, flat or raised, and with hair present or absent. • These naevi can occur at most sites of the body, with the palms, soles, and scrotum being exceptions. • All of the melanocytes are found within the dermis. • These naevi do not progress to malignancy.
Junctional naevi	• The melanocytes are distributed within the basal layer of the epidermis, with projections into the dermis. • They can vary in colour, ranging from light brown to black. • These naevi are mostly smooth, flat, and do not have any hair present. • They can occur anywhere on the body, including the soles, palms and genitalia. • These naevi do carry potential for malignant change.
Compound naevi	• These consist of features of both dermal and junctional naevi. • Clinically they appear similar to dermal naevi and therefore, it can be difficult to differentiate between the two.
Malignant melanoma	• See Insidious onset section.

Table 4.22: The classification of benign naevi and their features

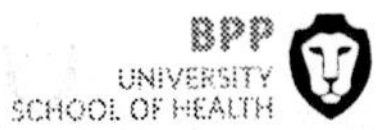

Lipoma

Epidemiology

Lipomas are the most common benign subcutaneous tumours, affecting 1% of the population. It can arise at any age but is often seen in adults between 40 and 60.

Aetiology

The aetiology is unknown.

Pathophysiology

These can be defined as benign tumours consisting of adipose tissue and can occur anywhere in the body where fat is present. They are the commonest type of benign tumour. Multiple lipomas are seen in a condition called Dercum's disease, which is a familial condition.

Large lipomas can develop into liposarcomas and calcification can also occur in the long term.

History/examination

- They are soft fluctuant swellings.
- They are usually painless.
- The swellings are mobile and not fixed to the overlying skin or deeper structures.

Investigations

This is usually a clinical diagnosis. However, investigations can be performed if the diagnosis is uncertain and a malignancy is suspected.

Imaging:

- USS: to delineate the macroscopic characteristics of the lump

Others:

- FNA: can provide histological diagnosis if lumps are considered suspicious. USS-guided FNA may increase the diagnostic yield of samples.

Management

- Excision of a lipoma is only considered if the patient is symptomatic and often a 'special circumstances' funding application must be made to the CCG.

Central nervous system	These lipomas can occur at any point within the extradural space, the spinal cord, and the brain.
Intraglandular	There have been cases of breast, pancreatic, and renal lipomas.
Retroperitoneal	The retroperitoneal tissue is a site for large lipomas. They are very rare.

Table 4.23: The classification of lipomas and their features

Type	Site
Subcutaneous	Often seen on the shoulders or back, but can occur anywhere.
Subfascial	They are seen under the palmar or plantar fascia. If left alone they can erode into the underlying bone.
Sub synovial	Commonly found in the knee and have often been mistaken for a baker's cyst.
Intra-articular	Commonly found in the knee and have often been mistaken for a baker's cyst.
Intermuscular	Rare benign lipoma originating from the joint synovium. Can restrict joint range of movement.
Parosteal	Common in the thigh and shoulders.
Subserous	These can be found under the pleura, and also in the retroperitoneal cavity.
Submucous	These are rare but can occur under the mucous membranes of the respiratory and gastrointestinal tracts, eg tongue, larynx, and intestine.

Table 4.24: The classification of cysts and their features

Neck

1. Lumps in the anterior triangle:
   i) Thyroglossal cyst
   ii) Dermoid cyst
   iii) Branchial cyst
   iv) Carotid body tumour

2. Lumps in the posterior triangle:
   i) Cystic hygroma
   ii) Cervical rib
   iii) Subclavian artery
   iv) Pancoast tumour

Thyroglossal cyst

Epidemiology

Thyroglossal cysts are a common congenital abnormality. They affect patients at all ages; however, almost 50% are diagnosed before the age of 20.

Aetiology

During embryological development the thyroid gland starts at the base of the tongue and descends to its final position at the lower midline aspect of the neck. Remnants of the thyroid can be left behind at any point and this is known as the thyroglossal cyst.

Pathophysiology

A thyroglossal cyst can occur:

- Under the foramen caecum
- In the floor of the mouth
- Suprahyoid
- Subhyoid
- On the thyroid cartilage
- At the level of the cricoid cartilage

History/examination

- The cyst is found in the midline of the neck and moves up when the tongue is protruded or on swallowing.

Investigations

This is a clinical diagnosis. However, if the diagnosis is uncertain and a malignancy is suspected:

Imaging:

- USS: to evaluate macroscopic structure

Others:

FNA: to aid differentiation of benign and malignant tumours

Management

- The cyst should be surgically excised due to the increased risk of infection – includes removal of the entire thyroglossal tract.
- Complications arise when the infected cyst is mistaken for an abscess and incised, which can result in a thyroglossal fistula.

Goitre

Epidemiology

Thyroid nodules are seen in approximately 5% of middle-aged women. They are more common in women than in men and can give rise to a goitre. Solitary nodules appear to be more common than multinodular goitres. Globally iodine deficiency is one of the leading causes of a goitre.

Anatomy

- The thyroid gland develops from the thyroglossal duct in the pharynx.
- The gland weighs about 20–25 g.
- The blood supply is extensive with many anastomoses between the thyroid arteries and branches of the tracheal and oesophageal arteries.

Aetiology

A normal thyroid gland should not be palpable. A goitre can be defined as a generalised enlargement of the thyroid gland and there are a number of different types.

Worldwide, simple goitres are the commonest and they are caused by a lack of iodine in the diet (particularly in mountainous areas such as the Himalayas and Alps, the Congo and Nile valleys and Derbyshire) and hormonal stimulation of the thyroid gland.

Diffuse hyperplastic goitres are seen in childhood and are found in the endemic areas with low dietary iodine. They also occur at times of increased metabolic need (eg pubertal goitre) and during stressful situations (eg pregnancy). Nodular goitres can consist of a single nodule, but more commonly contain multiple nodules. These nodules can be cystic, colloid, and haemorrhagic.

Pathophysiology

Diffuse hyperplasia of the goitre can occur as a result of continuous growth stimulation. The lobules of the thyroid contain follicles which are involved in the uptake of iodine. If the stimulation to the thyroid gland is stopped the goitre can regress. Occasionally, there is intermittent stimulation, which results in segments of active and inactive lobules of the thyroid gland. Active lobules develop and become increasingly vascular which may progress to haemorrhage and central necrosis. These necrotic lobules combine together and form colloid filled nodules. This process is repeated and a nodular goitre is formed.

Goitre	Features
Simple Goitre	• Diffuse hyperplastic eg physiological, pubertal, and pregnancy • Multinodular goitre
Toxic	• Diffuse eg Graves' disease • Multinodular • Toxic adenoma
Neoplastic	• Benign • Malignant
Inflammatory	• Autoimmune eg chronic lymphocytic thyroiditis, and Hashimoto's disease
Granulomatous	• De Quervain's thyroiditis
Fibrosing	• Riedel's thyroiditis
Infective	• **Acute eg bacterial and viral thyroiditis** • Chronic eg tuberculosis (TB)

Table 4.25: The features of the different types of goitres

History/examination

- Symptoms of thyroid disease (see Chapter 3).
- Retrosternal goitres may be asymptomatic or produce dyspnoea with cough and stridor, dysphagia, hoarseness, and neck vein engorgement.
- Any nodules tend to be visible and on palpation are smooth, firm, well circumscribed and not tethered to the skin but move on swallowing (as does a hyperplastic goitre).
- The goitre is painless.
- If the nodules are hard, painful, irregular and poorly circumscribed, suspicions are raised of a carcinoma.

Investigations

Blood tests:

- TFTs: serum thyroid hormones (T3 and T4) and TSH levels are detected.
- Autoantibody titres: to identify autoimmune thyroiditis.

Imaging:

- CXR: may illustrate a calcified mass and tracheal deviation.
- Isotope scan: the nodules can be referred to as 'hot' (overactive), 'warm' (active) or 'cold' (underactive) depending on whether they take up the radioactive isotope. This is not a first-line investigation.
- USS: this can be performed to identify any masses and illustrate some of the clinical features of the nodule/mass.

Management

- In endemic areas improvements have been seen with the introduction of iodised salt to the diet.
- Diffuse hyperplastic goitres can be reversed by giving thyroxine for a few months.
- Nodular goitres cannot be reversed. Most patients are asymptomatic thus surgery is not required. However, it may be performed for cosmetic reasons, if there is tracheal compression, toxic goitre or suspicion of malignancy.
  - A total thyroidectomy and lifelong thyroxine replacement can be offered.
  - A partial thyroid resection with conservation of functioning thyroid tissue is also possible.

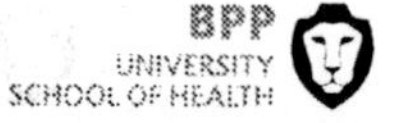

Branchial cyst

Epidemiology

They are the commonest congenital cause of neck lump and are bilateral in 2–3% of all cases. The exact incidence is unknown. The majority of patients present between the age of 15 and 25 years, but cases later in middle age have also been identified.

Aetiology

During foetal development at approximately five weeks, four branchial clefts (grooves) develop on each side of the neck. In between these clefts are branchial arches which contain a central cartilage. The first cleft progresses and becomes the auditory meatus. The second, third, and fourth clefts regress and normally disappear. Branchial cysts arise due to failure in this normal regression.

Pathophysiology

A branchial cyst, sinus or fistula usually develops from remnants of the second branchial cleft.

History/examination

- Site: branchial cysts are found on the upper and middle third of the anterior border of the sternocleidomastoid muscle.
- The swelling is fluctuant but may be difficult to palpate in the early stage.
- It may transilluminate.
- If there is a superimposed infection the swelling will be tender and erythematous.
- Failure of the distal branchial cleft fusion can result in a fistula or sinus. This appears as a small dimple on the skin, normally at the junction of the middle and lower third of sternocleidomastoid. It may intermittently discharge mucus.

Investigations

Largely a clinical diagnosis.

Others:

- FNA: can be performed on any swelling and if cholesterol crystals are visible the diagnosis is confirmed.

Management

- Surgical removal – the hypoglossal, accessory and mandibular branch of the facial nerves are in close proximity.
- If the cyst is not resected it is prone to developing recurrent infections.

Dermoid cyst

There are two different types of dermoid cysts known as inclusion and implantation cysts.

Type	Features
Inclusion dermoids	• These are congenital lesions and are found at sites of embryological fusion. Eg midline of the neck, root of the nose. • The lesions are described as swellings that are not attached to the overlying skin.
Implantation dermoids	• These lesions are associated with penetrating trauma. • They are usually seen in the hands as subcutaneous swellings. • These dermoids occur due to the introduction of epidermal tissue under the skin.

Table 4.26: The features of inclusion and implantation dermoid cysts

Pharyngeal pouch

Epidemiology

This is a condition that affects approximately 1 in 200,000 people in the UK. It is often seen in adults over the age of 60 years, with a greater prevalence in men than in women.

Anatomy

- The pharynx is in the upper part of the respiratory and oesophageal tract. It is a fibromuscular tube extending from the base of the skull to the sixth cervical vertebrae.
- It is divided into three different parts: the nasopharynx, oropharynx, and hypopharynx, with the latter leading into the oesophagus.

Aetiology

The true aetiology is unknown, but may involve increased lower oesophageal tone due to gastro-oesophageal reflux, or neuromuscular dysfunction.

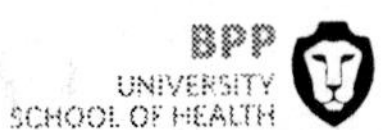

Pathophysiology

A pharyngeal pouch occurs as a result of the protrusion of the mucosa and submucosa through a weak area of the posterior pharyngeal wall, known as Killian's dehiscence.

Killian's dehiscence is located between the thyropharyngeus and circopharyngeus muscles. The fibres involved in this area of the wall and the upper oesophagus form the oesophageal sphincter.

History/examination

- Halitosis.
- Patients may feel like they have an object or lump in their throat.
- Dysphagia.
- Regurgitation on swallowing may occur.
- Occasionally liquid and food may aspirate resulting in aspiration pneumonia and lung abscess formation.
- At night patients may awake with a feeling of throat tightness or a coughing fit.
- With the pouch increasing in size patients will complain of:
  - Gurgling noises on swallowing
  - A swelling in the neck which gurgles on palpation (Boyce's sign)
  - Noticeable swelling on drinking
  - Weight loss

Investigations

Imaging:

- Barium swallow: to outline the pouch and upper oesophagus
- Video fluoroscopic study: will provide detail on the contraction waves of the pharynx, and the oesophageal sphincter
- CXR: to exclude aspiration pneumonia

Management

- Surgery is an option if the oesophageal sphincter has been affected and the patient has developed significant symptoms of dysphagia.
- This involves dissection and resection of the pouch through a cautious anterior approach, followed by several days' oesophageal rest using an NG tube.
- An alternative is endoscopic stapling/diathermy of the pharyngeal pouch (Dolman's procedure), but some literature suggests this method has a higher recurrence rate (5–7%).
- Complications of surgery include: infection, recurrent laryngeal nerve palsy (hoarse voice), pharyngeal fistula, oesophageal stenosis, and recurrence of the pharyngeal pouch.

Salivary gland neoplasm

Epidemiology

Salivary gland neoplasms account for approximately 1% of all head and neck tumours. The incidence is around 1.5 per 100,000 people and they normally present in the sixth decade of life.

Aetiology

There is currently no defined aetiology for salivary gland neoplasms. However, a clear association has been made with radiation therapy.

Pathophysiology

The salivary gland contains the parotid, submandibular, sublingual and other smaller salivary glands. Approximately 75% of salivary tumours are found in the parotid gland and of these 80% are benign (pleomorphic adenoma).

1. **Benign tumours:**
   i) Pleomorphic adenoma: 80% are found in the parotid region; however, they can also be present in the submandibular, sublingual, and accessory salivary glands. The patient may complain of a hard, well-defined, slow-growing lump in the parotid area. Treatment consists of wide excision of the tumour or complete removal of the salivary gland.
   ii) Adenolymphoma (Warthin's tumour): accounts for approximately 10% of parotid tumours. They are soft and have a cyst-like appearance. Local excision provides excellent results.

2. **Malignant tumours:**
   i) Adenoid cystic carcinoma: is the most common malignant tumour to affect the salivary glands. It arises more frequently in the smaller salivary gland and is slow growing. It often spreads along the nerve sheaths and can present with facial pain or facial nerve palsy. This type of tumour does not metastasise early and lymph node spread is uncommon.

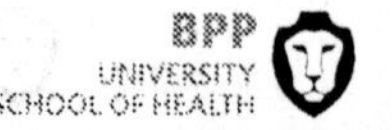

ii) Adenocarcinoma: 10% of submandibular and minor salivary gland tumours. In around 20% of cases, lymph nodes are involved at the initial presentation.
iii) Mucoepidermoid tumours: these are the commonest salivary neoplasm in children. They arise mainly in the parotid gland and metastasise to lymph nodes and later to the lungs and brain.

History/examination

- Slow-growing and enlarging painless lump
- Possible facial nerve paralysis
- Cervical lymphadenopathy which indicates metastasis

Investigations

Blood tests:

- FBC
- Inflammatory markers
- TFTs
- Antibodies: antibodies such as anti-Ro and anti-La should be used to rule out autoimmune disease such as Sjögren syndrome
- Rheumatoid and antinuclear factors: to rule out autoimmune causes

Imaging:

- CT or MRI: provides information on extra-glandular extension

Others:

- FNA: provides cytology, but is not definitive

Management

- The aim of surgery is to fully resect the tumour leaving a margin of macroscopically normal tissue, whilst preserving the facial nerve. Salivary gland tumours respond poorly to chemotherapy and it is only considered in palliative cases.
- Parotid tumours
  - Superficial parotidectomy: removal of the superficial parotid lobe only
  - Total conservative parotidectomy: complete removal of the parotid gland with preservation of the facial nerve
  - Total radical parotidectomy: complete removal of the parotid gland with the facial nerve
- Submandibular gland surgery: this follows similar principles to parotid gland surgery.
  - A small tumour can be removed by wedge resection. More extensive tumours require radical submandibular gland excision. If surrounding nerves (eg hypoglossal and lingual) are involved, they may need to be sacrificed.
- Neck dissection: this is required if there is nodal disease or a high grade tumour present.
- Post-operative radiotherapy is indicated if there is: residual disease, evidence of extra capsular lymph node spread, adenoid cystic tumour, surgery for recurrent tumours or high grade tumours.

Cystic hygroma

Epidemiology

Cystic hygroma is rare in the adult population; however, it is present in approximately 1 in 6,000 to 16,000 live births.

Aetiology

Cystic hygroma has an unknown aetiology. However, 90% are as a result of a congenital abnormality presenting in children less than 2 years of age.

Pathophysiology

A cystic hygroma is a lump identified in neonates or early infancy. It is commonly present at birth and on rare occasions causes obstruction during labour. It is a type of lymphangioma that occurs as a result of sequestration of the lymph sacs from the lymphatic system. These cysts contain clear fluid. Approximately 60% of cases involve the neck, but other sites affected include the axilla and chest wall.

History/examination

- Site: found in the posterior triangle or axilla
- It is a soft, non-compressible, transilluminable swelling that is superficial to underlying muscle
- When a child coughs or cries the swelling increases in size

Investigations

Imaging:

- USS: pre-natal diagnosis can be made during routine antenatal care of the mother
- CT: this is contraindicated in pregnancy and is therefore rarely used

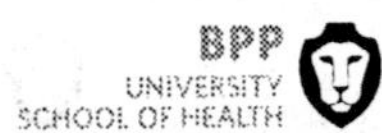

Management

- Cystic hygromas have been known to spontaneously regress
- If this does not occur the cystic hygroma should be surgically excised
- During the procedure care must be taken to avoid damage to surrounding structures, especially neurovascular structures

Groin and scrotum

Incompletely descended testis

Epidemiology

3% of all testicles at birth are undescended. The incidence falls to 1% after 1 year. Undescended testes are commonly seen in premature babies, who have an incidence of 30%.

Aetiology

Undescended testes commonly arise from a local defect during development.

Pathophysiology

An incompletely descended testis can be normal until the age of six years. After the onset of puberty the undescended testis develops poorly in comparison to intra-scrotal structures. Histological examination identifies immature tissue and destructive changes. This results in the absence of spermatogenesis and also increases the risk of developing testicular cancer.

History/examination

- Pain in the presence of trauma.
- Sterility is common in bilateral cases.
- Inguinal hernia resulting in torsion or epididymo-orchitis.
- If the testis is not palpable at any site on examination, further investigation is required.
- The testis may be found in the extraperitoneal cavity of the abdomen, just above the internal inguinal ring. It may also be situated in the inguinal canal, which can either be palpated or not or the superficial inguinal pouch.

Investigations

Usually a clinical diagnosis.

Imaging:

- USS or MRI: are used to identify the testes

Management

- All undescended testes will require surgery.
- An orchidopexy is not usually performed until the age of two years when it is safe to anaesthetise the child. This is usually a bilateral procedure.

Testicular torsion

Epidemiology

Torsion of the testis is relatively uncommon, as a normal fully descended testis should be secure and unable to rotate. It can occur at any age, but is commonly seen between the ages of 10 and 25 years. A higher incidence has been found in patients with an undescended testis.

Aetiology

Inversion of the testis is the most common cause of testicular torsion. The testis is found to be rotated and in a transverse position. If there is high attachment of the tunica vaginalis, the testis will hang within the tunica. The testis is often described as hanging like a 'bell-clapper' within the tunica vaginalis (intra-vaginal torsion). If the epididymis is separated from the body of the testis, torsion can occur. This type of testicular torsion does not involve the spermatic cord.

If any of the abnormalities above are present, activities such as straining, sexual intercourse, and lifting heavy weights may result in torsion.

Pathophysiology

Torsion of the testis prevents blood flow to the testis, resulting in infarction. Blood stained fluid exudes into the tunica vaginalis. There is irreversible infarction after a few hours without any treatment.

History/examination

- Sudden onset of severe groin and lower abdominal pain. The nerve supply for the testis is from the

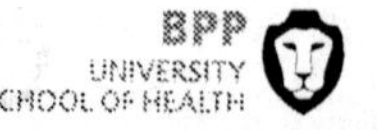

T10 sympathetic pathway, hence the abdominal pain.

- Vomiting.
- The testis may be swollen, tender and may be lying high.
- Thickened spermatic cord.
- The overlying scrotal skin becomes red and oedematous, which is a late sign.

Investigations

Testicular torsion is a urological emergency. Therefore the diagnosis is clinical without any formal investigations and the patient is prepared for emergency surgery.

Management

Within the first hour the testis may be manipulated gently. If this is successful, arrangements can be made for surgery to fix the testis in place, and prevent further episodes of torsion. However, if this is not possible surgical exploration of the scrotum is essential.

A scrotal incision is made to visualise the testis. The cord is untwisted and the testes are examined for viability. If viable the testis is fixed with non-absorbable sutures to the tunica vaginalis (scrotal wall). Alternatively the testis can be fixed with the creation of a dartos pouch and Jaboulay procedure, which entails everting the tunica vaginalis.

The opposite testis should also be fixed at the same time, due to the knowledge that most anatomical defects are likely to be bilateral.

If the testis is non-viable and completely infarcted it should be removed. If the testis is removed the patient can be counselled about prosthetic replacement, at a later date.

Hydrocele

This is an abnormal or excessive collection of serous fluid within the tunica vaginalis.

Epidemiology

A hydrocele is estimated to affect 1% of the male population.

Aetiology

Primary hydroceles are idiopathic and arise in children and the elderly. Secondary hydroceles are associated with an abnormal testis. The testis is surrounded by a serosal sac, which becomes filled with inflammatory or malignant exudates. Causes include:

- Trauma (Haemorrhagic)
- Epididymo-orchitis/Tuberculosis
- Testicular tumour
- Obstruction of the lymphatic drainage of the scrotum

Pathophysiology

There are four main types of hydrocele, ie vaginal, congenital, infantile and hydrocele of the cord.

1. **Vaginal hydrocele**
   i) A patent processus vaginalis is present but there is no communication with the peritoneal cavity.
   ii) The swelling is painless and therefore patients present late.
   iii) The testis may be palpable.
   iv) The swelling can be transilluminated.
   v) 5% of indirect inguinal hernias have a vaginal hydrocele on the same side.
2. **Congenital hydrocele**
   i) There is a connection between the patent processus vaginalis and the peritoneal cavity and therefore fluid from the hydrocele can drain back into the peritoneal cavity.
   ii) Most hydroceles are congenital and are noted in children aged one to two years.
3. **Infantile hydrocele**
   i) Found along the testis to the internal inguinal ring and do not enter the peritoneal cavity.
4. **Hydrocele of the cord**
   i) Rare.
   ii) There is a smooth swelling close to the spermatic cord and this is often mistaken for an inguinal hernia. If the testis is gently pulled down, the swelling moves downward.

Investigations

Imaging:

- USS: can assess for a hydrocele and identify an abnormal testis, which may require surgery.

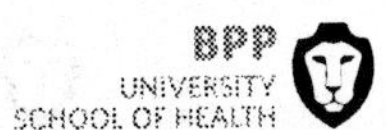

Management

- Most hydroceles resolve spontaneously and therefore can be conservatively managed in infants. Approximately 80% of newborn males have a patent processus vaginalis but most close within 12 months.
- Operative intervention will be required if the hydrocele has not resolved after one year.
  - Lord's operation: the tunica vaginalis is placated with interrupted absorbable sutures.
  - Jaboulay's procedure: the hydrocele sac is everted, with the opening secured with sutures.
- A hydrocele with a normal testis can be treated with aspiration; however, it may reoccur.

Varicocele

Epidemiology

Varicocele is defined as dilatation of the veins of the testis and arises in approximately 20% of the male population.

Anatomy

- The group of veins that drain the testis and the epididymis make up the pampiniform plexus.
- There are fewer veins along the inguinal canal and at the inguinal ring, which join together to form the testicular veins.
- The left testicular vein drains into the left renal vein and the right testicular vein drains into the inferior vena cava, just below the right renal vein.
- A collateral venous drainage system of the testes occurs via the cremasteric veins into the inferior epigastric vessels.

Aetiology

It has been found that 95% of cases are associated with the left side, as a result of the angle of the left testicular vein emptying into the left renal vein and the lack of anti-reflux valves. The dilated veins in the varicocele are the cremasteric veins. If the patient is diagnosed with a left renal tumour this can cause obstruction of the left testicular vein resulting in a varicocele.

History/examination

- Can be asymptomatic
- There may be an uncomfortable dragging sensation in the scrotum. The discomfort is worse when not wearing any underwear
- Usually associated with increased infertility and are commonly diagnosed following investigation for this
- On palpation with the patient standing, the scrotum feels like a 'bag of worms'
- The affected side may hang lower compared to the normal side
- On lying down the veins empty and the testis can be palpated

Investigations

Usually a clinical diagnosis.

Management

- Largely conservative treatment.
- Operative management if the patient is symptomatic with pain or unexplained infertility.
- A laparoscopic or open procedure is performed to ligate the testicular vein along the inguinal canal.
- Recurrence is common as a result of the collateral venous supply.
- Percutaneous embolisation of the internal spermatic vein via cannulation through the femoral vein is an alternative option. This is normally reserved for recurrent disease.

Epididymal cyst

Epidemiology

Epididymal cysts are common and are usually found in middle-aged individuals. These cysts are rare in children.

Aetiology

Epididymal cysts occur as a result of cystic degeneration of epididymal or para-epididymal structures.

Pathophysiology

The cysts are filled with clear fluid. They are typically found bilaterally, with multiple cysts present.

History/examination

- The cysts feel like a bunch of grapes on palpation.
- They are fluctuant and transilluminable.
- In most cases they are separate from the testis.

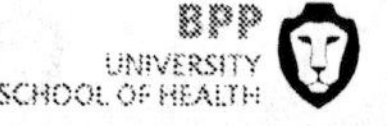

Investigations

Imaging:

- Scrotal USS: this will confirm the diagnosis of an epididymal cyst. Aspiration of fluid is occasionally performed; however, this is rarely useful.

Management

- Surgical removal is possible if it is causing the patient discomfort.

Epididymo-orchitis

Epidemiology

Males between the ages of 14 and 35 are commonly affected.

Aetiology

Epididymo-orchitis is inflammation of the epididymis and testis. The causes include the mumps virus, sexually transmitted infections (Chlamydia trachomatis and Neisseria gonorrhoea), complicated UTI, and following an operation involving the prostate or urethra.

Pathophysiology

The primary infection of the urethra, prostate or seminal vesicles spreads to the globus minus of the epididymis.

History/examination

- Fever
- Sweaty
- Urethral discharge
- Dysuria
- Swelling of the epididymis and the testis
- Tender on palpation
- The scrotum appears red and shiny
- This can progress to the formation of an abscess, with pus discharging through the scrotal skin

Investigations

Blood tests:

- FBC
- U&Es
- Inflammatory markers: CRP

Urinalysis:

- Urine dipstick
- MSU

Imaging:

- USS: to look for an abscess

Others:

- Urethral swab

Management

- In the acute phase bed rest is advised.
- A positive Chlamydia infection requires a course of doxycyline or a one-off dose of Azithromycin. If no organism has been identified a broad spectrum antibiotic (Levofloxacin or Ofloxacin) should be prescribed. A two-week course is usually sufficient, or until the inflammation has settled.
- Systemic illness warrants hospitalization and coverage with IV Ampicillin and Gentamicin.

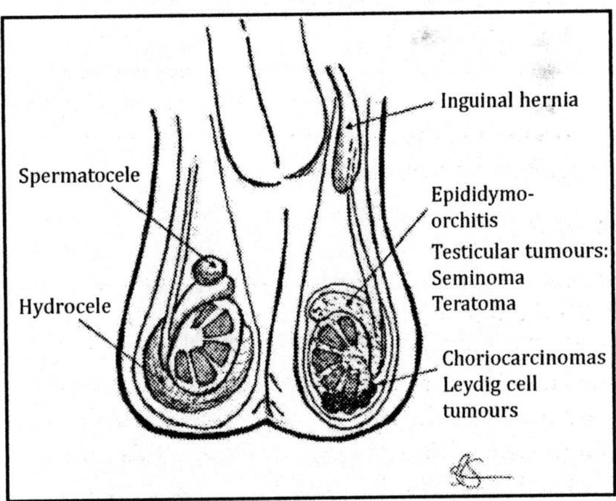

Figure 4.15: The common scrotal lumps

Hernias

A hernia is defined as the protrusion of a viscus through an abnormal defect in the wall of its containing compartment. Some hernias are more common than others. The most common are inguinal hernias (75%), umbilical hernias (15%), and femoral hernias (8%).

There are three parts to a hernia, the sac, the coverings, and the sac contents. The hernial sac is an out-pouching of the peritoneum comprising of a mouth, neck, body, and fundus. When the neck is narrow, strangulation of bowel can occur. However, the body of the sac varies in size and may or may not be occupied. The coverings are taken from the layers of the abdominal wall. It is through this that the sac passes. What occupies the sac is referred to as the contents. This may be omentum, intestine, a section of the bladder, ovary, diverticulum or peritoneal fluid.

Inguinal hernia

Epidemiology

The incidence of inguinal hernias in newborn babies is 4%. This increases to 30% in premature babies. Approximately 8–15% of patients with this hernia will present to the accident and emergency department with bowel obstruction and strangulation.

Anatomy

The inguinal canal:

- The inguinal canal is approximately 3.75 cm long and it extends downwards and medially from the deep inguinal to the superficial inguinal ring.
- It has four bordering structures:
  - The anterior wall consists of the external oblique aponeurosis and the internal oblique.
  - The posterior wall consists of the transversalis fascia and the conjoined tendon.
  - The roof of the canal contains the internal oblique which arches from front to back.
  - The floor of the canal represents the inguinal ligament.

The superficial inguinal ring:

- This is found in the external oblique aponeurosis.
- It is approximately 1.25 cm above and lateral to the pubic tubercle.

The deep inguinal ring:

- This is found 1.25 cm above the inguinal ligament, and is midway between the anterior superior iliac spine and the pubic tubercle (mid-point of the inguinal ligament).

Type of hernia	Features
Reducible	• The hernial sac can be returned to its original cavity
Irreducible	• The contents of the sac cannot be returned to its cavity • This is commonly a result of adhesions between the sac and its contents • Irreducibility predisposes to strangulation
Obstructed	• This hernia is irreducible and the lumen of the bowel is obstructed by the hernia neck • The blood supply to the bowel is not affected • On examination an obstructed hernia cannot be differentiated from a strangulated hernia
Strangulated	• The blood supply to the contents of the hernia has become compromised • Initially the venous system is occluded but with increasing pressure the arterial supply becomes compromised. In a very tight hernia neck the arterial supply can become directly occluded. The contents then become ischaemic and progress to gangrene formation • A femoral hernia is at a greater risk of strangulation due to its narrow neck
Sliding	• This is a type of hernia in which a segment of the sac is formed by the bowel
Richter's hernia	• This is identified as a hernial sac containing only a segment of the circumference of the intestine

Table 4.27: Classification of hernias

- At the posterior and medial aspect of the deep inguinal ring the inferior epigastric vessels will be found.

Aetiology

Inguinal hernias can either be congenital or acquired. Congenital abnormalities such as a patent processus vaginalis can predispose to hernias. The acquired causes all tend to produce a rise in intra-abdominal pressure. This will increase the chance of developing a hernia.

An increase in intra-abdominal pressure can be due to:

- Chronic cough
- Straining on defecation
- Prostatism or difficulty micturating
- Pregnancy
- Obesity
- Ascites
- Excessive or repetitive muscular effort

Previous hernia and hernia repairs tend to weaken the abdominal wall and hence predispose to developing hernias in the future. Smoking is also associated.

Pathophysiology

An inguinal hernia can be palpated above and medial to the pubic tubercle. They can be classified into a direct and indirect hernia.

History/examination

- Groin pain can be present, radiating to the testicle.
- When the patient coughs a bulge may appear.
- If palpated a cough impulse can be felt.
- It may often be best to examine the hernia with the patient standing as gravity enables the hernia to become visible.
- A hernia identified as being above and medial to the pubic tubercle is an inguinal hernia.
- Bowel sounds may be heard over the hernia.
- Always examine the scrotum to identify scrotal involvement.
- To differentiate between a direct and indirect hernia, the hernia is reduced and pressure applied over the deep inguinal ring. The patient is asked to cough or strain. If the hernia is controlled it is indirect and if it is revealed it is direct. However, the only definitive method of differentiating direct/indirect hernias is intra-operative examination.

Investigations

Usually a clinical diagnosis.

Management

If patients are fit to undergo surgery, an open or laparoscopic procedure can be performed.

1. **Inguinal herniotomy:**
   i) This is recommended in children.
   ii) The hernial sac is opened and the contents are reduced – no mesh is used.
2. **Inguinal herniotomy and repair (herniorrhaphy):**
   i) The hernial sac is excised.
   ii) The internal inguinal ring and transversalis fascia are repaired and the posterior wall of the inguinal canal is reinforced:
      - Shouldice repair: involves securing the transversalis muscle to the posterior wall with a nylon suture
      - Lichenstein repair: reinforces posterior wall with a synthetic mesh
   iii) Post-operatively patients require adequate analgesia, laxatives and scrotal support. They should refrain from heavy lifting/straining for four to six weeks.

Conservative management:

- Those patients who are unsuitable for surgical repair (eg elderly, other co-morbidities) may be prescribed a truss to support the hernia.
- However, such hernias can progress to strangulation and then require an emergency operation.

Direct hernia	Indirect hernia
• This hernia passes directly through the posterior wall of the inguinal canal • This is medial to the inferior epigastric vessels • This is a common hernia in the elderly population • These account for 35% of inguinal hernias • Direct hernias rarely extend to the scrotum	• This hernia passes through the internal ring, lateral to the inferior epigastric vessels • It can extend down the canal along the side of the spermatic cord into the scrotum • This is the most common type of hernia (65%) in the young adult • 55% are right sided and 12% are bilateral

Table 4.28: Features of direct and indirect hernias

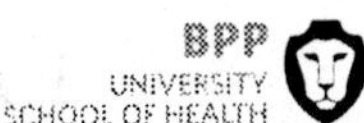

Femoral hernia

Epidemiology

These hernias usually occur in the middle-aged and elderly population. They account for almost 7% of all groin herniae. Approximately 50% of femoral hernias are diagnosed when they present to the accident and emergency department.

Anatomy

- The femoral canal is 1.25 cm long, and extends from the femoral ring to the opening of the saphenous vein.
- It contains fat and lymphatic vessels.
- The femoral canal is surrounded by a number of structures:
  - The anterior wall is composed of the inguinal ligament.
  - The posterior aspect is represented by Astley Cooper's ligament, the pubic bone, and the overlying pectineus muscle fascia.

Hernia	Key features in the history/examination	Management
Incisional	• Occurs through a previously acquired defect eg operative scar • Asymptomatic • Can be large and unsightly	• Conservative • Surgical repair eg mesh repair
Umbilical	• These are seen in infants • Congenital and acquired • Asymptomatic but unsightly	• 95% resolve spontaneously • Surgical repair after the age of three years
Para-umbilical	• These are seen in adults • Defect in the linea alba, above and below the umbilicus • Risk or irreducibility and obstruction	• Surgical repair with or without a mesh
Epigastric	• Defect in the linea alba • The hernia contains omentum • Pea-sized swelling • Risk of strangulation	• Operative repair with or without a mesh
Spigelian	• Rare • The hernia occurs through the linea semilunaris • The hernia is found between the abdominal wall layers	• Surgical repair
Obturator	• A lump can be felt within the femoral triangle • The hernial sac is found extending through the obturator canal • Risk of obstruction and strangulation • Referred pain can be felt over the medial aspect of the knee • Surgery can treat the obstruction	• The defect cannot be sutured
Lumbar	• Occur post-loin incisions	• Conservative methods eg corset • Surgical mesh repair
Sciatic	• The hernia is seen through the greater sciatic foramen • Presents as small bowel obstruction	• Surgical repair

Table 4.29: Classification and features of other hernia types

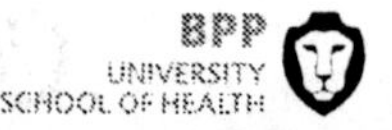

- The medial aspect consists of the lacunar ligament.
- The lateral aspect is composed of a thin septum which separates the canal from the femoral vein.

Aetiology

The causes are all acquired and are again associated with an increase in intra-abdominal pressure due to the causative features above.

Pathophysiology

The hernia passes down the femoral canal until the opening of the saphenous vein. Whilst inside the walls of the femoral canal, the hernia is narrow. However, once the hernia has passed through the saphenous opening it can dilate and distend. This increases the likelihood of an irreducible hernia which is at risk of strangulation.

History/examination

- Painless lump in the groin
- The lump is below and lateral to the pubic tubercle
- Often irreducible
- Severe pain if the hernia is strangulated and the lump will be hot, red, tender and irreducible

Investigations

Usually a clinical diagnosis.

Management

- All femoral hernias are treated surgically due to the risk of strangulation.
- A low approach (Lockwood) is taken where an incision is performed over the hernia. The femoral sac is excised and the repair is then performed which involves suturing the inguinal ligament to the pectineal ligament.
- In an emergency the femoral hernia is repaired using the high approach (McEvedy) with the incision being made over the inguinal region. This allows closer examination of the bowel which can be difficult with a low approach. The repair is performed as above.

Further reading and references

1. Aly, A., Devitt, P.G. and Jamieson, G.G. (2004) Evolution of surgical treatment for pharyngeal pouch. *Br J Surg* 2004; 91: 657–664.
2. Davenport, M. (1996) ABC of General Surgery in Children: Lumps and swellings of the head and neck. *BMJ* 1996; 312: 368–371.
3. Devendra, D., Hatton, R. and Patel, M. (2009) Thyroid swellings. *BMJ* 2009; 339: 563.
4. Ivaz, S., Lloyd-Hughes, H., Oakeshott, P., et al. (2009) Malignant melanoma. *BMJ* 2009; 339: 3078.
5. Mannu, G.S. and Odutoye, T. (2008) The pharyngeal pouch. *Student BMJ* 2008; 16: 616.
6. Jain, A., Mehanna, H.M., Morton, R.P., et al. (2009) Clinical Review: Investigating the thyroid nodule. *BMJ* 2009; 338: 733.
7. Mehta, M.R. (2000) Cystic Hygroma: Presentation of two cases with a review of the literature. *Indian Journal of Otolaryngology and Head & Neck Surgery* 2000; 52.
8. Pavlidis, T.E. (2009) Current opinion on laparoscopic repair of inguinal hernia. *Surgical Endoscopy* 2010.
9. Dannana, N.K., Prasad, K.C. and Prasad, S.C. (2006) *Thyroglossal duct cyst*: an unusual presentation. *Ear, Nose & Throat Journal* 2006.
10. Bhattacharyya, K., Gauray, K. and Purushotham, S. (2006) Pharyngeal pouch: associations and complications. *European Archive of Otorhinolaryngology* 2006; 263: 463–468.
11. Sandlow, J. (2004) Pathogenesis and treatment of varicoceles. *BMJ* 2004; 328: 967–968.

Organomegaly (Hepatomegaly/Splenomegaly)

Hepatomegaly

Epidemiology

The epidemiology is dependent on the aetiology.

Aetiology

The aetiology of hepatomegaly can be classified into five categories.

Pathophysiology

The pathophysiology is dependent on the aetiology.

Type	Diseases
Congenital	• Polycystic disease • Riedal's lobe
Cirrhosis	• Portal and biliary • Haemochromatosis
Inflammatory	• Alcoholic hepatitis • Viral hepatitis • Autoimmune hepatitis • Liver abscess • Leptospirosis (Weil's disease)
Haematological disease	• Hodgkin's and non-Hodgkin's lymphoma • Leukaemia • Polycythaemia
Metabolic conditions	• Amyloid • Gaucher's disease

Table 4.30: Classification of hepatomegaly

History/examination

- The enlarged liver is palpable below the right costal margin.
- Gross hepatomegaly is identified when the liver extends over to beneath the left costal margin.
- The liver moves with respiration and is dull to percussion.
- If a liver is palpable there may be associated splenomegaly and lymphadenopathy.

Investigations

Investigations should be tailored to individual differential diagnoses.

Blood tests:

- FBC
- U&Es
- LFTs
- Clotting
- Amylase
- Glucose
- Hepatitis screen
- Serology
- BNP – to exclude cardiac failure

Imaging:

- USS: of the liver
- CT: of the abdomen
- ECG and echocardiogram if cardiac failure is suspected

Others:

- Liver biopsy
- Urine dipstick: check for bilirubin

Management

- The indications for a liver transplant include:
  - Estimated survival of less than one year
  - Signs and symptoms such as ascites, lethargy, pruritus resulting in poor quality of life
- Some of the conditions suitable for a liver transplant include the autoimmune diseases, and hepatitis.
- Contraindications to liver transplant: Primary or secondary hepatic carcinoma or metastatic disease, current alcohol abuse, sepsis, cardiac, pulmonary and cerebral disease.

Splenomegaly

Epidemiology

The epidemiology is dependent on the aetiology.

Aetiology

The aetiology of splenomegaly can be classified into five categories.

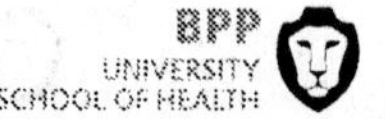

Type	Disease
Infections	• Viruses: glandular fever • Bacterial: typhoid and septicaemia • Protozoal: malaria, kala-azar, schistosomiasis • Parasitic: hydatid
Haemato-logical conditions	• Leukaemia: CML, CLL • Lymphoma: non-Hodgkin's and Hodgkin's lymphoma • Myelofibrosis: idiopathic thrombocytopenic purpura (ITP), polycythaemia rubra vera • Haemolytic disease: spherocytosis
Metabolic conditions	• Storage disease: Gaucher's disease, Niemann-Pick disease
Splenic masses	• Tumours • Cysts • Abscesses
Portal hypertension	• Cirrhosis • Hepatitis (rare) • Infection eg schistosomiasis • Portal vein thrombosis

Table 4.31: Classification of splenomegaly

Pathophysiology

The pathophysiology is dependent on the aetiology.

History/examination

- Mass palpable below the left costal margin, which is impossible to get above, is dull to percussion and descends on inspiration.

Investigations

This is dependent on the aetiology but a basic screen would be appropriate for all causes.

Blood tests:

- FBC
- Clotting
- Serology

Imaging:

- USS
- CT: of the abdomen

Management

- Each different cause can have varying presentations and require individual diagnostic tests. Specific management is dependent on the actual cause.
- However, a splenectomy may be the appropriate treatment if certain criteria are met:
  - Splenic rupture
  - Haematological disease eg haemolytic anaemia
  - Tumours
  - If required as part of another procedure eg radical gastrectomy for gastric carcinoma

Further reading and references

1. Poole, A. and Ramachandran, R. (2003) *Clinical Cases and OSCEs in Surgery (MRCS Study Guides)*. London: Churchill and Livingstone.

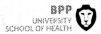

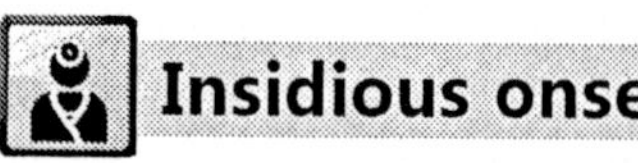

Insidious onset

Differential diagnosis

System/Organ	Disease
Skin	BCC (rodent ulcer) Bowen's disease SCC Malignant melanoma
Neck	Thyroid cancer
Breast	Breast cancer
Alimentary canal	Oesophageal cancer Colon cancer
Hepato-biliary	Hepato-cellular cancer (HCC) Cholangiocarcinoma Gallbladder cancer
Pancreas	Pancreatic carcinoma
Urological and groin	Renal carcinoma Bladder cancer Prostate cancer Testicular cancer

Table 4.32: Differential diagnosis of organ-specific diseases of insidious onset

Basal cell carcinoma (rodent ulcer)

Epidemiology

Basal cell carcinoma (BCC) is the commonest type of skin cancer, affecting adults between the ages of 40–79.

Aetiology

Sunlight exposure and irradiation are well-known predisposing factors.

Pathophysiology

90% of tumours are identified on the face, commonly around the eyes, nasolabial folds, and the scalp hairline. However, they can occur on any part of the body. Metastatic disease is very rare.

History/examination

- The tumour is a raised lesion with rolled edges. It is classically described as a pearly nodule with overlying telangiectasia.
- It is slow growing and results in long-term ulceration.
- Microscopically the involved cells arise from the basal layer. The tumour advances with surrounding tissue destruction. In some cases underlying bone and facial structures may be damaged and distorted.
- 26 types of BCC have been identified but often it is only 5 that are clinically diagnosed: nodular (50%); superficial (10%); cystic (8%); pigmented (6%); and morpheic (2%).

Investigations

- The diagnosis is usually made following clinical examination. However, a biopsy should be sent to confirm the diagnosis.

Management

- Treatment consists of complete surgical excision of the lesion with adequate margin resection.
- Surgery gives patients an 85–95% chance of a cure.
- In early cases or those unsuitable for surgery, superficial radiotherapy is offered with a success rate of around 90%.
- In advanced disease the only option is surgical removal.
- Follow-up is not usually necessary if histological margins are clear.
- Patients with the familial condition Gorlin's syndrome are predisposed to further BCCs, and therefore warrant close follow-up.

Bowen's disease

Epidemiology

The elderly population is typically affected.

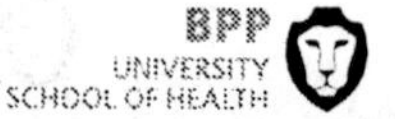

Aetiology

Defined as an intra-epidermal SCC. A viral aetiology has been suggested, due to the presence of HPV DNA identified in some lesions.

Pathophysiology

The lesions appear as flat, red, scaly, or crusted plaques. It is often difficult to clinically distinguish Bowen's disease from solar keratosis. If the lesion is left untreated 3–5% of patients will progress to malignancy.

Management

- If the diagnosis is uncertain a biopsy can be performed for histological confirmation.
- Local treatment involves cryotherapy or curettage and cauterisation.
- Radiotherapy and chemotherapy can be used.
- If local management of the superficial lesion fails to treat deeper structures, recurrence is often seen, which may eventually progress to invasive SCC.
- Treatment of choice is surgical excision.

Squamous cell carcinoma (SCC)

Epidemiology

SCC is a malignancy affecting the elderly and Caucasian population.

Aetiology

Solar keratosis and Bowen's disease are predisposing conditions to SCC. Other risk factors include sunlight/ultraviolet irradiation, infection with HPV (types 6, 11, 16, 18), exposure to carcinogens such as tar and soot, and chronic ulceration.

Pathophysiology

SCC is a malignant tumour arising from pre-malignant lesions. They are less common than BCCs, but are more malignant. The tumour spreads locally and via the lymphatic system.

History/examination

- Ulcerated lesion
- Raised and everted edges
- A central scab is present

Investigations

An incisional or punch biopsy is performed to confirm the diagnosis.

Management

WLE of the tumour is the treatment of choice. Radiotherapy is offered with inoperable tumours or post-operatively to ensure complete eradication.

Malignant melanoma

Epidemiology

Malignant melanoma accounts for 10% of all skin cancers. It affects the Caucasian population and is responsible for most deaths from skin cancer.

Aetiology

Exposure to ultraviolet radiation is a well-known risk factor. Skin conditions such as albinism and xeroderma pigmentosa are also associated with higher risk, as are patients with pre-existing junctional or compound naevi. There is also an association with a particular genetic mutation (V600) in the BRAF gene.

Pathophysiology

There are five different presentations of malignant melanoma: superficial spreading; nodular; lentigo maligna; acral lentiginous; and amelanotic. Malignant melanoma can spread to the lymph nodes, lungs, liver, and brain.

History/examination

Superficial spreading:

- The most common presentation.
- The lesion can occur anywhere on the body.
- Usually a palpable lesion, with an irregular border and varied pigmentation.
- Common sites include the legs in females and torso in males.

Nodular:

- Typically seen in the younger population, with lesions found on any part of the body.
- Considered the most malignant lesion.
- The naevi is a pigmented nodule, with a smooth surface, and irregular border.
- The nodule can bleed and ulcerate.

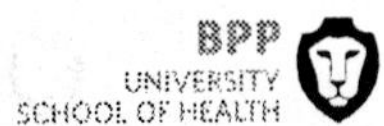

Lentigo maligna:

- Frequently seen in the elderly population
- Commonly seen on the face but can occur anywhere
- The lesion appears as a flat, brown and irregular pigmented patch

Acral lentiginous:

- Lesions are found on the extremities eg the palms and soles.
- Seen in dark-skinned races.

Amelanotic:

- Lesion appears pink with pigmentation at the base.
- May present with lymphatic spread.

Signs suggesting a malignant change of a melanoma include increases/changes in:

A – asymmetry/irregularity
B – loss of border definition/bleeding, ulceration, pain and itching
C – colour (increased/irregular pigmentation)
D – diameter
E – evolution ie a progressively changing lesion

Investigations

Clinical examination should arouse suspicion of a malignant lesion. Further investigations are required to confirm the diagnosis.

Others:

- Complete excisional biopsy: ensuring a 2 mm margin. The melanoma is then staged using the Clark's or Breslow thickness systems.

Management

- All patients should be managed with the support of a specialist skin cancer multidisciplinary team.
- Surgical resection is the first-line treatment – the lesion is completely excised with a minimum margin of 0.5 cm for stage 0 melanoma; 1 cm for stage 1 and 2 cm for stage 2.
- In certain cases the margins may be adapted for cosmetic or structural reasons.
- Topical imiquimod (a TLR-7 analogue that activates the innate immune system) may be used for stage 0 disease where incomplete histological resection is impossible.
- Immunotherapy with ipilimumab (CTLA-4 targeting mAb) may be offered to individuals with previously treated, advanced (unresectable/metastatic) disease.
- Patients with lymphadenopathy in the context of stage IIIB-C disease or nodal involvement on imaging should be offered a lymph node clearance.
- Dabrafenib or vemurafenib (B-raf inhibitors) may be offered for BRAF V600 positive, surgically inoperable metastatic disease.
- Palliative radiotherapy may be offered to those with metastatic disease, particularly involving the brain and cytotoxic chemotherapy may be considered if immunotherapy is unsuitable.
- Follow up:
  - A full skin and lymph node examination should be performed at every follow-up visit
  - **Stage 0:** discharge after completion of treatment
  - **Stage IA:** 2–4 visits for 1 year and then discharge
  - **Stage IB-IIB (or fully staged IIC):** every 3 months for first 3 years and then every 6 months for next 2 years. Discharge after 5 years
  - **Stage IIC (no SLNB) or stage III:** as per IB-IIB, with surveillance imaging if recommended by local MDT
  - **Stage IV:** personalised follow-up

Stage	Features
I	Involves the epidermis
II	The tumour goes through the epidermis and into the papillary dermis
III	The tumour invades the papillary dermis
IV	Reticular dermis is then invaded
V	The tumour finally invades the subcutaneous

Table 4.33: Clark's staging system for depth of tumour invasion in relation to the layers of the skin. The 5 year survival rate for stage II or less is approximately 90%

Depth (mm)	Five-year survival
<0.75	>95%
0.75–1.5	90%
1.5–4.0	70%
>4.0	<50%

Table 4.34: The 5 year survival rate according to the Breslow's staging system, which incorporates the thickness and depth of the tumour

Case Study: An unfortunate visit

Mr CW had not had an easy life. He had served overseas in Germany and Malta towards the end of the Second World War, and afterwards returned to the old family farm, where he had grafted for the next 60 years. His first wife died, very early in their marriage, and it had been nearly 40 years before he found someone else with whom to share his life. His new wife was nearly half his age, but had supported him through multiple heart problems, a stroke and treatment for his malignant melanoma. In return, Mr CW had been there all the way through the birth of their son and had supported the three of them for the last seven years on the farm's meagre outputs.

Follow-up for his melanoma had largely been uneventful. Two years after his surgery he came to an outpatient appointment three times a year, saw the specialist and left again. This time was a little different. As he walked into the appointment the surgeon struggled to understand what he was saying with his slightly slurred speech. He wobbled slightly and seemed much frailer than on previous visits, holding onto his wife's arm with a sense of fear that had never been evident before. Within an hour he had been through the CT scanner and admitted to hospital. Sadly, his scan revealed extension to the area previously damaged in his stroke, with much swelling and oedema and an MRI scan the following morning confirmed this was due to the presence of multiple metastatic deposits.

Mr CW sat silently while the news was broken to him, but his wife's fear was evident in her torrent of panicked questions. The distant dread of caring for an ageing husband and a young son on her own had suddenly become a horrible reality. Mr CW's story was a reminder of the destruction such diagnoses inflict on whole families, not just the patient. He died a few weeks later.

Thyroid cancer

Epidemiology

Thyroid neoplasms have an incidence of 3.7 per 100,000 per year. The relative incidences of thyroid carcinoma differ with each type of neoplasm.

Tumour	Incidence
Papillary carcinoma	70%
Follicular carcinoma	17%
Medullary carcinoma	5%
Malignant lymphoma	2–5%
Anaplastic carcinoma	1–2%

Table 4.35: The incidence of the different types of thyroid carcinomas

Aetiology

Papillary carcinoma is linked with accidental thyroid irradiation in childhood. Follicular carcinoma has been found to be prevalent in areas where goitres are endemic (eg populations with a low dietary iodine intake) or occur as a result of excess TSH activity. Medullary carcinoma has been associated with familial conditions and other malignancies including MEN 2, phaeochromocytoma, and neurofibromas. Malignant lymphomas are associated with autoimmune thyroiditis.

Pathophysiology

Papillary carcinoma is commonly seen in young adults and children. These tumours consist of papillary and colloid follicles and are slow growing and multifocal. Papillary carcinomas tend to invade locally and spread via the cervical lymphatics.

Follicular carcinomas are seen in middle-aged adults. They tend to be solitary and encapsulated and spread via blood to the lungs and bone. Lymph nodes are affected late in the disease.

Medullary carcinomas can occur in any age group. The tumours arise in para-follicular C-cells and can be multifocal. They secrete calcitonin which can be used as a tumour marker. Medullary carcinomas metastasise via the lymph nodes.

Anaplastic carcinoma is a carcinoma of the elderly population. It is rapidly growing and extremely aggressive. These tumours spread via local infiltration and the lymphatic system.

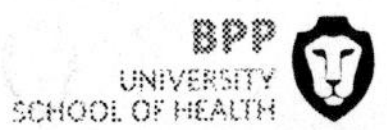

History/examination

- Thyroid swelling
- Enlarged cervical lymph nodes
- Hoarseness due to recurrent laryngeal palsy
- Dysphagia may occur if the tumour causes extrinsic oesophageal compression

Investigations

Most thyroid carcinomas are suspected on clinical examination. There is no investigation which is completely diagnostic of a carcinoma. This can only be achieved with surgical exploration and excision. However, some useful investigations should be considered:

Blood tests:

- Thyroid antibody titres: are sometimes raised in thyroid carcinoma
- Serum calcitonin: >0.08 ng/ml is suggestive of medullary carcinoma

Imaging:

- USS: commonly used but unable to differentiate benign and malignant nodules

Others:

- FNA: carried out in the outpatient setting under local anaesthesia. A minimum of three biopsies are recommended to minimise false-negative results. Diagnostic yields can be improved by using USS guidance.

Management

Papillary carcinoma:

- Total removal of the affected thyroid lobe
- Block lymph node dissection if lymph node spread or lesion >1 cm
- Thyroid suppression (reduce TSH) post-surgery with thyroxine
- Radioiodine for recurrent/metastatic disease
- Annual thyroglobulin measurements to identify recurrence

Follicular carcinoma:

- Thyroid lobectomy
- Total thyroidectomy if there is vascular invasion
- Radioiodine and thyroid suppression

Medullary carcinoma:

- Total thyroidectomy
- Lymph node clearance as involvement usually present
- Calcitonin measurements on follow up to detect recurrence/metastasis

Anaplastic carcinoma:

- A total thyroidectomy can be performed. However, most patients present late and have a mean survival of six to eight months.
- Palliative radiotherapy is performed in selected cases to de-bulk the tumour.
- If there is airway obstruction a tracheostomy or tracheal stenting may be required.

Post-operative complications:

Haemorrhage:
- Acute haemorrhage post-operatively can lead to airway obstruction, which can be life-threatening.
- Treatment involves removing the surgical clips and releasing the deeper sutures, followed by a return to theatre for further exploration.

Recurrent laryngeal nerve injury:
- The recurrent laryngeal nerve is located along the posterior aspect of the thyroid gland, where it is at particular risk during ligation of the inferior thyroid artery.
- Unilateral nerve injury can result in hoarseness.
- If both recurrent laryngeal nerves are injured this may cause acute airway obstruction.

Damage to the parathyroid glands:
- This can occur following accidental injury or reduced blood supply.
- If there is significant damage, hypocalcaemia will result and present as tetany. This can be demonstrated by Chvostek's sign (twitching of the muscles of the face when the facial nerve is tapped), and Trousseau's sign (the upper arm is compressed with a blood pressure cuff causing carpal spasm).
- Treatment is with oral calcium supplements or a slow infusion of calcium gluconate.

Hypothyroidism:
- Surgery can result in reduction of thyroid tissue, leading to hypothyroidism.
- Treatment is with levothyroxine replacement.

Breast cancer

Epidemiology

In the UK breast cancer affects 1 in 10 women, with approximately 20,000 new cases a year. The incidence of breast cancer continues to rise; however, a reduction in the mortality has been noted.

Aetiology

Previous breast cancer and a family history are strong risk factors. A first degree relative with breast cancer doubles the risk. The inheritance is autosomal dominant in 5–10% of cases, with causative mutations identified in the breast cancer 1 (BRCA1), breast cancer 2 (BRCA2) and p53 genes.

Oestrogen exposure is also a risk factor. This is noted in early menarche, late menopause, nulliparity, pregnancy after the age of 30 years or continued use of the combined oral contraceptive pill for more than 4 years or oestrogen-only hormone replacement therapy.

Other risk factors include obesity, exposure to radiation, smoking, alcohol intake and a diet high in saturated fats.

Pathophysiology

Breast cancer can be as *in situ* or invasive. If the cancer is *in situ* it carries a possibility of being curable as the ductal basement membrane has not been breached.

Non-invasive DCIS is a pre-malignant lesion. Mammograms classically show microcalcification. Uni-focal lesions may be treated with lumpectomy (localised excisions), but widespread lesions are commonly treated with a mastectomy. If left without any treatment the lesion can progress to invasive breast cancer. Non-invasive LCIS is less common than DCIS and is usually multi-focal.

Invasive ductal carcinoma is the commonest type of breast cancer. It is usually noted as a hard lump. Other cancers include invasive lobular carcinoma, invasive medullary carcinoma (which accounts for approximately 5% of all breast cancers and is seen in younger patients), and invasive papillary carcinoma.

Paget's disease presents as an eczema-type skin condition on the nipple, where the skin involved may ulcerate and bleed. This usually represents an underlying malignancy and therefore should be investigated further.

History/examination

- Firm, painless lump
- Breast asymmetry
- Nipple discharge
- Nipple retraction and breast tissue distortion/ skin tethering
- Peau d'orange (skin appearance)
- Fingating lesion
- Axillary/supraclavicular lymphadenopathy
- Bone pain, abdominal pain and hepatomegaly may represent metastatic disease

Investigations

All women who are referred with a breast lump receive a triple assessment, which aims to identify 95% of breast cancers. The assessment consists of a detailed history and examination, radiology (mammography and/or USS), and FNA cytology (or core biopsy).

Mammography:

- The breasts are compressed between two plates.
- Craniocaudal and oblique views of the breast are taken.
- Breast cancer will be illustrated as a white spiculated lesion with microcalcification.
- Approximately 10% of cancers are missed with mammography.
- The technique is only suitable for less dense breasts ie in older women.

Stage	Clinical features
Stage 1	• The growth is mobile • Confined to the breast • No lymph node involvement
Stage 2	• Clinical findings of stage 1 • Mobile axillary lymph nodes on the same side
Stage 3	• Tumour is fixed to the underlying muscle • The lymph nodes may have become fixed
Stage 4	• Tumour is completely fixed to the chest wall • Metastatic disease is present • There may be opposite breast involvement

Table 4.36: Classification of breast cancer staging

Ultrasound scan:

- This is used together with mammography or in denser breasts in younger women.
- It does not identify microcalcification.
- It can also be useful in identifying cysts.

Fine needle aspiration:

- If a lump has been identified FNA is performed.
- A 10 ml syringe and green needle is inserted into the lump and an aspirate is obtained.
- The results are divided into cytology codes.

Cytology code	Description
C1	Insufficient sample
C2	Benign cells
C3	Uncertain diagnosis
C4	Probable breast cancer
C5	Breast cancer

Table 4.37: The cytology codes

Core biopsy:

- If breast cancer is suspected and the FNA results are inconclusive (C1–C3), the lump may be removed or a core biopsy is performed.
- Patients return to clinic after a few days for the results.

Blood tests:

- FBC
- LFTs
- U&Es
- ALP

Imaging:

- CXR: to look for metastatic disease
- Liver USS: for staging
- Bone scan: for staging
- CT scan: for staging

Breast cancer treatment depends on: disease stage, patient morbidity and patient choice.

Operative management:

- Clinical stages 1 and 2 can be treated surgically.
- Surgery should be avoided in stages 3 and 4.
- WLE followed by radiotherapy is usually the common choice of treatment. This provides better cosmetic outcome.
- Mastectomy is preferred for larger tumours, multifocal disease or for patient preference.
- Survival rates are the same for WLE and mastectomy.
- It is important to identify lymph node involvement using axillary sampling eg sentinel lymph node biopsy to complete disease staging.
- If there is lymph node involvement, an axillary clearance is carried out, which involves removal of the nodes at different levels.
- Complications of lymphatic clearance include: wound infection, haematoma, seroma and lymphedema.

Medical management:

- Systemic treatment of early breast cancer can be adjuvant or neo-adjuvant (before surgery) therapy.
- This may consist of radiotherapy, chemotherapy, and endocrine treatment.

Staging of breast cancer:

Staging is carried out using the clinical staging process or the TNM classification:

- **Radiotherapy:** can be directed at the breast, chest wall, and/or axilla, depending on the clinical stage. It may also be used for palliative care.

TNM classification	Features
Tumour	T1: Tumour <2 cm T2: Tumour 2–5 cm T3: Tumour 5–10 cm T4: Tumour >10 cm, chest wall fixation and skin involvement
Node	N0: No nodes N1: Mobile lymph nodes on the same side of the breast lump N2: Fixed lymph nodes on the same side N3: Supraclavicular/ Infraclavicular lymph node involvement
Metastases	M0: No metastases M1: Metastatic disease (liver, bones, and lungs)

Table 4.38: The TNM staging of breast cancer

- **Chemotherapy:** Docetaxel is licensed as an adjuvant therapy in node-positive disease.
- **Hormone therapy:** Aromatase inhibitors such as anastrazole (or, if not tolerated, selective oestrogen receptor antagonists such as tamoxifen) can be used in oestrogen-receptor positive, invasive disease in post-menopausal patients for two to three years.
- **Biological therapy:** Trastuzumab (Herceptin) is a monoclonal antibody targets the HER2 and is licensed for those with HER2 receptor positive disease.

Management of advanced cancer (stage 3 and 4):

- Management depends on the disease status in each patient.
- Local recurrence is managed with radiotherapy, further excision and regional chemotherapy.
- Bone metastases will require analgesia, radiotherapy, and bisphosphonates.
- Brain metastases may be treated with radiotherapy, steroids and rarely debulking surgery.
- Palliative care input and appropriate support is essential.

Breast screening:

- Introduced to the UK in 1988 after publication of The Forrest Report.
- Women aged 50–70 are invited every 3 years to undergo a mammogram – this is currently being extended to include those between 47 and 73. Those over 73 may request ongoing screening but are not automatically invited.
- Triple assessment is subsequently performed if required.

Oesophageal cancer

The oesophagus is a muscular tube transporting food from the mouth to the stomach. It is approximately 25 cm in length, extending from the cricoid cartilage (C6) to the cardiac orifice of the stomach (T10). The epithelium of the oesophagus is stratified squamous up to the level of the gastro-oesophageal junction.

Epidemiology

Oesophageal cancer is the ninth commonest cancer in the UK with a lifetime risk of 1 in 64 for men and 1 in 116 for women. The disease tends to occur in people over 40. There is a higher incidence of cases in Russia and Asia, particularly China.

Adenocarcinoma	Squamous cell carcinoma
Barrett's oesophagus Gastro-oesophageal reflux (GOR) Obesity Cigarette smoking High alcohol intake	Tobacco use High alcohol Vitamin C & A deficiency Coeliac disease Oesophageal strictures Achalasia

Table 4.39: The associated risk factors of AC and SSC

Aetiology

There are two main histological types of oesophageal cancer: SCC and AC.

Pathophysiology

SCC tends to occur in the upper two-thirds and AC the lower third of the oesophagus. The incidence of SCC has remained relatively stable in the western population over the last two decades; however, AC has been increasing – thought to be related to trends in smoking, alcohol and obesity. The cancer metastasises initially to the peri-oesophageal lymph nodes and adjacent structures such as the tracheo-bronchial tree, aorta, and recurrent laryngeal nerve. The liver and lungs are affected late.

History/examination

- Dysphagia and/or odynophagia: patients normally give a history of progressive dysphagia initially with solid food and later progressing to liquids
- Retrosternal discomfort
- Aspiration pneumonia and coughing during ingestion
- Hoarse voice due to recurrent laryngeal nerve palsy
- Massive haematemesis
- Lymphadenopathy, in particular the supraclavicular
- nodes (Virchow's node)
- Systemic signs of malignancy: anaemia, weight loss, fatigue, night sweats
- Signs of metastatic disease eg hepatomegaly

Investigations

Imaging:

- Endoscopic USS: most sensitive at determining depth of tumour invasion and involvement of peri-oesophageal lymph nodes, allowing for TNM disease staging.
- CT chest and abdomen: provides important information on metastatic spread to lungs and liver

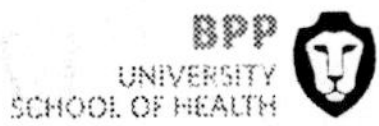

and gives information on tumour involvement with adjacent structures.

- Barium swallow: is sensitive at detecting oesophageal strictures and intra-luminal masses.
- PET scan: may identify metastatic spread.

Endoscopy:

- Oesophago-gastro-duodenoscopy: allows direct visualisation and biopsy to confirm histology.

Management

- Surgical resection is offered to all patients who are medically fit for surgery with no significant metastatic disease. Only about 30% of oesophageal cancers are appropriate for resection and the overall 5-year survival in the UK is approximately 25%.
- Patients with contraindications to surgery should be managed with palliative care. This includes those with:
  - Metastatic involvement to N2 nodes or solid organs
  - Invasion to adjacent organs such as the aorta, tracheo-bronchial tree or pericardium
  - Severe cardio-respiratory diseases

Surgical treatment:

- Surgical approach depends on tumour location and anatomy
- Ivor Lewis procedure (lower third oesophageal tumour):
  - An initial laparotomy to mobilise the stomach taking care to preserve the right gastro-epiploic arcade (now often performed laparoscopically).
  - The second part involves a right thoracotomy during which the tumour is resected and the stomach is brought up and anastomosed to the remaining oesophagus.
- Trans-hiatal approach (upper to middle third oesophageal tumour):
  - This involves an upper midline laparotomy and neck incision. The oesophagus is mobilised from above and below. A stomach conduit is brought up and an anastomosis is created with the cervical oesophagus.
- McKeown 3-stage procedure (upper third oesophageal tumour):
  - Similar to the Ivor Lewis procedure, but involves a third stage where a neck incision is made through which the stomach is brought up and anastomosed to the cervical oesophagus.

Palliative treatment:

- Stenting: self-expanding metal stent is inserted under endoscopic guidance. This keeps the oesophageal lumen patent and improves swallowing. It is particularly useful in the event of a tracheo-oesophageal fistula.
- Chemotherapy: particularly for AC.
- Radiotherapy: particularly for SSC.

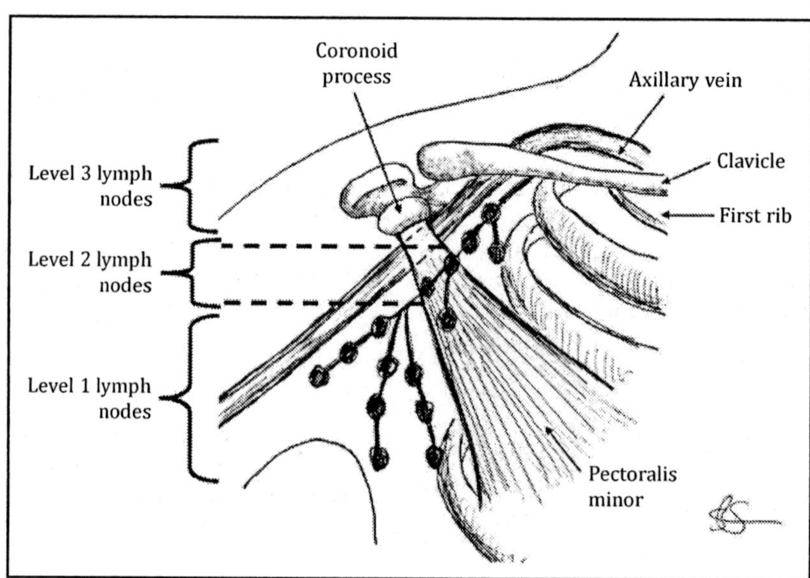

Figure 4.16: Axillary lymph nodes

- Laser therapy: Nd:YAG laser can debulk intrinsic tumours and improve swallowing.
- Appropriate palliative care input, support and advice.

Colon cancer

Epidemiology

Large bowel carcinomas are the second most common malignant cause of death in the UK. These tumours occur at all ages, with a peak incidence at 70–80 years. Females are affected more than males and the disease is more common in Western Europe than developing countries. Approximately 20% of cases present to emergency departments with intestinal obstruction or peritonitis.

Aetiology

Conditions including polyps and ulcerative colitis are predisposing factors for large bowel cancer. Similarly, inherited cancer syndromes such as FAP and HNPCC also increase the risk.

FAP accounts for 0.5% of all colorectal cancers. An autosomal dominant mutation in the FAP gene results in colorectal polyps, which frequently progress to malignany by age 40. HNPCC is another autosomal dominant mutation resulting in DNA mismatch repair. It accounts for 5% of colorectal malignancy and presents before the age of 50. There is also a strong association with ovarian, uterine, and gastric tumours.

A high fat and low fibre diet increases gut transit time, prolonging intestinal exposure to potential carcinogens. Similarly, pelvic irradiation also increases the risk of recto-sigmoid carcinoma.

Pathophysiology

Macroscopically the cancer is a colloid tumour that appears as a malignant ulcer with annular, infiltrating growth. Microscopically all tumours are adenocarcinomas. The aggressiveness normally correlates with the histological differentiation.

75% of lesions are located in the rectum and sigmoid colon. Patients with FAP and HNPCC have a higher incidence of right sided tumours. The severity of the

Grade	Features
I	Well differentiated
II-III	Moderately differentiated
IV	Anaplastic

Table 4.40: Grading of colon cancers

Stage	Features
A	The tumour is confined to the mucosa and submucosa of the bowel wall
B	The tumour has spread through the muscle layers and beyond the bowel wall
C	Regional lymph nodes are affected
D	Metastatic spread has occurred (eg to the liver or lungs)

Table 4.41: Dukes' classification staging system

cancer can be determined by tumour grade and disease TNM stage. Metastasis occurs via local, lymphatic, vascular (with subsequent liver and lung seeding) or trans-coelomic spread. The latter may result in malignant nodules throughout the peritoneal cavity which, if spread to the ovaries, become known as 'Krukenburg tumours'.

History/examination

- Anorexia and weight loss
- Symptoms of anaemia: lethargy, malaise, shortness of breath, and light headedness
- Alteration to normal bowel habit
- Rectal bleeding and mucus production
- Symptoms of intestinal obstruction: abdominal pain, absolute constipation, bloating, vomiting (a late feature)
- Right-sided tumours tend to have a mass on palpation in the right iliac fossa (or digital rectal examination for sigmoid/rectal/anal tumours). There may also be diarrhoea, rectal bleeding/mucous and anaemia
- Left-sided tumours tend to present early with abdominal pain and change in bowel habit.
- Signs associated with metastatic spread (eg hepatomegaly, ascites, and jaundice)
- Peritonism following perforation

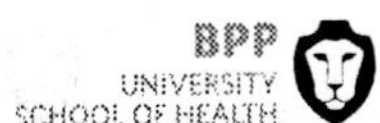

Investigations

Blood test:

- FBC: may reveal low Hb
- CEA – a bowel tumour marker

Imaging:

- Erect CXR: to exclude perforation and look for possible metastatic spread.
- AXR: shows intestinal obstruction acutely and to look for possible metastatic spread.
- CT: the investigation of choice in elderly patients who are unable to tolerate endoscopic investigation and those presenting with acute intestinal obstruction. CT-colonography has demonstrated a similar ability to colonoscopy in identifying bowel lesions for those unable to tolerate a pure colonoscopy.
- Ultrasound scan: for characterising liver metastasis. Used pre-operatively and in following up post-colonic tumour resection patients. Trans-anal USS can be used in staging rectal tumours.
- Barium enema (rarely used): can identify a growth or stricture ('apple core' appearance). A negative barium enema does not exclude a colonic tumour as small lesions can be missed.
- MRI: to stage ano-rectal tumours.

Endoscopy:

- Sigmoidoscopy: to identify rectal and sigmoid tumours and take a biopsy to confirm histology
- Colonoscopy: allows direct visualisation of the entire colon and facilitates biopsies of any lesions

Management

- All patients should be managed in a multi-disciplinary team setting.
- Patients need a thorough medical assessment to determine their operative suitability, as it is likely they have multiple co-morbidities.
- Determining the grade and disease stage (according to Dukes' classification and the TNM system) is important to guide management.
- The mainstay of treatment is surgical resection.
- Short-course pre-operative radiotherapy or chemoradiotherapy may be offered to patients with moderate or high-risk operable rectal cancer.

Surgical management:

- Acute bowel obstruction:
  - Patients with potentially curable left-sided tumours should be offered the option of entering a clinical trial to receive either colonic stenting or emergency resection (which may include a Hartmann's procedure if a primary anastomosis is impossible).
  - Patients with non-curable left-sided obstructing lesions should be treated with a colonic stent.
  - Patients with right-sided lesions should be offered a resection + primary anastomosis/ Hartmann's procedure.
  - Increased risk of anastamotic breakdown due to poor vascular supply may necessitate a defunctioning colostomy or ileostomy to protect the anastomosis.
- Non-acute presentations:
  - A pre-operative bowel preparation protocol is followed.
  - Treatment aims to resect the tumour, all bowel with the same blood supply and associated regional lymph nodes with a viable primary end-end anastomosis.

Adjuvant therapies:

- Following histological analysis of the resected lesions and discussion at the MDT, post-operative chemotherapy may be offered for early stage, histologically aggressive or later-stage tumours.

Site of tumour	Operation
Right colon	Right hemicolectomy
Transverse colon	Extended right hemicolectomy
Descending colon	Left hemicolectomy
Rectum	Anterior resection is where the rectal tumour is resected and the colon above is anastomosed to the rectal stump. A temporary stoma (which can be later reversed) may be produced to allow the primary anastomosis to heel. Abdominoperineal excision is performed for low rectal tumours

Table 4.42: Type of operation required for the different locations of colon cancer

Treatment for metastatic disease:

- In cases where metastatic spread has occurred, surgery is still an option for the palliative care of the patient. The obstruction is removed and a permanent colostomy may be required.
- Resection of any extra-intestinal metastases may be required if possible and palliative chemo/ radiotherapy may be helpful.

Prognosis

The five-year survival rates vary according to the stage of the tumour.

Stage of tumour	Five-year survival rate
Dukes A	80–85%
Dukes B	60%
Dukes C	30%
Dukes D	5%

Table 4.43: The five-year survival rate according to the tumour stage

Stomas

Definition: An artificial opening made into a hollow organ

- Right lower quadrant:
  - Usually an ileostomy
  - Normally spouted to protect the skin from irritant contents
  - May be an end ileostomy if patient has had a total colectomy or loop ileostomy to provide protection for a primary anastomosis
- Right upper quadrant:
  - Commonly a transverse colostomy
  - Continuous with the skin
  - Usually a temporary stoma to allow anastomosis to heal
- Left lower quadrant:
  - Can be end, loop or double-barelled colostomy
  - May be part of Hartmann's procedure following resection of sigmoid or rectum or permanent end colostomy after resection of anus and rectum (abdominoperineal resection)
  - A double-barrelled colostomy is performed when an anastomosis cannot be performed and both ends of the colon are brought out to the surface, such as following a mid sigmoid gut volvulus

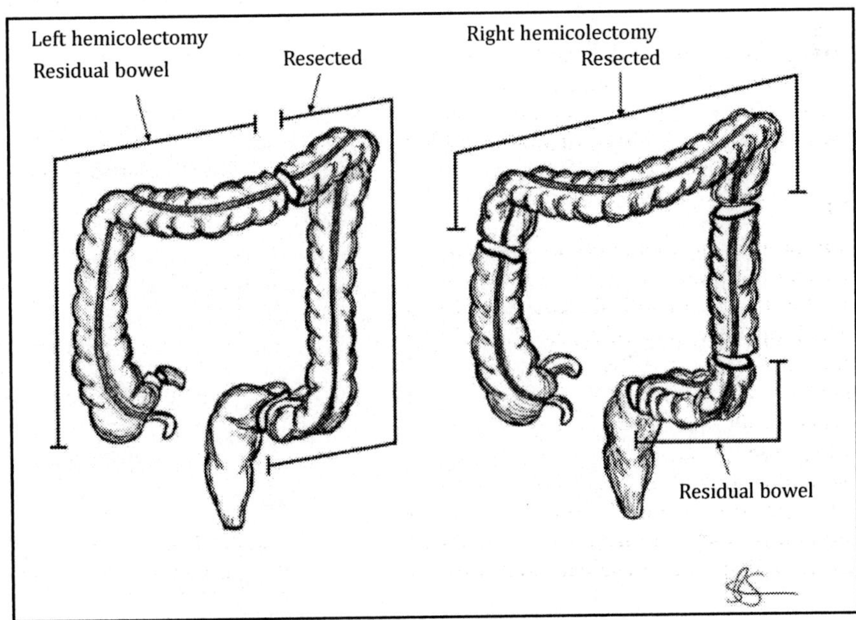

Figure 4.17: Left and right hemicolectomy procedures

  - A loop colostomy is constructed in cases where a resection has not occurred and the sigmoid colon has been brought out to the surface eg in patients with inoperable rectal tumours that are likely to obstruct
- Left upper quadrant stoma:
  - Stomas are not usually sited here – may be due to a technical issue with the surgical procedure

Hepatocellular carcinoma

Epidemiology

This is a common worldwide cancer (Africa and South-East Asia), but extremely rare in the UK.

Aetiology

80% of patients with hepatocellular carcinoma (HCC) have known liver cirrhosis. The common causes of liver cirrhosis progressing to cancer include HBV and HCV infection. In fact, HCC can develop 25 years after initial HCV infection.

Alcoholic liver disease and haemachromatosis are also common causes of cirrhosis leading to HCC and other risk factors include drugs (eg steroids), aflatoxin exposure and smoking.

Pathophysiology

Chronic inflammation within the liver leads to development of HCC. Macroscopically, there is a large solitary tumour with multiple lesions throughout the liver. HCC commonly metastasises to the lungs and bones.

History/examination

Patients will often be asymptomatic but can present with symptoms of chronic liver disease.

- Malaise and weakness
- Jaundice
- Upper gastrointestinal bleed
- Anorexia and weight loss
- Hepatomegaly
- Ascites
- Jaundice
- Decompensated liver disease leading to encephalopathy

Investigations

Blood tests:

- Serum AFP: is raised in HCC and cirrhosis

Case Study: An unfortunate skiing trip

The Reverend EK had been enjoying his retirement. Having taught religious studies for the last 30 years, he had loved renovating their 17th century home, tending the vegetable garden and even building a cider press to make the most of the vast orchard. A two-week skiing break with an old friend had seemed the ideal way to round off the first six months of freedom.

Two days into the trip Reverend EK began to feel a bit nauseous out on the slopes. He kept skiing for the next couple of days, but noticed he was becoming a little more bloated than usual. When he began to vomit, he decided it was time to seek some help. At the French hospital they went to the emergency department and the doctor asked when he had last opened his bowels. Rev EK realised he had not done so for many days.

A CT scan revealed a mass obstructing his lower colon and an emergency Hartmann's procedure was performed the following day. The surprise, speed of action and the language barrier all made it very difficult for Rev EK to accept his new stoma and he returned to the UK in considerable shock to begin several rounds of draining chemotherapy.

Fortunately, the histology report revealed a relatively low grade tumour with no extra-intestinal spread and 12 months later, chemotherapy completed, stoma reversed, the Rev EK was able to joke about the experience and laugh at the cause of his new-found momentum on the slopes. Five years later he remains disease-free, but it is a useful reminder of the insidious nature of these diseases and the sudden and unexpected presentations of many cases.

Imaging:

- USS/CT/MRI: can easily identify large tumours
- Small tumours (<1 cm) can be difficult to differentiate from cirrhotic nodules (may be distinguished using hepatic angiography)

Others:

- Liver biopsy: this will confirm the diagnosis. There is a 2% risk of tumour dissemination therefore this should be avoided if liver transplantation is a possibility.

Management

- Tumours not associated with cirrhosis and confined to a single lobe of the liver can be treated with a hemi-hepatectomy.
- Cirrhotic liver disease and HCC is difficult to treat as removal of liver substance will predispose the patient to post-operative liver decompensation and possible death.
- The final option is to undergo a liver transplant.

Prognosis

Patients with cirrhosis and HCC have a median survival of 12 months.

Cholangiocarcinoma

Epidemiology

The incidence of this bile duct carcinoma is increasing, with the disease predominantly affecting adults over the age of 50 years.

Aetiology

Cholangiocarcinoma is associated with inflammatory bowel disease, sclerosing cholangitis, congenital hepatic fibrosis, and a polycystic liver.

Pathophysiology

Macroscopically, cholangiocarcinoma is seen within the liver substance and in the extra-hepatic bile ducts. Common sites include the point at which the right and left hepatic ducts meet, the common hepatic duct, and the cystic duct.

Microscopically, the tumour is typically slow growing and is a mucin secreting AC. Tumours at the right and left hepatic ducts invade the liver parenchyma, and become fibrous. This results in the development of duct strictures. Tumours at the distal end of the bile duct are polypoidal and commonly obstruct the bile duct lumen. They both invade the lymphatic system.

History/examination

- Painless jaundice
- Dark urine and pale stools
- Weight loss
- Epigastric pain
- Steatorrhoea (foul smelling and difficult to flush away stool)
- Pallor
- Clinically jaundiced (yellow discolouration of the skin and sclera of the eye)
- Abdominal pain on palpation
- Hepatomegaly

Investigations

Blood tests:

- Serum CEA and carbohydrate antigen 19–9 (CA 19–9): are raised in approximately 20% of patients.

Imaging:

- USS: dilated intra-hepatic ducts
- MRCP: to visualise the the biliary tree
- Percutaneous transhepatic cholangiography: may identify filling defects in the bile ducts but can often be mistaken for bile duct stones
- CT guided needle biopsy

Endoscopy:

- ERCP: the bile duct stone will be identified and potentially removed. Bile cytology and brushings of the stricture may be performed

Management

- Cholangiocarcinomas are rarely curable.
- Surgical treatment is radical resection of the liver parenchyma and the affected bile duct.
- Palliative management can include endoluminal stenting with ERCP or a surgical bypass.

Prognosis

Very poor, with a 1-year survival of <20%.

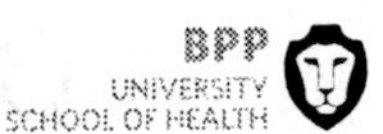

Gallbladder cancer

Epidemiology

Gallbladder cancer is commonly found in Central and South America, northern India, Japan, and central and eastern Europe. It usually presents between the ages of 50–60 with women being affected more than men.

Aetiology

The aetiology is unknown; however, an association has been made with gallstones. It is thought these may act as chronic irritants to the gallbladder mucosa. A calcified gallbladder, the 'porcelain' gallbladder has also been linked to the development of cancer.

Pathophysiology

90% of tumours are AC whilst 10% are SCC. The tumour usually spreads locally to the liver and its ducts.

History/examination

- Right upper quadrant pain
- Nausea and vomiting
- Weight loss
- Jaundice
- Right upper quadrant tenderness on palpation
- Palpable mass

Investigations

Imaging:

- CT: is the investigation of choice for staging
- Cholangiography: can aid with staging
- Hepatic angiography: can aid staging

Management

- Radical surgical resection can include resection of the gallbladder, right lobe liver parenchyma, and the biliary tree.
- Chemotherapy does not have a role.

Prognosis

There is a good prognosis in patients with tumour confined to the gallbladder mucosa. In advanced disease most patients are dead within a few months.

Pancreatic carcinoma

Epidemiology

Pancreatic carcinoma affects 10 per 100,000 of the population each year, and is the eighth commonest cause of death from cancer in the UK. The incidence is increasing and it frequently affects the elderly.

Aetiology

Risk factors include smoking, beta-naphthylamine (dye industry), benzidine, and an abnormality in drainage of the pancreas.

Pathophysiology

The majority (85%) of tumours are duct cell AC. Approximately 60% of tumours are found at the head of the pancreas, 25% in the body and 15% in the tail.

Macroscopically, the tumour appears irregular and hard. Microscopically, the cancers are usually undifferentiated. If an adenocarcinoma has been identified, it is typical to notice mucus secretion from the duct. However, an acinar cell carcinoma is a non-mucus secreting cancer, originating from the acinar cells.

Spread of the tumour can occur via direct invasion into the common bile duct, duodenum, portal vein, and the inferior vena cava or via lymphatic spread. Haematogenous spread can result in liver and lung metastasis whilst trans-coelomic spread results in peritoneal seeding and ascites.

History/examination

Pancreatic cancer can have different presentations:

- Anorexia and weight loss
- Painless jaundice due to compression of the bile duct
- Continuous epigastric pain that is dull in character
- Symptoms of diabetes (thirst, polyuria, polydipsia)
- Jaundice
- Epigastric mass on palpation
- Hepatomegaly and ascites suggestive of metastatic disease
- Courvoisier's law: 'Palpable painless mass in the presence of jaundice is unlikely to be a result of gallstones.' This law arises from the knowledge that recurrent gallstone attacks cause acute inflammation resulting in a thickened fibrosed gallbladder that does not distend easily

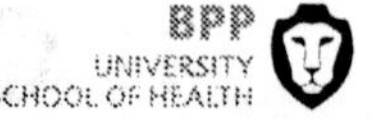

Investigations

Blood tests:

- FBC
- U&Es
- LFTs
- Clotting
- Amylase
- Glucose

Imaging:

- USS: will identify bile duct dilatation.
- CT: the tumour can be identified and allows guidance for a needle biopsy. If the tumour is less than 4 cm, confined to the head of the pancreas, and without metastatic spread the patient should undergo surgical treatment.
- ERCP: may identify bile duct obstruction. During this procedure a stent may be inserted to relieve the obstruction.

Management

Pancreatic cancer usually presents late, resulting in 90–95% of cases being unsuitable for operative management. Palliative treatment should be discussed with those inoperable cases.

Operative management:

- Patients with duct cell carcinomas (<4 cm) and no metastatic spread should be offered surgical treatment. The operation of choice is a pancreato-duodenectomy (Whipple's procedure) with preservation of the pylorus:
  - A cholecystectomy is performed.
  - The bile duct is dissected and lymphatic tissue removed.
  - The common hepatic artery is identified and the gastroduodenal branch divided to expose the portal vein.
  - The duodenum and right colon are mobilised, allowing dissection of the fourth part of the duodenum.
  - The jejunum is dissected and the proximal duodenum divided.
  - The pancreas is identified and divided.
  - Surrounding structures and tissues are separated from the mesenteric artery and vein until the bile duct is reached.
  - The bile duct is divided and the entire specimen is removed.

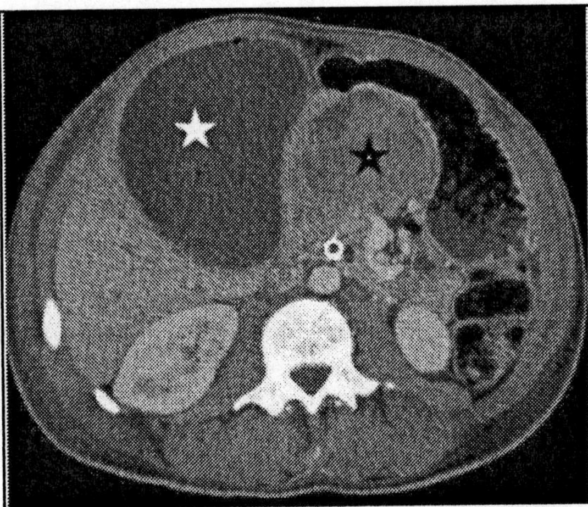

Figure 4.18: CT showing a large liver abscess (white star) in a patient with a big pancreatic malignant mass (black star)

  - Retroperitoneal lymph nodes are removed.
  - A subhepatic drain is placed.
  - Reconstruction includes:
    1. Choledochojejunostomy
    2. Pancreatojejunostomy
    3. Gastrojejunostomy
  - The procedure can take up to six hours.
  - Common post-operative complications include infection, bleeding and a pancreatic duct leak.

Palliative management

- Referral to a palliative care team is essential.
- If the duodenum becomes obstructed a gastrojejunostomy may be performed; however, if the patient presents late, insertion of a metal stent is considered to be more appropriate. Stenting may also be used to relieve obstructive jaundice.
- In patients who have an inoperable tumour diagnosed at laparotomy, a palliative bypass is considered (cholecysto or choledochoduodenostomy with gastrojejunostomy).
- Chemotherapy may induce remission in some duct cell AC.
- Appropriate management of general palliative symptoms: pain, nausea/vomiting, constipation, agitation, secretions etc.

Prognosis

- Median survival is 20 weeks.
- Less than 5% of patients will survive 5 years.

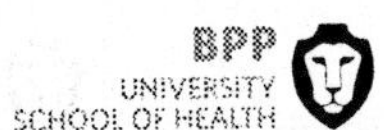

Prostate cancer

Epidemiology

Prostate carcinoma is the most common cancer in men. Its incidence increases with age, with 75% of cases found in those between the ages of 60–79 years.

Aetiology

The aetiology remains unknown; however, there are a few important predisposing factors associated with the disease. These include increasing age, changes in hormone levels such as oestrogen and testosterone, and exposure to carcinogens. A family history of prostate cancer in a first degree relative increases the risk by two-fold. The Afro-American population tend to have the highest risk of developing prostate cancer.

Pathophysiology

A layer of myoepithelial cells surrounds the prostate gland. Initially the basement membrane is lost and the cells appear less differentiated, but soon further layers of carcinoma cells are seen.

The cancer originates in the outer zone of the prostate gland, and later invades the entire gland. The carcinoma spreads initially to the peri-prostatic tissues, ie the bladder, urethra, and rectum. Further spread to the iliac and para-aortic nodes occurs via the lymphatic system.

Metastatic spread occurs through the blood stream via the vertebral venous plexus to the vertebra, skull, and pelvis. Macroscopically, the cancer appears hard, craggy, and pale. Microscopically, the cancer is an AC, and often moderately differentiated. The degree of differentiation is usually defined according to the Gleason grade of 2–10.

Staging

The carcinoma is staged using the TNM system.

History/examination

- Early stage can be asymptomatic
- Malaise and weight loss
- Pelvic pain
- Haematuria
- Symptoms of bladder outflow obstruction
- Bone pain
- Digital rectal examination:
  - Hard nodule
  - Enlarged and craggy prostate
  - The midline sulcus may have disappeared
  - There may be infiltration of the tumour on either side of the prostate into surrounding tissue

Investigations

Blood tests:

- PSA: is not a sensitive diagnostic marker in early disease. It is elevated in prostatitis, post instrumentation and UTIs. It is more useful as a marker of treatment response and recurrence.

Imaging:

- CXR/AXR: to visualise metastatic disease
- CT abdomen and pelvis: staging
- MRI: information on capsular invasion
- TRUS: can identify small tumours and it allows a needle-core biopsy to be taken from the prostate gland. However, complications include infection or prostatic abscess formation

Others:

- Trans-rectal biopsy: can be taken using an automated gun.
- TURP: can provide tissue for analysis as well as symptomatic relief.

TNM classification	Features
Tumour	TIS: Carcinoma *in situ* T1: Tumour found incidentally on needle biopsy or transurethral resection of the prostate (TURP) T2: Intracapsular palpable tumour T3: Tumour (mobile) spread beyond the capsule T4: Fixed tumour or locally invasive tumour
Nodes	N0: No lymph nodes N1–4: One or more lymph nodes
Metastasis	M0: No metastases M1: Metastatic spread

Table 4.44: The TNM classification for prostate cancer

- Isotope bone scan: will identify any 'hot spots' representing bony metastases

Management

Conservative management:

- Patients can be given the option to watch and wait as small, well-differentiated tumours have a ten-year survival rate without treatment.
- Close follow up with regular rectal examinations and PSA levels is required.

Medical management:

- Prostatic cancer is driven by androgens. Therefore, in locally invasive disease and metastatic disease the aim is to reduce androgen stimulation. This can be achieved with the following:
  - Oestrogens eg Stilboesterol: Now rarely used due to adverse side effects such as gynaecomastia, testicular atrophy, thrombosis and congestive cardiac failure
  - LHRH analogues eg Goserelin, which down-regulate the pituitary and inhibit release of the luteinising hormone, resulting in reduced testosterone
  - Anti-androgens eg 5a reductase inhibitors
- External beam radiotherapy: is the treatment of choice for bony metastases, providing symptomatic relief. It can supplement hormonal treatment to control disease progression.

Surgical management:

- Pre-operative counselling is necessary to warn patients of the following risks:
  - Retrograde ejaculation (occurs in 65% of men following the procedure)
  - Erectile impotence (5%)
  - 15% of patients will require a further procedure in 8–10 years
  - Mortality rate is less than 0.5%
  - Other complications include: urethral stricture, sepsis, haematuria, urinary incontinence, UTI and TUR syndrome
- TURP: should be performed if there are symptoms of bladder outflow obstruction.
- Radical prostatectomy is performed for T1 and T2 disease. It involves the complete removal of the prostate, seminal vesicles, and pelvic lymph nodes.
- Bilateral orchidectomy: is used for stage T3, T4 and metastatic disease, which achieves androgen ablation.
- Brachytherapy involves implanting radioactive iodine or palladium seeds within the prostate. This allows a higher dose of radiation than with external beam radiotherapy.

Testicular cancer

Epidemiology

Testicular cancers are rare and account for only 2% of all malignancies affecting the male population. However, it is the commonest malignancy affecting young adult males.

Aetiology

Predisposing factors include a family history of testicular cancer, previous contralateral testicular cancer, undescended testis (cryptorchidism), trauma and mumps.

Pathophysiology

Approximately 95% of testicular tumours are of germ cell origin. Most of the remaining 5% are sex-cord gonadal stromal tumours derived from Leydig cells or Sertoli cells. There are two sub-categories for germ cell tumours of the testicles:

1. Seminomas account for 60% of testicular germ cell tumours. They typically occur in males aged 15–35 years with 10% of cases occurring in patients with undescended testes. Seminomas arise from the cells of the seminiferous tubules. Macroscopically, the tumour appears large, smooth and solid. Microscopically, the cells are well-differentiated spermatocytes or undifferentiated round cells. Seminomas spread through the lymphatic system (para-aortic nodes) and rarely via the blood stream.
2. Non-seminomatous germ cell tumours (NSGCT) account for 40% of testicular germ cell tumours. They arise from primitive germ cells and contain embryonal stem cells. Therefore these tumours include embryonal carcinoma, teratoma (commonest), choriocarcinoma, and yolk sac tumour. Macroscopically the tumour has a cystic appearance and microscopically the cells differ greatly. The tumour can consist of bone, cartilage, fat, muscle and other tissue.

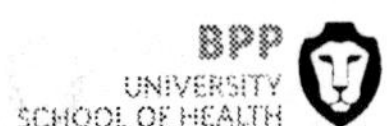

History/examination

- Enlarging testicular lump
- Pain can occur in 30% of patients
- Patients may complain of a sensation of scrotal heaviness
- The testis is smooth, enlarged, and heavy
- An associated hydrocele may be present
- Gynaecomastia is found in 5% of cases
- Shortness of breath suggests lung metastases
- Metastatic disease can present with abdominal lymph nodes and cervical lymphadenopathy, in particular supraclavicular lymphadenopathy

Investigations

Blood tests:

- AFP: is raised in 50–70% of NSGCT. The only NSGCT not to secrete this is a true choriocarcinoma.
- Beta-HCG is raised in 5–10% of seminomas and 40–60% NSGCT.
- LDH is a less specific marker for germ cell tumours but can be a gross marker of tumour burden.

Imaging:

- CXR: to look for metastatic disease
- Scrotal USS: to identify a solid tumour
- Abdominal CT: for staging

Stage	Features
I	The tumour is confined to the testis
II	Abdominal lymph nodes are affected
III	Supra-diaphragmatic and infra-diaphragmatic lymph nodes are affected
IV	Other metastatic spread eg lungs and liver

Table 4.45: The Royal Marsden classification for testicular cancer

Management

- Orchidectomy to excise the primary tumour
- Seminomas:
  - Stage I and II respond well to external beam radiotherapy.
  - Stage III and IV are treated with radiotherapy and chemotherapy (eg Cisplatin and Bleomycin).
  - Five-year survival for stage I disease is 98% and stage II disease is 85%.
- Non-seminomas:
  - Stage I is managed conservatively with monitoring of serum tumour markers.
  - Stage II, III, and IV are treated with chemotherapy.
  - 5-year survival of stage I and II disease is >85%.

Further reading and references

1. Nestler, G., Sagynaliev, E., Steinert, R., et al. (2006) Laparoscopic cholecystectomy and gallbladder cancer. *Journal of Surgical Oncology* 2006; 93: 682–689.
2. Cancer Research UK. *The UK testicular cancer incidence statistic.* [Online]. Available from: www.cancerresearchuk.org/health-professional/cancer-statistics/statistics-by-cancer-type/testicular-cancer/incidence [Accessed 7 November 2016].

Head injury

Differential diagnosis

Type of head injury	Differential diagnosis
Skull fracture	**Simple linear fracture** **Depressed skull fracture** **Base of skull fracture** Scalp laceration
Intracranial haemorrhage	**Extradural haemorrhage** **Subdural haemorrhage** **Subarachnoid haemorrhage** **Intracerebral haemorrhage**
Others	**Cerebral concussion** **Diffuse axonal injury** Seizure

Table 4.46: Differential diagnosis of head injury

It is estimated that approximately one million people in the UK present to the hospital with a head injury each year. It is one of the leading causes of mortality (40%) and morbidity.

Anatomy

The anatomy of the head can be divided into:

Scalp:

- The scalp is made up of skin, connective tissue, aponeurosis, loose areolar tissue and pericranium (SCALP itself is an acronym).
- The scalp is a vascular structure, and therefore a laceration can result in significant blood loss.

Skull:

- The cranial vault (calvaria) and the base are the two main structures.
- At the temporal regions the calvaria is thin and thus this area is protected by the temporalis muscle.
- The base of the skull has an irregular surface and therefore contributes to brain injury when there is movement of the brain during a head injury.
- The anterior, middle, and posterior cranial fossa make up the floor of the cranial cavity.
- In general the anterior fossa contains the frontal lobes, the middle fossa contains the temporal lobes, and the posterior fossa contains the brainstem, occipital lobe and the cerebellum.

Meninges:

- The meninges are a layer of membranous coverings over the brain and spinal cord, comprised of the dura, arachnoid and pia mater.
- The dura mater is firmly attached to the internal surface of the skull.
- Meningeal arteries, found between the dura and the internal surface of the skull, are often injured in skull fractures. The middle meningeal artery in the temporal region is particularly vulnerable.
- The dura is composed of two layers: the periosteal and meningeal dura. Between these layers, large venous sinuses are found, which are responsible for most of the venous drainage of the brain.
- The arachnoid lies beneath the dura mater, with the subdural space between them. This is a potential site for haemorrhage.
- The third layer is attached to the brain surface and is known as the pia mater.

Brain:

- The three main structures of the brain include the cerebrum, the brainstem and cerebellum.
- The cerebrum consists of a right and left hemisphere, which are divided by the falx cerebri.
- The brainstem consists of the midbrain, pons, and medulla. The latter contains the essential cardio-respiratory centres and extends caudally to form the spinal cord.
- The cerebellum is found in the posterior fossa and forms links with the spinal cord and brainstem.

Cerebrospinal fluid (CSF):

The choroid plexus in the roof of the ventricles produces CSF. CSF moves through the brain via a number of ventricles. The pathway starts at the lateral ventricles, moving through the foramen of Monro into the third ventricle. From there CSF flows through the aqueduct of Sylvius, and finally the fourth ventricle into the the subarachnoid space, from where it is eventually reabsorbed into the venous circulation.

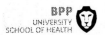

Types of brain injury

With any head injury there is a concern of underlying brain injury. Brain injury can be divided into primary and secondary types.

Primary brain injury:

This occurs at the time of the head injury and can be a result of direct or indirect injury to the brain. The strength and varying features of the applied forces determine the severity of damage.

Secondary brain injury:

This type of damage occurs at any point after the primary injury. The common causes include hypoxia, hypercapnia, intracranial bleeding, hypotension, and increased intracranial pressure. If these problems are managed early this can prevent and reduce secondary brain injury.

Physiological effects of head injury

The Monroe-Kelly doctrine:

The Monroe-Kelly doctrine assumes that the skull is a solid container in which the only contents are brain, CSF, and blood. It therefore follows that ICP is proportional to the volume of these contents. The formula is as follows:

$$ICP = V_{CSF} + V_{Blood} + V_{Brain}$$

This formula is the basis of the Monroe-Kelly doctrine which states that the ICP will increase if the volume of any of the three components increases. This increase in ICP can only be compensated to a certain degree by changes in the volume of the other components. An SOL of more than 100–150 ml exceeds the maximum compensation, resulting in a rise in the intracranial pressure.

A raised ICP has a number of consequences:

1. **Hydrocephalus:** occurs when the circulation of CSF is occluded. Most commonly seen with posterior fossa lesions.
2. **Cerebral ischaemia:** occurs due to a rise in ICP which eventually exceeds auto-regulation. The formula that describes the relationship between cerebral perfusion pressure, mean arterial pressure and ICP is:

Cerebral perfusion pressure = mean arterial pressure – ICP

3. **Brain herniation:** occurs when the ICP levels are high and therefore there is an increased risk of brain shift and resultant herniation. The herniation can occur through a number of sites. The commonly used term 'coning' actually refers to herniation of the midbrain through the tentorium.

Skull fracture

Simple linear fracture

- These appear as lucent lines on an SXR.
- Fractures increase the risk of an intracranial bleed.
- Patients should therefore be admitted for neurological observations.

Depressed skull fracture

- This type of fracture is common following blunt trauma.
- A segment of skull can be pushed down onto the brain tissue, resulting in laceration of the brain.
- Management may consist of elevation of the depressed segment if there are focal neurological signs.

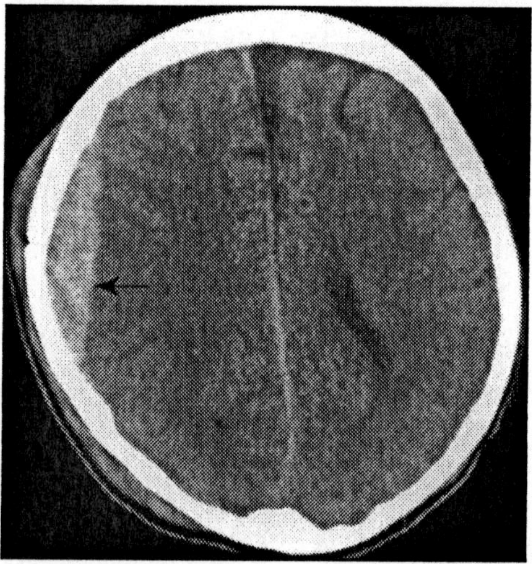

Figure 4.19: CT brain showing an area of increased density in the right parietal lobe (arrow), note the localised nature and internal convex border in keeping with an extradural haematoma

Base of skull fracture

- This fracture is not identified on an SXR.
- If fluid is seen in the sphenoidal sinuses this fracture can be present.
- Other clinical signs include rhinorrhoea and otorrhoea (CSF leaking from the nose and ears).
- Battle's sign (bruising around the mastoid process), haemotympanum, and Racoon eye sign (bruising around both eyes) may also be noted.
- This fracture is usually managed conservatively.

Intracranial haemorrhage

Extradural haemorrhage

- This is a bleed between the skull and dura mater, ie in the extradural space.
- It usually arises as a result of damage to the middle meningeal artery following a temporal bone fracture.
- Can also be associated with a parietal bone fracture.
- Patients initially experience a loss of consciousness, which is followed by a lucid interval.
- The haematoma continues to expand within the extradural space and the rise in ICP results in a second episode of reduced consciousness.
- The pupil on the affected side initially constricts and then later becomes fixed and dilated. A hemiparesis also develops on the same side.
- Investigations include an urgent CT scan, with early neurosurgical intervention for surgical removal of the clot if appropriate.
- If intervention is delayed the increase in ICP will eventually compress the brain and result in transtentorial herniation.
- There is a good prognosis with early treatment.

Subdural haemorrhage

- This results from a tear of the bridging veins between the dura and the cerebral cortex.
- Commonly seen following high velocity injuries.
- Chronic subdural haemorrhages can arise following trivial injuries. They are commonly seen in the elderly, as a result of shrunken brains with veins that are under tension.
- A subdural haemorrhage presents similarly to that of an expansile cerebral mass and causes a decline in conscious levels.
- Treatment involves removal of the clot via a craniotomy.
- The prognosis with this type of bleed is poor as a result of extensive brain trauma.

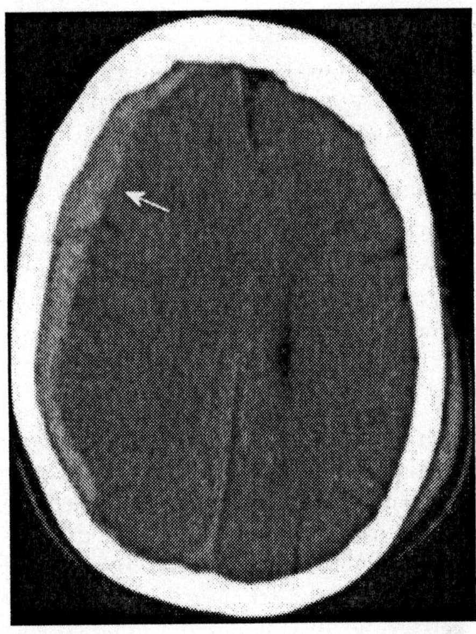

Figure 4.20: CT brain showing an area of increased density in the right parietal lobe (arrow), note the extension across the suture lines and concave internal border in keeping with a subdural haematoma

Subarachnoid haemorrhage

- Occurs as a result of trauma or spontaneously following rupture of berry aneurysms and vascular malformations.
- Patients present with signs of meningism, ie headache, neck stiffness, nausea and vomiting.
- In 50–60% of cases, the patient dies immediately and one-third suffer permanent disability due to hypoxic brain injury.

Intracerebral haemorrhage

- An expansile haematoma within cerebral tissue, arising as a result of contusions.
- Causes include hypertensive vascular disease (commonest), trauma and a bleeding tumour.
- Commonly seen in the frontal and temporal lobes.
- A CT scan will show lesions of increased density.
- A mass effect and midline shift may also be seen, necessitating evacuation of the haematoma.

Cerebral concussion

- If there is a temporary loss of neurological function following a head injury, it can be defined as concussion.
- The patient may complain of a headache, dizziness, and nausea, which subsequently resolve.
- If the history suggests loss of consciousness for greater than five minutes, the patient should be admitted for observation.

Diffuse axonal injury

- This occurs following a deceleration injury, in which the axons are torn and disrupted.
- It is a severe injury often with patients presenting in a coma, lasting from days to weeks.
- Patients also suffer autonomic dysfunction and therefore experience raised temperatures, sweating, and hypertension.
- Macroscopically, punctuate haemorrhages can be seen and microscopically, axonal damage and microglia clusters are visible in the white matter.
- There is a high mortality rate.

Clinical management of head injury

- ATLS guidelines should guide immediate resuscitation.
- Determine the GCS and manage as per the NICE guidelines.
  - GCS 13–15 is a mild head injury.
  - GCS 9–12 is a moderate head injury.
  - GCS 3–8 is a severe head injury.
  - GCS <8 is a coma state.

Investigations

Imaging:

- Cervical spine X-rays if the mechanism of injury involved a significant force
- CT: if the patient has decreased consciousness or an abnormal neurological examination, an urgent scan is required to exclude an intracranial bleed. NICE have clear guidelines on determining the need for a CT scan of patients with head trauma
- SXR: rarely performed

Management

- A basic neurological examination is important to continually assess the patient.
- If the patient meets the criteria for a CT scan, it should be performed and the results discussed with the medical and neurosurgical teams.

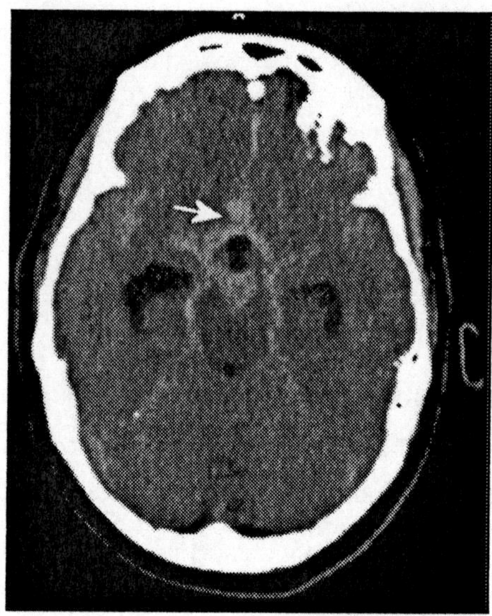

Figure 4.21: Non contrast enhanced CT brain showing increased density along the circle of Willis (arrow) in keeping with acute subarachnoid haemorrhage

- Patients, whom on clinical reassessment are fit to be discharged, should be sent home with head injury advice and be accompanied by a reliable adult.
- The patient should be admitted if the following apply:
  - CT evidence of intracranial pathology
  - Skull fracture
  - Reduced consciousness
  - Neurological signs and symptoms
  - Social circumstances eg lives alone
- Non-opiate analgesia in order to allow accurate regular neurological observations.

NICE guidelines for performing a head CT:

For adults with any of the following risk factors, a CT head scan should be performed within 1 hour:

- GCS less than 13 on initial assessment in the emergency department
- GCS less than 15 at 2 hours after the injury on assessment in the emergency department
- Suspected open or depressed skull fracture
- Any sign of basal skull fracture (haemotympanum, 'panda' eyes, cerebrospinal fluid leakage from the ear or nose, Battle's sign)
- Post-traumatic seizure
- Focal neurological deficit
- More than 1 episode of vomiting

	Response	Points
Eyes	Spontaneously	4
	Verbal command	3
	Pain	2
	No response	1
Verbal	Orientated	5
	Confused	4
	Inappropriate words	3
	Incomprehensible	2
	No response	1
Motor	Obeys commands	6
	Localises to pain	5
	Withdraws from pain	4
	Abnormal flexion	3
	Abnormal extension	2
	No response	1

Table 4.47: Calculating the GCS

Any of the following risk factors should warrant a CT scan within 8 hours:

- Age 65 years or older
- Any history of bleeding or clotting disorders
- Dangerous mechanism of injury (a pedestrian or cyclist struck by a motor vehicle, an occupant ejected from a motor vehicle or a fall from a height of greater than 1 metre or 5 stairs)
- More than 30 minutes' retrograde amnesia of events immediately before the head injury

When to involve the neurosurgeon

- All patients with new, surgically significant abnormalities on imaging
- Regardless of imaging, other reasons for discussing a patient's care with a neurosurgeon include:
  - Persisting coma (GCS ≤8) after initial resuscitation
  - Unexplained confusion for >4 hours
  - Deterioration in GCS after admission (particularly motor deterioration)
  - Progressive focal neurological signs
  - Seizure without full recovery
  - Definite or suspected penetrating injury
  - Cerebrospinal fluid leak

Further reading and references

1. Bulstrode, C.J.K., Russell, R.C.G. and Williams, N.S. (2000) *Bailey & Love's Short Practice of Surgery*. 23rd Edition. London: Arnold.
2. Calne, R., Ellis, H. and Whatson, C. (2002) *Lecture Notes on General Surgery*. 10th Edition. Oxford: Blackwell Publishing.
3. Goldberg, A. and Stansby, G. (2006) *Surgical Talk: Revision in Surgery*. 2nd Edition. London: Imperial College Press.
4. National Institute for Health and Clinical Excellence. (2007) *Head injury* (CG56). [Online]. Available from: www.nice.org.uk/guidance/cg56 [Accessed 7 November 2016].

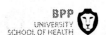

Chapter 5
Resuscitation

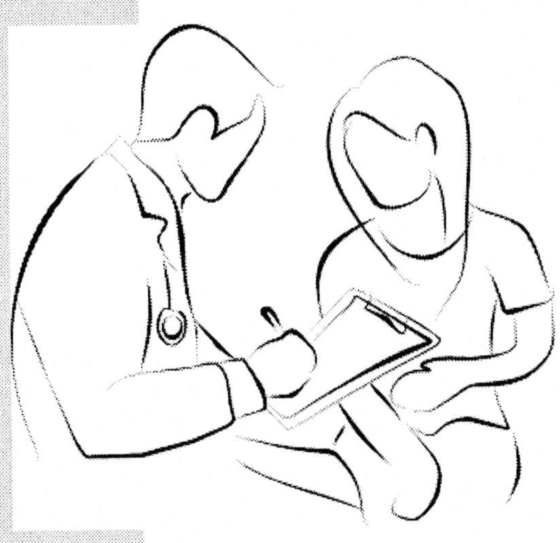

Chapter 5

Resuscitation

In nothing do men more nearly approach the gods than in giving health to men
Cicero (106BC–43BC)

Introduction

The information and algorithms in this chapter are correct at time of writing. Please consult the Resuscitation Council (UK)'s website for the latest guidance (www.resus.org.uk).

As a foundation doctor you will, at times, be reviewing critically unwell patients. You may be the first doctor to see the patient especially during ward cover shifts or on-call in the Emergency Department. At these times you will need to make a rapid assessment of the patient, formulate a problem list and initiate treatment, perhaps before senior support is able to reach you.

This can appear very daunting at first, but there are many training opportunities available to help in these situations. These include 'simulation training', the ALERT Course and courses offered by the Resuscitation Council (UK).

Many Foundation Schools sponsor F1 doctors through an ILS course and F2 doctors are expected to complete an ALS Provider course by the end of the year.

These courses teach a common approach to the assessment of the severely unwell patient. This is the 'A to E approach'. By using this, a comprehensive initial assessment can be made, initial interventions and potentially life-saving treatments started and then the patient can be reassessed using the same framework to check on progress.

There are, however, times when it may not be appropriate to initiate resuscitation attempts, where a DNAR order should be in place. The issues surrounding these orders will be discussed later in this chapter.

The A to E approach

Airway

Assessment of 'A'

1. Listening for any noises:
   talking = patent airway
   snoring/gurgling/stridor = partial occlusion
2. Paradoxical 'abdominal' breathing pattern

Management of 'A'

1. Open the mouth and look for obstructions.
2. Suction fluid matter using a yankauer sucker under direct vision.
3. Remove visible objects with forceps (leave close-fitting dentures in situ).
4. Maintain the airway using a head-tilt/chin-lift and jaw thrust manoeuvre (no head-tilt/chin-tilt if there is any uncertainty about C-spine injury).
5. Use adjuncts to help keep the airway patent – oropharyngeal and nasopharyngeal airways.

Breathing

Assessment of 'B'

1. Respiratory rate
2. Pattern of breathing: symmetry, use of accessory muscles
3. Cyanosis
4. Tracheal position
5. Percussion, auscultation, vocal fremitus
6. Pulse oximetry
7. CXR
8. ABG

Management of 'B'

1. **High flow oxygen should always be applied** as per British Thoracic Society (BTS, 2008) guidelines.
2. In the case of asthma or COPD a PEFR should be obtained, and initial management commenced: nebulised salbutamol and ipratropium and IV/oral steroids.

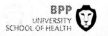

Circulation

Assessment of 'C'

1. Heart rate, rhythm, nature (peripherally – radial artery; centrally – carotid/femoral)
2. BP
3. Capillary refill time - press for 5 seconds over the sternum (normal <2 seconds)
4. Perfusion – warm and vasodilated or shut down?
5. Venous distension – is the neck collapsed or well filled?
6. 12-lead ECG and apply cardiac monitoring if available

Management of 'C'

1. Obtain IV access, preferably using a wide bore (green/orange or grey) cannula
2. Take bloods as indicated
3. Commence IV fluids

Disability

Assessment of 'D'

1. AVPU score (quicker than GCS – though latter should be calculated at later point)

   A – ALERT

   V – RESPONDS TO VOICE

   P – RESPONDS TO PAINFUL STIMULUS

   U – UNRESPONSIVE
2. Check pupil reactivity
3. Check limb movements and power
4. Capillary blood glucose

Management of 'D'

1. Correct any abnormalities in capillary blood glucose

Exposure

Assessment of 'E'

1. Fully expose the patient whilst being mindful of dignity and warmth.
2. Inspect fully, in particular checking for signs of haemorrhage, oedema, rash or any other injury.
3. Take the temperature.

At the end of the assessment the same framework can be used to reassess at a later point, particularly if treatments have been instigated, as well as to document the findings.

Foundation doctors should receive a high level of support when dealing with critically unwell patients. It is important to know who to ask for help, and **always ask for help early.**

More senior doctors are an obvious choice and in particular the on-call medical Registrar. However, care for the critically unwell is a multidisciplinary skill. Many hospitals have outreach teams, which may consist of ICU staff, specialist outreach nurses or resuscitation officers. They can often be contacted using 'triggers' such as Early Warning Scores (commonly the Modified Early Warning Score, MEWS).

Cardiac arrest

Cardiac arrests can and do happen anywhere within a hospital. No matter what the situation, the Resuscitation Council (UK) guidelines should be followed. These guarantee a standardised approach to treating a cardiac arrest and are taught on the ILS and ALS courses. It is important for you to be up to date with the current guidelines.

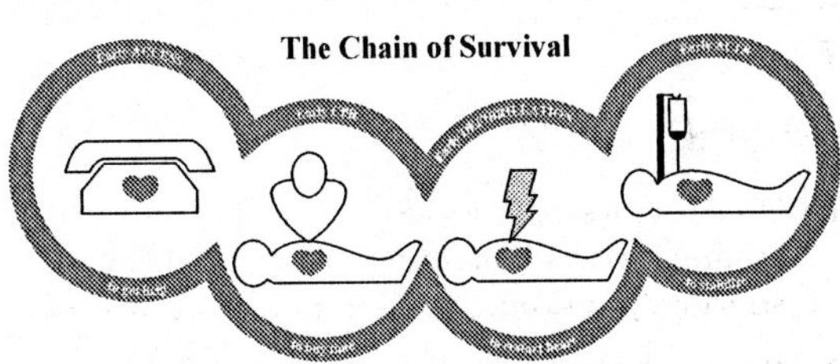

Figure 5.1: Chain of Survival highlighting the four important factors in reducing mortality during a cardiac arrest. Courtesy of Laerdal Medical Ltd. Reproduced with permission (www.resus.org.uk)

A foundation doctor would be expected to identify and confirm cardiac arrest, call for help and ensure the cardiac arrest team is called by dialling 2222 in hospitals and initiate resuscitation in the absence of a more senior experienced member of clinical staff. The chain of survival is important to know and to instigate (see Figure 5.1).

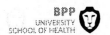

The resuscitation team

Cardiac arrests require a team to work together to provide the patient with the best possible chances of survival. The team should comprise people with specific skills including advanced airway management, defibrillation, chest compressions and drug administration. It is also usual to have a scribe who also monitors timings and can explain to any observers such as family or students what is happening.

The team should be clearly led by a leader, who is often the medical registrar but may be the Emergency Department consultant/registrar or Resuscitation Officer. Typically, the foundation doctor will be directed by the team leader to perform tasks such as inserting cannulae, taking bloods and blood gases and performing chest compressions. Evidence shows that good quality chest compressions are important to maintain coronary perfusion pressure and maximise the chances of survival. They should take place at a rate of 100 per minute and depth of 4–5 cm. Care should be taken to minimise interruptions in chest compressions.

It is essential to ensure that all team members are up to date with their resuscitation training and most trusts provide regular update courses for staff.

The Universal Algorithm

The Universal Algorithm (see Figure 5.2) is the standard approach to a cardiac arrest and is the one taught on Resuscitation Council (UK) courses. All individuals involved in resuscitation should be aware of the steps involved.

The initial action to be taken is to open the airway and confirm cardiac arrest, by **looking, listening** and **feeling** for respiratory effort and pulse for not more than ten seconds. On confirmation of cardiac arrest, basic life support should begin whilst the cardiac arrest team is called. A defibrillator should be obtained as soon as possible.

Once the patient is connected to the defibrillator the rhythm must be analysed to ensure that the correct pathway of the algorithm is followed. The rhythm can be analysed by an automated external defibrillator or manually by a person competent to do so. There are only four possible rhythms associated with cardiac arrest, with which you should be familiar:

Shockable rhythms (requiring defibrillation)

1. **Ventricular fibrillation:** absence of a pulse and chaotic electrical activity
2. **Pulseless ventricular tachycardia:** organised broad complex (QRS greater than 3 small squares or 0.12 seconds) tachycardia and the absence of a pulse

Defibrillation should be followed by immediate chest compressions and administration of the following drugs:

> ADRENALINE 1 mg 1:10,000 BEFORE THE THIRD SHOCK AND THEN EVERY OTHER CYCLE
>
> AMIODARONE 300 mg BEFORE THE FOURTH SHOCK

Non-shockable rhythms (no defibrillation)

1. **Asystole**: No pulse and no electrical activity
2. **Pulseless electrical activity**: absence of a pulse, but some electrical activity

Chest compressions should be initiated and the following drugs administered.

> ADRENALINE 1mg 1:10,000 EVERY OTHER CYCLE
>
> ATROPINE 3mg ONCE ONLY FOR ASYSTOLE AND PEA WITH A HEART RATE <60 bpm

It is important to make sure you are familiar with the particular kind of defibrillator used in your trust. All Resuscitation Officers offer induction training to new staff and you should ensure that you attend to familiarise yourself with the equipment and energy levels used.

Reversible causes (4Hs and 4Ts)

Whilst resuscitation is underway, any possible reversible causes of cardiac arrest should be considered. There are eight recognised reversible causes – the four Hs and four Ts – and whilst the presenting complaint, past medical history, observation charts and physical assessment of the

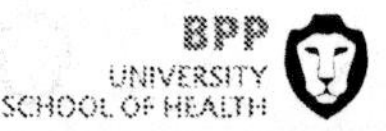

patient may provide information about which is the most relevant, all should be considered to avoid missing an intervention. It should be noted that more than one reversible cause might be present in the same patient.

1. Hypoxia

Hypoxia should be considered in all patients.

Interventions

- Insert a definitive airway (laryngeal mask, oropharangeal airway or endotracheal intubation depending on the skills available).
- Administer 15 litres of oxygen using a bag valve mask – 2 breaths every cycle of 30 chest compressions.
- ABG but it should be remembered that patients in cardiac arrest will be hypoxic due to lack of spontaneous respiration unless adequate artificial ventilation is provided.

2. Hypovolaemia

Hypovolaemia should be considered in patients where there is a suspicion of fluid loss. Note that a patient in cardiac arrest will not have a blood pressure so other means will need to be used in order to establish whether the patient may be hypovolaemic. The patient should be examined for signs of active bleeding and previous vital signs and fluid balance charts should be checked.

Interventions

- Cannula in both antecubital fossae
- Give a bolus infusion of fluids

3. Hyper/hypokalaemia

Hyper/hypokalaemia and other metabolic disorders should be considered in patients with relevant past medical history. Recent blood results should be reviewed and a sample should be sent for rapid analysis. Many ABGs provide results of important electrolytes.

Interventions

- Correct any identified electrolyte disturbance.
- Treat hypokalaemia with intravenous potassium at a maximum rate of 2 mmol/min for 10 minutes followed by 10 mmol over 5–10 minutes.
- Treat hyperkalaemia by:
  - Protecting the myocardium with 10 ml of 10% calcium chloride
  - Shifting the potassium into the cells using a dextrose/insulin infusion (10 units of actrapid with 50 ml of 50% dextrose)
  - Removing the potassium from the body using calcium resonium or haemodialysis
- Treat severe acidosis or renal failure with a rapid infusion of 50 mmol of sodium bicarbonate.

4. Hypothermia

Hypothermia should be particularly considered in patients who have sustained out-of-hospital cardiac arrests. A core temperature should be taken.

Interventions

- Administer intravenous warmed fluids, warmed oxygen and lavage the major body cavities with warmed fluids.

5. Tension pneumothorax

Tension pneumothorax should be considered in patients who have sustained trauma or who have respiratory conditions such as asthma and COPD. Identification of a tension pneumothorax is through clinical examination – hyper-resonance on percussion and reduced air entry on the affected side with late tracheal deviation away from the pneumothorax.

Interventions

- Needle decompression using a wide bore cannula on the affected side in the second intercostal space in the mid clavicular line
- Insertion of a chest drain if resuscitation is successful

6. Toxic

Toxic causes should be considered for inpatients taking medications as well as for out-of-hospital arrests, particularly those in which the collapse was unwitnessed. Ambulance crews who attended the scene should examine the patient for signs of drug use such as track marks and for any packages or articles that may provide clues as to the drugs that may have been involved.

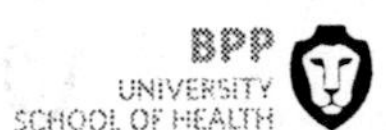

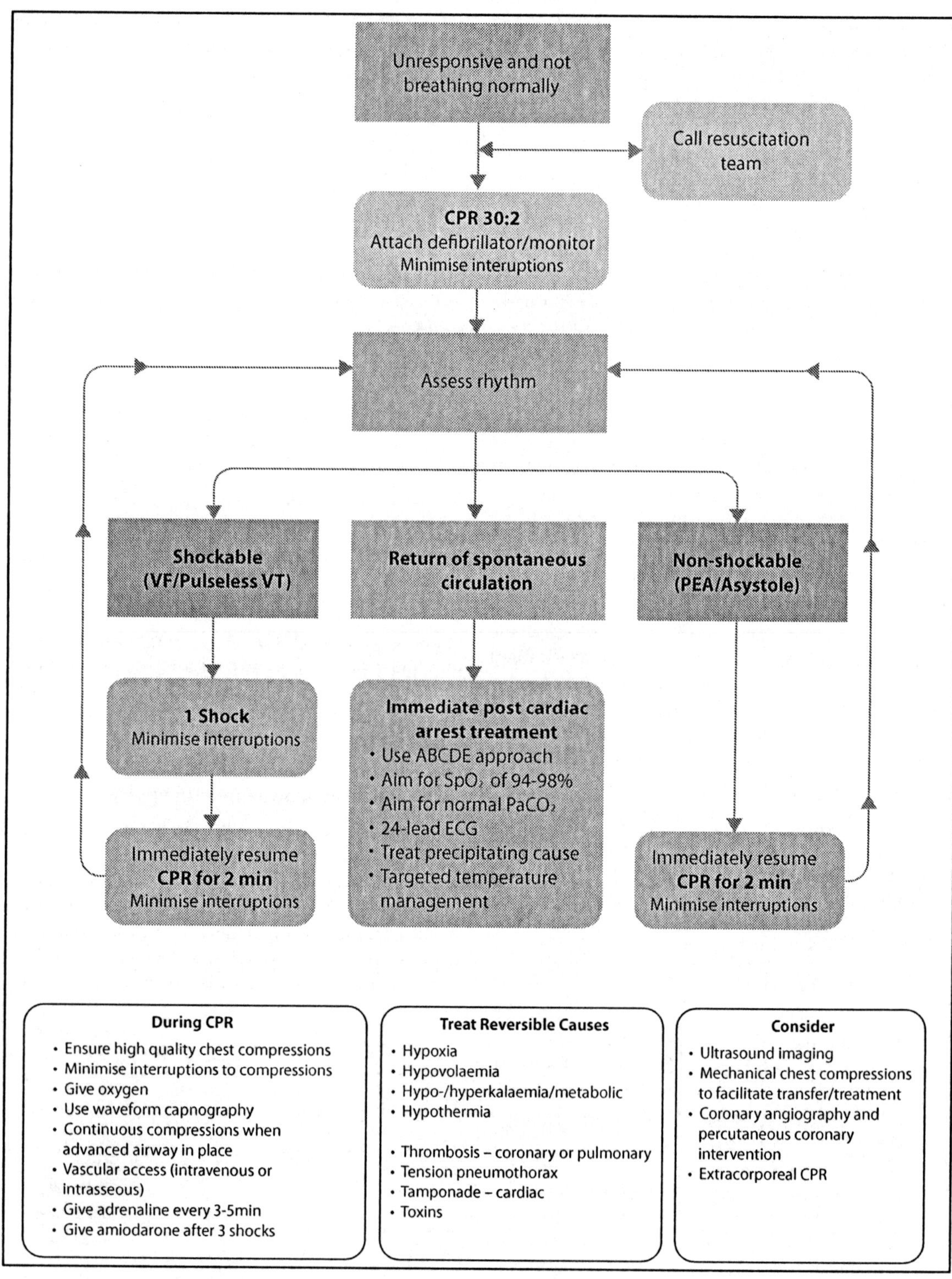

Figure 5.2: The Adult Advanced Life Support Algorithm. Courtesy of the Resuscitation Council UK. Reproduced with permission

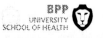

Interventions

- Give any appropriate antidote if it is possible a toxin may have contributed to the cardiac arrest

7. Tamponade

Tamponade should only be considered where there is reasonable suspicion that fluid (such as blood) has accumulated in the pericardial space either through cardiothoracic surgery, trauma to the chest, or more rarely post-myocardial infarction. There is no way of diagnosing tamponade in cardiac arrest unless you have immediate access to a portable ultrasound machine.

Interventions

- Insertion of a pericardiocentesis needle to the left of the xiphisternum at an angle of 45 degrees pointed towards the left scapula. This should be done by seniors only!

8. Thromboembolism

Thromboembolism should be considered in all patients with relevant history, such as ischaemic heart disease, previous stroke, recent prolonged period of immobility, previous thromboembolism or hypercoagulability. There may be evidence to suggest a thromboembolic cause in the events preceding the cardiac arrest – for example chest pain.

Interventions

- Thrombolysis – if given during cardiac arrest the arrest must be continued for sufficient time to allow the thrombolysis to work, which may mean continuing the resuscitation for a period of up to 90 minutes.

Post-resuscitation care

Resuscitation does not stop on ROSC. At this point the patient is likely to be very unstable and requires a full examination and stabilisation of their condition. The A to E approach should be used to assess the patient and guide ongoing treatment. Almost all patients require intensive support following cardiac arrest, with many requiring ventilation and inotrope support and some may need definitive treatment such as surgery. Invasive monitoring may be needed, such as a central venous catheter, arterial line and urinary catheter. Full and regular observations should be recorded and bloods sent including FBC, U&Es, LFTs and serial ABGs. An ECG and chest X-ray should be performed. Prior to transfer, patients should be stabilised and lines secured.

Therapeutic-induced hypothermia should be considered for patients sustaining out of hospital VF cardiac arrests. This has been demonstrated to have a neuroprotective effect and improve outcomes and involves reducing the patient's core temperature to 32–34°C for 24 hours post-arrest. A number of methods can be used, ranging from cooling jackets and helmets to the use of cooled fluids – the exact method will depend on the local Intensive Care Unit policy.

Documentation and audit

During a resuscitation attempt it is important to ensure that there is a member of the team keeping a written record of what has occurred. Many patients undergoing resuscitation will need to be referred to the Coroner's Officer and be the subject of a post-mortem examination, therefore it is useful for the Coroner to be able to identify drugs and procedures that the patient had during the arrest. Most hospitals will have an audit form on which a record of the resuscitation is made, which allow identification of good practice and can highlight issues within local services as well as being used nationally and internationally for research and comparisons into the outcomes of cardiac arrest.

Decision to stop resuscitation

The majority of resuscitation attempts are unsuccessful and a decision to stop will have to be made. The decision to stop should be a team decision and all members of the team have a right to have their say. When the team is in agreement for the attempt to be stopped, resuscitation is terminated and the time recorded. If the team is not in agreement the team leader should lead a discussion to explore the underlying reasons and to reach an agreement. During this discussion resuscitation should continue.

Relatives witnessing resuscitation

Relatives observing resuscitation remains a contentious issue for many healthcare professionals. It is common practice for parents to be present during the resuscitation of their child yet frequently relatives of adult patients are excluded from the resuscitation. Relatives may have been present when their loved one collapsed, are likely to be the first person to have attempted to resuscitate the patient and will have witnessed pre-hospital resuscitation attempts. A large body of evidence has demonstrated that relatives who witness the resuscitation of loved ones find it easier to accept the outcome and generally have fewer concerns regarding alternative treatment that could have been attempted to save their relative.

It is important that relatives that are witnessing resuscitation attempts should be supported by a member of staff who is able to explain to them exactly what is happening. This person should be experienced in resuscitation. It is important that certain ground rules are established early in the resuscitation process. The relative should agree that they stand back and allow the team to work on the patient and that if the team request the relative should leave the room. At any time should the relative wish to leave they must be accompanied by a staff member.

Many find the presence of a relative a stressful experience for a variety of reasons. Resuscitations can be very stressful for the team and members may feel their skills are under scrutiny particularly if they are not very experienced. For this reason, all members of the team should be happy with the relative being present.

Breaking bad news

Cardiac arrests often end in a patient's death and this news must be broken to the next of kin and family members in a compassionate manner. The best person to break bad news is someone who had some prior interaction with the next of kin. This may not always be possible and in that case someone who knows exactly what happened, often the team leader, should break the news. Foundation doctors should not routinely be expected to inform the next of kin that their relative has died. However, you may wish to observe a colleague breaking the news or break the news yourself because you knew the patient and their family well.

Whenever bad news is being broken there are specific principles that should be followed to ensure that the message is communicated sensitively and effectively:

- **Setting**

  Ensure privacy, provide comfortable seating, make sure that the room is well lit and have access to a telephone and tissues. It is important that whoever is breaking the news ensures that they are not going to be disturbed; this may mean handing a bleep to another member of staff and ensuring that mobile phones are switched to silent.

- **Personnel**

  No one should break bad news alone; reactions to upsetting news can range from stunned silence, through to uncontrollable crying, through to violent and aggressive outbursts.

- **Language**

  The language used should be clear and unambiguous. Phrases such as 'gone to a better place' and 'gone to rest' should be avoided and words such as 'died' and 'dead' should be used as early as possible.

- **Information**

  It is important to explain what will happen next and wherever possible provide the information in a written format including relevant contact details such as the hospital bereavement office, local support networks and the Coroner's Office. Many hospitals have this information pre-printed in a booklet.

- **Questions and closure**

  It is important to allow the family and next of kin to ask any questions and give them the opportunity to view their deceased relative if they so wish.

Aftermath

Cardiac arrests and resuscitation attempts are stressful for all those involved. Other patients may ask you questions about what happened and it is important that you are honest with them without breaching patient confidentiality. Student nurses and medical students may not have witnessed a resuscitation attempt before and it is important that they have an opportunity to ask questions and discuss how they are feeling. Treating a patient in cardiac arrest or being with a patient as they arrest can be very traumatic. This is especially the case for allied healthcare professionals such as therapy or administration staff who are not generally exposed to critically unwell patients. You can never predict how a resuscitation may affect you and it may depend on the circumstances of the arrest and your own personal circumstances. Debriefs with the team can be useful, allowing a review of what happened and understanding areas that could be improved. These can either be informal, shortly after

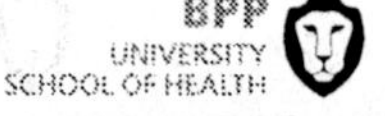

the event or more formal at a later stage. Hospital chaplains are good resources when there has been a traumatic resuscitation and many hospitals also provide counselling services through the Occupational Health department.

Decisions not to attempt resuscitation

There are some patients who are not suitable for resuscitation as attempts would be futile. This decision ultimately lies with the consultant responsible for the patient's care. A DNAR should be discussed with the patient (where possible), their next of kin, members of the medical team and the nursing staff. The discussion and subsequent decision should be clearly documented in the medical notes and communicated to all parties following Resuscitation Council Guidelines issued in 2009. Hospitals will have local policies regarding DNAR forms and foundation doctors should be familiar with them.

A DNAR decision does not mean that the patient should not be actively treated if their condition deteriorates. It only stipulates that in the event of cardio-respiratory arrest no treatment should be instigated.

Advance directives and capacity

There are some patients who are very clear about the treatment that they do or do not wish to receive, should their condition deteriorate. A competent person may not wish to be resuscitated, and this is a reason for completing a DNAR form. Alternatively, under the Mental Capacity Act (2005), a nominated person with lasting power of attorney can make medical decisions on behalf of those now lacking capacity to decide on resuscitation.

Legally binding advance directives are becoming more common and generally these are used by patients in the terminal stages of a disease process. A valid legally binding advance directive has to be made whilst a person is deemed to have capacity to give consent.

Just because we can doesn't mean we should, and just because we should doesn't mean we can

Anon

Resuscitation – the FACTS

Out of Hospital Cardiac Arrests (OHCA)

- In 2013, the UK Emergency Services attempted to resuscitate approximately 28,000 cases of OHCA. An estimated 60,000 cases of OHCA occur each year in the UK.
- The average overall survival of these 28,000 cases to hospital discharge was 8.6%.
- When someone has a cardiac arrest, every minute without CPR reduces their chances of survival by 7-10%.

In Hospital Cardiac Arrests (IHCA)

- In April 2014-March 2015 there were 15,779 reported IHCA.
- Of those, 32.7% occurred in inpatients aged 75-84 and 23.6% in those aged 85 or older.
- Return of spontaneous circulation was achieved in 46.6%, with one-third of those patients being taken to ICU/HDU post-arrest.
- 80.1% of those initial survivors achieved a cerebral performance score of 1 (good cognitive performance, able to work with possible mild cognitive or psychological deficit).
- 18.0% of those initial 46.6% survived to hospital discharge.

Tip:
When counselling patients about resuscitation or DNAR decisions, it is important to make these numbers meaningful.

- **Almost half of people who undergo CPR will initially survive, but only 1 in 5 will leave hospital.**
- **1 in 5 (or more) of those who undergo CPR will not have normal cognitive function afterwards.**
- **The older you are, on average all outcomes are likely to be worse.**

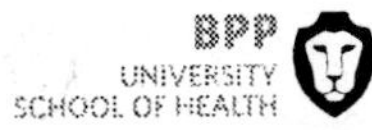

 Advanced Trauma Life Support

In cases of suspected traumatic injury, a slightly different systematic approach is used, based on ATLS principles. This involves conducting an 'A to E' Primary Survey, followed by a Secondary Survey once the patient has been stabilised. Assessment and interventions for A-E are as for resuscitation above, but there are some additional injuries that must not be missed and management steps to treat them.

As an F2 doctor you may be a member of the 'trauma team' and have to participate in trauma calls. The basic principles of ATLS are outlined below.

Primary survey

'A' – Airway and C-spine stabilisation

As above with triple immobilisation of the C-spine in a neutral position using side head supports, semi-rigid cervical collar and strapping.

'B' – Breathing and ventilation

Six life-threatening thoracic conditions that must be identified and managed are:

- Airway obstruction – **definitive airway**
- Tension pneumothorax – **needle thoracocentesis**
- Massive haemothorax – **chest drain**
- Open pneumothorax – **three-sided dressing**
- Flail chest segment with pulmonary contusion – **analgesia**
- Cardiac tamponade – **pericardiocentesis**

'C' – Circulation and haemorrhage control

As above for detection of circulatory instability and gaining intravenous access. A cross-match request should be made immediately if bleeding is suspected.

Anatomical sites where bleeding may occur can be remembered as 'on the floor and four more' – ie abdomen, pelvis, chest and long bones. A Focused Assessment with Sonography for Trauma (FAST) may be used to identify blood in the perisplenic, perihepatic, pericardial or pelvic regions and definitive management for this will involve pericardiocentesis or surgery.

Measures to address more superficial bleeding include pressure dressings and elevation and application of pelvic binders or limb traction.

The major haemorrhage protocol (MHP) should be activated (this will be a hospital-specific process, but can often be achieved through the switchboard). Group O (Rh –ve blood for childbearing age females) is often available in A&E and theatres, but activation of the MHP alerts the haematology lab to urgently prepare cross-matched blood, platelets, fresh frozen plasma and cryoprecipitate. A haematologist should be available to advise on this.

'D' – Disability

As above. Similarly to ALS, it is imperative to exclude hypoglycaemia as a cause of altered consciousness. In patients with suspected head injuries, a Glasgow Coma Score should be calculated along with the AVPU score rating. This is based on motor, verbal and eye responses and has a score of 3–15.

Motor:

1 – no respponse
2 – extends to pain
3 – flexes to pain
4 – withdraws from pain
5 – localises to pain
6 – obeys commands

Verbal:

1 – none
2 – incomprehensible
3 – inappropriate
4 – confused
5 – normal conversation

Eyes:

1 – none
2 – opens to pain
3 – opens to voice
4 – opens spontaneously

As soon as the patient is stable and the primary survey completed they should be taken for a 'trauma series' of images, which is most often a 'head-to-thigh contrast-enhanced multi-detector CT scan, which will identify any intracranial pathology.

'E' – Exposure

The patients' garments all need to be removed in order for a full examination to take place. However, it is important to ensure hypothermia does not develop and the patient should be kept in a warm environment and infused with warmed intravenous fluids.

Secondary survey

As soon as the primary survey is completed, the patient is stabilised and observations are normalising, the secondary survey can begin. This is a complete head-to-toe evaluation of the patient, including a full history and examination. A log-roll (if not already completed during the primary survey) should be undertaken to identify any posterior injuries and if at any point the patient deteriorates, the primary survey should recommence until they have been adequately stabilised. Follow-up for trauma patients is as for those who have undergone ALS treatment.

Further reading and references

1. A Joint Statement from the British Medical Association, the Resuscitation Council (UK), and the Royal College of Nursing. (2007) *Decisions relating to Cardiopulmonary Resuscitation.* [Online]. Available from: www.resus.org.uk/dnacpr/decisions-relating-to-cpr/ [Accessed 7 November 2016].
2. Adams, S., Bloomfield, P., Whitlock, M., et al. (1994) *Should relatives watch resuscitation?* BMJ 1994; 308: 1687-9.
3. Ambulance Service Association. (2006) *National Out-of-Hospital Cardiac Arrest Project 2006.* [Online]. Available from: http://bmjopen.bmj.com/content/5/10/e008736.full [Accessed 7 November 2016].
4. Awoonor-Renner, S. (1991) I desperately need to see my son. *BMJ* 1991; 302: 351.
5. British Thoracic Society. (2008) Guideline for emergency use of oxygen in adult patients. *Thorax* 2008; 63.
6. British Thoracic Society and Scottish Intercollegiate Guidelines Network. (2008) *British Guideline on the management of asthma.* [Online]. Available from: www.brit-thoracic.org.uk/document-library/clinical-information/asthma/btssign-asthma-guideline-2008/ [Accessed 7 November 2016].
7. Hanson, C. and Strawser, D. (1992) Family presence during cardio-pulmonary resuscitation: Foote Hospital ED nine year perspective. *Journal of Emergency Nursing* 1992; 18:104-106.
8. Martin, J. (1991) Rethinking traditional thoughts. *Journal of Emergency Nursing* 1991; 17: 67–8.
9. Resuscitation Council (UK). (2008) *Advanced Life Support.* 7th Edition. [Online]. Available from: www.resus.org.uk [Accessed 7 November 2016].
10. Resuscitation Council (UK) and Intensive Care National Audit & Research Centre. (2015) *Key Statistics from the National Cardiac Arrest Audit 2014/15.* [Online]. Available from: www.icnarc.org/Our-Audit/Audits/Ncaa/Reports/Access-Our-Data/2015/10/15/Key-Ncaa-Statistics-201415 [Accessed 7 November 2016].
11. Resuscitation Council (UK). (2006) *Should Relatives Witness Resuscitation?* [Online]. Available from: www.resus.org.uk/archive/archived-cpr-information/should-relatives-witness-resuscitation/ [Accessed 7 November 2016].
12. Royal College of Nurses. (2002) *Witnessing Resuscitation. Guidance for nurses.* [Online]. Available from: www2.rcn.org.uk/__data/assets/pdf_file/0006/78531/001736.pdf [Accessed 7 November 2016].
13. Royal College of Radiology. (2015) *Standards of practice and guidance for trauma radiology in the severely injured patient.* [Online]. Available from: www.rcr.ac.uk/system/files/publication/field_publication_files/bfcr155_traumaradiol.pdf [Accessed 7 November 2016].
14. Cretin, S., Larsen, M.P., Roe, D.J., et al. Estimating effectiveness of cardiac arrest interventions: a logistic regression survival model. *Circulation* 1997; 96:3308-3313.
15. Ambulance Quality Indicators, www.england.nhs.uk/statistics/stasistical-work-areas/ambulance-quality-indicators/.

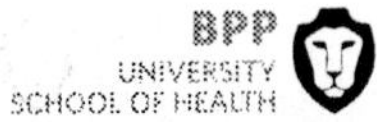

Chapter 6
Fluid management and shock

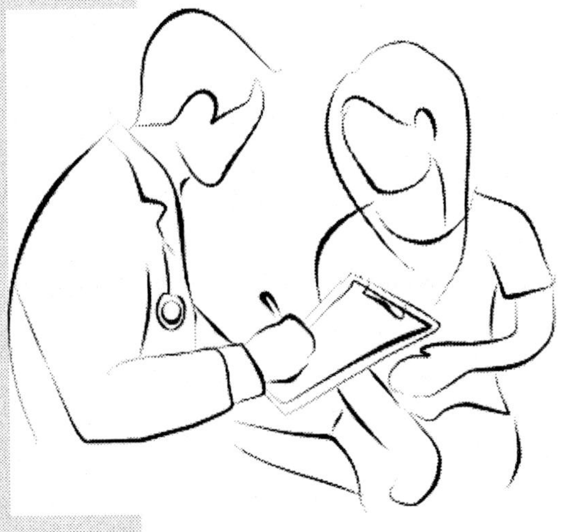

Chapter 6

Fluid management and shock

Endeavour to play easy pieces well and with elegance; that is better than to play difficult pieces badly.
Robert Schumann 'Advice to Young Musicians'

Fluid management

'Doctor, will you just write up some fluids please?' is probably one of the commonest requests you will face during your foundation years. From day one you will have to prescribe intravenous fluids on a patient's fluid/drug chart. It seems a very simple task – and it can be. However, incorrect or careless fluid prescription also kills patients. It is estimated that one in five patients suffer adverse complications as a result of inappropriate fluids or electrolyte replacement prescription. Therefore, don't underestimate this task but treat it with the diligence and caution you would any other prescription.

Compartments of the human body

The human body consists of approximately two thirds (60%) water. This is present in two physiological compartments as: intracellular fluid (ICF) and extracellular fluid (ECF). The pathological 'third space' arises when there is a mismatch in the normal homeostatic mechanisms within the two compartments.

For the average 70 kg man:

Physiological		Pathological
Intracellular fluid (30L)	**Extracellular fluid (15L)**	**Third space**
2/3 of total body water Within cells	1/3 of total body water Plasma (3.5L) Interstitium (8.5L) Lymph (1.5L) Transcellular (1.5L) Separated by a layer of endothelium	Fluid accumulates here in disease Not readily exchangeable with the rest of the ECF causing dehydration

Table 6.1: Fluid distribution for an average 70 kg male

Osmolality

Fluid can move between compartments as a result of the balance between osmotic pressures. The distribution is determined by Starling's forces: hydrostatic pressure (ie force of fluid against the vessel walls) and oncotic pressure (force exerted by the presence of large solutes – mainly proteins).

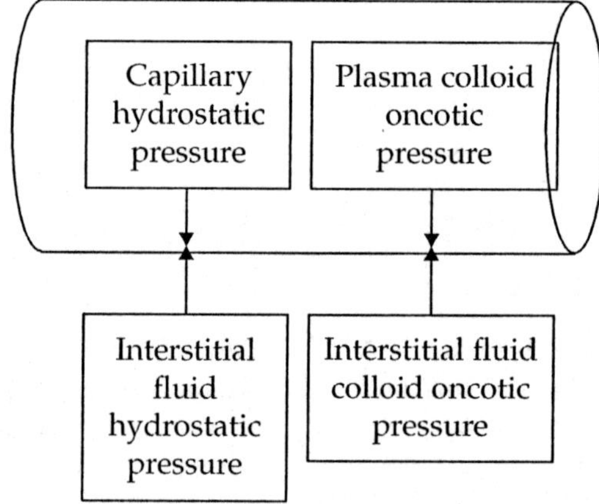

Figure 6.1: Balance between hydrostatic and oncotic pressures in determining fluid distribution between compartments

Osmolality is the total particle concentration, which is the same in all body compartments.

Isotonic fluid has the same osmolality as plasma, therefore when placed in plasma this fluid will not enter the ICF compartment.

The distribution of extra-cellular fluid between plasma and the interstitial space is regulated by the capillary and lymphatic system:

> ECF = [Capillary hydrostatic pressure + Tissue oncotic pressure] – [Tissue hydrostatic pressure + Capillary oncotic pressure]

Electrolyte distribution/requirements

Electrolyte distribution within each compartment differs:

- ICF: K+ and Mg2+ main cations, phosphate and proteins, main anions
- ECF: Na+ main cation, chloride and bicarbonate main anions

Individual requirements:

- 2 mmol/kg/24 hrs of Sodium (approximately 140 mmol)
- 1 mmol/kg/24 hrs of Potassium (approximately 60 mmol)

Normal input/output values (for 70 kg male/24 hrs):

Input (ml)		Output (ml)	
Oral fluid	1,500	Urine	1,500
Fluid in food	750-1,000	Faeces	300
Water of oxidation	300	Lung	500
		Skin	500
Total	280		2,800

Table 6.2: Normal fluid input and output for an average 70 kg male

Prescribing fluids

When to prescribe fluids?

- Replacement of abnormal fluid losses eg diarrhoea, vomiting, burns
- Normal fluid requirements for a patient who is NBM
- Pre-operative resuscitation
- Post-operative resuscitation
- Electrolyte imbalance

What fluids to prescribe?

There are three main types of fluid: crystalloid, colloid and blood. However, in the majority of clinical settings, only the former tend to be prescribed, supplemented as required by blood.

- **Crystalloids**
  - Electrolyte solutions
  - Move through a semi-permeable membrane, therefore distribute themselves throughout the fluid compartments
  - Examples include normal saline, dextrose saline and Hartmann's solution
  - Typically used as maintenance or replacement fluids

- **Colloids**
  - Contains high molecular weight molecules, therefore cannot move through a semi-permeable membrane
  - Remains in the vascular compartment for longer
  - Examples include albumin, Gelofusin and HES fluid
  - Used primarily in intensive care or resuscitation settings for intravenous volume expansion

- **Blood**
  - Remains in the intravenous compartment, so effective volume expander
  - Cross-matched is best – takes one hour
  - Type-specific (ABO and Rh) takes ten minutes
  - O negative can be used in a haemorrhagic emergency

Practical prescribing

The average adult daily requirements are 2–3 litres of water, 100 mmol sodium and 60 mmol potassium.

If the patient is losing additional fluid (eg vomiting, diarrhoea or has an NG tube), they will require extra fluid replacement.

1. Assess the fluid balance
2. Assess their fluid needs
3. Start a fluid balance chart (with catheter insertion if appropriate)
4. Prescribe a fluid challenge or fluids as per calculated requirements
5. **Review**

Crystalloid composition

- **0.9% normal saline (mmol/L):**
  - 154 sodium
  - 154 chloride

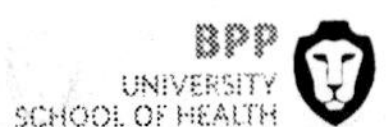

- **Hartmann's solution:**
  - 129 sodium
  - 109 chloride
  - 29 lactate
  - 5 potassium
  - 2 calcium

- **5% dextrose solution:**
  - 5% dextrose in 95% 0.9% sodium chloride

A typical 24 hour fluid regime may be:

> **3x 1L Hartmann's solution +/- electrolyte replacement (eg 20 mmol KCl) as required**
>
> **or**
>
> **1x 1L 0.9% NaCl + 2x 1L 5% dextrose +/- electrolyte replacement (eg 20 mmol KCl) as required**

Fluid balance

When prescribing any fluid it is important to assess the fluid status of a patient through clinical examination, urine output and CVP.

- **Clinical examination**
  - Signs of dehydration: dry mucous membranes, sunken eyes, low BP and postural hypotension, raised pulse rate, low JVP, and confusion
  - Signs of fluid overload: pulmonary/peripheral oedema

- **Urine output**
  - This should be at least 0.5 ml/kg/hr (ie 35 ml/hr for a 70 kg man)

- **CVP**
  - Invasive and accurate monitoring possible only if a patient has a central venous catheter ie intensive care or possibly intra-operatively
  - Trends are more important than absolute values

- **Response to a fluid challenge**
  - Administering a 250 ml or 500 ml bolus based on patient age, size and co-morbidities and assessing the haemodynamic response may indicate fluid status

> **Top tips for the ward round**
>
> 1. Check that catheter is still in place
> 2. Check that catheter is not blocked – flush using 50 ml bladder syringe and sterile water
> 3. Palpate the bladder to identify or rule out urinary retention

Post-operative fluid therapy

Post-operatively a number of hormones (catecholamines, ADH, cortisol, and aldosterone) increase as a result of the stress involved in surgery. Over 24–48 hours this results in the conservation of salt and water, and increased losses of potassium and hydrogen ions by the kidneys. With this water retention it is sensible to reduce the daily intake of water to 2L 24 hours post-operatively. Potassium supplements are often not given due to the increased release of potassium following tissue injury during surgery.

In patients who have undergone abdominal surgery a bowel ileus may develop (from mechanical handling or general anaesthetic), resulting in third space losses, as fluid in the bowel is not reabsorbed. These patients require additional fluid replacement which is prescribed according to urine output/nasogastric tube aspirates. On day two or three post-operatively the patient will experience a sudden diuresis, which signifies recovery of the bowel. Fluid therapy can be best guided by checking serum electrolytes.

> **Top tip:**
>
> As with much medical practice, the most effective way of managing fluids is to make your best assessment based on clinical and observational findings, instigate a therapy based on that assessment and then **review, review, review!!**

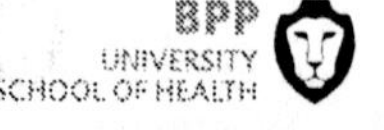

Case Study: A balancing act...

Mrs Griffiths was 89 years old and, like many nearing their tenth decade of life, enjoyed a daily diet of seemingly thousands of pills. She took pills for her heart failure and puffy legs, blood pressure, irregular heartbeat and poor kidneys. She took pills to lower cholesterol, prevent a stroke, ease her angina and finally, she took pills to ease the side effects of all the other pills – antihistamines and the occasional anti-emetic. 'I takes so many pills I rattles,' she would gleefully recount, repeating the old joke a pharmacist had once told her, before bursting into guffaws of laughter that ended in a huge coughing fit as her congested lungs gave up and resumed their drowning.

As well as providing much mirth for the patient, Mrs Griffiths' pills damaged her kidneys. Every day they fought against the onslaught of her 'medicines' sometimes working better, sometimes worse. Every day on the ward round, the consultant would go through the same actions: he looked at the fluid chart, pressed the swollen legs, listened to the crackling chest and the latest blood test results and he would sigh. 'Mrs Griffiths, Mrs Griffiths, what are we going to do with you. Let's give you a slow bag of fluid – a **slow** one, mind you – and increase the diuretics as well. Those kidneys of yours don't like us drying you out, but your heart and lungs are drowning. What **are** we going to do?' Mrs Griffiths smiled toothlessly – she hadn't put her dentures in yet – and patted his arm, 'whatever you tells me to do, doctor,' she said. She never made it out of hospital.

Shock

Shock is inadequate perfusion of vital organs and tissue oxygenation.

Classification of shock

- Hypovolaemic:
  - Haemorrhagic shock is the most common
  - Diarrhoea and vomiting
- Septic
- Anaphylactic
- Cardiogenic
  - Blunt injury
  - Cardiac infarct
  - Cardiac tamponade
- Neurogenic
  - Spinal injuries

There are four stages of hypovolaemic shock, defined on clinical parameters and classified according to the percentage of blood loss (see Table 6.3).

Management

1. ABC and initial resuscitation (get appropriate help ASAP – trauma/resus team, senior colleagues, ITU support/anaesthetists, haematology advice etc)
2. All patients require fluid resuscitation
   i) 2 x large bore cannulae
   ii) Bloods: FBC, U&Es, cross-match (2 samples often needed), glucose
   iii) 2L crystalloid to commence STAT (according to ATLS protocol)
3. Catheter + hourly urine output monitoring
4. Request emergency O negative blood and cross-matched units ASAP and commence transfusion immediately if shock is due to blood loss
5. Depending on setting, a CVP line may be possible, otherwise monitor haemodynamic response non-invasively
6. Instigate definitive management ie antibiotics, surgery etc

Response to fluid resuscitation

Initial fluid resuscitation can lead to three different types of response:

Rapid response:

- <20% fluid loss
- Rapid response to fluid replacement
- Patients remain haemodynamically stable when fluids are slowed or stopped

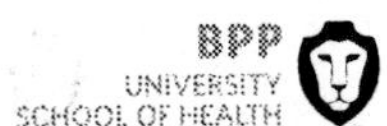

Transient response:

- 20–40% of fluid loss
- A small initial response to fluid therapy may be seen
- If the fluids are slowed they rapidly deteriorate and become haemodynamically unstable indicating inadequate fluid resuscitation or continuous haemorrhage
- These patients may require surgical management

No response:

- >40% of fluid loss
- Little or no response to fluid resuscitation
- Indicates severe haemorrhage which requires urgent blood replacement. Typically type-specific is used, which takes about ten minutes to prepare
- Urgent surgical intervention needed to control the haemorrhage
- There may be non-haemorrhagic causes of shock such as cardiac tamponade, which will not respond to fluid resuscitation
- Depending on the severity of shock and the degree of organ ischaemia, high level input (ie inotropic support and close monitoring (with arterial line and CV pressures) may be required on HDU or ITU

Stage	Blood loss (%)	Blood loss (ml)	Heart rate	BP	RR	Conscious state	Urine output	Fluid replacement
I	0–15	750	Normal	Normal	Normal	Mild anxiety	Normal	Crystalloid
II	15–30	750–1,500	>100	Normal	20–30	Agitated	20–30	Colloid
III	30–40	1,500–2,000	>120	Decreased	30–40	Confused	5–15	Colloid +/- Blood
IV	>40	> 2,000	>140	Decreased	>35	Drowsy/lethargic	0	Colloid +/- Blood

Table 6.3: Fluid distribution for an average 70 kg male

Further reading and references

1. Bulstrode, C.J.K., Russell, R.C.G. and Williams, N.S. (2000) *Bailey & Love's Short Practice of Surgery*. 23rd Edition. London: Arnold.
2. Calne, R., Ellis, H. and Whatson, C. (2002) *Lecture Notes on General Surgery*. 10th Edition. Oxford: Blackwell Publishing.
3. Goldberg, A. and Stansby, G. (2006) *Surgical Talk: Revision in Surgery*. 2nd Edition. London: Imperial College Press.
4. NICE. (2013) *Intravenous fluid therapy in adults in hospital* (CG174). [Online]. Available from: https://www.nice.org.uk/Guidance/CG174 [Accessed 7 November 2016].

Chapter 7

Clinical radiology

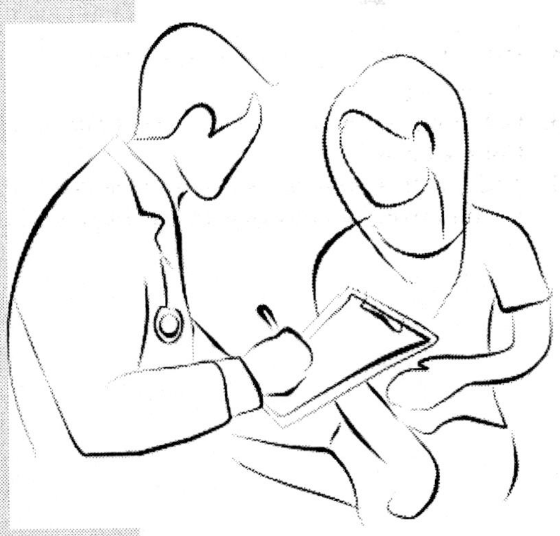

Chapter 7

Clinical radiology

When you no longer know what headache, heartache, or stomachache means without cistern punctures, electrocardiograms and six X-ray plates, you are slipping
Martin H. Fischer (1879–1962)

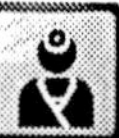

Introduction

The radiology department occupies a pivotal role in every medical institution. The majority of patients attending the outpatient or inpatient services of a hospital utilise their facilities.

Radiologists not only aid with a diagnosis but also offer valuable therapeutic services. For these simple reasons, it is paramount that you foster a congenial relationship with the radiology department.

Different imaging techniques

A radiologist has different imaging techniques in their armoury to answer a relevant clinical question. The selection of the appropriate technique is guided by multiple factors, some of which are:

- The clinical question
- Age of the patient
- Patient mobility
- Amount of radiation exposure
- Availability of facilities

In the UK, clinical radiation exposure of patients is guided by the basic principle of keeping all radiation exposures 'As Low As Reasonably Practical' (ALARP).

Plain film (X-ray/radiographs)

Plain films tend to be the first-line investigation of many common clinical presentations. Radiographs are performed relatively quickly and are available 24 hours a day and can even be done by the bedside of the patient in emergencies. These are useful in imaging patients presenting with cardiothoracic, musculoskeletal and gastrointestinal problems.

Fluoroscopy

Fluoroscopy is based on the same principles of radiographs and allows continuous, ie live, monitoring of the area of interest. Common procedures utilising fluoroscopy include: contrast examinations such as barium swallow/enema, IVP, etc (see Figure 7.1) and interventional procedures such as angiography, hepato-biliary or colonic stenting.

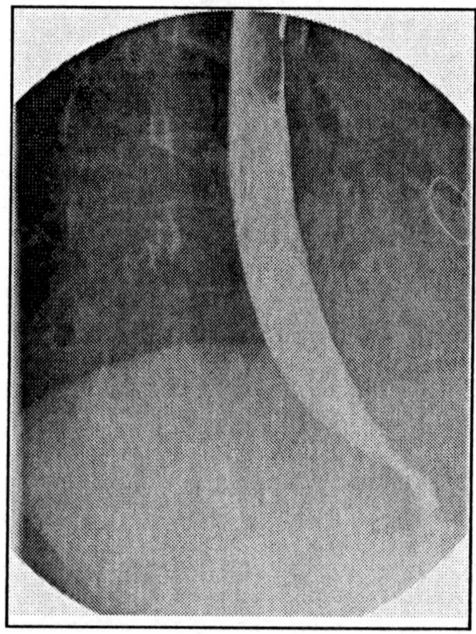

Figure 7.1: Static image from a barium swallow examination showing a normal distal oesophagus

Some of the contrast examinations are either being complemented or supplemented by other imaging techniques such as CT.

Ultrasound scans (USS)

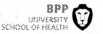

Ultrasound is perhaps the safest and most widely available imaging modality. USS does not involve any ionising radiation so it can be used for imaging pregnant women, children and young adults. USS works on the same principle as sonar used by submarines, ie sound waves are reflected back by tissues to form an image. As a Foundation Year (FY) doctor, you would be expected to organise a multitude of ultrasound scans in your day-to-day practice. The current clinical utilities of USS include:

- Imaging abdominal viscera
- Imaging chest/thorax for pleural effusions
- Visualising vascular abnormalities in DVT and strokes
- Imaging of soft tissues such as breasts
- Imaging of joints eg shoulder, wrist

USS guided interventions are also available such as biopsies and drain insertion. Recent BTS and NICE guidelines advocate the use of ultrasound imaging for inserting all central venous catheters and chest drains.

Computed tomography

Recent technological advances in CT have revolutionised the world of medical imaging. The current generation MDCT allows rapid acquisition of a significant amount of data in a single breath hold. MDCT imparts a relatively higher dose of radiation than plain films and fluoroscopy, hence extra care should be taken prior to requesting an MDCT examination. MDCT is commonly used for diagnosing pathologies of the chest, abdomen, pelvis and brain (see Figure 7.3).

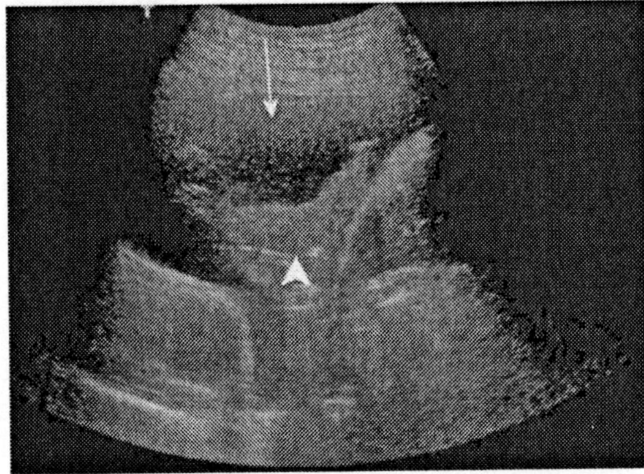

Figure 7.2: USS image of right chest showing a moderate sized effusion (arrow) and the underlying collapsed lung (arrowhead)

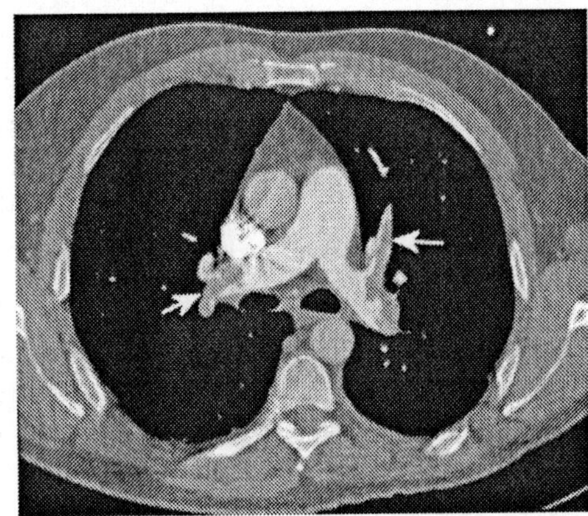

Figure 7.3: Computer tomography pulmonary angiogram (CTPA) showing filling defects (arrows) that can be seen as dark areas in the pulmonary arteries in keeping with pulmonary embolus

Magnetic resonance imaging (MRI)

MRI is another modality that has come on in leaps and bounds in the last decade due to technical advances. MRI is based on magnetic properties of the hydrogen nuclei found within the hydrogen atom. Given that the majority of the body consists of fluid, which is made of hydrogen atoms and nuclei, nearly every part of the body can be imaged with MRI. The relative advantages and disadvantages of MRI are shown in Table 7.1.

MRI is widely used for imaging brain, heart, liver and musculoskeletal pathologies. It has two basic imaging sequences, T1 and T2. In T2 sequence fluids CSF, effusion, ascites etc) appear bright and it appears dark on T1 sequence. T1 sequences are good at depicting the anatomy while T2 are good at highlighting areas of inflammation (see Figure 7.4).

Advantages	Disadvantages
Lack of exposure to ionising radiation	Longer scan times
High quality detailed images	Expensive equipment
Ability to produce images in all three planes (axial, coronal and sagittal)	Significant contraindications including defibrillators/ some pacemakers, metallic neurosurgical clips

Table 7.1: The advantages and disadvantages of MRI

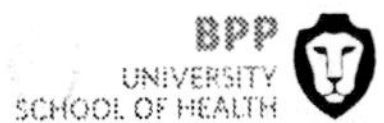

Radionuclide imaging

Radionuclide imaging makes use of radioactive isotopes for the diagnosis of diseases. The radiation dose from isotope studies can vary depending on the isotope used and the part of the body imaged.

Most common nuclear studies that you might come across are shown in Table 7.2.

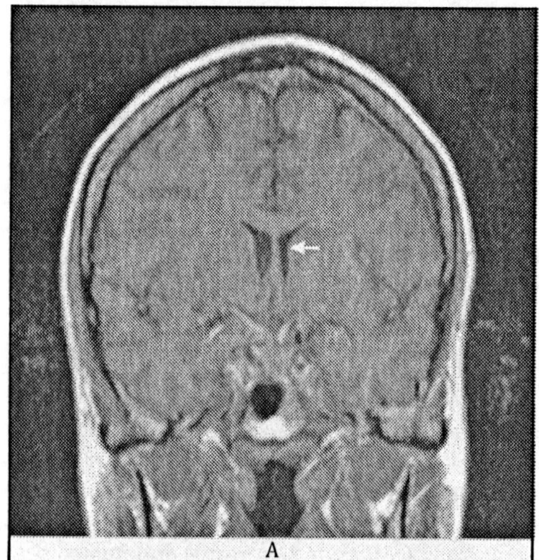

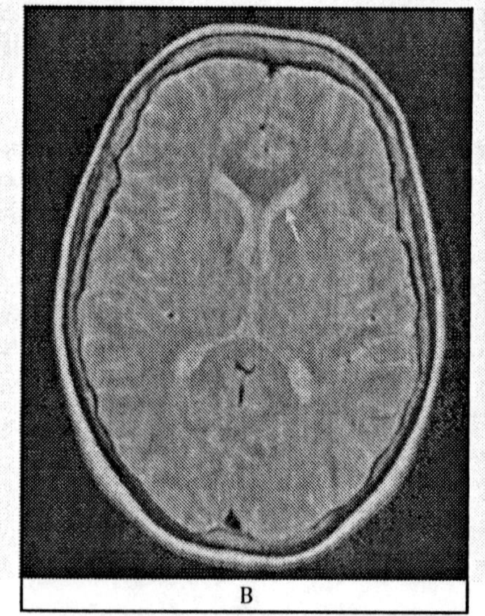

Figure 7.4: (A) MRI of the brain in coronal plane showing dark CSF (arrow) in keeping with T1-weighted image. (B) MRI of the brain in axial plane pointing at CSF (arrow) that is bright, in other words T2-weighted image

Radionuclide imaging technique	Indication
Ventilation Perfusion (V/Q)	Detecting pulmonary embolism for patients who cannot have CT
Bone scan	Detect metastasis
Renal isotope study	Assess function and anatomy
Cardiac and oncology imaging (see Figure 7.6)	Analyse molecular and functional data

Table 7.2: Types of radionuclide imaging techniques and their indications

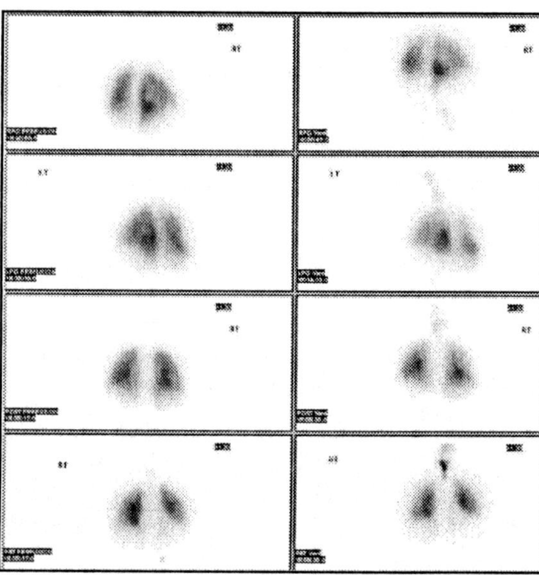

Figure 7.5: Normal V/Q scan of the chest. Images on the left depict the perfusion of lungs while the ones on the right depict ventilation

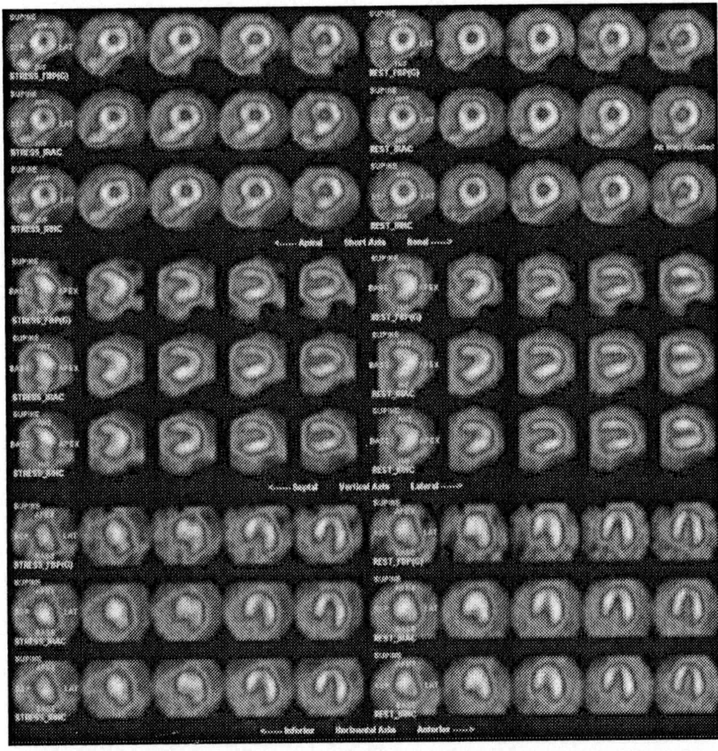

Figure 7.6: Image of a normal myocardial radionuclide perfusion study. The lighter areas denote the uptake of tracer material by viable myocardium implying adequate perfusion. Images can be reconstructed in different planes (short, vertical and horizontal axis) and are acquired at both rest and stress to demonstrate stress induced perfusion defect

Modality	Equivalent period of natural background radiation
X-ray/radiography	Days to months
Chest X-ray (CXR)	3 days
Abdominal X-ray (AXR)	4 months
Fluoroscopy/angiography	Months to years
Barium swallow	8 months
Barium enema	3.2 years
CT	Months to years
CT head	10 months
CT chest	3.6 years
CT abdomen or pelvis	4.5 years
Radionucleotide imaging	Months to years
V/Q	7 months
Cardiac perfusion	2.7 years
Positron emission tomography (PET) of the head	2.3 years

Table 7.3: Different imaging techniques with respective equivalent background natural radiation. (RCR 2007) (Hart & Wall 2002)

Radiation dosage

All clinicians should aspire to keep radiation exposures as low as reasonably practical in accordance with 'ALARP'. This is important as excessive radiation exposure can cause serious physical and genetic damage. Table 7.3 outlines the commonly used imaging studies with their respective equivalent radiation dose compared to the natural background radiation. This information should help you in weighing the risk/benefit ratio of each test prior to requesting it.

How to read X-rays

Chest X-ray

1	Confirm the identity of the patient
2	Confirm the date of the examination
3	Confirm which size is left and right
4	Confirm whether the investigation is antero-posterior (AP) or postero-anterior (PA)
5	Confirm whether the film is technically adequate
6	Identify any iatrogenic structures
7	Examine the trachea and bronchi
8	Examine hilar structures
9	Examine the lung fields
10	Examine the heart and mediastinum
11	Examine the diaphragm and area immediately below it
12	Examine any soft tissues and bones

Table 7.4: Systematic approach to examining a CXR

This is perhaps the most common investigation that a foundation doctor will come across. In order to avoid making unnecessary errors of interpretation, especially early on, emphasis should be on 'things not to miss' rather than 'what is the diagnosis'. To successfully achieve this, a systematic approach is suggested for reviewing a CXR (see Table 7.4).

AP or PA

A CXR can be acquired by passing the X-ray beam from front to back (AP), from back to front (PA), or from side to side (lateral). Patients who are bedbound tend to have AP films while patients who are mobile have PA films taken. An AP film will usually have an annotation (supine, AP), which should make it easier to decide (see Figure 7.7). Only PA films allow you to accurately assess the size of the heart.

Technical adequacy

In order to facilitate accurate interpretation, there needs to be:

- **Non-rotation**: the spinous processes located midway between the two medial clavicle heads
- **Adequate inspiration**: the diaphragm should be intersected by the 5th–7th anterior ribs in the mid-clavicular line
- **Appropriate exposure**: the vertebrae should be just visible behind the heart

Identify any iatrogenic structures

ET tube tips should lie about two inches above the carina, nasogastric (NG) tubes should be below the level of diaphragm, and central venous catheter (subclavian or internal jugular) tips should be at the level of second costo-chondral junction ie superior vena cava (see Figures 7.7, 7.8 and 7.9).

The location of chest drains will vary depending on the clinical indication for drainage. For example the tip of the drain should ideally be at the base for pleural effusions. The draining holes need to be in the thoracic cavity rather than subcutaneous layer, as the latter will lead to extensive subcutaneous emphysema.

Trachea and bronchi

Is the trachea centrally located between the two medial clavicle heads? This may be important in differentiating simple from tension pneumothoraces and is also useful if soft tissue masses are present. Follow the trachea to the carina (level T4/5) and the bronchi into the lungs. Is there any obvious deviation or obstruction?

Hilar structures

Each hilar contains the pulmonary vessels and primary bronchi. There are also some lymph nodes located here that are not usually visible on CXR. Commonly the left hilum is slightly higher than the right, but both should be a similar size and density – if they are not, it is suspicious.

Lungs

Spend time looking at each lung from the apex to the base. In a pneumothorax, you would see the pleural margin and there will be a lack of vascular markings beyond this margin. Tension pneumothorax is a medical emergency whereby there is contralateral mediastinal shift due to increasing pressure, ie size of pneumothorax (see Figure 7.9).

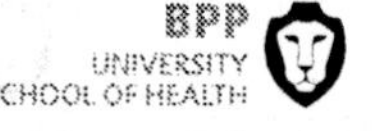

Pleural effusions will appear different depending on how the film was taken. On an erect CXR, the effusion gravitates to the lung bases and therefore it is seen as a white opacity with a meniscus (see Figure 7.10). On the other hand, if the patient was in a supine position during the CXR, then the fluid gravitates to the posterior lung and the lung would appear hazy and whiter compared to the other side with no obvious meniscus (see Figure 7.11).

Consolidation on a CXR is essentially pulmonary. In most cases, consolidation secondary to fluid replacement can be differentiated from that due to tissue replacement with the help of clinical history and the CXR as the latter tends to be more focal and well defined (see Figure 7.12).

Lobar collapse is seen as increased opacity in a lung with loss of volume and ipsilateral shift of the mediastinum. The affected lobe can be localised by simple silhouette principles, for example: if the opacification is caused by replacement of air in the distal air spaces by fluid (transudate, exudate or blood) or tissue (carcinoma, lymphoma). If the opacity obscures the right heart border then the involved lobe is the middle lobe of the right lung, whereas if the left heart border is obscured it is the lingula part of the left upper lobe that is involved. In a similar fashion, if the diaphragm is obscured by the opacity then the affected lobe is the lower lobe (see Figure 7.13).

Heart and mediastinum

Trace the outline of the great vessels and heart. These should be clearly defined and the cardiophrenic angles should be visible. If they are not, it is suggestive of consolidation in the lungs or an effusion.

Calculate the caridiothoracic ratio. This is the proportion of the thorax occupied by the heart and, if greater than 50%, is considered abnormal. As mentioned above, this is only accurate if the film is PA as an AP view exaggerates the heart size (see Figure 7.14).

The mediastinum contains the heart and great vessels (middle mediastinum) and potential spaces in front, behind and above the heart (anterior, posterior and superior mediastinum). These spaces are not usually defined on an X-ray, but an awareness of their position can help identify and describe disease processes.

Identify the aortic knuckle, aorto-pulmonary window and the right paratracheal stripe. These represent the left lateral edge of the aorta, which may be enlarged in aneurysmal disease; a potential space between the arch of the aorta and pulmonary arteries where lymph nodes may enlarge; and the right edge of the trachea.

Review areas

Review the diaphragm and the area immediately below it. Any free air here is indicative of a possible ruptured viscera (see Figure 7.16).

Look for any obvious soft tissue abnormalities, which may include areas of swelling (often only noticed because they distort other structures) and surgical emphysema.

Finally, look for any bony abnormalities. Examine any visible long bones, the ribs, clavicles etc. It is all too easy to miss something if you do not deliberately look for it.

Be careful you do not miss any obvious abnormalities in your desire to be systematic. When asked to present an X-ray, a suggested format would be:

'This is:

- An AP/PA plain chest radiograph
- Of [Patient's name]
- Taken on [date]
- It is technically adequate [or why not]
- The most obvious abnormality is...
- On further examination I note a central trachea, normal lung fields, normal cardiac and mediastinal structures and diaphragm. There are no obvious bony or soft tissue abnormalities (if there are any abnormalities then state what they are)'

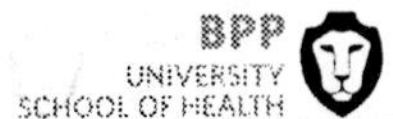

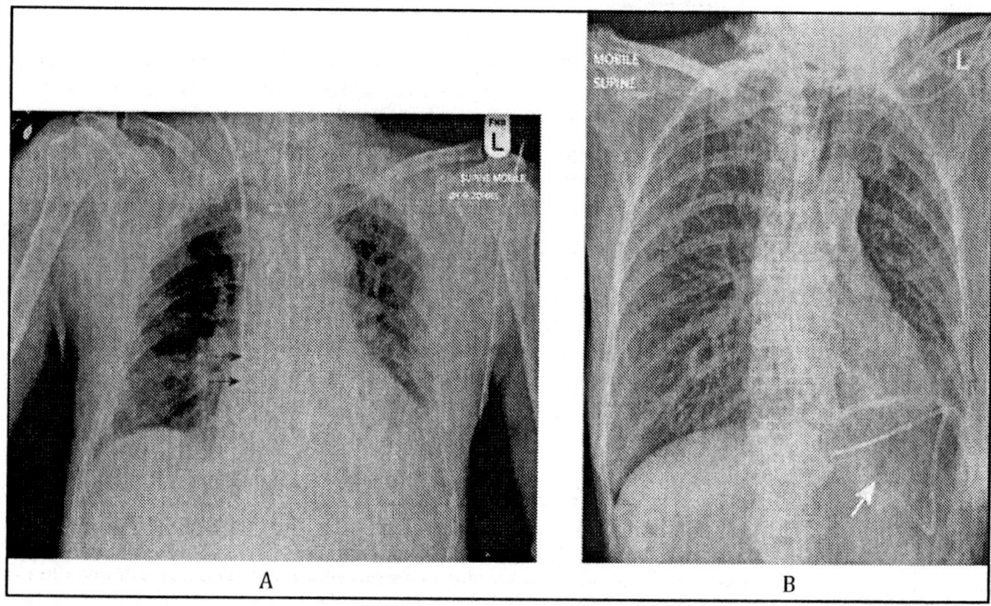

Figure 7.7: (A) Supine CXR with an Endo Tracheal tube (white arrow with ball) and a Swan Ganz catheter (black arrow) with its tip in the pulmonary artery. In the background you can also see a prosthetic valve and mediastinal drain. (B) CXR showing a NG tube coiled in the stomach below the diaphragm (white arrow)

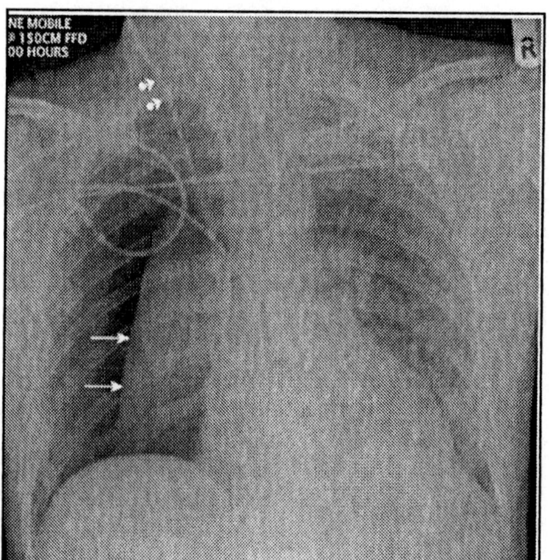

Figure 7.8: CXR showing the collapsed lung edge (white arrow) in a large right tension pneumothorax following an internal jugular line insertion (arrow with ball)

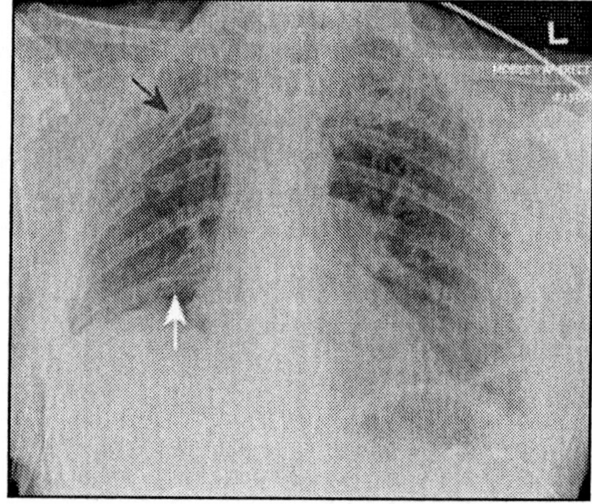

Figure 7.9: AP CXR of a patient with an apical (black arrow) and basal (white arrow) chest drain

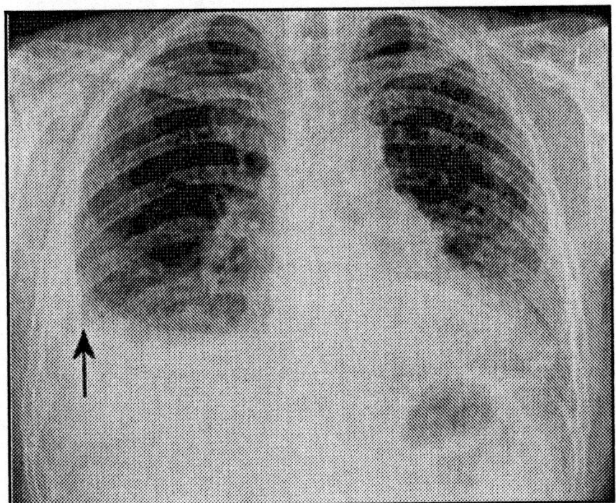

Figure 7.10: Moderate sized right pleural effusion with the meniscus sign (arrow) on an erect CXR

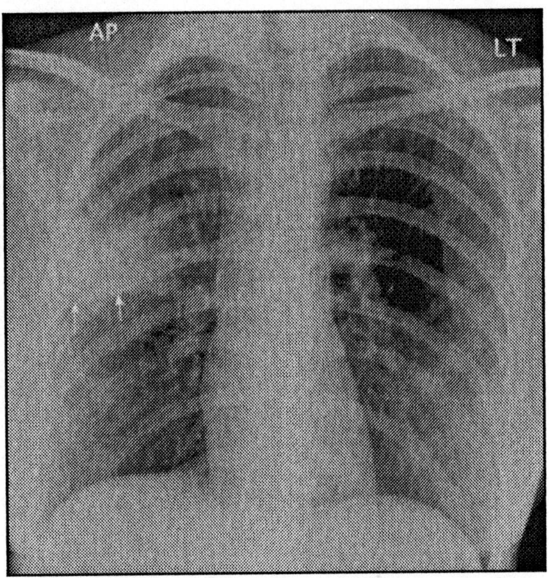

Figure 7.12: AP CXR with increased opacity in the right mid zone in keeping with consolidation. The horizontal fissure is clearly visible (arrows) confirming the involvement of the right upper lobe

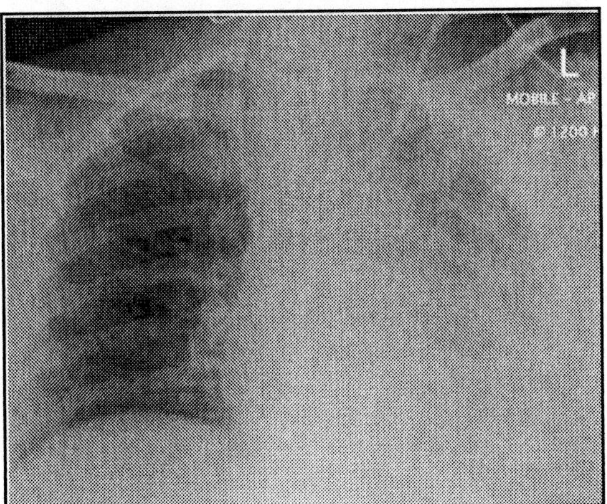

Figure 7.11: Mobile AP supine CXR, note the diffuse increased opacification of left lung compared to the right due to underlying pleural effusion

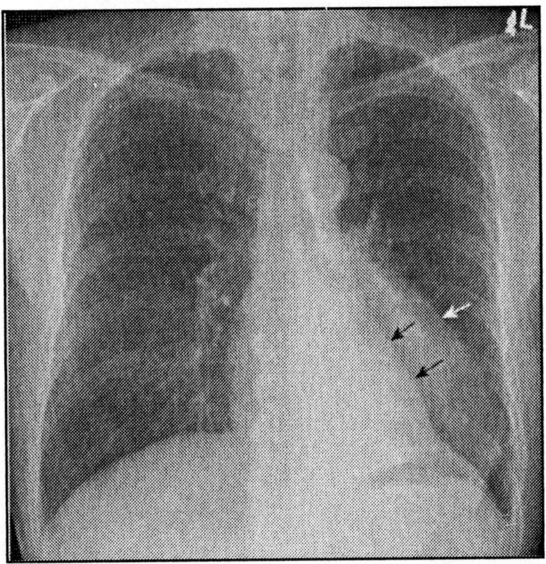

Figure 7.13: Left lower lobe collapse on a CXR. Note the obscured medial aspect of the left hemidiaphragm due to collapsed lung (black arrow), which is projected behind the heart (white arrow)

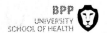

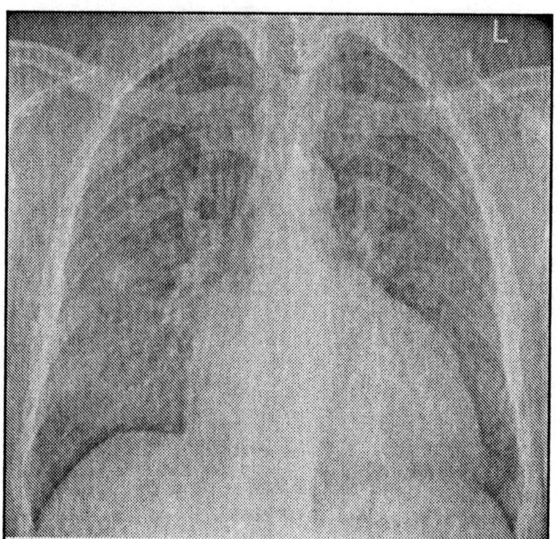

Figure 7.14: PA CXR in a patient with cardiomegaly where cardiac shadow is more than 50% of the thoracic width. This is secondary to dilated cardiomyopathy

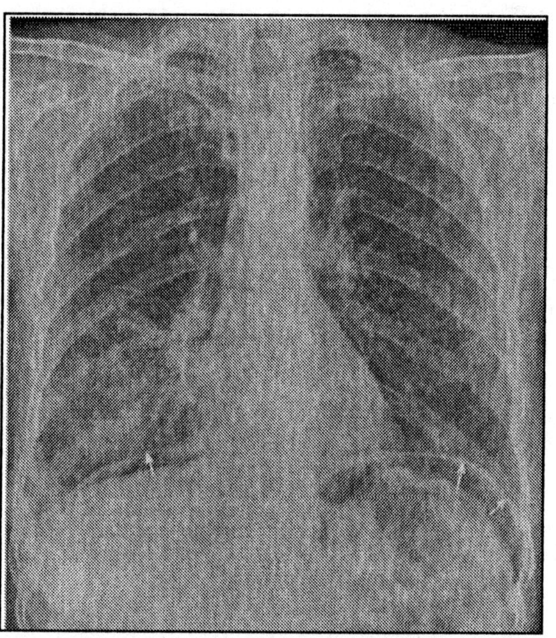

Figure 7.16: CXR of a 55-year-old man who presented with central chest pain. Note extensive free intra-peritoneal air under the diaphragm (arrows) in keeping with abdominal viscera perforation

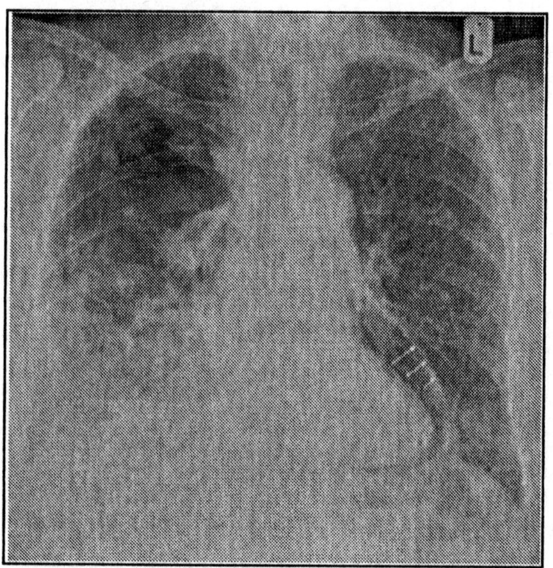

Figure 7.15: CXR following right pleura resection shows opacification in the right lower zone in keeping with recent surgery and extensive air outlining the pericardial surface (arrows) in keeping with pneumo-mediastinum

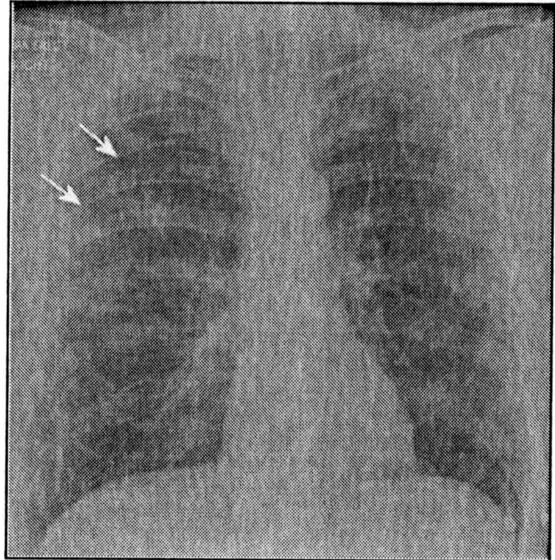

Figure 7.17: Erect CXR of a patient who presented at the chest outpatient department with cough. A small right apical pneumothorax (arrows) is seen but this can be easily missed if not reviewed thoroughly

Abdominal X-ray

The most common indications for AXRs are suspected small bowel obstructions or suspected large bowel obstructions. AXR is not the investigation of choice if a hollow viscera perforation is suspected. An erect CXR is more likely to pick up free air than an AXR. In a normal AXR, air is within the stomach, in two to three loops of small bowel and the distal large bowel (sigmoid and rectum) (see Figure 7.18).

Small bowel obstruction

Central distended loops of bowel with very little gas in the colon, especially rectum, is suggestive of small bowel obstruction. The valvulae (intra-luminal markings) extend from one end of the lumen to the other (see Figure 7.19).

Large bowel obstruction

Peripheral distended loops of bowel where haustral markings do not extend from wall to wall is suggestive of large bowel obstruction (see Figure 7.20). The rectum and sigmoid colon might not have any air if the obstruction is proximal to the sigmoid colon. The central small bowel loops may or may not be dilated depending on the competency of the ilio-caecal valve. Sigmoid and caecal volvulus appear as extensively distended loops of large bowel.

Ileus

An ileus is commonly seen in patients with reduced mobility during the post-operative period or in intensive care patients. There is distension with air in both small and large bowel including the rectum (see Figure 7.21). This is a clinico-radiological diagnosis and correlation with biochemical profile, especially potassium, levels are necessary.

Hollow viscera perforation

Free intra-peritoneal air can be difficult to detect on an AXR. When present, you will be able to see a clear outline of the bowel wall due to the presence of air on either side of it (Rigler sign). This is a surgical emergency (see Figure 7.22).

Renal calculi

Renal calculi can be present in the kidney, bladder or along the ureters and are seen as high-density foci. Non-contrast CT has a better sensitivity and specificity, compared to plain film, in detecting renal

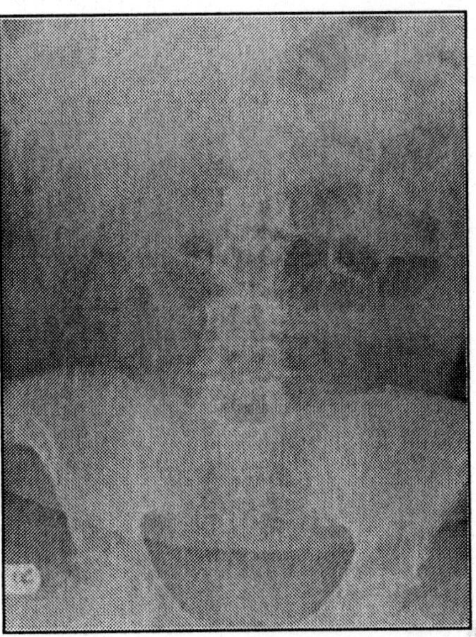

Figure 7.18: A normal AXR of a young female patient showing normal small and large bowel loops

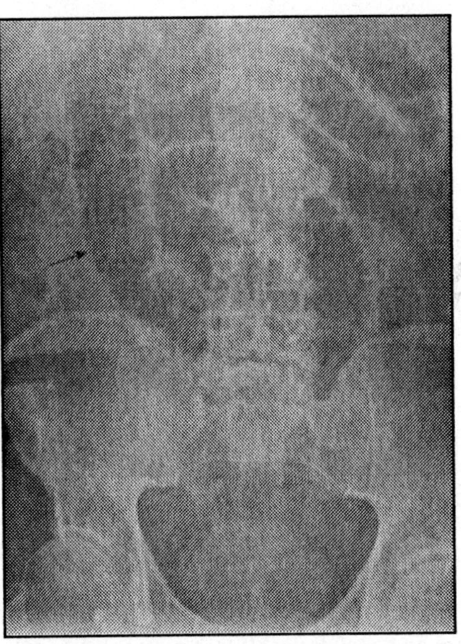

Figure 7.19: AXR of a 70-year-old man who presented with abdominal pain, vomiting and distension. There is extensive dilatation of central small bowel loops (arrow) with very little air in distal large bowel, in keeping with small bowel obstruction

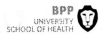

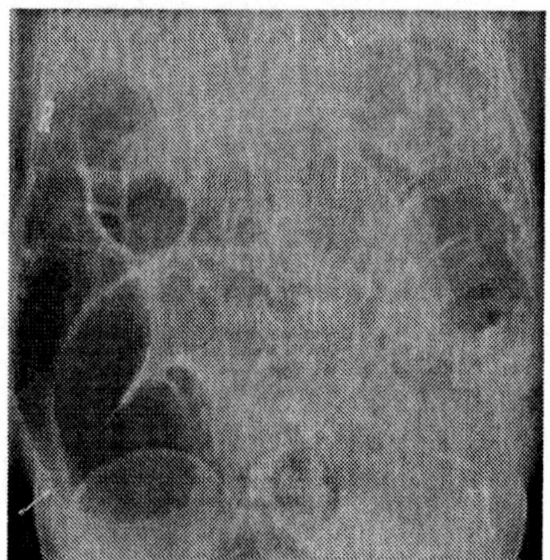

Figure 7.20: AXR of an 80-year-old woman who presented with abdominal distension and constipation. Note dilated peripheral loops of bowel (arrows) with a lack of complete haustral markings in keeping with large bowel obstruction

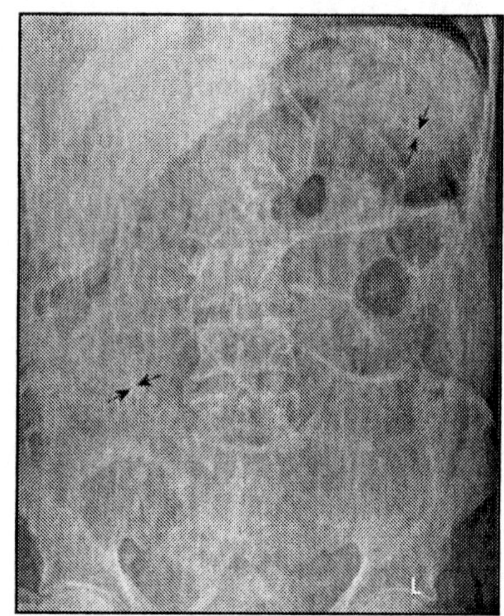

Figure 7.22: AXR demonstrating central small bowel obstruction in a patient who presented with abdominal pain. In this film it is possible to delineate both sides of the bowel wall (arrow), compared to Figure 7.21 where only the internal aspect of the wall is clearly seen, in keeping with free intra-peritoneal air (Rigler sign)

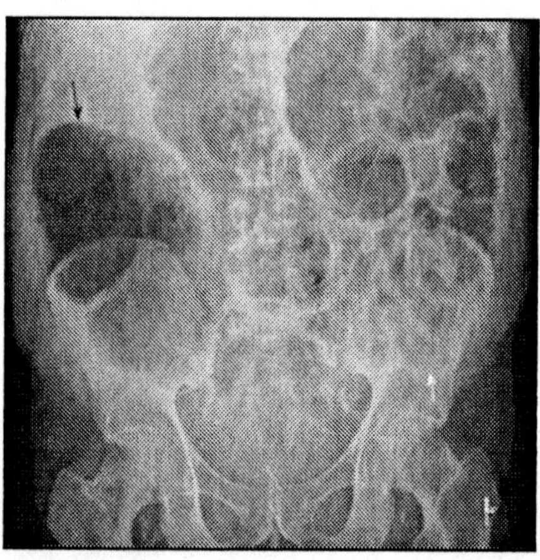

Figure 7.21: AXR demonstrating dilated small (white arrow) and large bowel (black arrow) loops with some air in the rectum in a patient post-sternotomy

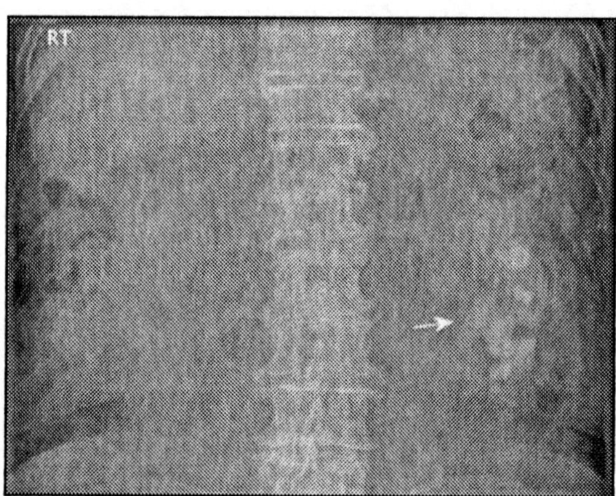

Figure 7.23: Focused AXR of the kidneys demonstrating extensive calcification filling the pelvic calyceal system of the left kidney (arrow) in keeping with a Staghorn calculus

stones but may not be the first-line investigation in your centre (see Figure 7.23).

CT head

In line with the NICE guidelines, a significant number of patients with head injury are investigated with a CT scan of the head. As an FY doctor you might be quizzed or asked to review a CT head scan but in routine practice a radiologist reports these. Some examples of common acute pathologies found in such scans have been described.

Stroke

The different types of stroke and their appearance on CT are summarised in Table 7.5.

Extradural haemorrhage

Extradural haemorrhage is usually due to an arterial bleed secondary to trauma. It is seen as a localised peripheral area of hyper-density (blood) that has a convex internal margin and does not cross suture lines. This is a surgical emergency as there is usually associated midline shift to the contralateral side with increasing risk of coning/brain herniation (see Figure 7.26).

Type of stroke	Appearance on CT
Ischaemic	Usually seen as area of hypodensity (dark) in one cerebral hemisphere (see Figure 7.26)
Haemorrhagic	Haemorrhage is seen as an area of hyper-density (bright) (see Figure 7.27). Haemorrhagic stroke has areas of both hyper- and hypodensity and is one of the main contraindications for thrombolysis.

Table 7.5: The different types of stroke and their imaging appearance

Subdural haemorrhage

Subdural haemorrhage is secondary to a venous bleed and is commonly seen in elderly patients. In the acute phase it is seen as a hyper-dense peripheral area that has concave internal margins. The management can either be conservative or surgical depending on the size of the haemorrhage and the patient's clinical condition. In subacute and chronic stages the haemorrhage tends to decrease in density and become isodense to the brain parenchyma (see Figure 7.27).

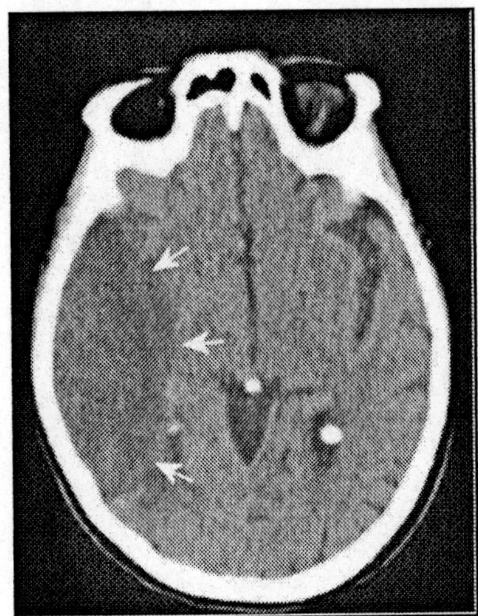

Figure 7.24: Non-contrast CT head showing a large area of hypodensity in the right temporo-parietal lobe (arrows) in keeping with an acute ischaemic infarct in the middle cerebral artery territory

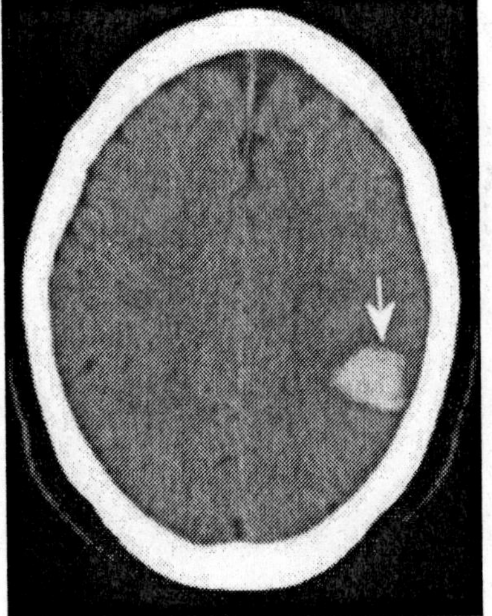

Figure 7.25: CT head showing focal area of increased density (arrow) in the left parietal lobe with minimal surrounding hypodensity

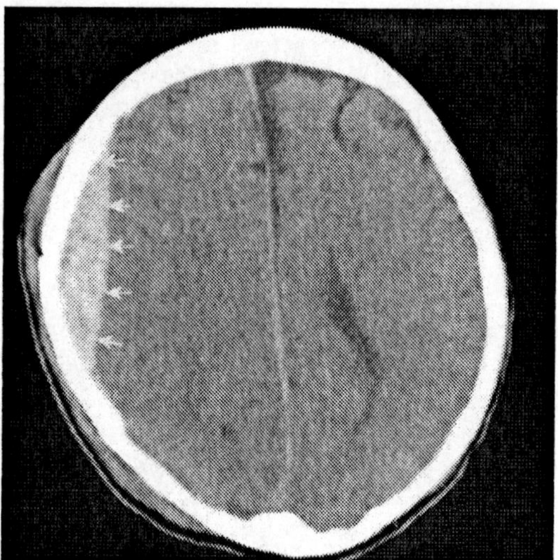

Figure 7.26: Non-contrast CT head showing a peripheral hyper-dense area in the right cerebral hemisphere. Note the convex internal outline (arrows) in keeping with an acute extradural haemorrhage

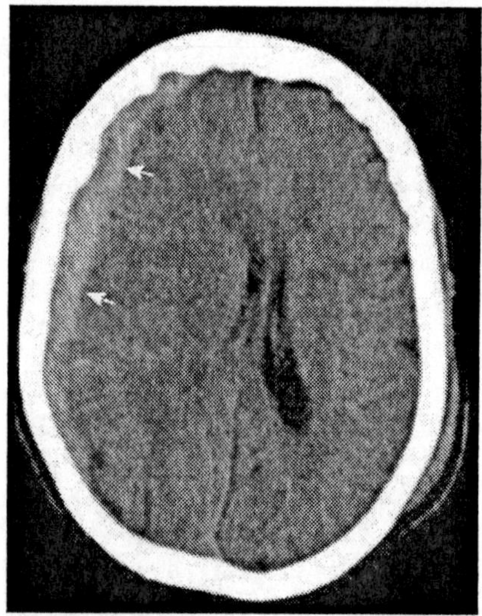

Figure 7.27: Non-contrast CT head showing the relatively hyper-dense region outlining the right cerebral cortex; this has an internal concave outline (arrows) in keeping with an acute subdural haemorrhage

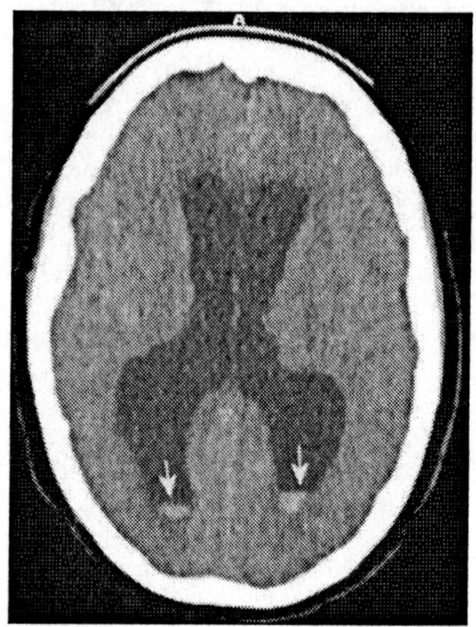

Figure 7.28: Non-contrast CT head showing dilated lateral ventricles with layering of hyper-dense blood in the occipital horns (arrows). This patient had a subarachnoid haemorrhage with intra-ventricular spread and secondary hydrocephalus

Cerebral contusion/haemorrhage

Cerebral contusion/haemorrhage is seen as a focal area of increased density. These are usually seen secondary to head injury, underlying brain malignancy or coagulopathy (see Figure 7.24 and 7.25).

Hydrocephalus

Hydrocephalus is secondary to blockage of CSF outflow in the ventricles. It can be secondary to multiple pathologies and is usually seen as dilated ventricles, especially the temporal horn of the lateral ventricles (see Figure 7.28).

Skull fractures

CT is the investigation of choice as skull X-rays are no longer used to diagnose skull fractures.

Pelvic and hip radiographs

Hip fractures are unfortunately becoming increasingly common given the changing demographics in society, resulting in an increasing proportion of elderly individuals prone to falling.

Such patients tend to present with an inability to weight bear, tenderness on palpation and movement of the affected hip joint and a shortened, externally rotated leg. However, beware the compacted, easily missed fractures, which tend just to present with tenderness and a difficulty weightbearing. AP pelvic and lateral hip X-rays are the best investigations for assessing any patient with a suspected hip fracture, with a CT or MRI scan being second line if there is any uncertainty about the diagnosis.

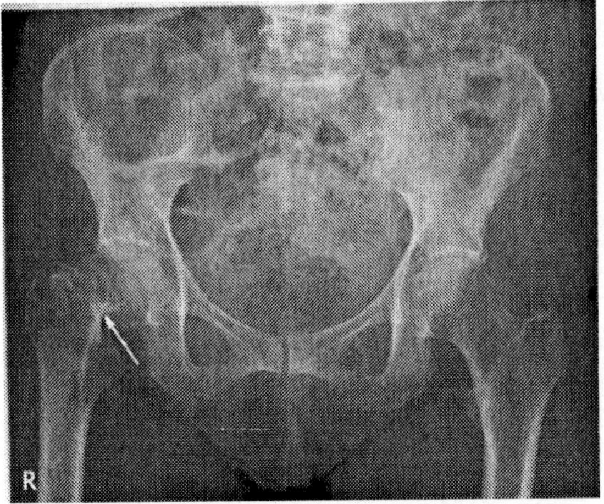

Figure 7.29: Displaced intracapsular hip fracture

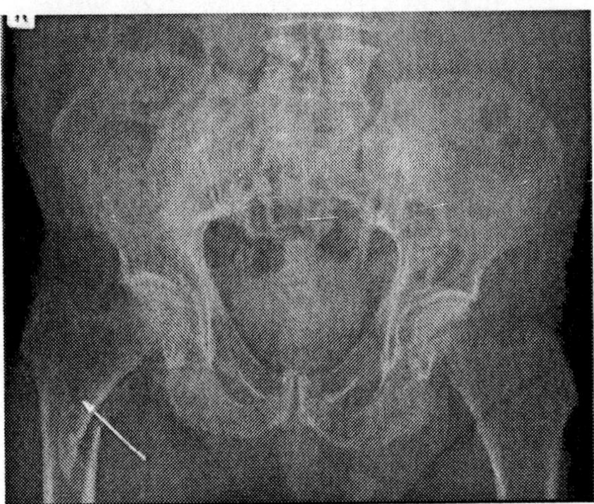

Figure 7.30: Displaced Intertrochanteric hip fracture

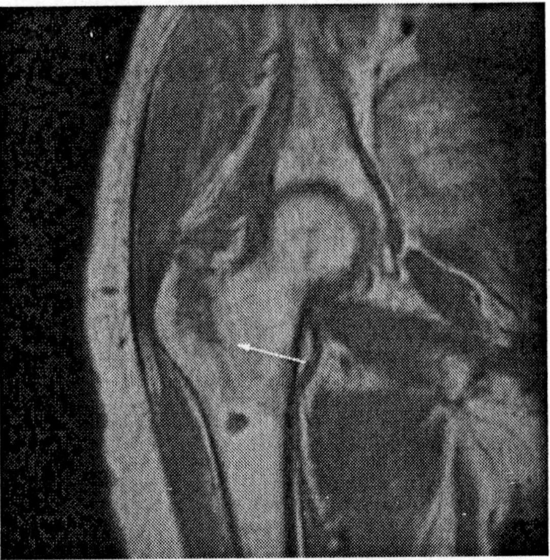

Figure 7.31: MRI showing non-displaced intertrochanteric hip fracture

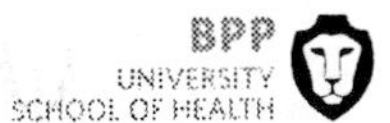

Communicating with the radiologist

A foundation doctor is responsible for the organisation and co-ordination of essential imaging investigations for inpatients. Many of these will be performed on the basis of the clinical information you provide either on the request card or during your discussion with the radiologist. Some of the points you should consider while requesting a radiological investigation are described below:

- **Has this test been done already?** Every attempt should be made to avoid repeating tests by getting previous images and reports.
- **Do I need it?** The results of some tests are unlikely to affect patient management because either they are unexpected or they are irrelevant.
- **When do I need it?** If it is not required for urgent management, do **not** request it urgently. However, if it is needed as soon as possible then discuss the investigation with the on-call radiology team.
- **Is this the best investigation?** If in doubt discuss with a radiologist. Prior to any discussion with a radiologist ensure that you have gone through the clinical notes and are aware of the differential diagnosis.
- **Have I explained the problem?** Make sure your handwriting is legible, all the relevant clinical details are provided and relevant questions asked. If irrelevant clinical details are provided the reports are likely to be clinically irrelevant. In other words, 'garbage in, garbage out'.

Head-to-toe case-based imaging

Knowing what radiological tests to do and when to do them will not only aid patient care but will also reduce unnecessary time wasting for all. Table 7.7 gives examples of the most appropriate imaging techniques for the patient's presenting symptoms.

Clinical presentation	Primary imaging test	Secondary/definitive imaging test
Head injury (vomiting, focal neuralgia, headache, etc)	CT head	–
Headache, vomiting, visual disturbance (query subarachnoid haemorrhage)	CT head	Lumbar puncture
Acute stroke, transient ischaemic attack (TIA)	CT head	MRI
Neck pain (road traffic accident (RTA))	Cervical spine X-ray	CT cervical spine
Chest pain (pulmonary emboli (PE), aortic dissection, acute coronary syndrome (ACS))	CXR	CT, MRI, V/Q
Cough, fever (pyrexia of unknown origin (PUO))	CXR	CT chest
Haemoptysis, weight loss (malignancy)	CXR	CT chest
Upper abdominal pain (gallstones, pancreatitis)	Erect CXR	USS, CT, MRI
Loin to groin pain (renal colic)	X-Ray kidneys-ureters-bladder (KUB)	USS, CT KUB
Acute loin pain, hypotension (abdominal aortic aneurysm)	USS	CT abdomen and pelvis
Abdominal pain, distension and constipation (small or large bowel obstruction)	Erect CXR, AXR	CT abdomen and pelvis
Change in bowel habit, weight loss (large bowel malignancy)	Colonoscopy	CT abdomen and pelvis
Acute limb ischaemia	CXR	Angiography
Swollen calf (query DVT)	USS	CT, venography

Table 7.6: Appropriate imaging techniques for the patient's presenting symptoms

Further reading and references

1. Agramunt, M., Coronel, B., Errando, J., et al. (2004) Suspected ureteral colic: plain film and sonography vs. unenhanced helical CT. A prospective study in 66 patients. *European Radiology* 2004; 14: 129–36.
2. Bankier, A.A., Hansell, D.M., MacMahon, H., et al. (2008) Fleischner Society: glossary of terms for thoracic imaging, *Radiology* 2008; 246(3): 697–722.
3. Duffy, J., Laws, D. and Neville, E. Pleural Diseases Group, Standards of Care Committee, British Thoracic Society. (2003) BTS guidelines for the insertion of a chest drain, *Thorax* 2003; 58 Suppl 2: ii53–9.
4. Hart, D.H. and Wall, B.F.W. (2002) *Radiation exposure of the UK population from medical and dental X-ray Examinations. Didcot: National Radiological Protection Board.* [Online]. Available from: http://cloud.medicalphysicist.co.uk/nrpb_w4.pdf [Accessed 7 November 2016].
5. Health and Safety Executive. (1999) *Ionising Radiations Regulations.* Statutory Instrument 1999 No. 3232.
6. Khoo, T.K., Lin, M.B. and The, H.S. (2001) Flank pain: is Intravenous Urogram necessary? *Singapore Medical Journal* 2001; 42(9): 425–7.
7. Ly, J.Q. (2003) The Rigler sign. *Radiology* 2003; 228(3): 706–7.
8. National Institute for Health and Clinical Excellence. (2002) *Guidance on the use of ultrasound locating devices for placing central venous catheters* (TA49). [Online]. Available from: www.nice.org.uk/guidance/ta49 [Accessed 7 November 2016].
9. National Institute for Health and Clinical Excellence. (2007) *Head injury. Triage, assessment, investigation and early management of head injury in infants, children and adults* (CG56). [Online]. Available from: www.nice.org.uk/guidance/cg56 [Accessed 7 November 2016].
10. RCR. (2007) *Making the best use of clinical radiology services – Referral Guidelines.* 6th Edition. London: Royal College of Radiologists.

Chapter 8

Practical prescribing

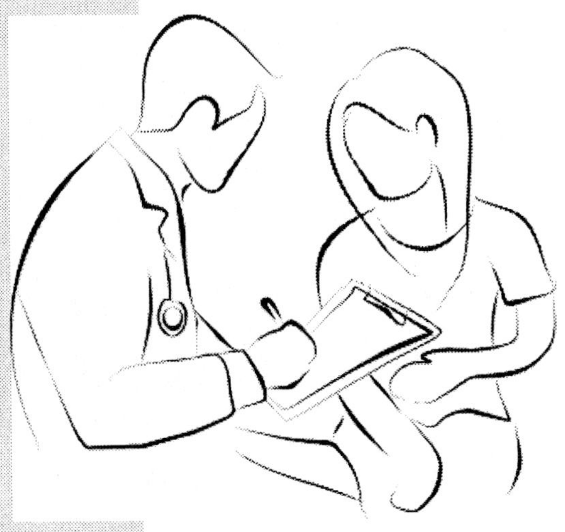

Chapter 8

Practical prescribing

All who drink of this remedy recover in a short time, except those whom it does not help, who all die. Therefore it is obvious that it fails only in incurable cases

Galen, 2nd century

Introduction

Prescribing mishaps make a major contribution to hospital adverse events and medico-legal activities. It is estimated that 7% of hospital admissions are related to medication problems, which may rise to 30% in the typical elderly medical intake, and these account for 4,000 to 7,000 deaths per year in the UK. The financial implications of this for the NHS are also great. The leading cause of medical injury in hospital practice is adverse drug events, about half of which are error-related, whilst reports from independent insurers show that injuries caused by drugs are the most common reason for procedure-related malpractice claims.

Many of these mishaps are blamed on FY doctors even though the chain of events usually includes someone else. Adverse events, a term officially used to describe any kind of mishap without attributing blame, nearly always involves several people, each of whom could have prevented the event if they had been on top form that day. It is therefore essential that when prescribing you do not assume someone else will cover for any of your errors.

However, prescribing is not just about avoiding errors but also achieving the best for patients. This chapter outlines some important features of prescribing in general and then details a few specific areas that are known to trouble new prescribers.

Prescribing is about communicating

It may sound obvious, but the act of prescribing is to communicate the prescriber's intentions for a patient to the persons who will dispense or administer the drugs and to the patient themselves. For this to work properly, the very minimum information required is the drug name, form (liquid, cream, patch, etc), dose, route, and frequency of administration. There are also legalities such as signature, date and additional instructions which might include duration of treatment, precautions or limitations such as 'only if diastolic blood pressure >60 mmHg', or other notes.

In surveys in Thames Valley hospitals, 21% of inpatient drug prescriptions lacked even the basic information and 32% were endorsed by a pharmacist to provide the necessary warnings and advice for the nurses to administer the drug safely. 80% of patients had their charts endorsed by pharmacists.

Remember that you are not the only person who gets tired on duty. Even nurses can lose concentration or fail to read your mind accurately in the absence of a clear prescription!

Avoiding errors

1. Complete every box.
2. Write in BLOCK CAPITALS. Once you get into the habit it does not slow you down too much and it does prevent a lot of confusion. There are numerous cases of poor handwriting leading to the wrong drug being given and the patient suffering.
3. Do not use unorthodox abbreviations. Patients who should have had zidovudine have been given azathioprine because someone wrote 'AZT' on a chart, thinking everyone would know what it meant.
4. The dose should be specified clearly in appropriate units. Never abbreviate the word 'units' to 'U' because it looks too much like an extra zero and many patients have had a ten-fold overdose of insulin or heparin as a result. 'Micrograms' and 'nanograms' should never be abbreviated. Doses less than 1 mg are more likely to be given correctly if written as micrograms eg DIGOXIN 125 micrograms rather than 0.125 mg.
5. Do not write several routes down eg IV/IM/oral, unless the dose is the same for each route. If you do want to give nurses the option, make it clear which is the preferred route.

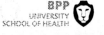

6. Make sure the dosing frequency and times of administration match and the times suit the nursing procedures as well as the patient's needs.
7. If writing a *prn* drug make the indication clear, for example when prescribing Codeine make sure to indicate whether it is for pain or diarrhoea. If prescribing two *prn* analgesics, which one should the nurse give and in what circumstances?
8. Specify any restrictions very clearly. Heart failure drugs may be required even if the blood pressure is low whereas the same drug given for hypertension is contraindicated when the pressure drops. Consider what you write in the patient's notes as well as on the chart; will a cover doctor know what to do when the nurse calls them on the weekend?
9. The differences between brands of the same medication are closely controlled by the licensing authorities and are often not important; the pharmacy will buy and supply the best deal, which may not be the cheapest brand. The ease of administration and other practical issues would have been taken into account. Therefore you should use generic (non-proprietary) names for most prescribing. In some cases, however, the differences between brands can matter and the BNF advises the use of brand names for some drugs including anti-epileptic and transplant medication. When patients bring in their own medication, make sure you do not duplicate items by prescribing some with brand names and some with generic names; analgesics are a particular problem in this respect.

There is good advice on prescribing at the front of the BNF; the hospital will most likely have specific protocols and your ward pharmacist should be able to provide advice if required.

Communication issues

When a patient arrives

Good communication is not only important when a patient is in the hospital, it is vital when the patient moves from community into hospital and back again.

Getting an accurate drug history when a patient arrives is notoriously difficult, particularly if the patient is too unwell to tell you, or does not know, what medicines they are taking. Most GPs can provide a list of what has been prescribed, but there is no guarantee that this is what the patient is actually taking. Furthermore, no GP practice is open at 3 o'clock in the morning!

There are national moves to try and improve this situation. For example the NHS Spine Summary Care Record is an online patient record, which includes basic and more detailed information (including medication prescriptions) based on patient preference for data sharing.

In most hospitals, medical admissions will be checked by a pharmacist within the first day or so of their stay and several sources of information will be used to create an accurate drug history. Surgical patients will often have been seen in a pre-admission clinic where medicine-taking can be checked.

If in doubt about a patient's medication when they arrive, follow the principle of 'first do no harm'. Many medications can be stopped safely for a period while checks are made or progress is observed. Some of these problems are due to non-adherence but some are due to adverse reactions. However, stopping medications without careful consideration would not be wise for anti-epileptic medications, many cardiac medications, transplant immunosuppression medication, anti- psychotic drugs, and bronchodilators.

During their stay

Communication about medication between different healthcare professionals – particularly doctors and the nursing staff who must administer the medications – and teams is a vital part of an inpatient stay. Hospital pharmacists provide a vital service, reducing prescription errors and drug interactions, as well as suggesting options for improved efficacy and economy.

However, many trusts are also moving towards electronic prescribing systems. These have numerous advantages, including real-time validation of a prescription, which will be complete and legible; easy access to protocols, 'powerplan' prescriptions

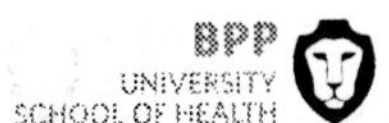

and the hospital formulary with automatic alerts for allergies or drug interactions. Nurses are easily able to change administration rates and directly request medications from pharmacy and there is an automatic and accurate administration record.

Negative elements include the possibility of making errors due to lack of familiarity with trade/generic drug names and frustration that often arises with automated systems. Moreover, programmed prescriptions may not be suitable for all patients and nurses may be unable to change administration times etc.

When a patient leaves

When a patient leaves your care they may be looked after by a lay carer or relative, a residential home assistant or no one. It is essential that your intentions regarding medication are clearly communicated. For example, if prescribing antibiotics or other short courses, including steroids for asthma or post ACS anti-platelet agents, make sure the stop date is clear.

A number of discharge situations require advance planning on your part. Try to insist that your seniors give you a clear plan for each patient so that you are not taken by surprise when they say 'the patient can go now'! All drugs need to be dispensed or checked for discharge and the patient needs to have counselling on their medication, both of which take time. If the patient is not clear on what to do, or is not happy with it, you will be seeing them again. The BTS guidelines recommend that patients on respiratory medication should use their exact discharge prescription for 24 hours in hospital before discharge to establish that it is indeed the appropriate prescription.

If the patient needs a special administration system, eg a Dossette box, to help them adhere to their prescription the pharmacy will need advance notice to make arrangements with a community pharmacy and the GP to continue the supply without interruption. A carer may need to be instructed on how to deal with such devices and some medications are part of shared care agreements between primary and secondary care, which must be managed according to agreed protocols. Therefore it is helpful to try and predict the discharge prescription well before the patient goes home.

Some common issues

One chapter cannot cover all the issues that will arise in prescribing. The BNF and the BNF for Children have deserved worldwide reputations for their detailed guidance and should be consulted frequently. The NHS has set up a 'one-stop' website for accessing guidelines on all sorts of medical issues from organisations such as the NICE and the Scottish Inter-collegiate Guidelines Network (SIGN). What follows are some brief hints on a few areas known to give concern to foundation doctors.

Adverse drug reaction

All drugs cause adverse reactions and it is illegal in the UK to advertise a medicine as safe. Some adverse effects are consequences of their intended action, known as Type A, eg hypotension from an ACE inhibitor. These are easy to detect and can be treated simply by omitting or removing the offending medication. Others are due to a different mechanism, known as Type B, eg hepatotoxicity with isoniazid and these are much harder to isolate and treat. Finally, there may be immune-mediated complications such as anaphylaxis.

Dealing with a possible reaction

1. Take a thorough history. Note all the drugs the patient has consumed (suspect or not, prescribed or not, conventional or alternative, legal or illicit) in the relevant period. Check at what times they were taken and whether they were actually consumed and not just prescribed by using the nurses' administration chart. Ask if the patient has ever had a similar reaction; what caused/ alleviated/resolved it? Has anything else changed recently eg diet, cosmetics, food supplements or minor illnesses?
2. Write a thorough description of the reaction: time and nature of onset, progression, relieving or aggravating factors.

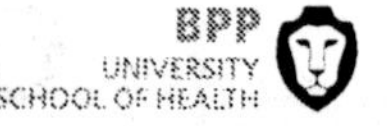

3. Consider any relevant laboratory tests that should be done eg renal and hepatic function tests. Consider spirometry for a wheeze and photograph any rash to help describe it in dermatology-speak.
4. Consult pharmacy's medicines information department on the likelihood of this reaction being attributable to any of the listed drugs. The temporal link will be crucial to attributing blame; some reactions occur immediately on exposure, some take a standard period eg a few days or a few weeks, and some require a long exposure.
5. Stop the most likely drug (or several drugs if safe to do so) and observe the patient. However, do not forget to deal with the condition for which the drug was prescribed originally.
6. Do not make a re-challenge without senior support; some reactions are much more intense, even life-threatening, on re-challenge.

Commonly prescribed medications

Cardiology medications

The young physician starts life with 20 drugs for each disease, and the old physician ends life with one drug for 20 diseases.

William Osler (1849–1919)

Cardiology is an ever-expanding area, with a strong evidence base for many of the interventions used. When prescribing for patients with cardiovascular disease, it is essential to check both the diagnosis and the latest prescribing guidance for the condition as many drugs can be used for multiple indications, at different doses, and the guidelines are frequently updated in line with latest evidence.

Arrhythmias, commonly atrial fibrillation, are often present in sick or elderly patients. The management involves identifying and treating the underlying cause, rather than relying on pharmacological interventions against the arrhythmia. Sepsis, electrolyte disturbances, especially hypokalaemia, hormonal imbalances such as hyperthyroidism, stimulants such as caffeine and alcohol and prescribed medications can all cause such rhythm abnormalities, as well as cardiac disease. Treatment for arrhythmias associated with the latter are most often managed by electrical interventions eg pacing, cardioversion, and ablation in specialist units.

All anti-arrhythmic drugs are also pro-arrhythmic. Beta-blockers, diuretics, antidepressants and anti-histamines can all cause arrhythmias and the latter can also prolong the corrected QT interval and render the patient at risk of the dangerous ventricular arrhythmia, Torsade de Pointes. This is most often a problem when they are combined with an anti-arrhythmic such as Amiodarone or with a cytochrome enzyme inhibitor such as Erythromycin. Carefully reviewing the drug charts of all patients with new rhythm irregularities is an essential part of their management.

Blood pressure regulation normally requires chronic management; however, there are a couple of urgent situations, which require careful, acute interventions. Acute hypertensive emergencies require senior input as there is a need to balance the risks of high blood pressure with the dangers of lowering too rapidly and precipitating a central hypoperfusion. Similarly, patients who have suffered a cerebrovascular incident tend to have volatile blood pressures acutely and thus caution should be taken in the first seven to ten days not to treat their hypertension too zealously.

Patients with ischaemic heart disease often respond to nitrate treatment for anginal symptoms; however, asymmetric dosing is required to prevent the development of tolerance. A 'nitrate free' period each day (at least 14 hours between doses of isosorbide mononitrate tablets) should be arranged, eg by dosing at 8am and 2pm. Caution should also be taken when initiating and stopping any beta-blocker therapy in those with respiratory diseases, diabetes and ischaemic heart disease as abrupt withdrawal can lead to rebound ischaemia.

ACE inhibitors and angiotensin receptor blockers are used in lower doses in heart failure than in hypertension. They must be initiated much more cautiously in heart failure to avoid first dose hypotension, especially in elderly patients. Patients should be appropriately counselled regarding hypotensive risks when initiating and increasing dose. It may be appropriate to give initial doses at bedtime if the patient is unlikely to need to get out of bed until normal waking hours, but nocturnal diuretic prescription should be avoided.

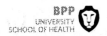

Anticoagulants/Antiplatelets

Poisons and medicine are oftentimes the same substance given with different intents.

Peter Latham (1789–1875)

The number of patients taking some kind of 'blood-thinning' medication seems to be continually increasing. Recommendations for which drug may be used for treatment, primary or secondary prevention therapeutic regimens are based on the latest clinical guidelines, which are constantly being updated (see Chapter 3 for further details). However, there are a few generic prescribing issues that should be considered.

Prescription of anti-platelet agents, most notably aspirin, should be kept to a minimum effective dose to reduce the risk of gastrointestinal bleeding. Vulnerable patients such as the elderly, patients with prior history of bleeding or dyspepsia, or patients with concomitant use of steroids should be co-prescribed a proton-pump inhibitor.

Traditional anticoagulants including warfarin, heparin and low molecular weight heparin molecules cause more avoidable mishaps than any other agents and must be regularly monitored (using the INR or APTT ratios) to maintain the balance between under- and overdosing. Infections or new medications for inpatients may disrupt their normal metabolism and cause dangerous alterations to anticoagulant levels, therefore vigilance is essential. The BNF gives lists of interacting drugs and of target values for INR and APTT in various clinical circumstances.

New Oral Anticoagulants (NOACs) include direct thrombin inhibitors such as dabigatran and factor Xa inhibitors such as rivaroxaban and apixaban. These are oral agents that have been licensed for some patients with atrial fibrillation or for prophylactic prevention or treatment of venous thromboembolic events. These oral agents are: highly efficacious in preventing stroke in non-valvular AF; have a lower incidence of major bleeding in trials; are convenient to use, with minimal drug and food interactions; and have predictable pharmacokinetics, rapid onset/offset of actions, a short half-life and no need to be monitored regularly. However, they are costlier, there is no specific antidote and should not be used in patients with severe hepatic or renal disease.

Antiglycaemic agents

We are overwhelmed as it is, with an infinite abundance of vaunted medicaments, and here they add another one.

Thomas Sydenham (1624–1689)

Thomas Sydenham's quote feels particularly apt in the world of diabetic medicine – there always seems to be a new oral antiglycaemic or insulin available and non-specialists struggle to keep up. Luckily most hospitals have specialist nursing teams who will be able to provide assistance, but again there are a few key points of which to be aware.

Diabetics are particularly vulnerable to changes in prescribing, especially on arrival at hospital or around surgery when a nil-by-mouth regimen is used. Sliding scales for insulin are common and every hospital has a local version in which insulin is diluted in normal saline and infused at a rate determined by frequent blood glucose measurements. The prescriber must ensure that the scale is written clearly and in the units which the nurse will use when adjusting rates. For example, if the infusion device is calibrated in ml/hour then the prescription must be in ml/hour with the concentration of the insulin solution specified. The nurse should not be expected to convert the rate from units/hour or units/kg/hour or anything else. Such mental conversions are a major source of error.

A sliding scale should be set up for all diabetics who are undergoing surgery even if they are not normally insulin-dependent. However, well-controlled patients undergoing short procedures may not need any insulin. Diet-controlled diabetes patients do not usually need any specific intervention before surgery.

Patients on short-acting sulphonylureas should omit the morning dose on the day of operation but longer-acting sulphonylureas should only be stopped two to three days before surgery to prevent peri-operative hypoglycaemia. Patients may be converted to a short-acting sulphonylurea or insulin.

Metformin should be stopped at least 48 hours before elective surgery and not restarted for at least 48 hours post-operatively to prevent lactic acidosis. For radiological studies metformin should be discontinued, preferably 24 hours before the time of the test and for 3 days after the procedure.

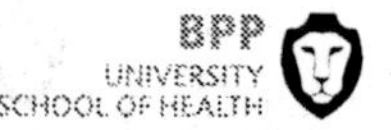

Thiazolidinediones should be omitted on the morning of surgery and restarted once the patient is eating and drinking post-operatively.

Regular insulin is given by a variety of regimens but most include a fast-acting insulin and a medium or long-acting insulin. Brand-name prescribing is essential because of the variation in effect due to subtle changes in insulin preparations. Again the BNF is a good source of information, and if in doubt – ask!

Antibiotics

New medicines, and new methods of cures, always work miracles for a while.

William Heberden (1710–1801)

Increasing bacterial resistance, 'super-bug' outbreaks and treatment failure have been widely blamed on poor prescribing. Government action has strengthened microbial surveillance and there is a strong impetus to control antibiotic prescribing. Such measures emphasise avoiding unnecessary prescribing and selecting the right drug and route for the severity of illness. Therefore, you should familiarise yourself with your hospital's antibiotic policy. This will be in place to reduce the incidence of resistance and hospital-acquired infection and will take local resistance patterns into account.

Always take samples for microbiology before starting treatment; monitor the duration of antibiotic course and in simple infections specify and complete the full course. Review IV antibiotics regularly to avoid the risks associated with IV cannulae and have a low threshold for discussing any questions or queries with the microbiology team.

Analgesia

A desire to take medicine is, perhaps the great feature which distinguishes man from other animals.

William Osler (1849–1919)

Analgesia has classically been under-prescribed and patients have been brushed off with words like 'discomfort'. To promote the proper use of opiate analgesia, the WHO published an Analgesic Ladder in 1996. It is applicable to chronic pain where it builds up from Paracetamol to Morphine. For acute pain, including surgical pain, the ladder is reversed and prescriptions start with major analgesics and step down as time permits.

Paracetamol is the starting point for treating all chronic pain and should continue through all stages of management at the maximum dose – either orally, intravenously or per rectum. NSAIDs may be used in addition, but these all have risks of gastrointestinal damage and bleeding as well as renal impairment in dehydrated patients, heart failure patients or patients taking ACE inhibitors. If using in vulnerable patients, a proton-pump inhibitor should be co-prescribed.

The second step is to add an oral mild opiate such as Dihydrocodeine. Codeine is not metabolised to the active metabolite (morphine) in some patients and should be exchanged for an alternative if it does not seem to be effective. Laxatives, eg Lactulose and senna, should be prescribed prophylactically for regular use, not just after constipation is evident.

The third step is to use Morphine instead of Dihydrocodeine. Morphine does not have a dose-ceiling and may be increased as required. Laxatives are essential and anti-nauseants/emetics may be required. The UK is one of only two countries in the world to license diamorphine but apart from increased solubility, which makes it easier to use in a small portable syringe, it has no advantage over morphine.

When prescribing opiates, ensure that they are given regularly at intervals that suit the formulation eg 12-hourly for modified release tablets. In addition, always make provision for break-through pain. If using tablets or intermittent injections, prescribe a prn dose that is one-sixth of the daily dose in current use; if using a continuous infusion allow for boluses to be given at the equivalent of 30–60 minutes' infusion.

Review opiate prescriptions at least once a day to adjust up or down according to the patient's use of break-through medication.

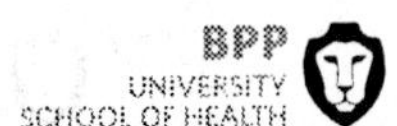

Further reading and references

1. James, S., Meakin, S., Pirmohamed, M., et al. (2004) Adverse drug reactions as cause of admission to hospital:prospective analysis of 18820 patients. *BMJ* 2004; 329: 15-19.
2. Cassan, S., Floutard, E., Peyriere, H., et al. (2003) Adverse drug events associated with hospital admission. *Ann Pharmacother* 2003; 37: 5-11.
3. Brennan, T.A., Laird, N.M., Leape, L.L., et al. (1991) Incidence of adverse events and negligence in hospitalized patients: results of the Harvard Medical Practice Study I. *NEJM* 1991; 324: 370–6.
4. Karch, F.E. and Lasagna, L. (1975) Adverse drug reactions: a critical review. *JAMA* 1965; 234: 1236–41.
5. Shakur, R. and Scott, D. (2008) The art of prescribing. *Br J Hasp Med (Lond)* 69(5): M72-3.
6. Barber, N., Dean, B., Schachter, M., et al. (2002) Causes of prescribing errors in hospital inpatients: a prospective study. *Lancet* 2002; 359: 1373–8.
7. Evidence search, www.evidence.nhs.uk.

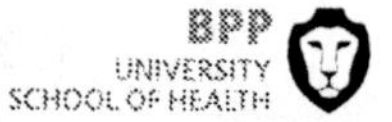

Chapter 9

DOPS assessments – core procedures

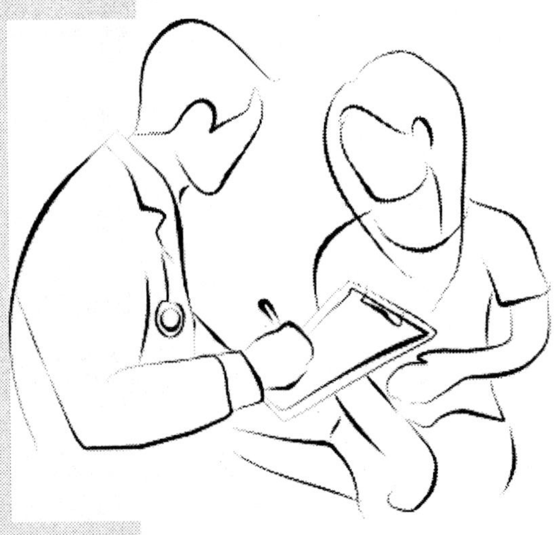

Chapter 9

DOPS assessments – core procedures

Introduction

I tell a student that the most important class you can take is technique. A great chef is first a great technician. 'If you are a jeweler, or a surgeon or a cook, you have to know the trade in your hand. You have to learn the process. You learn it through endless repetition until it belongs to you.'

Jacques Pepin (1935–)

There are 15 core procedures that foundation doctors must demonstrate competence in to progress through FY1. In addition, further procedures may be observed as a DOPS, which is a type of supervised learning event (SLE). Whilst core procedures are relevant to the majority of medical and surgical placements, DOPS cover a wide variety of procedures and can be used to demonstrate a foundation doctor's interests and aid applications for speciality training.

This chapter aims to cover the theoretical aspects behind the core procedures, and selected additional skills, that should be learnt during the Foundation Programme.

The theory covered in this chapter will not replace practical experience on the wards but will address the indications, contraindications, relevant anatomy and complications of each procedure. Where appropriate there will be a brief guide to the interpretation of results gained from performing the procedure.

Core procedures
1. Venepuncture
2. IV cannulation
3. Prepare and administer IV medications, injections and fluids
4. Arterial puncture in an adult
5. Blood culture (peripheral)
6. IV infusion including prescription of fluids
7. IV infusion of blood and blood products
8. Injection of local anaesthetic to skin
9. Subcutaneous injection
10. Intramuscular injection
11. Perform and interpret an ECG
12. Perform and interpret peak flow
13. Urethral catheterisation (male)
14. Urethral catheterisation (female)
15. Airway care including simple adjuncts

Table 9.1: Core procedures requiring competency sign-off for completion of FY1

Top tip:

As an F1 you will be performing these procedures so often yet most people still leave them too late! Try to complete the easy ones early leaving your time to focus on other things. Ask nurses if you can help them on the evening Dalteparin rounds to cross off subcutaneous injections. When you request an ECG ask if you can do it with the nurse!

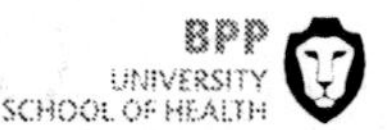

Core procedure essentials

Core procedures should be observed by an assessor, who can be a more senior doctor or a nurse, and recorded in the e-portfolio. They assess a range of aspects, from knowledge and technical ability, to communication skills and professionalism.

Common themes

Primo non nocere. A cardinal rule in medicine is to 'first do no harm'. In all cases procedures should only be performed when you have sufficient competency, or adequate support. Observing seniors and practice in a skills lab can be useful.

Preparation

Preparation is frequently the key to success in all procedures. Consent should be obtained and consideration given as to where to carry out the procedure, and the need for additional staff to assist. This will often depend more on who the patient is rather than the procedure.

Collect all of the necessary equipment required before beginning the procedure and consider whether any analgesia may be beneficial. Take your time, there is no rush.

Aseptic Non-Touch Technique

The majority of core procedures require an aseptic ('as clean as possible') non-touch technique (ANTT). The basis of ANTT is avoiding touching key parts that may come into contact with key sites of a patient, eg venipuncture wound or site of catheter insertion. This prevents the spread of pathogens. Using this technique properly avoids the need for sterile gloves or a sterile field.

Ensure you use ANTT when performing all procedures in this chapter unless stated otherwise. As always, do not forget to wash your hands!

Consent

Undertaking a procedure without consent is legally known as 'battery'. Consider what form of consent is required (implied/verbal/written). Some trusts may require formal consent forms to be completed for certain procedures. For consent to be valid the patient must be adequately informed, meaning the indication, the procedure and the complications (common and rare) have been explained to them. Does the patient have capacity? This means are they able to understand and retain the information, weigh up the pros and cons and communicate their decision. If the patient lacks capacity, the doctor can proceed if acting in the patient's best interests. If a second party holds lasting power of attorney, consent will need to be obtained from them. In any case, if a patient lacks capacity it is considered good practice to discuss the procedure with a relative, especially if there are potentially serious implications. When explaining potential complications consider the circumstances specific to the patient ie risk of bruising when taking blood.

Post-procedure management

Clear up sharps and dispose of biological waste promptly and appropriately. Arrange for follow-up of results and for further management. See individual procedures for specific details.

Documentation

Accurate documentation is important in all areas of medicine. When documenting, consider the need to document all aspects of the procedure including consent, sterility, details of equipment (eg size), important stages that prevent or limit complications (eg replacement of foreskin after urethral catheterisation), any complications encountered and ongoing management issues.

Communication skills

Prior to the procedure, and as part of consent, explain to the patient what will happen and what to expect during and after the procedure. In addition, remember to communicate effectively with other professionals, be it professionals involved in the procedure itself or those who will manage the patient's post-procedural care. For example, explain to nursing staff clearly how to care for a patient's chest drain and what parameters would warrant a cause for concern.

Professionalism

As with all aspects of medicine, a professional approach is essential. In addition to the points outlined previously, patient dignity should be maintained at all times. All doctors should recognise their own limitations in performing a particular procedure and should not be afraid to seek senior assistance when concerned.

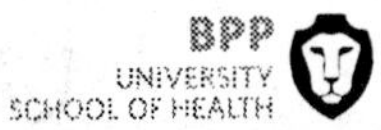

1. Venepuncture

Indications

- Diagnostic testing of blood
- Monitoring of physiological and pharmacological parameters

Contraindications

- Cellulitis
- Avoid in limbs post-local/regional lymph node dissection
- Avoid in injured limbs
- IV infusions if running in same limb could affect results

Relevant anatomy

Common sites of venepuncture include the antecubital fossa, small veins of the hand, forearm and the femoral vein.

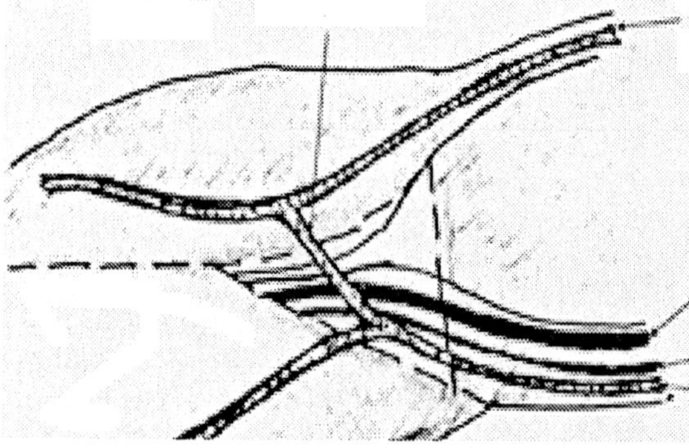

Figure 9.1: Antecubital fossa is a common site for venepuncture

Equipment required

Tourniquet, gloves, chlorhexidine/alcohol swab, needle, vacutainer/butterfly/needle and syringe, cotton wool/gauze, tape, connectors and appropriate blood bottles.

Procedure

Closed vacutainer systems are the preferred method for blood collection as they reduce the risk of needlestick injuries and minimise the number of samples rejected by the lab.

1. Apply tourniquet and identify suitable vein
2. Prepare skin by wiping with chlorhexidine/alcohol swab for 30 seconds and allow to dry by evaporation
3. Fix vein using a spare finger (especially important in elderly patients or dorsal hand veins)
4. Insert the needle at a 30–45 angle into vein
5. Take sample:
    i) When using a needle and syringe or butterfly needle a flashback will be seen as the needle enters the vein; once this is seen draw back the syringe to collect sample or connect sample bottles.
    ii) No flashback will be seen with a vacutainer. If needed, adjust the position of the needle beneath the skin until blood is collected in the bottle. Once the vacuum has been lost the sample bottle cannot be reused.
6. Remove tourniquet before removing needle to reduce bruising
7. Apply pressure to puncture site with cotton wool/gauze. If appropriate, tape in place
8. Dispose of any sharps in the sharps bin
9. Label blood bottles immediately
10. Document in the notes

Top tip:
In peripherally shut down patients, particularly during resuscitation, it may be more appropriate to obtain blood from the patient's femoral vein or artery.

The femoral vein lies just medial to the femoral artery, which can be palpated immediately inferior to the mid-inguinal point.

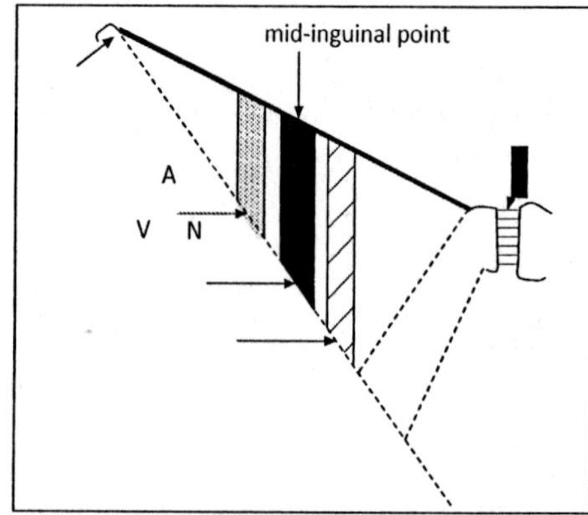

Figure 9.2: The location of the femoral vein

2. Intravenous cannulation

Indications

- Administration of IV fluids, medications and blood products

Contraindications

- There are no absolute contraindications.
- Avoid cannulation in areas of cellulitis and in injured limbs or limbs post lymph node dissection.

Relevant anatomy

Common sites of IV cannulation include the antecubital fossa and small veins of the hand and forearm. The long saphenous vein and dorsal foot veins may also be useful in children and the elderly.

The antecubital fossa is often easier to cannulate but is not comfortable for patients, who must keep their arms straight. The larger veins here are often most appropriate to use in times of resuscitation.

Equipment required

Tourniquet, gloves, chlorhexidine/alcohol swab, cannula, adapter system (single or double lumen, flushed with saline), 10 ml syringe, 10 ml 0.9% saline, cannula site dressing and gauze.

Procedure

1. Apply tourniquet
2. Identify suitable vein
3. Clean skin using chlorhexidine / alcohol swab
4. Fix vein using a spare finger
5. Insert cannula at a 10–15° angle into vein
6. When flashback is observed flatten the cannula and advance it further into vein, whilst slowly withdrawing the needle
7. Remove tourniquet
8. Depress vein to prevent bleeding and remove needle completely. Dispose of needle in sharps bin
9. Place adapter system onto end of cannula
10. Flush with 5–10 ml of 0.9% saline
11. If blood sampling also required connect syringe or vacutainer to cannula and remove sample prior to flushing
12. Apply dressing and label with date of insertion
13. Document completion in notes and complete a Visual Infusion Phlebitis (VIP) score

Post-procedure management

Monitor for signs of phlebitis and regularly reassess need for continued IV cannulation.

After three to five days the cannula site should be changed to minimise the risk of phlebitis. Once a patient no longer requires IV fluids or medications their cannula should be removed.

Complications

- Infection
- Bleeding, bruising and haematoma

Top tip:

Choosing the right vein is key to success. Spend time examining the patient before your first attempt – failure is frustrating when you realise you missed a large vein on their other hand!

There are many techniques you can use if you are finding it difficult to find a vein or they are peripherally shut down:

1. Use gravity to your advantage
2. Try lightly tapping on the back of their hand
3. Immerse their hand in warm water or fill a glove with warm water and hold it to the back of their hand

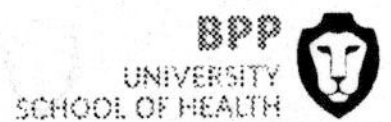

3. Arterial puncture and interpretation of arterial blood gases (ABG)

Indications

- To assess respiratory and metabolic status, including pH, PaO_2, $PaCO_2$, HCO_3-, BE and lactate
- To obtain rapid measurement of electrolytes, glucose and haemoglobin
- Allows calculation of the anion gap and alveolar-arterial gradient

Contraindications

- No collateral circulation through ulnar artery (as determined by Allen's test) would contraindicate this procedure in the radial artery. However, arterial puncture of the femoral artery could be performed
- History of severe artery spasm following previous puncture

Relevant anatomy

The most common site for ABG sampling is the radial artery, just lateral to the tendon of flexor carpi radialis. The femoral artery is another common site for arterial puncture, and is a more appropriate choice during cardiac arrests.

Equipment required

Chlorhexidine/alcohol swab, gloves, heparinised ABG syringe, gauze, tape, 25 gauge orange needle for radial artery (a longer needle would be more suitable for femoral puncture).

Procedure

1. Locate artery and identify area of maximum pulsation
2. Perform Allen's test to ensure adequate collateral circulation if using the radial artery
3. Clean skin with alcohol swab
4. Ensure syringe plunger is partially retracted
5. Insert needle perpendicular to skin into the artery with the wrist extended
6. Observe for pulsation of blood into syringe. When enough blood has been drawn ensure it is mixed with heparin to prevent clotting
7. Remove needle and dispose in sharps bin
8. Apply cotton wool / gauze with pressure for at least three to five minutes
9. Take sample for analysis
10. Document results and procedure in notes, including what concentration of oxygen the patient was on (FiO_2)

Complications

- Bleeding, brusing and haematoma
- False aneurysm
- Prolonged arterial spasm, which may result in pain and numbness
- Arterial occlusion
- Damage to local structures

Allen's test

Arterial puncture carries the risk of causing arterial occlusion. Therefore, Allen's test is performed prior to radial artery puncture to ensure adequate ulnar collateral supply.

1. Elevate the patient's hand and ask them to clench their fist for at least 30 seconds
2. Apply pressure to the ulnar and radial arteries
3. Ask patient to open their fist; their hand should appear blanched
4. Release pressure from their ulnar artery and observe for blood flow back into their hand:
   i) If blood returns in 5–15 seconds the test is positive and ulnar collateral flow is sufficient
   ii) If blood does not return in 5–15 seconds the test is negative and it is not safe to perform radial artery puncture

Top tip:
Taking your time is crucial. Firstly, ensure that both you and the patient are comfortable and that their wrist is well supported and hyperextended at the wrist. Palpate the artery with two fingers, one distal and one proximal, to give you a feel for the direction of the artery. Inserting the needle between your fingers will ensure you hit the artery.

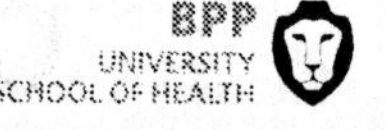

Interpretation

ABGs provide a lot of information if you can interpret them correctly. This brief guide should cover the results in common medical situations.

Respiratory failure:

Type I: PaO_2 <8 kPa on air
Type II: PaO_2 <8 kPa on air and $PaCO_2$ >6 kPa

Acid-base balance:

1. Check the pH. Does the patient have an acidosis (pH <7.35) or alkalosis (pH >7.45)?
2. Check whether the $PaCO_2$ and HCO_3^- are low, normal or high. A low $PaCO_2$ increases the pH causing alkalosis; a high $PaCO_2$ decreases the pH causing acidosis. HCO_3^- counters the effect of CO_2. Therefore, a low HCO_3^- increases the PH causing acidosis and a high HCO_3^- decreases the pH causing an alkalosis.
3. Match the pH to the $PaCO_2$ and HCO_3^- to determine the cause of the acid-base disorder.
4. Check for compensation. If the $PaCO_2$ or HCO_3^- go in an opposite direction to the pH then that system is compensating. If the pH is within the normal range then full compensation is present; if outside the normal range then it is partial compensation.

Anion gap:

The anion gap can be determined in metabolic acidosis to help with diagnosis. The anion gap is calculated using the following equation:

$$\textbf{Anion gap} = [Na^+ + K^+] - [Cl^- + HCO^-]$$

Normal anion gap = 10–18

The anion gap measures the difference between measured cations (Na+ and K+) and measured anions (Cl and HCO-). Not all anions and cations are measured and therefore the equation does not equal zero.

The anion gap is raised if there are excess anions in the blood eg lactate (lactic acidosis), ketones (DKA or starvation), urate (renal failure), and exogenous acids such as salicylates and methanol.

Metabolic acidosis with a normal anion gap is due to the loss of bicarbonate eg renal tubular acidosis or diarrhoea.

Disorder	pH	pCO_2	HCO_3	Base excess
Acute respiratory acidosis	Low	High	Normal	Normal
Chronic compensated respiratory acidosis	Normal	High	High	Positive
Acute on chronic respiratory acidosis	Low	High	High	Positive
Acute respiratory alkalosis	High	Low	Normal	Normal
Acute metabolic acidosis	Low	Normal or Low (Respiratory compensation)	Low	Negative
Acute metabolic alkalosis	High	Normal or high (Respiratory compensation)	High	Positive
Mixed respiratory and metabolic acidosis	Low	High	Low	Negative

Table 9.2: Common acid-base disturbances

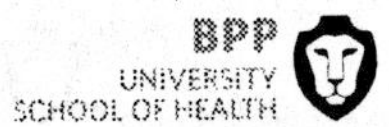

4. Blood cultures from peripheral and central sites

Indications

- Sepsis (forms part of the 'Sepsis 6')
- Suspected infection – to identify organisms and test sensitivity of antibiotics

Contraindications

- No absolute contraindications exist
- Choose site with care as you would for venepuncture

Relevant anatomy

Blood cultures are taken from the same sites as for venepuncture. Samples from multiple sites may be required eg if infective endocarditis suspected.

Equipment required

The same equipment as for venepuncture with anaerobic and aerobic blood culture bottles.

Procedure

1. Blood cultures can be taken using the techniques described previously for venepuncture. There are a few important differences to note to minimise the risk of contamination:
   i) Use a fresh venepuncture site for blood cultures (do not draw blood from cannulas)
   ii) Avoid femoral puncture, due to increased risk of contamination
2. Before filling the bottles with blood remove the caps and wipe each clean with a fresh alcohol wipe
3. Fill the aerobic bottle first, then the anaerobic bottle
4. Remove bar code sticker from blood culture bottle and put in notes

Taking blood from central line

The following technique can be used to draw blood from a central line for blood cultures.

1. Put on sterile gloves
2. Remove cap of the central line port
3. Clean tops of blood culture bottles with alcohol wipe as above. Clean central line port with a fresh alcohol wipe
4. Connect a 10 ml syringe and aspirate 5–10 ml
5. Discard this syringe
6. Connect a new syringe and aspirate a further 10 ml
7. Connect a needle to this syringe and empty it into the culture bottles
8. Dispose of sharps
9. Flush the central line with 10 ml 0.9% saline
10. Replace the cap

Top tip:
Blood cultures should be taken prior to the administration of antibiotics. However, do not delay antibiotic prescribing whilst waiting to take blood cultures if you cannot take them immediately. Patients with sepsis should have antibiotics within the first hour!

Take extra care with your ANTT technique as contamination will give you false-positive results. Do not palpate the vein before venepuncture, once you have cleaned it.

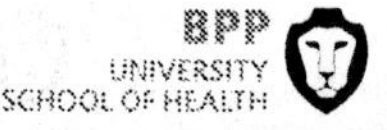

5. Subcutaneous, intra-muscular and intravenous injections

For all three different injection routes a needle, syringe, alcohol swab and appropriate medication are required.

It is important when administering drugs by any route that you first check the patient's details, check the medications you are about to administer against the prescription chart, ask about allergies and ensure the medication is within its expiry date. After administering the medication you should record details on the drug chart and sign for it.

Subcutaneous injections

Indications

- Drug delivery
- May be suitable alternative route if IV access is difficult or inappropriate (eg palliative patients)

Contraindications

- No absolute contraindications; however, choose site with care
- Obesity may reduce bioavailability of the drug due to poor absorption

Relevant anatomy

Three common sites for subcutaneous injection are the abdomen, the back or side of the upper arm and the anterior thigh. Ensure you pick a site so as to inject into the subcutaneous tissues and not muscle.

Procedure

1. Draw up the medication into a syringe or use a specifically designed injector pen
2. Clean skin with alcohol swab
3. Pinch the skin to pull the skin and subcutaneous tissues away from the underlying muscle
4. Inject the medication into the subcutaneous tissue at a 90° angle (use a shallower angle if necessary to avoid injecting into muscle)
5. Once the medication has been injected dispose of the needle and syringe into the sharps bin
6. If necessary apply light pressure to the injection site with cotton wool

Complications

It is important to rotate injection sites to prevent complications such as lipodystrophy; this is mainly an issue for diabetics requiring frequent insulin injections. Avoid using dextrose in subcutaneous injections as skin irritation can occur; use 0.9% saline instead.

Intra-muscular injections

Indications

- Drug delivery
- Allows rapid delivery of mediation without the need for IV access

Contraindications

- Thrombocytopenia
- Coagulation disorders

Relevant anatomy

There are five potential sites for IM injection. As always avoid any site with evidence of infection or injury.

1. **Deltoid** – Inject within the centre of an upside down equilateral triangle with the acromion process as its base to avoid the axillary nerve.
2. **Dorsogluteal** – Inject in the upper outer quardrant of the buttock, avoiding the sciatic nerve in the lower medial quadrant. Be careful to inject into muscle rather than fat.
3. **Ventrogluteal** – Place the palm of your hand on the greater trochanter of the femur with your index finger extending along the iliac crest. Your middle finger is placed medially creating a triangle within which you can inject.
4. **Vastus lateralis** and **5. rectus femoris** – lateral and medial thigh respectively.

Absorption is fastest in the arm and slowest in the buttock.

Procedure

1. Draw up the medication into a syringe
2. Select a needle long enough to reach the muscle
3. Wipe skin with an alcohol swab

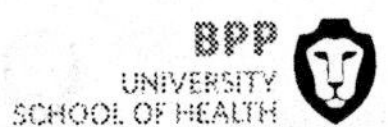

4. Slide the skin and subcutaneous tissues 2–3 cm in any direction and hold taut
5. Insert the needle perpendicular to the skin into the muscle
6. Pull back on the syringe, if blood is aspirated alter the position of the needle and try again
7. Inject medication slowly (<1 ml / 10 seconds)
8. Release skin
9. Remove needle and dispose in sharps bin

Intravenous injections

Indications

- Rapid drug delivery

Contraindications

- None

Relevant anatomy

Intravenous medications should be administered through a cannula.

Procedure

1. Examine cannula for signs of infection
2. Clean cannula port with alcohol swab
3. Ensure cannula is patent by flushing with 5–10 ml normal saline
4. Administer drug as directed (some medications require slower injections)
5. Flush again with 5–10 ml normal saline to ensure all medication has been delivered to patient and is not in cannula's dead space

6. Intravenous infusions and fluid prescription

Medications can be delivered intravenously by injection (as discussed in the previous chapter) and by infusion. Intravenous infusions of medications are administered in the same way as intravenous fluids.

Equipment required

Fluids, giving set, alcohol swab, saline flush and working cannula.

Procedure

1. Open fluid bag and check for any leaks or precipitate in fluid
2. Unwrap giving set and close adjustable valve
3. Insert giving set into the bag outlet
4. Hang fluid bag on drip stand
5. Prime the giving set by half filling the giving set chamber
6. Slowly open the valve and allow fluid to flow to the distal end of the giving set
7. Close the valve and check for air bubbles in the giving set. If present run them out
8. Connect the giving set to the cannula
9. Adjust the valve to set the appropriate flow rate

Determining the flow rate of the infusion

The flow rate of the infusion is determined by adjusting the number of drips per minute into the giving set chamber. It is important to know the number of drops in 1 ml; in a standard giving set this is 20 drops.

This formula can be used to calculate the drip flow rate:

Flow rate (gtts/min) =
volume (ml) × drop factor (gtts/ml) / time (min)

Beware of any occlusions in the line or of rising pressures as monitored by the infusion pump, which may be a sign of cannula failure.

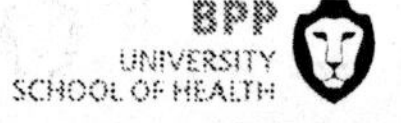

7. Prescription of blood and blood products

The technical steps needed for blood transfusion are similar to those for the infusion of fluids, except using specific giving sets. The most important difference is the surrounding safety steps that ensure the transfusion proceeds safely and that the correct blood is given to the correct patient. It is also important to be aware of the various reactions and adverse events that can occur following blood transfusion.

Indications

- Major haemorrhage
- Symptomatic anaemia
- Peri-operative transfusion

Thresholds for blood transfusion will change depending on where you work so be led by local guidelines.

Safe prescribing

Trusts will have different protocols to ensure safe blood transfusions; there are a number of generic things to be aware of.

1. Positively identify patient and confirm patient's details match those on wristband
2. Label blood bottles at patient's bedside
3. Ask about previous transfusion history
4. Identify need for special blood products

Special transfusion requirements

When you make transfusion requests you will be asked about special requirements and you should be aware of the indications for this blood:

CMV negative:

- HIV infection
- Many bone marrow / stem cell transplant patients

Gamma irradiated:

- Hodgkin's disease
- Congenital immunodeficient states
- Patients treated with purine analogues eg fludarabine
- Many bone marrow / stem cell recipients
- Bone marrow donors over time of harvest

Monitoring

Vital signs should be recorded routinely before starting the transfusion, after 15 minutes, and at the end of the transfusion. Additional observations should be made as clinically necessary.

> **Top tip:**
> You will sometimes see a furosemide bolus prescribed alongside packed red cells. Packed red cells are a colloid and therefore increase the intravascular volume, which could cause symptoms of fluid overload in vulnerable patients.

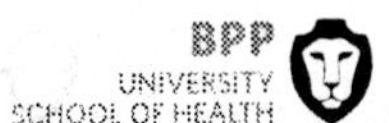

Complication	Clinical features	Management
Acute haemolytic transfusion reaction Cause: ABO incompatibility resulting in intravascular haemolysis mediated by IgM and complement activation.	Symptoms occur within minutes of starting transfusion: fever, rigors, anxiety, flushing, chest/lumbar pain, dyspnoea, hypotension haemoglobinuria and renal failure. Disseminated intravascular coagulopathy (DIC).	Stop transfusion. Return donor units to lab. Take new blood sample from patient for cross-matching. Transfuse compatible RBCs. Maintain blood pressure and renal function with IV fluids.
Delayed haemolytic transfusion reaction Cause: Allo-immunisation by previous transfusions/pregnancies results in IgG-mediated extravascular haemolysis.	Jaundice, fever and symptoms of anaemia develop one week after transfusion. Patient may be asymptomatic.	Take new blood sample for direct antiglobulin test (Coombs test), which should be positive. Monitor Hb. Give further transfusions for symptomatic anaemia.
Febrile non haemolytic reaction Cause: Anti-leucocyte antibodies in allo-immunised recipients reacting against leucocytes in transfused blood. Cytokines released from donor leucocytes in platelet concentrates.	Symptoms tend to develop towards end of infusion: fever, rigors, flushing, tachycardia. Becoming less common with use of leucocyte-depleted blood products.	Mild: slow transfusion, give Paracetamol, increase observations. Severe: stop transfusion, seek advice from transfusion laboratory. Call haematologist.
Urticaria Cause: Auto-antibodies in recipient reacting with donor plasma proteins.	More common during transfusion of platelets or plasma than red cells. Symptoms occur during transfusion and include urticaria and itch.	Slow transfusion, give 10 mg Chlorpheniramine IV, increase observations.
Anaphylaxis Cause: tends to occur in patients lacking IgA. Anti-IgA reacts with IgA in transfused blood.	Life-threatening features of anaphylaxis including airway compromise and circulatory collapse.	Stop transfusion immediately. Maintain airway (call anaesthestist and consider endotracheal intubation). Give 0.5 mg 1:1,000 Adrenaline IM as per ALS algorithms. Give 10 mg chlorphenamine IV. Prevent recurrence by using washed red cells or blood from IgA deficient donors.
Infective Shock Cause: bacterial contamination of blood products eg *Yersinia, S.aureus.*	Symptoms usually develop during infusion of first 100 ml. Fever, rigors, tachycardia, hypotension, DIC. Very high mortality.	Manage septic shock with IV antibiotics and fluids (maintain BP and urine output).
Transfusion-related acute lung injury (TRALI) Cause: reaction antibody in donor plasma with leucocytes of recipient.	Symptoms develop during or soon after blood transfusion: fever, shortness of breath. Typical appearances on chest X-ray. Can be life-threatening.	Maintain airway. Manage as for acute respiratory distress syndrome. Give ventilatory support if necessary.

Table 9.3: Complications of blood transfusions

8. Local anaesthetics

In your foundation years you are required to demonstrate competence in administering local anaesthetics to skin eg prior to excision biopsy or wound closure. Local anaesthetic can also be used for other purposes such as nerve blocks, which is not covered in this chapter.

Indications

- To anaesthetise surgical area for minor procedures under local anaesthetic only
- To provide pain relief post-op for patients following general anaesthetic

Contraindications

- Previous hypersensitivity reactions

Relevant anatomy

Local anaesthetics can be administered topically or via an injection. If an injection is required, take into consideration the site and depth of injection required. If injecting into digits do not use adrenaline.

Equipment required

Local anaesthetic, gloves, needle, syringe, alcohol swab

Procedure

1. Draw up local anaesthetic into a syringe. Check drug, dose and expiry date.
2. Warn patient of a stinging sensation during administration; be aware that they may withdraw – caution with the needle. (Discomfort can be reduced by adding bicarbonate, warming the solution, injecting slowly and through already anaesthetized areas; using the minimum volume required).
3. Aspirate before injecting to avoid inadvertently inject into a blood vessel. Should you aspirate blood, alter the position of the needle and re-aspirate until satisfied you are not in the vessel.
4. Use a small 25G (orange) needle to raise a bleb under the skin initially and then change to a larger needle.
5. Insert larger needle through bleb once anaesthesia has been achieved to anaesthetise deeper structures / larger areas of skin.

Topical application

A range of topical local anaesthetics are available:

- Creams for cannulation/venepuncture (especially in paediatrics)
- Gel for urethral catheterisation
- Mouth spray for pre-endoscopy / trans-oesophageal echocardiography

Top tip:

You can move larger needles under the skin whilst injecting to anaesthetise larger areas. Provided you maintain movement you do not need to re-aspirate continuously as any movement through a vessel will be transient.

Properties and doses

Different local anaesthetics have different properties. It is important to be aware of, and calculate, the maximum safe dose of local anaesthetic before administration. The maximum dose of local anaesthetic may affect the feasibility of performing a procedure.

The concentration of local anaesthetic is given as a percentage, where 1% = 10 mg/ml, 2% = 20 mg/ml etc.

Name of local anaesthetic	Onset of action	Duration of action	Maximum dosage
Lidocaine	Fast: 1–2 mins	Medium: 30–60 minutes	3 mg/kg without adrenaline 7 mg/kg with adrenaline
Bupivacaine	Medium: 5–10 mins	Long 4–6 hrs	2 mg/kg

Table 9.4: Comparative properties of commonly used local anaesthetics

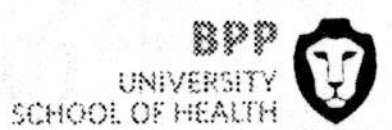

Conventional wisdom advises that adrenaline should not be used on appendages or digits as vasoconstriction can result in ischaemic necrosis; however, actual surgical practice varies.

Complications

Inadvertent intravascular administration can cause the following:

- Hypersensitivity reactions: mainly with esterified local anesthetics (benzocaine, cocaine, procaine, tetracaine)
- Cardiovascular side effects (hypotension, conduction defects, arrhythmias, asystole)
- CNS effects (light-headedness, sedation, twitching, and if severe seizures and coma)
- Symptoms of mild toxicity include peri-oral tingling, metallic taste, tinnitus, visual disturbances and slurred speech

9. Performing and interpreting an electrocardiogram (ECG)

Indications

- Patients with active chest pain, syncope, palpitations, shortness of breath etc
- Provide baseline measurements pre-operatively

Contraindications

- None

Relevant anatomy

An ECG provides a 3D representation of the electrical activity of the heart. Consequently, accurate lead placement is essential in enabling interpretation and subsequent management. Consistent placement of leads also allows accurate monitoring of ECG changes. Locations for lead placements are below.

Lead	Onset of action
V1	4th intercostal space right sternal edge
V2	4th intercostal space left sternal edge
V3	Between V2 and V4
V4	5th intercostal space mid-clavicular line
V5	5th intercostal space anterior axillary line
V6	5th intercostal space mid-axillary line
Limb leads	1 electrode is placed on each of R wrist, L wrist, L ankle and R ankle (on bony points). Alternatively use bony prominences of shoulder / hip

Table 9.5: Leads used for performing an electrocardiogram

Procedure

1. Expose patient's chest and, if necessary, shave any excessive hair
2. Apply ECG electrodes and connect leads as described in above table
3. Ensure machine is calibrated (speed 25 mm/sec, voltage 1 mV/cm)
4. Ask the patient to lie still
5. Record the trace

Interpretation

Normal values:

PR interval = 0.12–0.2 ms

QRS complex <0.12 ms

QTc interval = 0.30 – 0.44 (0.45 in women)

The QT interval depends on the heart rate; a corrected QT (QTc) can be calculated using:

$$QTc = \frac{QT}{(\sqrt{RR})}$$

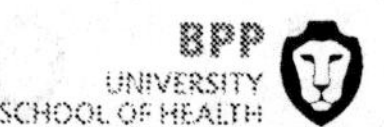

Approach ECG interpretation logically and consistently so that you do not miss anything:

Ask yourself	Are details correct? • Right patient: name, DOB, hospital number? • Right date and time? What is the clinical setting? What were the patient's symptoms at time of ECG?
Check	Calibration • Speed (25 mm/sec) • Amplitude (1 mV/cm)
Rate	Normal, bradycardia, tachycardia?
Rhythm	Regular, regularly irregular or irregularly irregular?
P waves	Present? Morphology? Relation of P waves to QRS?
PR interval?	Pacing spikes?
Axis	Normal, left, right?
QRS complexes	Pathological Q waves? (>2 mm depth >1 mm width) Narrow or wide? (< or > than 3 mm (0.12 sec)) Pattern? eg LBBB/RBBB Size? eg LVH/RVH
ST segment	Isoelectric, depressed, elevated Pattern of depression/elevation Site in relation to coronary artery territory Shape (eg saddle, high take off, reverse tick)
T waves	Inversion?
Corrected QT interval	Causes of elongation?
Anything else?	Any particular patterns synonymous with a particular syndrome? ie Brugada syndrome
Comparison with old ECGs	Are there any dynamic changes? Are ECG changes old?

Table 9.6: Systematic approach to interpreting the electrocardiogram

10. Performing and interpreting peak flow

The peak flow is a useful lung function test that measures the fastest rate of air a patient can blow out (peak expiratory flow). Normal values depend on a patient's sex, age and height.

Indications

- Diagnosis and monitoring of asthma (although spirometry is preferred to confirm diagnosis)
- Assessing severity of acute asthma attacks

Contraindications

- None

Equipment required

Peak flow meter, mouthpiece, normogram of predicted values

Procedure

1. Ensure peak flow meter marker is at zero
2. Attach a new mouthpiece to meter
3. Ask patient to stand if able
4. Instruct patient to take a deep breath in, seal their lips around the mouthpiece of the spirometer, and blow out as hard and fast as possible
5. Record the best of three readings
6. Compare to patient's usual PEF or calculate as a percentage of their predicted value

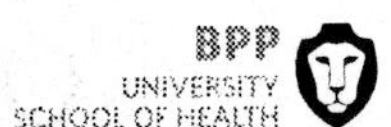

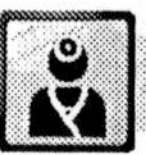

11. Airway care

Indications

- Reduced conscious level causing obstruction of airway by tongue and other soft tissues
- Intra-luminal obstruction eg vomit, blood, foreign body
- Swelling of airway eg anaphylaxis, angio-oedema
- Laryngospasm eg epiglottitis
- Exogenous compression eg tumour
- Trauma
- Pre-emptive anticipation of airway difficulty eg facial burns

Airway compromise is a medical emergency and if complete can rapidly result in death. When suspected, seek senior help immediately. Foundation doctors should be familiar with simple manoeuvres and adjuncts for maintaining an airway. In clinical practice use only the techniques you feel adequately trained in and competent with.

When managing an acutely compromised airway give high flow oxygen. You should continually reassess the patient's airway after implementing any of the following manoeuvres/adjuncts, or if there is any change in the patient's condition.

Recognising a compromised airway

Look:

For chest wall movements, cyanosis, signs of respiratory distress

Listen:

For breath sounds, stridor, choking, gurgling, snoring, inability to speak in full sentences

Feel:

For air movement

If the airway obstruction is complete you may observe paradoxical respiration. Here there is a see-saw pattern of breathing: as the diaphragm moves down in inspiration there is abdominal distension and in-drawing of the inter- and subcostal muscles. The reverse is seen with expiration and the upward movement of the diaphragm.

You should assume the airway is compromised, or potentially compromised, in patients with a Glasgow Coma Scale score of <8.

Simple manoeuvres

Open mouth:

1. Look for any obstructions.
2. If any obstructions are found they should be removed under direct vision:
    i) McGill's forceps can be used to remove any defined objects.
    ii) A wide bore, rigid (Yankauer) sucker is useful to remove liquids, eg blood/vomit.

Head tilt / chin lift:

1. Tilt the head back, extending the airway and reducing compression by anterior structures.
2. With fingertips beneath the anterior mandible, lift the chin forward.

Jaw thrust:

1. With index and other fingers of each hand behind the angle of the mandible, lift ('thrust') the mandible anteriorly and support it with sustained pressure

Adjuncts

When considering using adjuncts consider where within the airway the obstruction is and which parts of the airway the adjunct will support.

Oropharyngeal (Guedel®) airway

A curved flattened tube that can be inserted to lie between the tongue and hard palate.

Indications:

- Useful in unconscious patients in protecting them from posterior displacement of the tongue

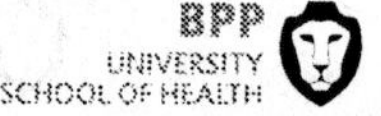

Contraindications:

- Patients with an intact gag reflex; may lead to vomiting or laryngospasm
- Maxillofacial injuries

Procedure:

1. Estimate size of the Guedel® required by holding different dizes parallel to the head. The correct size should reach from the incisors to the angle of the jaw
2. Open the mouth and remove any foreign material as above
3. Initially insert the Guedel® upside down. As it hits the palate rotate it 180° so that the curve is lying over the curve of the tongue
4. Reassess the patient

Nasopharyngeal airway

A flexible tube that is inserted through the nose to the oropharynx.

Indications:

- Useful in patients with reduced levels of consciousness but with intact gag reflexes

Contraindications:

- Known or suspected base of skull fracture
- Grossly abnormal nasal anatomy
- Severe maxillofacial injuries

Procedure:

1. Examine the nasal bridges and ethmoid sinuses to rule out any inflammation or trauma before proceeding. Check there are no obstructions in the nasopharynx.
2. Estimate the size required. The diameter has traditionally been estimated by using a size correlating to the size of the patient's little finger (6–8 mm are commonly used in adults).
3. New models have a flange to prevent the airway slipping into the nose. In older models place a safety pin across the end to prevent this.
4. Lubricate the pointed end of the airway without obstructing the lumen.
5. Insert airway into the larger nostril after examining for obstructions (eg septal deviation, polyps).
6. Advance directly posteriorly (not superiorly) until the flange lies against the nostrils.

Advanced airways

A number of more advanced airways are available, including laryngeal mask airways, iGel®, and laryngeal tubes. These should only be used when one is adequately trained. A cuffed endo-tracheal tube is the only definitive airway.

Tracheostomy tubes

A tracheostomy is a procedure that creates a direct opening into the trachea, creating a surgical airway. The patency of this surgical opening is maintained by the placement of a tracheostomy tube.

Tracheostomy tubes come in a variety of different sizes. When first inserted, a tube with a lumen roughly three-quarters of the size of the patient's tracheal lumen should be used. As the patient is weaned off their tracheostomy, the size of the tube may be decreased to allow increased movement of air through the upper airways.

Indications:

- Upper airway obstruction
- Prolonged mechanical ventilation in patients with respiratory failure
- Severe trauma and/or burns around the head and neck area

Contraindications:

- None – this is frequently a life-saving procedure

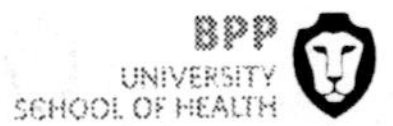

Tracheostomy tubes

Tracheostomy tube	Description
Cuffed	• Allows positive pressure mechanical ventilation and protects against aspiration of gastric contents. • Cuff pressures should be monitored meticulously and cuffs deflated regularly to reduce risk of tracheal stenosis.
Uncuffed	• Should be used in preference to cuffed tubes if the cuff is not necessary. • Allows movement of air around tracheostomy tube to facilitate speaking and weaning.
Fenestrated	• Additional opening in body of tube to allow air to pass through tube when external opening is plugged ie for speaking and weaning. • Fenestrations are often not in the correct place and can cause irritation and granulation of the tracheal mucosa.
Double-cannula tube	• This consists of an outer (permanent) tube and an inner tube which can be removed for short periods of time to be cleaned (or replaced). • It maintains patency of tracheostomy lumen for longer.
Single-cannula tube	• Single-lumen tube without an inner cannula. • They need to be changed more frequently to maintain patency of airway.

Table 9.7: Different types of tracheostomy tubes

Tracheostomy care

Whilst you will not be expected to know how to create a tracheostomy, you may have patients on the ward with tracheostomies and you should have an understanding of how to care for them.

Suctioning:

Suctioning of tracheostomy tubes is required when build-up of respiratory secretions within the tube lumen occurs. The frequency of suctioning varies with the ability of the patient to clear their secretions through expectorating. Luminal obstruction increases the work of breathing and causes respiratory distress.

1. Open sterile suctioning catheter and attach to the suction tubing using principles of ANTT
2. Insert suction catheter gently into tracheostomy tube to approximately one-third of the catheter length
3. Start suctioning as the catheter is removed by placing thumb over suction port
4. Suction should not be applied for longer than ten seconds to avoid hypoxia
5. If further suctioning is required a fresh suction catheter should be used
6. Repeat until airway is clear
7. Observe and document the amount of secretions, their colour and their consistency

Changing a tracheostomy tube:

Tracheostomy tubes need to be changed when the lumen becomes blocked with secretions in order to maintain airway patency. When single-cannula tracheostomies become blocked with secretions, the whole tube needs to be removed and a new tracheostomy tube placed through the stoma. This should be done with two people present and only by someone who is adequately trained.

Double-cannula tracheostomies have an inner tube which can be removed and either cleaned or replaced with a new inner tube, whilst the outer tube remains in situ. The inner tube should be removed during exhalation and replaced within 15 minutes.

Top tip:

Airway care can be a difficult core procedure to get signed off during daily clinical practice as using these skills will often not be planned in advance. Be proactive in using simulation sessions as an opportunity to demonstrate your skills on models.

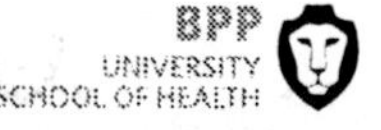

12. Urethral catheterisation

Indications

- To relieve urinary retention (acute or chronic)
- To accurately monitor urine output

Contraindications

- Established or suspected urethral trauma

Relevant anatomy

The male urethra consists of three main parts, the spongy urethra, membranous urethra and prostatic urethra. The prostate gland can prevent passage of the catheter if hypertrophic. The female urethra is shorter and straight. The external urethral meatus in females is immediately anterior to the vagina within the vestibule.

Equipment required

Sterile gloves (x2), catheter pack (contains sterile drape, gallipot, cotton wool, gauze, kidney dish, forceps), sterile saline, Foley catheter, local anaesthetic gel (eg Instillagel®), 10 ml syringe, 10 ml sterile water, catheter bag.

Catheter types:

Male catheters are longer than female catheters due to the greater length of the urethra. Catheter sizes are quoted in French gauge; larger diametre catheters have a larger number. In most cases a 12–14G is appropriate for males. Catheters used for intermittent self-catheterisation are usually narrower and do not have a balloon.

Top tip:

If unable to pass a catheter try again with a larger size and adjust the positioning of penis.

If struggling to identify the urethral meatus in females, warn the patient, insert index finger into vagina to elevate the anterior vulva and guide the catheter along the finger into the urethra.

Do not force the catheter in against resistance – you risk creating false passages and making future attempts more difficult.

Short-term catheters are latex and should be removed or changed after 2 weeks. Long-term catheters can remain in situ for up to 12 weeks.

Patients with clot retention, or who are at risk of clot retention (eg post-urological surgery), should have a triple lumen (three-way) catheter inserted. The third lumen allows for irrigation of the bladder.

Other types of catheter include Caudé catheters, which have an angled tip to aid passage of the catheter through an enlarged prostate.

Procedure

1. Prepare equipment on clean trolley
2. Expose the patient
3. Put on two pairs of sterile gloves
4. Place drape around genitalia
5. Place gauze around the shaft of the penis so that it can be held easily, retract the foreskin with one hand and clean glans with sterile normal saline, starting centrally
6. Insert local anaesthetic gel into the external urethral meatus and hold the penis upright for one to two minutes to limit leakage of gel
7. Remove outer pair of gloves (alternatively, wear one pair of gloves initially and change them at this point)
8. Insert Foley catheter into urethra whilst holding the penis taught and perpendicular to the body. Insert it up to the bi/trifurcation
9. Once inserted urine should start to drain from the catheter into kidney dish
10. Inflate balloon with 10 ml sterile water, whilst observing patient for evidence of pain (pain at this stage may indicate balloon inflation in the urethra – if this occurs stop and deflate the balloon)
11. Withdraw catheter until resistance is felt
12. Connect catheter to catheter bag
13. Replace foreskin
14. Document the procedure, including the volume of water in the balloon, the residual volume and that you have replaced the foreskin

Female catheters can be directly inserted following cleansing of the external urethral meatus and with

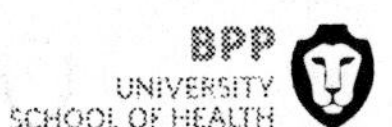

either simple lubrication of the catheter or local anaesthetic gel lubrication.

Complications

- Infection
- Bleeding
- Paraphimosis (if foreskin not replaced)
- Urethral perforation
- Creation of a false passage
- Urethral stricture (with long-term use)

Chapter 10

Mini Clinical Evaluation Exercise (Mini-CEX)

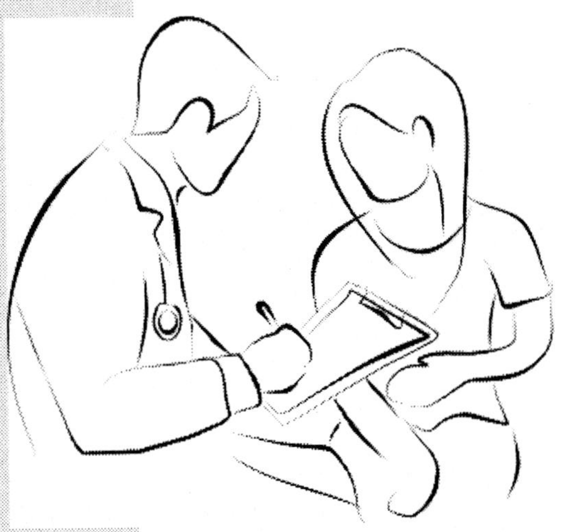

Chapter 10

Mini Clinical Evaluation Exercise (Mini-CEX)

All of the details that most of us memorize in medical school - you don't have to learn those things. They're going to be in your computer

Leroy Hood (1938–)

Introduction

Mini-CEX assessments are designed, unlike knowledge-based medical school examinations, to assess the important, practical aspects of a doctor's performance in a particular clinical encounter. These can vary from taking a history and performing specific examinations, to discussing diagnosis and/ or management plans with patients or their relatives.

Such work-based assessments are designed to help you develop post-graduate learning techniques whereby feedback enables you to identify personal areas of weakness and devise strategies to improve them.

This chapter aims to cover the basic structures of history taking, common examinations and a simple guide to basic communication skills. Further aspects specific to certain cases and conditions are discussed in the CBD chapters.

	Activity
Communication skills	Basic communication skills Communication in Mini-CEX settings Special cases
History taking	Basic structure and concepts
Medical examinations	Cardiovascular system Respiratory system Gastrointestinal system Peripheral nervous system Cranial nerve examination (speech, Parkinson's Disease, cerebellum) Musculoskeletal screening examination Locomotor system
Pre-operative	Pre-operative assessment Taking consent
Surgical examinations	Pre-operative examination Lumps (hernia, thyroid) Varicose veins Peripheral vascular system

Table 10.1: Examples of possible situations for carrying out Mini-CEX assessments

Mini-CEX assessments

Mini-CEX assessments require completion of a web-based assessment form by an assessor. The assessments can range from history taking to clinical judgement, professionalism, organisation and efficiency. The exact content depends on the nature of the encounter.

Communication skills

Basic communication skills

How to talk to people

Most of your time as a junior doctor will be spent communicating with patients, relatives, nurses, fellow colleagues, and other healthcare professionals. Remember that most complaints about doctors are not about mistakes, but about communication failure. Modern medical schools place a huge emphasis on communication skills, so you may be feeling confident about your ability to deal with communication problems. This confidence may evaporate the second you are faced with an angry relative, or when having to break bad news to a patient or relative. More often these intense communication situations occur when the ward is busy, or when there are a number of people present. Relatives will want to know 'what is going on with mum', without telling you who 'mum' is, or without allowing you time to collect your thoughts. They will expect you to know all of the medical information with regards to their family member, and it is in these pressured situations where you are in danger of forgetting your training and making communication errors.

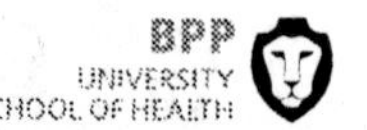

As with all skills, communication is something that you will improve on over time, and with practice. There is no substitute for this; however, this does not mean your communication skills will be poor! Some people are natural when it comes to communicating, others are less so. The most effective communicators are those that are able to explore the patient's knowledge, thoughts and expectations, and at the same time obtain the information required to complete the assessment. Listening to the patient, asking both open and closed questions and ensuring the conversation is a two-way process will almost inevitably lead to a positive outcome. Communication skills are part of Mini-CEX assessments, and a description of how they fit in is included later. The following are some useful tips that will help you whilst communicating:

Top tips:

- Be prepared
- Get off to a good start
- Find the agenda
- Be polite and caring
- Be clear
- End your conversation
- Have an exit strategy

Be prepared:

If you have time before initiating a conversation, always try to have all of the information to hand. An appropriate setting ensuring privacy with a chaperone is important, for example a private room, or often on the ward drawing the curtains of the cubicle.

Read the notes, look at any reports and blood tests, and ensure you are clear about the management plan. By having all of this information you will avoid the embarrassing situation of seeming to know very little about the patient in question, or worse, giving inaccurate information. Common questions often asked by patients include, do you have a firm diagnosis? If you do not, how are you planning on reaching one? What is my prognosis? How long will I stay in hospital? If you are prepared and have the answers to these questions, you will more likely be taken seriously.

Have an exit strategy:

Never start a conversation that you are unable to finish. Always know what your intended outcomes are: do you want to give the family some information, or do you want some information from them? Usually it will be a mixture of these.

You must also consider if you have sufficient time to continue a particular conversation. For example, if you are being approached for a 'quick word' on a hospital ward, and you are in the middle of looking after an acutely unwell patient, politely explain that this is not the best time and try to arrange a specific time, or for another member of the team to talk to the person in question. Consideration should also be given to whether you are the right person to be talking to this patient or relative.

Get off to a good start:

Make an effort to look smart, and dress appropriately. The rest is simple: introduce yourself, make direct eye contact with everyone involved in the conversation and ensure you know who you are talking to. Smile if it is appropriate.

Find the agenda:

Rarely do people just want to have 'a chat'. Usually there is another motive to people wanting to speak with you. It is your job to find out what the other issues are, in order for you to address any of their concerns. There is no fixed method to achieve this, but there are some ways to make the situation easy for you. Start the conversation with the patients or relatives with an open statement inviting them to express their expectations. Try:

'How may I help you?'

or

'Is there anything you would like to know?'

Let the person you are talking to do most of the talking to start with. This will allow you to get a feel for what they want out of the conversation. Sometimes agendas are hidden, and will take all of your skill, and potentially more than one conversation, to elicit. People have to trust you before they tell you their deepest secrets and concerns, so give them time and space to talk.

Be polite and caring:

Again, this sounds obvious, and something you would normally do, but there is a special sort of politeness that helps with communicating with patients and relatives. Your aim should be to actively listen and ensure the patient feels they have your complete attention. Making people feel like they are your number one priority will make them feel their concerns are valued, and that you genuinely care for them. Try not to break off from a conversation until it is obviously finished. In situations where you are explaining delicate and potentially difficult information, make sure you hand over your bleep to a colleague, and ensure you have a nurse present.

Be clear:

Always say exactly what you mean, in a manner that your audience will understand. Avoid medical jargon, abbreviations or technical terms. People will remember only a fraction of what you are saying, so do not be afraid to repeat the important facts. If you have any doubts as to whether you are being clear, ask the person directly: 'Does that make sense?' or 'Am I being clear?' Ask them to summarise or repeat back to you what you have said, therefore confirming that they have understood the information.

End your conversation:

Ending the conversation can sometimes be difficult; however, there are a number of ways to do this; the easiest way is to summarise the conversation and then ask the other person if they agree. Finally thank them for their time and leave. Other, more subtle, techniques are just as effective. Try listening for a while whilst crouching or kneeling at the bedside, and then standing up when you want to end the conversation. Your actions can be interpreted as 'stretching your legs', but it gives a sense of movement to the conversation. Always ensure the patient is happy to end the conversation, and that they have been able to ask all their questions.

Communication in Mini-CEX assessments

Mini-CEX are observed encounters with patients. They may take the form of any interaction of the doctor and the patient, but are often stereotyped encounters, where a senior watches you take a history from a patient or perform a clinical examination. There are separate sections for history taking and communication skills, although these are often closely linked in the actual clinical event.

Treat the assessment as you would any simple interaction with a patient. There should be nothing different done just because someone is watching you, and the following is good practice for any clinical encounter.

Generic history

Introduce yourself and explain who you are in the team. Apologise for the presence of your assessor and explain that they are watching to make sure that you are doing the right things. Confirm with the patient they consent to this.

Find out who anyone else around the patient might be (partner, friend, or taxi driver) and check if the patient wants them to stay whilst you talk to them, or if they would rather be on their own.

Start with some open questions; find out what the patient is worried about most and why they are in hospital/your office. Try to spend the first third of the conversation saying as little as possible.

Then move on to asking some closed questions. By now you should have a good idea about which system is troubling the patient. If you don't, you haven't let the patient say enough early on. Focus on a system and ask the patient some specific questions. These questions are covered in the history taking Mini-CEX below.

Ideas, concerns and expectations

Explain what you are going to do next (examine patient, take blood etc) and ask the patient if they have any questions they might like to ask. Use specific signpost questions, so your assessor can tick this box:

- 'Tell me about what you think is causing your symptoms?'
- 'What do you think might be happening?'
- 'What are your main concerns?'
- 'Is there anything particular or specific that you are concerned about?'
- 'What do you think might be the best plan of action?'
- 'How might I best help you with this?'

Closing the encounter

When you have finished your clinical encounter, thank the patient for their time, and ask them again if they have any questions. Tell them what your plan is and ensure they understand what will happen next. Try to give them a feel for how long they might have to

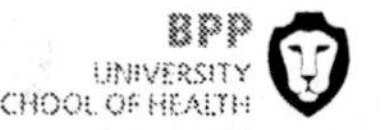

wait, and what sorts of outcomes they might expect. Give them a way of getting hold of you again, even if it is just telling them that the nurses can bleep you if needed.

Special cases

There are a few special situations where all your skills will be tested, and it is a good idea to have a strategy for dealing with them. Here we will discuss dealing with an angry person, and breaking bad news.

Talking to angry people

People get angry because they cannot control the situation they are in. They might be afraid, or in pain, or have unrealistic expectations that have not been met. They have resorted to anger because they cannot get what they want through more peaceful means. Different people resort to anger at different times, but the basic formula is the same.

Usually you will be called to see an angry patient or relative because they are angry, for example at the nursing staff, and they have decided they need your help to deal with it. Alternatively the person themselves have demanded to see a doctor, because they think you will be able to give them what they want. Sometimes they will approach you directly.

Remember when dealing with angry people that if they are verbally or physically threatening or abusive, you simply do not have to talk to them. Warn them that they are overstepping the mark, and if they continue to be aggressive, walk away stating they are being hostile, therefore you will not discuss anything further and will call security.

Usually, people are angry within the limits of social acceptability. In these cases, your aim should be to diffuse the situation, and then identify with them exactly what it is making them angry. The following may assist you in achieving this:

1. Diffuse the situation by remaining calm yourself.
2. Never lose your composure.
3. Use 'open' body language; do not fold your arms or stand over people's beds.
4. Use slow, deliberate and open gestures.
5. Ensure appropriate eye contact and tone of voice.
6. Simply listening to an angry person for a few minutes is usually enough to calm the situation.
7. If it is possible to apologise for the problem, do so. This is not an admission of guilt or fault, but it will help placate the person and show that you are trying to be constructive and not defensive. For example, 'I am really sorry that you feel that the nurse/doctor did not get your mother the analgesia when she asked. I can see that this has really upset you'.
8. Once the situation has become calm, enquire about the exact nature of why the person is angry.
9. They may have lots of different complaints, and therefore may not seem all that focused, in which case try to get them to tell you what is mostly upsetting them.
10. Ask them for their opinion on how the problem can be resolved. If this is possible, go ahead and do it. However, if it is not possible, calmly explain the reason why this is, and offer an alternative solution.
11. Sometimes, people will be directly angry at you, or at something you have done. Again, if they are threatening or abusive, walk away from the situation. If they are willing to listen and remain calm, try to explain your reasoning and thoughts with regards to the incident they are angry about.
12. If you are genuinely to blame for an incident, then apologise and take their criticism on board.
13. Patients and relatives should be made aware of the PALS if they wish to lodge an official complaint.
14. After the situation has resolved, speak to your consultant to discuss the event and acknowledge any important learning points from the incident. At the same time write a short piece known as reflective practice to insert into your learning portfolio, which again will help you to identify both positive and negative aspects about the incident, and help you to identify areas to improve on when faced with similar situations in the future.

If during the interaction you feel out of your depth, request a senior to deal with the problem. Remember the NHS has a zero tolerance policy on violence or abuse of any of its staff.

Breaking bad news

Telling someone bad news is always difficult. There are a number of different methods used, and you may have heard of some of these strategies before. This is simply a general guide to the sorts of things that you will need to consider when breaking bad news.

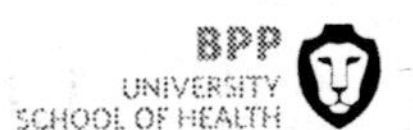

Placement:

1. Explain that you want to have an important discussion, and ask the patient if there is anyone they would like to have around when this discussion takes place.
2. If there is, you can arrange a time for you to meet them.
3. Try to meet in a quiet place where there is a low chance of being interrupted.
4. Take a nurse with you.
5. Ideally the person breaking the bad news should be a senior doctor, but this is not always the case.
6. Hand your bleep to a colleague to ensure you will not be disturbed.

Information:

1. Again, enter this encounter armed with as much information as you can.
2. Usually, patients will want not only to know the piece of bad news, but what this means for them.
3. You should aim to know the prognosis for the condition in question, and what the immediate management will be.
4. Talk to your seniors about this if you have the chance.

Prior knowledge:

1. Ask directly what the patient knows, and what sort of news they are expecting.
2. They may tell you that they are worried about the specific piece of bad news you are bearing.
3. They may have completely unrealistic expectations, in which case you can explain that their understanding is not quite accurate, and slowly introduce a more realistic view.

Be direct:

1. When the time comes to tell your patient the news, do so clearly and without medical jargon or euphemism.
2. Allow this information to sink in, and answer any questions to the best of your ability.
3. If there is information that you do not have – admit it, and promise to find out.
4. Offer the services of the hospital counsellors or the bereavement team.
5. Leave the way open to talk to a senior doctor at a later time.

Prognosis:

1. Patients will want a prognosis.
2. You can never provide an exact answer.
3. Describe prognosis if your seniors have mentioned one, or explain that more tests will be required before a prognosis can be made.

Documentation:

1. Record in the multidisciplinary notes what was discussed and who was present at the meeting.
2. Document what the patient wanted to know and what their expectations were, as well as a description of their reaction.
3. Ensure that the date, time, signature, name and designation are clearly documented.

Confidentiality

Breaking confidentiality is illegal and unprofessional. Confidentiality is often broken through carelessness, rather than malice, so be on your guard. Simple measures, like refraining from discussing patients in public (including the corridors of the hospital, lifts, on the bus) should ensure you never breach confidentiality. Never leave your 'patient ward list' lying around. Always be careful about carrying patient data around on electronic devices such as USB memory sticks. Ensure these are encrypted if you do use them.

Relatives:

Relatives have no absolute right to information. They can only be told about your patient's condition if your patient agrees to this. The 2005 Mental Capacity Act has been put in place to protect those individuals who do not have the capacity to make decisions for themselves (eg patients with dementia, head injuries and learning disabilities). Sometimes this can lead to difficulties with relatives, especially those of elderly people. If someone is not deemed capable of giving consent for this, then talking to their relatives can be done under the 'doctrine of necessity', if you determine that the conversation is in the patient's best interest.

Telephone conversations are often difficult, as you are never quite sure who you are talking to. Best practice is to ask the person on the phone to come

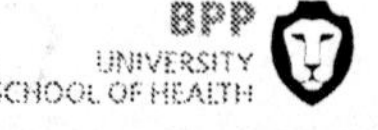

in and speak to you in person, and at the same time take the patient's consent to speak about them with this person.

Children:

Talking to parents is not considered to be a breach of confidentiality unless the child is 'Gillick' or 'Fraser' competent and expresses the wish that their parents are not informed. Children under the age of 16 are considered to be 'Gillick' or 'Fraser' competent if they have the ability to sufficiently understand the information given to them, and fully understand what is being proposed. Obviously, this requires a judgement to be made, so if you identify any potential problems, call a senior early on.

History taking

Observe, record, tabulate, communicate. Use your five senses. Learn to see, learn to hear, learn to feel, learn to smell, and know that by practice alone you can become expert.

William Osler (1849–1919)

A good, well-structured, and accurate history is often the key to successful diagnosis, and appropriate management. All histories should include certain common elements, although the exact structure may vary depending on the clinical setting.

Always consider why you are asking the questions and what you aim to gain from the history. This allows you to target your questions and interpret the significance of the answers. For instance, the significance of smoking is different for a patient being assessed pre-operatively, to a patient presenting with possible lung cancer. The typical format and structure of a history is as follows:

1. **Presenting complaint:** Why has the patient presented, and what is the main problem?
2. **History of presenting complaint:**
   i) What/Where/When
   ii) Events before/during/after
   iii) Associated/exacerbating/relieving factors
3. **Past medical history:**
   i) Medical, surgical (anaesthetic), possibly obstetric or psychiatric background, including recent hospital admissions, procedures or chronic medical conditions
   ii) Screen for common conditions (**most relevant in bold**):
      M – previous MI (or CV disease)
      J – jaundice (or hepatic disease)
      T – TB
      H – hypertension
      R – rheumatic
      E – epilepsy
      A – asthma (resp diseases)
      D – diabetes
      S – stroke or CVA, PE/DVT
4. **Drug history:**
   i) Regular medications (dose, time, indication)
   ii) PRN medications
   iii) OTC (over-the-counter) medications
   iv) Drug allergies (what happens, timing in relation to drug, any alternatives tried)
5. **Family history:**
   i) First, second degree relative
   ii) Treatment and outcomes
   iii) Any known genetics
6. **Social history:**
   i) Where the patient lives and with whom
   ii) Any extra support from family or carers
   iii) Occupation(s): current and past
   iv) Activities of daily living
   v) Other activities/hobbies
   vi) Pets

1 pack year = 20 cigarettes/day for 1 year

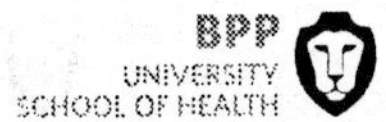

vii) Smoking history: define what is/has been smoked in pack years if possible

viii) Illicit drugs – ask directly

$$\text{Number of units} = \frac{\text{Volume}(\text{ml}) \times \text{strength}(\%)}{1{,}000}$$

ix) Alcohol history: volume and type of alcohol (calculate weekly units). 1 unit = 10 g pure alcohol

Roughly:

- 750 ml (13.5%) bottle of wine = 10 units
- 1 large shot (35 ml) of spirits = 1.4 units
- 1 pint 3.5% beer/lager/cider = 2 units
- 1 pint 5.2% beer/lager/cider = 5 units
- 275 ml 5.5% alcopop = 1.5 units
  - Pattern of drinking: regular, binge
  - Features of alcoholism: formal CAGE criteria:

    C – Do you think you should cut down?

    A – Do you get angry when people try and discuss drinking?

    G – Do you feel guilty about your drinking?

    E – Eye-opener: Do you need a drink in the morning?

7. **Systemic enquiry:**

   Any other symptoms:

   i) **Cardiovascular system:** chest pain, palpitations, dyspnoea, orthopnoea, paroxysml nocturnal dyspnoea, syncope

   ii) **Respiratory system:** shortness of breath, cough, sputum, haemoptysis, pleuritic chest pain

   iii) **Gastrointestinal system:** constipation, diarrhoea, rectal bleeding, nausea and vomiting, jaundice, haematemesis, change in appetite, abdominal pain or lump, change in bowel habit

   iv) **Musculoskeletal system:** joint pain, stiffness, rash

   v) **Central and peripheral nervous system:** headache, collapse, seizures, dizziness, limb weakness or numbness

   vi) **Genitourinary system:** frequency, dysuria, nocturia

   vii) **General:** fatique, weight loss, lethargy

Once the history has been taken, this naturally progresses to performing a clinical examination after obtaining consent from the patient.

Medical examinations

Common principles

The importance of the 'end-of-the-bed-ogram' cannot be overstated! Similarly, building a good rapport with your patient through a calm, reassuring and professional manner and communicating your findings succinctly and logically are also of great importance and require practice.

General structural overview (non-musculoskeletal or neurological examinations)

- Inspection
- Palpation
- Percussion
- Auscultation

Cardiovascular system examination

1. **Introduction**

   i) Wash your hands

   ii) Introductions (name and role)

   iii) Explanation and consent

   iv) Exposure (maintain dignity)

   v) Establish any current discomfort or patient concerns (ask if they would like a chaperone if appropriate)

   vi) Position at 45 degrees

2. **Peripheral examination**

   i) General appearance: unwell, in pain, pale, obvious scars, mitral facies, marfanoid features

   ii) Hands: clubbing, stigmata of infective endocarditis (splinter haemorrhages, Osler's nodes, Janeway lesions)

   iii) Capillary refill <2s (press nail bed 5s)

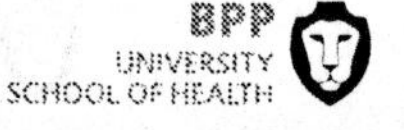

iv) Radial pulses together: rate, rhythm, pattern (eg collapsing – AR, slow-rising – AS); and radio-radial delay (coarctation of the aorta)

v) Measure blood pressure accurately

vi) Examine the JVP level (vertically from the sternomanubrial joint) including the hepatojugular reflex

vii) Palpate the carotid pulse for character

viii) Eyes: pale conjunctiva, corneal arcus and xanthelasma, jaundice

ix) Mouth: cyanosis, dentition, high arched palate (Marfan's syndrome)

3. **Central examination**

   i) Expose the chest and inspect the precordium for scars/PPM and axillae for thoracotomy scars

   ii) Palpate the position (should be fifth intercostal space, mid-clavicular line) and character of the apex beat

   iii) Palpate for heaves (LVH) and thrills (palpable murmur)

   iv) Auscultate: all four praecordial areas, left axilla and carotids

   v) Auscultate in mitral area with patient in left lateral position in inspiration and at the left sternal edge with the patient leaning forwards in expiration. The former accentuates mitral murmurs and the latter aortic (identify the character of the two heart sounds, any additional sounds, any murmurs)

   vi) Auscultate the lung fields

   vii) Examine for peripheral and sacral oedema and leg scars consistent with venous harvesting

4. **Completing the examination**

   i) Examine observation chart and ECGs; offer to examine for AAA and the peripheral vascular system

   ii) Reposition the patient to ensure dignity and comfort. Thank the patient

   iii) Present positive findings and salient negatives in a logical and appropriate manner

Characterising murmurs

The following features of any murmur should be noted:

- **Character:** ejection/pansystolic
- **Timing:** systolic/diastolic; early/mid/late

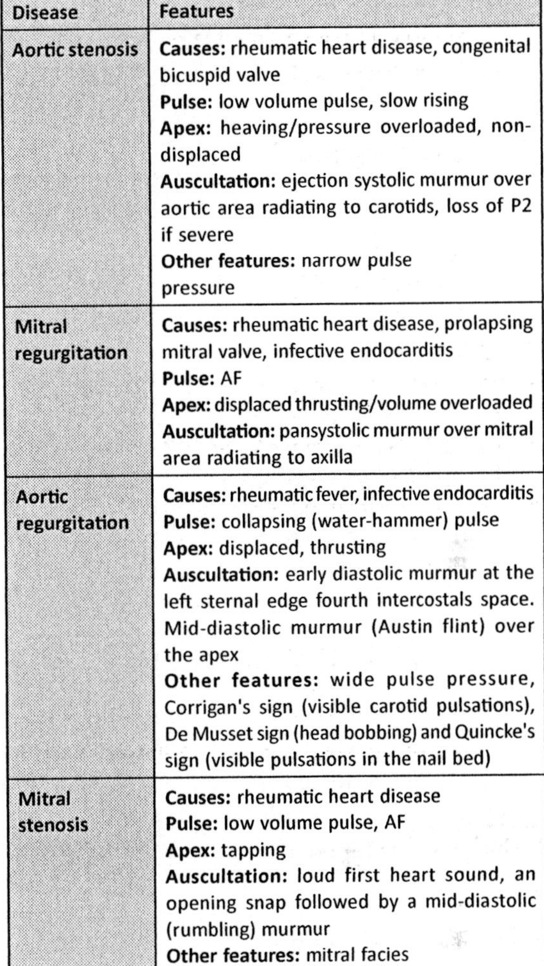

Disease	Features
Aortic stenosis	**Causes:** rheumatic heart disease, congenital bicuspid valve **Pulse:** low volume pulse, slow rising **Apex:** heaving/pressure overloaded, non-displaced **Auscultation:** ejection systolic murmur over aortic area radiating to carotids, loss of P2 if severe **Other features:** narrow pulse pressure
Mitral regurgitation	**Causes:** rheumatic heart disease, prolapsing mitral valve, infective endocarditis **Pulse:** AF **Apex:** displaced thrusting/volume overloaded **Auscultation:** pansystolic murmur over mitral area radiating to axilla
Aortic regurgitation	**Causes:** rheumatic fever, infective endocarditis **Pulse:** collapsing (water-hammer) pulse **Apex:** displaced, thrusting **Auscultation:** early diastolic murmur at the left sternal edge fourth intercostals space. Mid-diastolic murmur (Austin flint) over the apex **Other features:** wide pulse pressure, Corrigan's sign (visible carotid pulsations), De Musset sign (head bobbing) and Quincke's sign (visible pulsations in the nail bed)
Mitral stenosis	**Causes:** rheumatic heart disease **Pulse:** low volume pulse, AF **Apex:** tapping **Auscultation:** loud first heart sound, an opening snap followed by a mid-diastolic (rumbling) murmur **Other features:** mitral facies

Table 10.2: Features of common valvular heart conditions

- **Loudness:** (note: the 6 point Levine grading scale exists, but is rarely used in practice)
- **Location:** site where the murmur is the loudest
- **Radiation:** axilla or carotids
- **Accentuating manoeuvres:** inspiration accentuates right-sided and expiration left-sided murmurs

Respiratory system examination

1. **Introduction** (as per cardiovascular examination)
2. **Peripheral examination**

   i) General appearance: unwell, in pain, pale, obvious scars, respiratory effort (accessory muscles, nasal flaring, cyanosis, oxygen in situ)

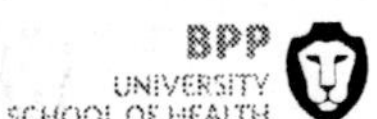

ii) Respiratory rate
iii) Hands: clubbing, tar stains, small muscle wasting, CO_2 retention flap and tremor
iv) Radial pulse
v) JVP level
vi) Eyes: Horner's syndrome (meiosis, ipsilateral partial ptosis, enophthalmos, and ipsilateral anhydrosis)
vii) Conjunctival membrane: anaemia
viii) Mouth for central cyanosis/poor dentition from smoking

3. **Central examination**
   i) Tracheal position and apex beat
   ii) Cervical, supraclavicular, axilliary lymphadenopathy
   iii) Expose the chest and examine the precordium for deformities and scars and axillae/back for thoracotomy scars
   iv) Measure chest expansion, assessing for symmetry
   v) Percuss anterior chest, identifying hypo- or hyper-resonance and auscultate in same positions
   vi) Repeat for the posterior chest (can also palpate for tactile fremitus and auscultate for either vocal resonance or whispering pectoriloquy)
   vii) Examine for peripheral and sacral oedema
4. **Completing the examination**
   i) Examine: observation chart, drug chart, peak flow readings and any sputum samples
   ii) Reposition the patient to ensure dignity and comfort. Thank the patient
   iii) Present positive findings and salient negatives in a logical and appropriate manner

Abdominal examination

1. **Introduction** (as per cardiovascular examination)
2. **Peripheral examination**
   i) General appearance: unwell, in pain, pale, obvious scars, jaundice, dehydrated
   ii) **Hands:** signs of chronic liver disease (clubbing, leukconychia, koilonychia, palmar erythema, dupytren's contracture, liver flap)
   iii) Radial pulse
   iv) Arms: tattoos, needle marks, scars/intravenous drug marks and dialysis fistulae
   v) Eyes: anaemia, jaundice and xanthelasma
   vi) Mouth: angular cheilitis (iron or B vitamin deficiency), foetor hepatica, candidiasis, leukoplakia, glossitis (B12 deficiency) or ulcers (possible Crohn's disease)
   viii) Palpate the supraclavicular lymph nodes (Virchow's node)
   ix) Chest: gynaecomastia, loss of axillary hair
3. **Abdominal examination** (lie the patient flat for this part)
   i) Inspect for abdominal striae, scars, body hair distribution, dilated veins, shape, and obvious swellings/masses/hernias

Disease	Features
Consolidation	**Mediastinum:** central **Ipsilateral chest wall movement:** decreased **Percussion:** dull **Auscultation:** bronchial breathing, reduced breath sounds, coarse crackles **Vocal Resonance/Whispering Pectoriloquy/ Tactile Vocal Fremitus:** increased
Collapse	**Mediastinum:** shifted towards collapse **Ipsilateral chest wall movement:** decreased **Percussion:** decreased **Auscultation:** reduced breath sounds
Effusion	**Mediastinum:** shifted away from effusion **Ipsilateral chest wall movement:** decreased **Percussion:** stony dull **Auscultation:** reduced breath sounds Crackles and/or bronchial breathing just above the effusion **Vocal Resonance/Tactile Vocal Fremitus:** reduced
Simple Pneumothorax	**Mediastinum:** central **Ipsilateral chest wall movement:** decreased on affected side **Percussion:** resonant **Auscultation:** reduced breath sounds
Tension Pneumothorax	**Mediastinum:** shifted away from affected side **Ipsilateral chest wall movement:** decreased on affected side **Percussion:** hyper-resonant **Auscultation:** reduced breath sounds

Table 10.3: Examination findings of common respiratory conditions

ii) Ask the patient to breathe in (to exaggerate masses/organomegaly) and to cough (to exaggerate hernias)
iii) Kneel down to the level of the patient's abdomen – check for visible pulsations (aneurysms) and visible peristalsis (small bowel obstruction)
iv) Ask if there is any pain in abdomen and look at the face throughout the examination
v) Palpate gently all four quadrants of the abdomen (starting away from any pain)
vi) Check for tenderness on superficial and deep palpation, guarding, masses/lumps and bumps
vii) Palpates the liver, starting at the right iliac fossa (RIF) and asking patient to breathe in/out until the inferior margin is palpable
viii) Percuss the liver, from the nipple line down to the RIF; if enlarged, assess size, tenderness, regularity and pulsatility
ix) Palpate for the spleen, starting at the RIF and asking patient to breath in/out
x) If enlarged, assess size and surface
xi) Balott both kidneys and if enlarged, assess size, surface and consistency
xii) Palpate for an AAA
xiii) Check for shifting dullness
xiv) Listen for bowel sounds and any aortic or renal bruits

4. **Completing the examination**
   i) Offer to perform a digital rectal examination, dipstick the urine (urinalysis), examine for hernias and the external genitalia (in a male). Look at the observation and drug charts
   ii) Reposition the patient to ensure dignity and comfort and thank the patient
   iii) Present positive findings and salient negatives in a logical and appropriate manner

Peripheral nervous system examination

It is important to remember that this examination requires a patient to perform some 'strange' and complicated manoeuvres. Being well rehearsed in the routing yourself and knowing what you are going to say to describe the movements is extremely important.

Always remember to compare one side to the other and follow the structure:

- Special tests
- Tone
- Power
- Reflexes
- Sensation
- Co-ordination

Upper limb

1. **Introduction** (as per cardiovascular examination – ensure adequate exposure, including shoulder)
   i) General inspection: look for obvious deformities, wasting, fasciculations (UMN lesion) and resting tremor
   ii) Pronator drift: arms stretched fully out, palms up, eyes closed – and pronation (possibly UMN lesion)
2. **Tone**
   i) Ensure the patient is relaxed. Flex and extend the elbow and pronate and supinate at the wrist looking for hypotonia or rigidity – 'clasp-knife' or 'leadpipe'. Look for 'cogwheeling' at the wrist. If it is suspected ask the patient to perform any other distracting movement to reinforce the effect.
3. **Power** (demonstrate actions required and oppose them with the same muscles as those being tested when possible)
   i) Shoulder abduction and adduction: 'Make wings with your arms and don't let me push them up or down.' (Note – this will not test supraspinatus)
   ii) Elbow flexion and extension: 'Hold your arms in front of you with the elbows bent. Pull me towards you. Push me away.'
   iii) Wrist flexion and extension: 'Hold your fists out in front of you. Don't let me push them down.'
   iv) Grip strength (long and short finger flexors): 'Squeeze my fingers as hard as you can'.
   v) Thumb abduction: 'Hold your hands out, palm upwards and thumbs to the sky. Don't let me push it down'.
   vi) Finger abduction: 'Spread your fingers. Don't let me close them'.
   vii) Finger extension: 'Hold your fingers out straight, don't let me bend them'.

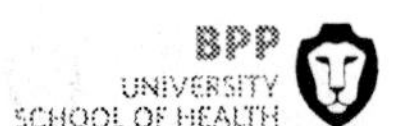

viii) Finger adduction: 'Put this paper between fingers and don't let me pull it out'.

4. **Reflexes** (if initially absent, use reinforcement)
   i) Biceps (C5/6)
   ii) Triceps (C7)
   iii) Supinator (C5/6)
   iv) Finger – positive Hoffmann's sign in UMN lesions
5. **Sensation**
   i) Light touch: Ask the patient to close their eyes and demonstrate light touch with some cotton wool over the upper part of the sternum.
   ii) With the upper limbs in the anatomical position, randomly touch them in every dermatome (C5-T2) and specific innervating nerve areas, asking the patient to say 'yes' whenever they feel you (note: axillary, radial, median and ulnar nerves are tested in the regimental patch region, anatomical snuffbox, radial index and ulnar little fingers respectively).
   iii) Repeat for pin-prick and ideally temperature.
   iv) Vibration: Use a 128 Hz tuning fork. After demonstrating on the sternum, start on the thumb and if unable to distinguish the vibration work proximally on bony prominences on the wrist and elbow.
   v) Joint position sense: Gripping the thumb by the sides ask the patient to close their eyes and demonstrate an up movement and a down movement. Then move the thumb up or down and ask the patient which direction you have moved it. If unable to tell reliably, move up a joint and test the wrist.
6. **Co-ordination**
   i) Past-pointing with the 'finger-nose' test
   ii) Dysdiadochokinesis

Movement/action	Muscle	Innervation
Shoulder abduction (first 60)	Supraspinatus	C5
Shoulder abduction	Deltoid	C5
Shoulder adduction	Pectoralis muscles	C5-C8
Elbow flexion	Biceps	C5/C6
Elbow extension	Triceps	C7
Wrist flexion	Flexor Carpi Radialis Flexor Carpi Ulnaris	Median nerve Ulnar nerve
Wrist extension	Long extensors	Radial nerve
Power grip (finger flexion)	Long and short flexors	C8–T1
Thumb abduction	Abductor Pollicis Brevis	Median nerve
Finger abduction	Dorsal Interossei	Ulnar nerve/T1
Finger extension	Long extensors	Radial nerve/C8
Finger adduction	Palmar Interossei	Ulnar nerve/T1

Table 10.4: Movements/actions of the upper limb and the muscle and nerves involved

Lower limb

1. **Introduction** (as above with exposure as dignity permits)
2. **Special tests**
   i) If they are able, ask the patient to stand and walk and examine their gait.
   ii) Heel-to-toe walking.
   iii) Romberg's test 'Stand with your feet together. Now close your eyes.' Ensure you reassure the patient that they won't fall and that you lightly support them at the shoulders.
3. **Tone**
   i) Ensure the patient is relaxed and not trying to 'help' you. Roll the leg from side to side, looking at the toes to help decide on abnormal tone. Quickly lift under the knee and release.
   ii) Check for ankle clonus (up to four beats is normal).
4. **Power**
   i) Hip flexion/extension: 'keep your leg straight and lift it off the bed. Do not let me push it down. Now push down against my hand'.
   ii) Knee flexion and extension: 'bend your legs. Pull your ankle towards your bottom. Now push out against my hand'.
   iii) Ankle dorsiflexion and plantar flexion: 'stop me pushing your foot down. Now push down against my hand'.
5. **Reflexes**
   i) Knee (L3/4)
   ii) Ankle (S1)

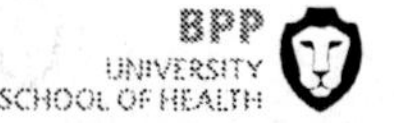

iii) Plantar – Babinski sign (upgoing in upper motor neurone lesions)

6. **Co-ordination**
   i) Heel-shin test
7. **Sensation**
   i) Light touch: Ask the patient to close their eyes and demonstrate light touch with some cotton wool over the upper part of the sternum. Then randomly touch the lower limbs in every dermatome.
   ii) Pin-prick.
   iii) Vibration: Use a 128 Hz tuning fork. After demonstrating on the sternum, start on the great toe then, if absent there, move proximally to the medial malleolus, knee and iliac crest.
   iv) Joint position sense: Gripping the great toe by the sides ask the patient to close their eyes and demonstrate an up movement and a down movement. Then move the toe up or down and ask the patient which direction you have moved it.
   v) Note: sensory loss may be in a dermatomal pattern, but much more commonly it is in a 'stocking' distribution – if so, delineate the level.

Movement/action	Muscle	Innervation
Hip flexion	Iliopsoas	L1/L2
Hip extension	Gluteal muscles	L4/L5
Knee flexion	Hamstring muscles	L5/S1
Knee extension	Quadriceps	L3/L4
Dorsiflexion of the ankle	Tibialis anterior and long flexors	L4/L5
Plantar flexion of the ankle	Gastronemius	S1
Extension of the great toe	Extensor Hallucis Longus	L5

Table 10.5: Movements/actions of the lower limb and the muscle and nerves involved

0	Complete absence of movement
1	Flicker of movement
2	Movement when gravity eliminated
3	Movement against gravity but not against resistance
4	Movement against resistance but not full power
5	Normal power

Table 10.6: MRC power scale

8. **Completing the examination**
   i) Examine: observation chart, drug chart. Ask to examine central nervous system
   ii) Reposition the patient to ensure dignity and comfort. Thank the patient
   iii) Present positive findings and salient negatives in a logical and appropriate manner

Reflexes are conventionally graded:

–	No response. Abnormal
+	Slight response. May be normal
++	Brisk response. Normal
+++	Very brisk response. May be abnormal
++++	Clonus or abnormal

Table 10.7: Reflex grading scale

Patterns of peripheral weakness

Upper motor neuron (UMN):

- Increased tone/spasticity (note: acute stroke may have hypotonia)
- Pyramidal pattern of weakness: all muscles are weaker but the arm flexors are stronger than the extensors and the leg extensors are stronger than the flexors
- Hyper-reflexia
- Upgoing plantars
- Typical causes: stroke, demyelination, and spinal cord damage

Lower motor neuron (LMN):

- Wasting and fasciculations
- Flaccid tone
- Weakness
- Hypo-reflexia
- Typical causes: radiculopathy, mononeuropathy and damage to a peripheral nerve

Neuromuscular junction:

- Symmetrical weakness
- Fatigability: muscles become weaker with ongoing activity
- Typical cause: myasthenia gravis

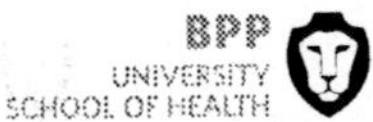

Muscle weakness:

- Symmetrical weakness
- Usually proximal
- No other neurological signs
- Typical causes: muscular dystrophy, Cushing's syndrome, paraneoplastic, polymyositis
- Note: Myotonic dystrophy is atypical and causes distal weakness. Polymyalgia rheumatica causes pain and stiffness but not weakness

Abnormal gaits

Spastic:

- Foot turned inward
- Hip tilts upwards to lift the affected foot off the floor
- Look for hemiplegia and UMN lesion

Cerebellar:

- Foot turned outwards
- Wide based, and unsteady
- Lurching from side to side
- Look for other cerebellar signs

Ataxic:

- Wide based
- Stamping
- Patient looks at the floor to see where their feet are
- Check Romberg's sign and proprioception

High stepping:

- Knee lifted high to lift the forefoot from the ground
- Foot drop
- Common peroneal nerve palsy

Parkinsonian:

- Difficulty instigating movement
- Short and shuffling steps ('festinant gait')
- Loss of arm swing
- Look for other signs of Parkinson's disease

Waddling:

- Wide gait
- Weight shifted from side to side
- Look for proximal neuropathy

Nerve palsies

Median nerve:

Causes of lesions:

- Carpal tunnel syndrome: idiopathic, rheumatoid arthritis, hypothyroidism, acromegaly, occupational eg those who suffer repeated wrist vibrations/ pressure
- Trauma to the wrist
- Supracondylar humeral fracture
- Mononeuropathies

Clinical features:

- Thenar wasting
- Tinel's and Phalen's signs
- Test with thumb abduction and opposition
- Sensory loss to the area supplied
- May need nerve conduction studies prior to any surgical decompression of the carpal tunnel

Ulnar nerve:

Causes of lesions:

- Trauma or arthritis at the medial epicondyle of the elbow
- Wrist trauma
- Compression against the pisiform and hamate bones of the hand. This is commonly seen in occupations with prolonged pressure to the outer part of the palm such as road workers using vibrating drills
- Mononeuropathies

Clinical features:

- Generalised wasting of the hand with sparing of the thenar eminence
- Dorsal guttering
- Froment's sign (flexion of IPJ due to FPL compensation when asked to grip a piece of paper between thumb and index finger)
- Low lesion (at the wrist): claw hand due to paralysis of the lumbricals causing hyperextension of the MCP joints. At the same time, the intact flexor digitorum profundus (FDP) flexes DIP joints
- High lesion (at the elbow): the less pronounced claw hand (the ulnar paradox) as the FDPs are also paralysed
- Sensory loss to the area supplied

Radial nerve:

Causes of radial nerve lesions:

- Fracture of humeral shaft: the nerve runs along the radial groove on the lateral border
- Saturday night palsy: sleeping with the arm over the back of a chair

Motor	Sensory
Motor to 4 muscles – 'LOAF' • Lateral 2 lumbricals • Opponens pollicis • Abductor pollicis brevis • Flexor pollicis brevis	Sensation to thumb and lateral 2 ½ fingers

Table 10.8: Motor and sensory innervations of the median nerve

Motor	Sensory
Motor to all the other intrinsic muscles of the hand.	Sensation to the little and medial border of the ring finger.

Table 10.9: Motor and sensory innervations of the ulnar nerve

Motor	Sensory
Motor to the forearm extensors (extends the wrist).	Sensation to the anatomical snuff-box.

Table 10.10: Motor and sensory innervations of the radial nerve

- Trauma to brachial plexus (Klumpke's paralysis – lower roots)
- Mononeuropathies

Clinical features:

- Wrist drop: test power of wrist extension
- Reduced grip strength as wrist extension is required for full strength
- Sensory impairment in the area supplied

Central nervous system examination

1. **Introduction** (as per peripheral nervous examination – patient should be seated, facing examiner)
2. **Cranial nerves**
   i) Examine face for any obvious abnormalities eg facial droop
   ii) **CN I (olfactory):** ask about any changes in taste/smell; can be formally tested with scents if required
   iii) **CN II (optic):**
      - Acuity: Snellen chart if possible/book or newspaper if not. Test each eye independently. If acuity too poor to read, use finger movement or ability to detect light.
      - Visual fields: 1 m separation between examiner and patient. Use confrontation approach, with patient and examiner

Case Study: A salutary lesson

Mr AJ was, as he was quick to point out, currently between jobs. Sadly, it was not hard to imagine why this might be. The sight of the young man lying swathed in hospital blankets, with his right arm bandaged to the shoulder and his left leg in plaster, gave him a temporary air of vulnerability; an air that swiftly evaporated as he described in vivid detail the speeds he had reached in his thrilling car chase, before his wheel had clipped a curb and the car flipped – repeatedly. His eyes shone as he recalled how the police car had been unable to catch him and he brushed away his damaged limbs. In many ways he was lucky – he was alive, anyway. Unfortunately, his right arm, which had been hanging out of the open window at the time the car somersaulted, had been severely crushed in the crash. On exploration in the operating theatre, full transections of both ulnar and radial nerves were found, and whilst the median remained intact, all three had been severely battered and damaged. The plastic surgeon managed to repair them as best she could, but made it very clear to Mr AJ that the road to recovery would be long, and she could not predict where it would end. Mr AJ again brushed her concerns aside. However, when he returned to clinic six months later, with his police escort, his expression was more sober. His right arm was almost completely useless to him, despite the combined efforts of the surgeon, splints and physiotherapists. It hung limply by his side and he struggled to limp along with a stick clasped tightly in his left hand. His prognosis was not good. Nerve grafts and other procedures were all possible, but none guaranteed recovery, or even improvement. He still had six months of his sentence to serve, but it seemed likely that on release, he would remain indefinitely 'between jobs'.

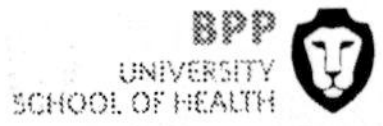

covering mirroring eyes and examine ability in four quadrants to detect moving finger/red hatpin.

- Accommodation: ask the patient to look at a far object and then a close finger.
- Reflexes: shine light into one eye and look for direct reflex, and again, observing the other for the consensual reflex (this is also testing the efferent oculomotor pathway to the other eye). Also perform the 'swinging light test' for relative afferent papillary defect.
- Fundoscopy (particularly important to be able to detect blurred optic disc margins).

iv) **CN III, IV and VI (oculomotor, trochlear and abducens):**

- In an oculomotor lesion, the pupil appears 'down and out'. There is ptosis with or without papillary involvement.
- In an abducens lesion the eye is unable to abduct on the affected side.
- The patient should keep their head still and follow your finger in an 'H' configuration. Look for blurred/painful vision, nystagmus and pursuit movement.
- Test saccadic movement and look for internuclear opthalmoplegia.

v) **CN V (Trigeminal):**

- There are three divisions: ophthalmic, maxillary and mandibular
- Test light touch bilaterally in three divisions
- Check masseter power by asking patient to 'bite your teeth'
- Offer corneal and jaw jerk reflexes

vi) **CN VII (facial):**

- Inspect for any obvious droop. Note: forehead sparing in UMN and involvement in LMN lesions
- Ask patient to raise eyebrows, puff cheeks, show their teeth (test power against resistance)

vii) **CN VIII (vestibulocochlear):**

- Screening test involving whispering a number in each ear whilst occluding the other.
- Perform Rinne and Weber tests using a 512Hz tuning fork.
- Rinne's test: Place the tuning fork both behind the ear on the mastoid bone and in the air next to the ear. Ask which is loudest. Air conduction is better than bone conduction normally but this pattern is also seen with sensorineural hearing loss. In conductive hearing loss, bone conduction is better.
- Weber's test: Place the tuning fork on the centre of the forehead. Sound will localise to the deaf ear in conductive deafness, but will localise to the contralateral ear in sensorineural loss.

viii) **CN IX and X (Glossopharyngeal and Vagus):**

- Look in the mouth and ask the patient to say 'AAAHHHH'. Observe palatal movement and look for deviation of the uvula (towards the lesion)
- Offer to perform the gag reflex

ix) **CN XI (Accessory):**

- Test power of patient shrugging their shoulders against resistance
- Test sternocleidomastoid power against resistance (palpate the contralateral muscle)

x) **CN XII (Hypoglossal):**

- Inspect tongue for wasting, fasciculations and deviation (way from the lesion)

3. **Completing the examination**

i) Examine: observation chart, drug chart; ask to examine peripheral nervous system

ii) Reposition the patient to ensure dignity and comfort. Thank the patient

iii) Present positive findings and salient negatives in a logical and appropriate manner

Pupils

Causes of nydriatic (large) pupil:

- Third nerve palsy
- Holmes-Adie pupil. Classically reacting to accommodation but slowly to light
- Traumatic iridoplegia
- Drugs: Tropicamide, cocaine and amphetamines

Causes of miotic (small) pupil:

- Horner's Syndrome
- Argyll Robertson pupil. Classically bilateral, reacting to accommodation but not to light

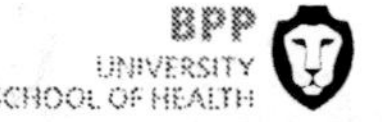

- Age related and are bilateral
- Anisocoria: asymmetric pupil size

Ptosis:

- Horner's syndrome: there is usually partial ptosis.
- Third nerve palsy: usually complete ptosis. The eye is 'down and out' with a large pupil.
- Myasthenia gravis: may be unilateral or bilateral. The pupils are normal. It is associated with fatigability and complex opthalmoplegia.
- Myotonic dystrophy: usually bilateral. The pupils are normal. It is associated with cataracts, frontal balding and myotonia.

Visual field defects:

Site of lesion	Visual field defect
Optic Nerve	Unilateral blindness
Optic Chiasm	Bitemporal hemianopia
Optic Tract	Contralateral homonymous hemianopia
Optic Radiation – parietal lobe	Contralateral homonymous quadrantanopia (inferior)
Optic Radiation – temporal lobe	Contralateral homonymous quadrantanopia (superior)
Occipital Cortex	Cortical blindness

Table 10.11: Summary of visual field defects

Internuclear opthalmoplegia:

- The abducting eye is seen to move smoothly but the adducting eye is slow to move. A brief nystagmus is seen in the abducting eye.
- This results from damage to the medial longitudinal facsiculus which co-ordinates uniform horizontal gaze movements.
- Most commonly from demyelination as seen in multiple sclerosis.
- If found, look for the five signs of optic nerve damage:
  - Central scotoma
  - Decreased visual acuity
  - Decreased colour vision
  - Relative afferent papillary defect
  - Optic atrophy

Horner's syndrome

- Due to a lesion in the sympathetic chain
- Causes:
  - Interruption to the supply from the hypothalamus to the synapse in the spinal cord
    - o Stroke
    - o Demyelination
    - o Syrinx
    - o Space occupying lesion
    - o Spinal cord trauma
  - Interruption to preganglionic neurones running from the cord to the superior cervical ganglion
    - o Pancoast's tumour
    - o Cervical rib
    - o Neck surgery
  - Interruption to post ganglionic neurones running to the pupil
    - o Carotid artery dissection or aneurysm
- **Clinical features (all ipsilateral)**
  - Miosis (reduced innervation to pupillodilators)
  - Partial ptosis (levator palpabrae supplied both by the sympathetic but also the parasympathetic chain)
  - Anhydrosis
  - Enophthalmosis

Facial nerve palsy

- **Facial nerve anatomy:**
  - Exits brainstem at the cerebellopontine angle
  - Enters the internal auditory meatus
    - o Gives off the Greater Petrosal Nerve which is secretomotor to the lacrimal gland
  - Enters the facial canal
    - o Gives off the nerve to the Stapedius
    - o Gives off the Chorda Tympani which gives parasympathetic innervation to the submandibular and sublingual glands as well as supplying taste to the anterior two-thirds of the tongue
  - Exits via the stylomastoid foramen
  - Splits as it transverses the parotid gland
- **Causes of facial nerve palsy:**
  - Bell's palsy
  - Ramsay Hunt syndrome (post-viral)

- Parotid swelling/tumour
- Stroke
- Demyelination
- Cerebellopontine angle tumour eg acoustic neuroma
- Bilateral Facial Nerve palsy neurosarcoid, lyme disease, Guillain-Barré syndrome

- **Clinical features:**
  - Unilateral facial weakness
  - Inability to completely close the eye
  - Loss of naso-labial fold
  - Mouth droop

Bulbar and pseudobulbar palsies

- **Bulbar:**
  - LMN lesion
  - Flaccid, nasal speech
  - Feels as if the tongue is too big and keeps getting in the way
  - Salivary pooling
  - Caused by a unilateral lesion
- **Pseudobulbar:**
  - UMN lesion
  - Spastic speech: 'Donald duck', 'hot potato', 'high pitched'
  - Tongue feels tight and moves very little from the floor of the mouth
  - Caused by bilateral lesions: demyelination or bilateral internal capsule strokes

Cerebellar examination

Signs of cerebellar dysfunction can be recalled using the mnemonic DANISH:

- **D**ysdiadochokinesis (the inability to make rapidly alternating movements)
- **A**taxia
- **N**ystagmus
- **I**ntention tremor (coarse, 4Hz tremor which increases in amplitude with target-directed movement
- **S**lurred speech
- **H**ypotonia (subtle and difficult to elicit)

Unilateral lesions cause ipsilateral signs.

The cerebellum is composed of three major functional divisions:

1. **Spinocerebellum:**
   i) Receives proprioceptive input from the spinocerebellar tracts, dorsal columns and trigeminal nerve and projects to rubrospinal, vestibulospinal, reticulospinal tracts and cortex.
   ii) Important in adaptive motor co-ordination, as it can predict the position of a body part during movement.
2. **Flocculonodular lobe:**
   i) Receives input from the vestibular system and visual input and projects to the vestibular nuclei to regulate balance.
3. **Neocerebellum:**
   i) Receives inputs from the contralateral cortex for fine motor control and sends efferents to the cortex via the thalamus.
   ii) Involved with planning and timing movements.

Examination of the cerebellum should take the following form:

1. **Introduction (as above)**
   i) Inspect for monitoring, medications and paraphernalia of neurological disease (walking aids, visual aids, etc).

2. **Examination**
   i) Examine the patient at rest. Lesions affecting the midline (spinocerebellum) cause truncal ataxia, which may be noticeable when sitting and cause titubation. Lesions of the cerebellar hemispheres (neocerebellum) tend to produce appendicular ataxia.
   ii) Examine for clues to the underlying diagnosis; any evidence of: arteriopathy, head trauma, lesions at multiple CNS locations, as in MS, stigmata of chronic liver disease and/or alcohol abuse in Wernicke's encephalopathy, antiepileptic toxicity? Young patients with hearing impairment, pacemakers, scoliosis, pes cavus and diabetes may have Freidreich's ataxia.
   iii) Ask the patient to stand with their hands crossed over their chest. Is there evidence of truncal ataxia, with unsteadiness on standing?
   iv) Ask the patient to walk. Lesions of the vermis may result in a wide-based gait, whilst one

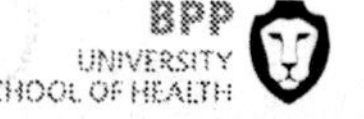

affecting the cerebellar hemispheres will cause the gait to veer towards that side. Then ask the patient to tandem-walk back, 'as though on a tight-rope'. This will reveal a subtler lesion.

v) Perform Romberg's test (as above).

vi) Test smooth pursuit (as above) – looking for disrupted, jerky pursuit and square wave jerks, which may occur at rest and nystagmus (fast phase in the direction of the lesion).

vii) Test saccades by holding the index finger of one hand in front of the patient and a curled fist at the periphery. Ask them to rapidly alternate gaze between finger and fist. Dysmetric saccades are often seen in midline lesions.

viii) Test speech by asking the patient to repeat 'baby hippopotamus', 'West Register Street', and 'British constitution'. Cerebellar speech is often dysarthric, indistinct and slow as the patient tries to co-ordinate palatal and lingual movements, often with explosive elements interspersed.

ix) Verbal dysdiadochokinesis can be elicited by asking the patient to repeat phonemes 'buh-buh-buh', 'kuh-kuh-kuh', and more complex word forms 'fa-ba-da, fa-ba-da, fa-ba-da'.

x) Test for 'Riddoch's sign', ie cerebellar rebound. Ask the patient to close their eyes and extend their arms, palms up. Press their arms down and ask them to return their arms to their previous positions. The ipsilateral arm will 'rebound' and come to lie higher.

xi) Assess the tone in the arms (may be reduced on the ipsilateral side).

xii) Test for dysmetria by holding your finger arm's reach away from the patient and ask them to alternate touching your finger with their nose as rapidly as possible. Patients will initially overshoot and need to make adjustments to reach the target. They will also show an intention tremor; that is, a tremor that increases in amplitude as the target is approached. Test both sides and in the lower limbs using the heel-shin test.

xiii) Dysdiadochokinesis is best elicited in two stages. First, ask the patient to clap the palm of their left hand with their right. Patients with cerebellar lesions clap arrhythmically and with variable amplitude. Then ask the patient to alternate between clapping with the palmar and dorsal surface of the hand. Patients may be unable to make rapid alternating movements. This can also be tested in the lower limbs by assessing rhythmicity of toe tapping).

xiv) Assess tone in the lower limbs.

3. **Completing the examination**

   i) Offer a formal speech examination.

   ii) Further investigations: MRI, lumbar puncture, FBC and CRP (exclude infection), ANA, ANCA, vitamin E, anti-Yo, anti-gliadin and anti-GAD antibodies, nerve conduction studies (Freidreich's ataxia).

Causes of cerebellar pathology

- Vascular: Ischaemic or haemorrhagic stroke.
- Infective: Encephalitis, meningitis (Varicella zoster has a predeliction for the cerebellum).
- Trauma.
- Autoimmune: Vasculitis, SLE, anti-GAD associated ataxia.
- Metabolic: Wernicke's encephalopathy (thiamine deficiency, with opthalmoplegia, confusion and ataxia); vitamin E deficiency. Gluten ataxia is believed to be an abnormal immune response to gluten, associated with anti-gliadin antibodies.
- Neoplastic: Mainly metastases, occasionally primaries. Anti-Yo antibodies are associated with lung, ovarian and breast cancers, among others, and cause Purkinje cell death.
- Congenital: Spinocerebellar ataxias can be recessive, dominant or X-linked. They present at different ages and are associated with different cerebellar and extra-cerebellar features. Freidreich's ataxia is possibly the best characterised. It is caused by a trinucleotide repeat in the Frataxin gene on chromosome 9 and affects the spinocerebellar and corticospinal tracts, the peripheral motor neurons, the dorsal columns and other tissues. Presentation is below the age of 25 with nystagmus, ataxia, tremor and dysarthria, as well as optic nerve atrophy, pyramidal weakness and arreflexia with upgoing plantars, impaired fine touch and proprioception, pes cavus, scoliosis, cardiomyopathy and diabetes. Ataxia-telangectasia is another recessive spinocerebellar ataxia.

- Other congenital metabolic/mitochondrial diseases can affect the cerebellum, including Kearns-Sayre syndrome, mitochondrial epilepsy with ragged red fibres, Refsum's disease and cerebrotendinous xanthomatosis.
- Drugs: Alcohol, phenytoin, carbamazepine, cancer treatments.
- Degenerative: Multiple sclerosis, multisystem atrophy.

Speech examination

Disordered speech is not an uncommon finding. There is a temptation to label such a patient as 'confused', rather than identifying underlying pathology.

Speech also depends on language and adaptations will need to be made if the patient does not speak English.

1. **Introduction** (as above)
2. **General speech**
   i) Ask a few general questions to get the feel of the speech eg what the patient had for breakfast
3. **Comprehension**
   i) Stick your tongue out
   ii) Close your eyes
   iii) Can increase complexity to two-step commands
4. **Expression**
   i) Name
   ii) Age
   iii) Address
5. **Naming**
   i) Watch
   ii) Pen
   iii) Tie
6. **Articulation**
   i) British constitution
   ii) West register street
   iii) Baby hippopotamus
7. **Specific structures involved in speech**
   i) Lips: 'me me me'
   ii) Tongue: 'la la la'
   iii) Palate: 'k k k'
8. **Completing the examination**
   i) As above
   ii) Proceed to the appropriate neurological examination

Speech problem	Lesion	Features
Expressive Dysphasia	CNS lesion in Broca's area in the inferior part of the dominant frontal lobe	Inability to verbally express despite adequate comprehension. Patient knows what they want to say but are unable to so. This can be very frustrating
Receptive Dysphasia	CNS lesion in Wernicke's area in the superior temporal lobe	Inability to understand speech. Fluent speech but not related to the conversation
Nominal Dysphasia	CNS lesion in posterior part of the dominant superior temporal gyrus	Inability to name objects. Usually part of a wider dysphasia
Global Dysphasia	CNS lesion in Wernicke's area and Broca's area	Inability to comprehend or express
Dysarthria	Cerebellar disease, extrapyramidal lesions including Parkinson's disease and dystonias, bulbar palsy, pseudobulbar palsy, myasthenia, oral ulceration or severe oral candidiasis	Inability to articulate but no underlying disorder of speech content. See individual sections for further detail

Table 10.12: The different types of speech disorders and the features and lesion associated with them

Parkinson's examination

Parkinson's disease is one of several akinetic rigid syndromes. It is characterised by the triad of bradkinesia, tremor and rigidity. Unlike most other akinetic rigid syndromes it is asymmetrical.

1. **Introduction (as above)**
2. **General**
   i) Look around for medications (eg an apomorphine pump or tablets), monitoring and paraphernalia (walking aids, writing aids etc).
   ii) Inspect the patient at rest. Look for a stooped posture, scars of deep brain stimulation on the scalp, hypomimia and an asymmetric resting tremor. Choreiform movements may be an effect of L-Dopa. Check for dysarthria,

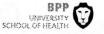

dysphonia and monotonous speech during your introduction.

3. **Gait**
   i) Assessing standing – do they 'rev up'.
   ii) Assess gait. Patients will typically have a stooped posture, delayed initiation, festination (small, shuffling steps), an asymmetrical loss of arm swing (in idiopathic Parkinson's disease), turning 'en bloc' (turning with multiple, small, shuffling steps) and, rarely, freezing.
   iii) Offer the retropulsion test (the righting reflexes are lost in akinetic rigid syndromes). The examiner will usually advise you not to perform this due to the risk of injury. To perform the test, stand behind the patient and gently pull their shoulders back towards you. Patients stagger backwards and start to fall unless they are caught.
4. **Central examination (work from forehead to feet)**
   i) Glabellar tap: gently use a finger to tap repeatedly on the patient's forehead. In Parkinson's disease the blink reflex is not extinguished, ie Myerson's sign positive.
   ii) Opthalmoplegia: ask the patient to focus on your finger as you move it in the shape of an H, pausing at extremes of gaze. Vertical gaze palsy is a key feature of progressive supranuclear palsy, while nystagmus may be a feature of multiple system atrophy.

Differential	Pathology	Features
Vascular	Lacunar infarcts in the subcortical white matter and basal ganglia.	Little tremor. Bilateral bradykinesia and rigidity. Cognitive impairment/personality change. Marche a petit pas. May have upper motor neurone signs. Vascular risk factors.
Post-encephalitic	Neurofibrillary tangles in the basal ganglia following viral infection. Largely associated with Spanish influenza in the early 20th century.	Young age of onset. May have oculogyric crisis, opthalmoplegia and/or pupil abnormalities. History of acute headache, fever and somnolence, which may precede parkinsonism by several years.
Pugilistic	Chronic traumatic encephalopathy following recurrent concussive or sub-concussive head trauma. Often affects multiple brain regions.	May present with some or all of dementia, ataxia, disinhibition or parkinsonism.
Wilson's disease	Mutation in *ATP7B* gene on Chr 13 leads to inability to conjugate copper and caeruloplasmin leading to accumulation in the liver, kidneys, eyes and brain.	Neurological (movement disorders including parkinsonism and psychosis) and non-neurological (cirrhosis, Kayser-Fleischer rings and sunflower cataracts, haemolytic anaemia, renal tubular acidosis type 2, pseudogout, cardiomyopathy, hypoparathyroidism). Onset in teens and twenties.
Drug-induced	Anti-dopaminergic drugs cause bradykinesia and rigidity with little tremor.	
Multiple system atrophy	α synuclein deposits in the substantia nigra and striatum, cerebellum and autonomic neurons.	Varying degrees of parkinsonism, cerebellar features and autonomic dysfunction. Usually symmetrical. Little or no Parkinsonian tremor. May be MSA-P (parkinsonism dominant) or MSA-C (cerebellar dominant). May have mini-polymyoclonus. Falls are an early feature. Onset around 55. Not responsive to dopaminergic drugs.
Corticobasal degeneration	Tauopathy associated with astrocytic plaques, mainly causing neuronal loss in the frontal and parietal lobes as well as the basal ganglia asymmetrically.	Asymmetric bradykinesia and rigidity, alien arm syndrome, ideomotor apraxia and gait disturbance, dystonia, myoclonus, non-fluent aphasia and cognitive impairment. Onset around 60. Little response to dopaminergic drugs.
Progressive supranuclear palsy	Tauopathy with neurofibrillary tangles in the basal ganglia, brainstem, dentate nucleus and frontal cortex.	Vertical gaze palsy, slow saccades and interrupted smooth pursuit, personality change, dementia, bradykinesia and rigidity, dysarthria and dysphagia, falls, neck dystonia.

Table 10.13: Differential of akinetic rigid syndromes

iii) Tremor: ask the patient to rest their hands in their lap and observe any tremor. Parkinson's disease is characterised by an asymmetrical 4-6Hz 'pill rolling' tremor at rest. The tremor is worsened by distraction and stress and is re-emergent. To test for these features ask the patient to subtract serial 7s from 100. Ask the patient to hold their hands out in front of them (parkinsonian tremors emerge after a delay, whereas postural tremors present immediately). Then ask the patient to bring their hands to their nose. The same pattern of re-emergent tremor should be seen.

iv) Tone: assess the arms by randomly flexing and abducting the shoulder; flexing and extending the elbow; and flexing, extending and rotating the wrist. Compare both arms. Ask the patient to trace a star in the air with their left hand while you re-examine tone in the right arm and vice versa. Parkinsonism is characterised by rigidity, rather than spasticity (see below), and is often described as 'cogwheel' due to the superimposed tremor. Tone increases with distraction (as when the other arm traces a pattern in the air, ie Froment's manoeuvre).

v) Test for decriment of movement (a sign of bradykinesia) by asking the patient to rapidly pronate and supinate both arms simultaneously/make repetitive pincer movements. Amplitude will decrease over time.

vi) Test for functional impairment by asking the patient to draw a spiral. Ask the patient to fasten a button.

vii) Offer to measure lying and standing blood pressure (a postural drop may be seen in multiple system atrophy), assess cognition with an MMSE or MOCA (to exclude Lewy body dementia), and to assess construction apraxia (a feature of corticobasal degeneration). Offer a speech and language assessment.

5. **Completing the examination**
   i) As above
   ii) Proceed to any other appropriate examinations

Musculoskeletal system screening examination

The musculoskeletal system can be assessed using a screening history and examination. This screening system is known as the GALS assessment (gait, arms, legs, and spine).

Screening questions

1. Do you have any pain/stiffness in your joints or muscles?
2. Are you able to walk up and down stairs without any problems?
3. Can you undress/dress yourself without any difficulty?

Screening examination

1. **Introduction (as per previous examinations)**
2. **Examination**
   i) Gait
      - Inspect the patient as they get up from a sitting position
      - Inspect the patient as they walk
      - Inspect the patient as they turn whilst walking

   ii) Spine
      - Inspect the spine from the back and each side of the patient
      - Ask the patient to bend and touch their toes
      - Ask the patient to flex their neck laterally (touch each ear to each shoulder)

   iii) Arms
      - Ask the patient to stand with both hands by their sides, then out in front of them, palms down
      - Ask the patient to turn hands over and make a fist
      - Touch the tip of each finger to the thumb
      - Squeeze the second and fifth metacarpal joint to assess for pain
      - Ask the patient to place both hands behind their head

   iv) Legs
      - Inspect the legs from the front and back with the patient standing
      - With the patient lying flat inspect the legs more closely
      - Flex each hip and knee whilst holding the knee
      - Passively perform internal and external hip rotation

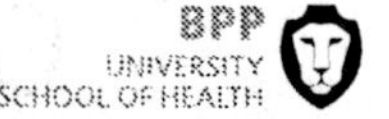

- Whilst straightening each leg feel for crepitus
- Palpate the knee for tenderness and any swelling
- Press across the metatarsal joints to identify any tenderness
- Inspect the soles of the feet for any callosities

3. **Completing the examination**
   i) As above
   ii) If indicated, examine any particular joint in more detail

Locomotor system examination

Joint examinations follow the following structure: inspect, palpate, move, special tests. Compare one side with the other. Specific joints will follow particular patterns.

1. **Introduction (as per previous examinations, with patient standing for upper limb and supine at 45 degrees for lower limb, with adequate exposure)**
2. **Inspection (think about skin, soft tissue and bone)**
   i) Skin changes
   ii) Swelling/effusion
   iii) Muscle wasting
   iv) Deformity (fixed or mobile)
3. **Palpation**
   i) Swelling – assess for consistency (bony/soft tissue), fluctuance
   ii) Test for effusions
   iii) Palpate joint margins and surrounding structures for pain/deformities
   iv) Temperature (with the dorsum of your hand)
   v) Neurovascular status
4. **Movement**
   i) Degree of active and passive movement from a neutral position
5. Examine joint above and below, and look at an antero-postero and lateral X-ray

Examination of the hand

1. **Inspection**
   i) Inspect the hands of the patient on a flat surface in front of you.
   ii) Look for skin changes, swelling, deformity and nail changes.
   iii) Ask the patient to turn over their hands to allow inspection of the palms.
   iv) Look for any tendon thickening or callosities.
   v) Identify any muscle wasting.
2. **Palpation**
   i) Check if the patient has any pain anywhere
   ii) Systematically palpate each 5 MCPJs, 4 PIPJs, 1 IPJ and 4 DIPJs.
   iii) Identify any swelling, nodules, and deformities.
   iv) Osteoarthritis: Heberden's nodes on the DIPJs, Bouchard's nodes on PIPJs.
   v) Warmth.
   vi) Any palmar pain – possible flexor sheath involvement.
   vii) Sensation – the radial and ulnar digital nerves in each finger; median, ulnar and radial nerve specific areas.
   viii) Capillary refill, radial and ulnar pulses if concerned about vascular status.
3. **Movement**
   i) Extent of active and passive flexion and extension and thumb flexion, extension and opposition. Perform against resistance.
   ii) Ask the patient to adduct and abduct the fingers and resist.
   iii) Test FDP/S and FPL each finger and thumb. Test extension against resistance. Pain on resisted tendon testing suggests possible partial injury.
4. **Function**
   i) Ask the patient to do up a button, write their name, turn a key.
   ii) Ask if anything the patient is unable to do because of their hand.

Pre-operative history

1. **Introduction**
   i) Set the scene and explanation about the importance of pre-operative preparation
2. **Presenting complaint**
   i) Check the patient's comprehension of the procedure they are about to undergo
   ii) Symptoms
   iii) Clinical journey through diagnosis, investigations/previous procedures
3. **Past medical/surgical history**
   i) Importantly: hypertension, respiratory diseases, diabetes, previous CVAs, cardiovascular

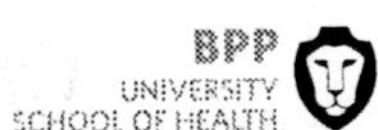

disease, previous venous thromboembolic events and any other pertinent conditions

ii) Previous operations: any complications

iii) General anaesthetics: any complications/family history of complications

iv) ITU admissions

v) Duration of hospital stay

4. **Drug history**

i) Current prescribed/over the counter medication (importantly: anticoagulants/platelets)

ii) Illicit drugs

iii) Allergies

iv) Previous transfusions

5. **Family history**

i) Any familial conditions

6. **Social history**

i) Functional level (activities of daily living)/mobility

ii) Any assistance required/difficulties experienced

iii) Support network/package of care (to aid with post-operative recovery/ability of patient to cope in pre-operative environment)

iv) Alcohol/smoking history

7. Review of systems to exclude/identify conditions that may affect the anaesthetic/operation or recovery

8. **Summary**

i) Ask if the patient has any questions

ii) Provide any useful patient information leaflets

iii) Address any concerns

iv) Inform the patient of the plan for the day of surgery including starving instructions and when/where to arrive

Consent

Informed consent is an important principle in medicine and determining whether a patient has the capacity to give consent, and whether they have done so, is a crucial skill to develop.

As an F1 doctor with provisional registration, you are unable to take formal consent for procedures, whilst at F2 level and higher, a doctor is only allowed to consent a patient if they themselves can perform the procedure, or have received specific training in how to take consent for it. However, even as an F1 doctor you will be performing simple procedures on patients, and it is important to have an understanding of the skills involved in consenting, as you will need to gain a patient's verbal consent to take their blood, insert catheters or cannulas and order investigations for them etc.

Capacity

The first step in taking consent is establishing whether a patient has capacity to give it. This is a decision and time-specific assessment and a patient's capacity can fluctuate.

Capacity depends on a patient being able to:

- Understand information being given to them
- Retain the information long enough to make a decision
- Weigh up the information to make the decision
- Communicate that decision

Information to be discussed

Consent is not the signing of a form; it is a process that begins with the very first discussion about an intervention potentially being offered. When taking consent (verbal or written) for a particular procedure, the following areas should be discussed:

1. The patient's condition and likely prognosis
2. What the procedure will entail
3. Alternative options, including no treatment
4. Aim and potential benefits of the procedure
5. Possible risks and complications, however small – both of the procedure and alternatives
6. The healthcare professionals involved in the different options

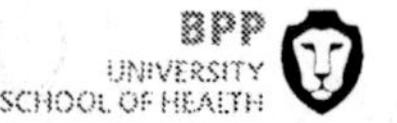

7. The likely future treatment pathways and prognosis depending on the different treatment options.
8. Other: permission for tissue samples, medical student presence, photographs etc.

If you do not feel happy to consent a patient, do **not** do it – the patient deserves to discuss their procedure with somebody who is confident to do so.

Surgical examinations

General pre-operative examination

1. **Introduction (as per previous examinations)**
2. **Cardiovascular examination**
   i) As described previously
   ii) Important to identify AF and establish anticoagulant use, any murmurs, signs of heart failure, carotid bruits, aortic aneuryms or hypertension
   iii) Compare current ECG to any previous traces available
   iv) Consider need for an echocardiogram, carotid Doppler, abdominal ultrasound or anaesthetic review
   v) Ideally, in collaboration with the patient's GP, antihypertensive management should be optimised prior to surgery
3. **Respiratory examination**
   i) As described previously
   ii) Identify any clinical signs of lung disease, any cigarette use
   iii) Consider need for pre-operative CXR, lung function tests and baseline ABG
4. **Abdominal examination**
   i) As described previously
   ii) Identify any hepatomegaly, splenomegaly, abdominal masses – investigate as indicated
5. **Neurological examination**
   i) Baseline AMTS for all elderly patients:
      - Date of birth
      - Age
      - Year
      - Recognition
      - Place
      - Address recall
      - Year of WW2
      - Prime Minister
      - Time
      - Count backwards from 20 down to 1

   A score of eight or less should warrant further investigation with the MMSE.
6. **Anaesthetic assessment**
   i) Can the patient fully flex and extend the neck?
   ii) Any history of arthritis in the neck?
   iii) If either, the patient should be discussed with the anaesthetist
   iv) The anaesthetist will examine the patient and will gain a more definitive idea of airway difficulty, but the Mallampati classification can be used to establish a general idea based on features seen on mouth opening
7. **General points throughout**
   i) Establish a good rapport by being polite, professional and ensuring the patient's dignity is maintained at all times
   ii) Offer the patient the opportunity to raise any concerns or ask any questions they may have
8. **Baseline measurements**
   i) BP, pulse rate and peak flow
   ii) Calculate BMI
   iii) ECG
   iv) Bloods
      - FBC: anaemia, infection, and platelets
      - U&Es: renal function, any electrolyte imbalances
      - LFTs: if deranged may require further investigation
      - Coagulation screen if on anticoagulants
      - Group and save (or cross-match) if patient likely to require transfusion

Lump examination

When examining any lump or mass it is important to have a systematic approach and ensure a thorough assessment is performed. Document the following:

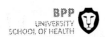

- Site
- Size
- Shape
- Surface
- Colour
- Contour
- Consistency
- Temperature
- Tenderness
- Transilluminance
- Tethering
- Pulsatility
- Auscultation

Hernia examination

1. **Introduction** (as previously, patient should initially be standing for examination and exposed as dignity allows from the waist down – ensure a chaperone is present)
2. **Brief history**
   i) Is there a lump in the groin?
   ii) Tender?
   iii) How long/any changes eg increasing in size/pain?
   iv) Can the patient reduce the lump?
   v) Any associated symptoms eg nausea and vomiting
3. **Examination**
   i) Inspect for: swellings (and characterise), scars, skin changes, signs of infection or hernia strangulation
   ii) Palpate for: lump characteristics
   iii) It is then perfectly acceptable (and may be easier) to perform the rest of the examination with the patient supine
   iv) Ask the patient to reduce and observe where this occurs (ie deep or superficial inguinal rings)
   v) Feel for a cough impulse over the lump
   vi) Determine the type of hernia by placing a finger at the pubic tubercle and asking the patient to cough. Inguinal hernias are found superior and medial and femoral hernias inferior and lateral to the pubic tubercle
   vii) Reduce the hernia and place pressure over the deep inguinal ring (mid-point of the inguinal ligament – pubic tubercle to ASIS). The patient is then asked to cough. If the hernia is controlled this is an indirect hernia, and if the hernia is revealed it is a direct hernia. This is clinically accurate in only 20–30% of cases
   viii) Auscultate for bowel sounds
   ix) In male patients examine the scrotum to identify hernia extension. If a mass in the scrotum is present and you cannot get above it, then the likely diagnosis is a hernia
   x) Any scrotal lump should be formally examined
4. **Completing the examination**
   i) Examine the contralateral side
   ii) Examine for any lymphadenopathy
   iii) Examine the abdomen
   iv) Present positive and salient negative findings in a logical and appropriate manner

Thyroid examination

Examination of the neck includes examination of all swellings, lymph nodes and the thyroid gland. Having an understanding of the possible aetiologies of neck swellings will assist you in performing a focused examination. It is also important to look for other stigmata of diseases manifesting with lump swellings, particularly thyroid disease or malignancy.

1. **Introduction** (as previously with patient seated, exposed to supraclavicular fossae)
2. **Brief history**
   i) When did the patient first notice the lump?
   ii) Has the lump changed over time?
   iii) Any associated symptoms – particularly pain, dyspnoea or dysphagia
   iv) Any family history of thyroid problems or neck lumps?
3. **Examination**
   i) **General inspection:** agitation, restless, sweating, low weight, heat intolerance (hyperthyroidism); overweight or myxoedematous, peaches and cream complexion, dry skin/hair, pretibial myxedema, cold intolerance, low mood (hypothyroidism)
   ii) **Neck:** examine from front and side, looking for: lump position, number of lumps, overlying skin changes (tethering in malignancy, erythema with inflammation), asymmetry, scars. Ask the patient to swallow some water. If the lump ascends on swallowing then it is

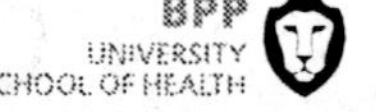

associated with the thyroid gland; if it moves on tongue protruberance a thyroglossal cyst is likely

iii) **Hands:** warm, sweating, tachycardia/AF, palmar erythema, fine tremor (hyperthyroidism); bradycardia, dry palms, cold, slow capillary refill (hypothyroidism); thyroid acropachy (Graves' Disease)

iv) **Eyes:** exophthalmos/proptosis (abnormal projection of the eyeball), opthalmoplegia (limited eye movement) or chemosis (conjunctival oedema), lid lag or retraction are all seen in autoimmune thyroid disease and Graves' Disease

v) **Lump:** palpate the lump from behind, after ascertaining if there is any pain. Ensure trachea is central then palpate isthmus, lateral lobes of thyroid gland and any other swellings (a normal thyroid gland is not palpable). Ask the patient to swallow again and extrude tongue whilst palpating to confirm lump movements

vi) Percuss anterior chest wall for any retrosternal extension and auscultate for any bruits (increased vascularity)

vii) **Lymphadenopathy:** examine the anterior and posterior cervical chains, submandibular, submental, pre-auricular, post-auricular and occipital regions for any palpable nodes

viii) Get patient to stand without using arms to assess for proximal myopathy and test reflexes (brisk in hyperthyroidism and slow relaxing in hypothyroidism)

ix) Offer but **do not** test for Pemberton's sign (distended neck veins and stridor on elevation of both arms above the head due to vena caval compression by a mediastinal mass ie a large retrosternal goitre)

4. **Completing the examination**

i) Thank the patient and present findings in a logical and appropriate manner

ii) Possible further investigations include thyroid function tests, ultrasound scan of thyroid gland/neck, a radionuclide scan of thyroid or a lymph node biopsy

Varicose vein examination

1. **Introduction** (as per previous examinations; patient should be standing, exposed, as dignity allows, from the groin down)
2. **Brief history**

i) How long have the varicose veins been present?

ii) Symptoms (pain, itching, bleeding)

iii) Any associated risk factors? (Obesity, pregnancy, abdominal masses)

iv) Any associated symptoms? (Ulcers, pain, pruritis, discolouration)

v) Have the veins changed over time?

vi) Any previous varicose vein or vascular surgery?

3. **Examination**

i) Inspection: dilated tortuous veins (long/short saphenous distribution).

ii) Palpate for a dilated sapheno-femoral junction (2.5 cm below and lateral to the pubic tubercle) and check for a cough impulse – positive indicates incompetent SFJ.

iii) Special tests (Trendelenburg, Perthes and Tap test) have largely been replaced by Doppler assessment, but may arise in an unpleasant exam situation!

iv) Trendelenburg test – a tourniquet test to assess the site of valve incompetence in the superficial veins of the legs. Leg is raised with patient on their back and tourniquet applied just below SFJ. Patient stands and if veins remain empty, SFJ is incompetent and the cause of superficial venous reflux. If the tourniquet allows the veins to fill, the test can be repeated down the leg to find the site of valvular incompetence.

v) Perthes test assesses the patency of the deep venous system. With the tourniquet still on ask the patient to walk around and stand up and down on their tiptoes. If the veins improve the deep system is intact. If the calf veins become engorged and there is increasing calf discomfort the deep venous system is occluded.

vi) Tap test – the visible vein is tapped proximally and felt distally for a percussion wave. If this is present, an incompetent valve lies between the two sites (this is a particularly unreliable test).

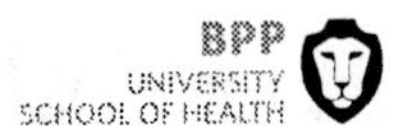

vii) Check all foot pulses – compression stockings are contraindicated if there is lower limb arterial insufficiency

viii) Auscultate over the vein for bruits – may indicate arteriovenous fistulae, often mistaken for varicosities

4. **Completing the examination**

   i) Thank the patient and allow them to redress

   ii) Present positive and salient negative findings in a logical and appropriate manner

Peripheral vascular examination (lower limb)

1. **Introduction** (as previously; patient should be standing and exposed from the groin down as dignity allows)

2. **Examination**

   i) General inspection: mottling, uskiness, necrosis and missing toes

   ii) Ulceration: site, size, shape, edge, slough, venous (painless, varicose veins, eczema) or arterial (painful with punched out lesions)

   iii) Hands: discolouration (tar stains etc), temperature, capillary refill

   iv) Any scars from previous surgery

   v) Palpation: temperature (back of your hands, comparing both sides); tenderness; capillary refill time, peripheral pulses (work distal to proximal and check both sides): dorsalis pedis, posterior tibial, popliteal, femoral; feel for an abdominal aortic aneurysm

   vi) Auscultate for femoral and aortic bruits

   vii) Buerger's test – raise the leg and identify the angle where it becomes white:

   - ≥90° = Normal angle
   - 20° – 30° = Ischaemic leg
   - <20° = Severe ischaemia

   The leg is then hung over the side of the bed and observed:

   - Foot stays pink = normal
   - Turns pink slowly with reactive hyperaemia = ischaemic leg
   - Takes 30s to turn pink = severe ischaemia

   viii) Calculate the ABPI – the ratio of the systolic blood pressure in the legs to that in the arms. The latter should be slightly higher. Both dorsalis pedis and posterior tibial pulses are measured on both legs using a Doppler probe and the highest values used. The brachial pulses are measured on both arms in the same way and the ratio between the two ie brachial/highest lower limb pulse calculated

3. **Completing the examination**

   i) Observe the patient's gait

   ii) Perform a neurological and locomotor examination

   iii) Present positive and salient negative findings in a logical and appropriate manner

Further reading and references

1. Douglas, D., Nicol, F. and Robertson, C. (2009) *Macleod's Clinical Examination.* 12th Edition. London: Churchill Livingstone.
2. Cookson, J., Epstein, O. and Perkin, G.D. (2008) *Clinical examination.* 4th Edition. Maryland Heights: Mosby.
3. Hall, T. (2008) *PACES for the MRCP: With 250 Clinical Cases.* 2nd Edition. London: Churchill Livingstone.
4. National Institute for Health and Clinical Excellence (2006). *Parkinson's Disease. National clinical guideline for diagnosis and management in primary and secondary care* (CG35). [Online]. Available from: www.nice.org.uk/guidance/cg35/evidence/full-guideline-194930029 [Accessed 7 November 2016].

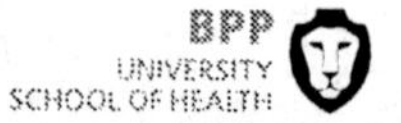

Chapter 11

Foundation Year 2 and beyond

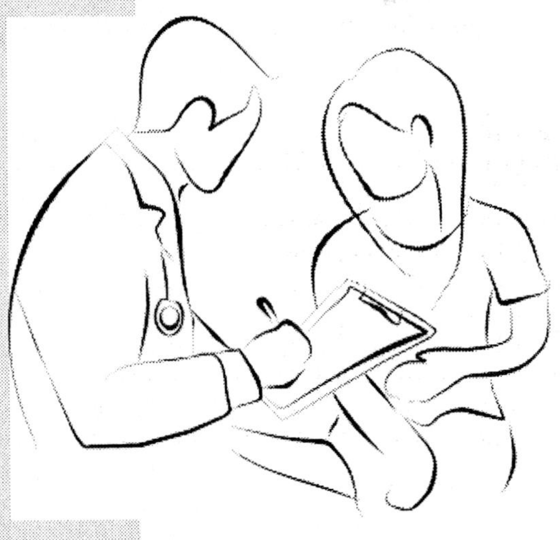

Foundation Year 2 and beyond

Introduction

With my career I want to either make something or make an impact. Writers both make something, and make an impact.
Jarod Kintz – *This book is Not FOR SALE* (Amazon Media 2011)

The first year of the Foundation Programme has been designed to provide the newly qualified doctor with a range of rotations in general medicine and surgery, during which they can gain valuable practical skills and experiences. Following successful completion of this year a doctor is eligible for full registration with the GMC. This entitles a doctor to practise independently, outside of the supervision of a Foundation Programme – importantly allowing them to take up temporary locum or non-training posts.

In contrast, the aim of FY2 rotations is to expose the doctor to a range of clinical specialties. Although you may work in a speciality for which you do not have a particular interest, it is still a valuable experience to work with such teams and experience the pros and cons of the specialist environment. If there is a speciality you would like to experience that you do not have as a rotation during your foundation years, it is often possible to arrange a few taster days with a local team. You are entitled to approximately 30 days' study leave in most trusts (10 must be used for formal FY2 teaching) and it is important to plan early how you would like to use this – courses, taster days or particular projects would all be suitable.

FY2 is clearly **not** a comprehensive overview of all possible specialties or career options. While you may be keen to apply directly for a speciality training post if you know there is a route you would like to pursue, it is also important not to feel pressurised to do so. There are many options that will offer you a broader range of experiences should you need more time to explore other career possibilities and these will be reviewed in a number of case studies later in this chapter.

FY2 speciality rotations

The brief reviews of the specialties below are not designed to be comprehensive, nor is the list exhaustive. They are designed as brief introductions, to give you an overview and insight into the kind of placements you may be able to undertake at an FY2 level.

When it comes to speciality training applications, it is highly beneficial – and will enable you to have a better idea of whether or not you do seriously want to apply – if you have completed a rotation during your Foundation years in that speciality. It is therefore important to think about which specialties you might like to experience and try and facilitate these in your Foundation Programme application – although this may be easier said than done!

Hospital specialties

Paediatrics

A rotation in Paediatrics (Paeds) will allow you to participate in the care of children up to the age of 16, with the potential for greater experience within a particular subspeciality eg neonatal medicine, community paediatrics. You will be involved in work on the children's ward neonatal unit, outpatient clinics, children's day unit and paediatric accident and emergency. You will also have the opportunity to see and assess new patients and suggest a possible management plan, before confirming this with the team.

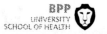

In addition to providing a valuable insight into paediatrics as a speciality, the rotation will offer you training on neonatal and paediatric life support, performing newborn examinations and completing practical procedures as well as opportunities to take part in audit cycles, teaching and clinical presentations, which will allow you to satisfy the requirements of the Foundation Programme.

Obstetrics and gynaecology

Obstetrics and Gynaecology (Obs and Gynae) encompasses the care involved in 'women's health' and, attractively, manages to combine the fields of medicine and surgery in one speciality.

An Obs and Gynae rotation involves exposure to gynaecology theatre, labour ward, early pregnancy unit, and outpatient clinics (antenatal clinic, gynaecology clinic and urodynamics), allowing you to develop your specialist knowledge – very useful for both an Obs and Gynae or GP career path) and gain practical skills. You will also be offered the opportunities to fulfil the Foundation Programme competencies, and may be able to attend certain courses, such as Basic Surgical Skills or Advanced Life Support in Obstetrics.

Surgical specialties

ENT, Oral and Maxillofacial Surgery, Plastic Surgery and Opthalmology are all surgical specialties to which you may be exposed as an FY2. Whilst all of them will largely entail general ward and on-call work, there will also be opportunities to take part in outpatient and acute clinics and participate in some theatre lists. You will gain a broad exposure to the conditions seen within that particular speciality and may receive dedicated specialist teaching sessions. This is a good opportunity to discover how a more specialist surgical unit manages both clinical cases and patient throughput, as well as providing an insight into these specialties as potential career choices.

When considering career routes, it is essential to look at the roles of both trainees and consultants – it is no good doing a job you like for 10 years only to hate the role you end up doing for the next 30, but equally, it is important to enjoy your years as a trainee and not have to keep thinking, 'it will get better in the end; it must get better in the end'.

Other hospital specialties to which you may be exposed as an FY2 doctor include: A&E; Pathology; Microbiology; Radiology; ITU; Public Health Medicine, Clinical Genetics and other specialist areas of medicine. All will allow you to gain insight into career pathways in these fields as well as developing specialist knowledge and practical skills.

Psychiatry

Psychiatry combines multidisciplinary teamwork in hospital and community settings, in order to address the psychological and social aspects of a patient's mental health condition and the impact this has on the lives of patients, their friends and families.

During an FY2 psychiatry placement, you will participate in routine ward work, outpatient clinics, reviewing patients in the community, attending multidisciplinary meetings and sometimes assessing patients in A&E. This can sometimes be an emotionally challenging experience as, like in General Practice, the patient is often not removed from the context of their illness, and it is possible to see the life-changing impact of such diseases.

General practice

A better name for the general practitioner might be 'multispecialist'
Martin H. Fischer (1879–1962)

In 2015, the well-known Scottish GP Dr Margaret McCartney wrote an article in the *BMJ* entitled, 'General Practice is the best job in the world'. In it, she wrote that:

> *General Practice encompasses health and sickness, benefit and harm, living and dying. You are a prescriber, diagnostician and font of evidence – but also advocate and avoider of medical harm.*

There is much in this statement, all of which you will experience as an FY2 doctor in General Practice.

Primary Care is a very different environment to hospital medicine, with a far greater emphasis on continuity of care. Depending on how the practice you are placed in organises FY2 rotations, you will be working largely independently, with the supervision of a GP tutor. You will be intimately involved in the initial presentation of a patient, any investigations, referrals and follow-up as well as working with the various healthcare professionals involved in their care. This involvement in the care pathway will allow you to gain a greater insight into an individual patient's experience of illness and how both health and sickness fit into the context of their everyday lives.

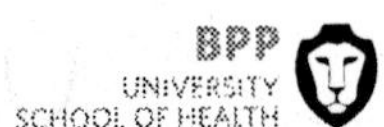

Academic placements

Academic placements allow an FY2 doctor to gain a broader exposure to education, teaching or research whilst maintaining a clinical role. There are a number of different placements available and interested participants must complete a separate, parallel application process, including a selection interview if shortlisted, when they apply for their Foundation Programme place.

Different Foundation Programmes arrange their placements in various ways; however, all offer the possibility of combining an individual, supported research project with clinical work. Many Foundation Programmes will also offer some teaching research methodology or the possibility of attending academic courses or conferences. This provides an excellent initial basis for an Academic Clinical Fellowship, MA or MD/PhD application, should you decide to pursue an academic route.

A 'portfolio' career is becoming increasingly popular amongst doctors and this placement offers an excellent opportunity to experience the reality of a clinical-academic or clinical-educational career.

Life beyond Foundation Year 2

As you come towards the end of your Foundation years, the future can seem both exciting and daunting. Perhaps you are about to step onto the training path for a long dreamt of speciality job; maybe you are about to return to student-hood to complete a further qualification, or take some time out to explore medicine and career options in other parts of the world. These are all possible, indeed popular, options.

'Modernising Medical Careers', introduced in 2005, was designed to streamline specialist training, allowing doctors to 'progress more quickly and in a more structured way to their desired career, reducing time spent in unnecessary or inappropriate training' (2009). However, many foundation doctors simply do not know what their 'desired career' may be after just one year of professional experience and this has contributed to a year-on-year decline in the number of trainees progressing directly into specialist training posts. In 2015, only 52% of successful FY2 doctors chose to apply to a specialist training programme.

It is vital to recognise the breadth of options after FY2 and spend some time in FY1 exploring different opportunities and what would be required to realise them. You should not feel pressured to choose any particular path but try and pursue the one that feels best for you at this time – it is always possible to change directions later and no experience is ever wasted!

Speciality training programmes

Run-through training

A number of specialities consist of run-through programmes ie no further applications for further training posts are required once you are accepted onto the schemes. Currently these include: Chemical Pathology; Clinical Radiology; Community Sexual and Reproductive Health; General Practice; Histopathology; Neurosurgery; Obstetrics and Gynaecology; Opthalmology; Paediatrics and Child Health and Public Health. Some areas are also trialling Cardiothoracic and Oral and Maxillofacial surgery as run-through programmes.

If you have always been interested in a speciality and know that you will want to apply to that training programme, it is essential to show your commitment early – either at medical school or during FY1 as recruitment applications and interviews will take place early in FY2. This may manifest in relevant audit or quality improvement projects, attending (and ideally presenting) at speciality conferences, participating in advanced training courses or taking part in research projects relating to that speciality. It is always a good idea to seek the advice and mentorship of senior doctors within a speciality of interest, as they will be able to guide you as to the best routes forward – and will often be delighted that you are thinking of joining them!

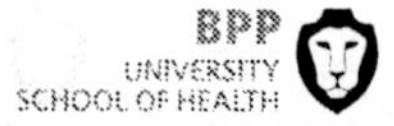

Case Study: Core Medical Training

This year I am completing year 1 of Core Medical Training, hoping to pursue a career in Neurology. It is a branch of Medicine that is going to expand rapidly with new imaging/genetic/computational techniques. It's a very exciting time, and there are lots of opportunities for research. However, it is pretty competitive and any applicant needs publications, presentations, research and, ideally, a PhD (which I do not have).

The training has been varied – four months on Respiratory medicine was intensely stressful dealing with very sick patients in a failing trust with inadequate staffing. The on-calls in this hospital were terrifying, with only 1 doctor looking after all the medical patients on 20+ wards with the single SpR trying to run acute admissions with a skeleton staff. People were often demoralised and overwhelmed.

I have since spent four months on the Neurology ward in a tertiary centre at a DGH. It was an absolute dream. I feel I learned a lot and was exposed to a vast range of pathologies whilst being very well supported by registrars.

My latest job has been Neuro/Stroke Rehab. We are hideously understaffed, patients are often unfit for transfer to a non-acute ward, we have one consultant ward round a week, and have received no teaching. The on-calls have been interesting, as the hospital is smaller and there is more time for discussion, teaching, reviewing sick patients etc.

In short, CMT is a mixed bag. Try to get a range of jobs that will set you up for being the SpR on-call (Cardio, Neuro, Resp, ITU etc), but try to get in at least one less taxing job (Derm, ID etc).

Non run-through training

A number of other training routes consist of two years of core training in related specialties, followed by further speciality applications at ST3 level or above. These include the: acute care common stem (ACCS) and core anaesthesia, medicine, psychiatry and surgery training programmes.

ACCS is a two-year programme in anaesthesia, emergency medicine and intensive care, which subsequently feeds trainees into those – and other related – specialties. The other core programmes are designed to provide trainees with basic skills for future careers in the relevant specialties, and may be general or themed in nature. Applications are through national recruitment rounds, where candidates will be offered their preference of posts based on rankings devised from written application and interview performance.

Again, seeking advice from more senior trainees and consultants about the training pathways and further speciality applications etc is vital. It is important to remember that you will be a junior doctor in a training programme for a considerable amount of time, and these years need to be enjoyable in order to be sustainable – understanding what is really involved, before you make the application, will help minimise later disappointment and disillusionment.

Academic training

Academic Clinical Fellow posts are NIHR or locally funded training schemes, which combine 75% clinical with 25% dedicated research time. They provide an excellent grounding in a combined academic-clinical career and are designed to lead onto a successful PhD/MD or Academic Clinical Lectureship application. Applications are made for specific posts through national recruitment rounds and any interviews and offers are made locally.

It is also possible to take time out after the Foundation Programme to directly enter an MA/PhD or MD programme. However, the competition for those posts combining clinical work is fierce.

Case Study: Core Surgical Training CT1 with ACF GP and MPH application

I started core surgical training in August, working in a tertiary centre plastic surgery department. I assisted at theatre lists once or twice a week, completed minor operations (minor ops) lists with a registrar and spent the rest of the days on call. This involved answering GP referrals, completing the minor injuries clinic and seeing any patients in A&E.

After six months in plastics I started trauma and orthopaedics, but resigned after two months and worked as a locum for the remainder of my CT1 year.

During my plastics rotation I decided I wanted to apply for an academic general practice job and a Master's in Public Health at Harvard. The former involved an application to the national GP recruitment scheme, with an online application, knowledge test and interview with written task and clinical scenarios. I also had a separate academic interview. The latter involved an online application, verification of all my certificates and qualifications and sitting the GRE (a selection examination required for all US graduate schools). I had to pay for all of these and the total process cost around £500.

What I had to do to get there:

I completed my MRCS A&B prior to applying for Core Surgical Training through the national recruitment scheme, although this is not expected. I submitted the online application by the deadline in late November during my first F2 rotation and then attended national selection interviews in London in January. These involved three ten-minute clinical, management/leadership and portfolio stations. I then received my job offer two to three weeks later.

Why I chose this path:

Having carried out my elective in plastics in Groote Schuur, Cape Town, I was enthused and was keen to experience more of the speciality. I had done a few taster days during F1 and wanted to learn whether developing the surgical skill required to be a good surgeon would be sufficient job satisfaction for me to want to do it long term. Plastics is a competitive speciality, therefore if I did want to do it as a career I wanted to make myself as attractive as possible, hence the early MRCS completion.

Advantages:

I had the opportunity to participate in some amazing operations and certainly developed my surgical skills and confidence. I think when you start in a proper training role (as opposed to a foundation job) you get a much better idea of what the job (and training pathway) will actually be like. This helps you to gain a better understanding of whether this is something you want to pursue longer term. In my experience, everybody has been very supportive of my decision to change career paths, seeing my additional year of training as a positive experience.

Disadvantages:

There are significant financial implications to starting any training scheme – you are expected to pay for the online portfolio websites and book and attend training courses. If I ever wanted to come into surgery again, it may be more difficult to do this, having started but not completed a training programme.

Top piece of advice:

Have a go at anything you want to try, but if you don't like it, don't be afraid to change.

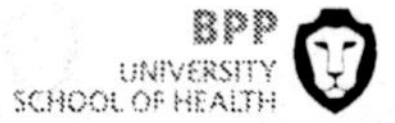

Career breaks

Further qualifications

Many doctors decide to take a career break after the Foundation Programme. Further qualifications are a popular option, which may allow for some time spent in locum work and travelling, whilst also developing your experience and building your curriculum vitae. The London School of Hygiene and Tropical Medicine (LSHTM) offers a very popular diploma in infectious diseases, for doctors who may be interested in working or volunteering overseas – indeed it (or an equivalent) is often a requirement with many aid agencies.

Further taught Master's programmes may also be attractive. These are diverse, both in field, structure and cost. Popular choices include MA degrees in clinical education; public health; Business Administration (MBA) or Health Research (MRes). It is sometimes possible to gain funding support for these courses, but this is limited and it is important to research these options early and be sure about the benefits successful completion will add to a career.

Part-time or online courses are another option, which may allow individuals to continue some clinical work at the same time and may range from certificate through to diploma and Master's degree level. The structure and duration of these qualifications is highly variable, but they may be more viable financially than the full-time options.

Clinical Fellow posts

Clinical Fellow posts exist in particular specialties and combine a reduced level of clinical work with research or teaching activities in order for a doctor to gain more experience or expertise in that area. In addition, there are specific schemes, such as the National Medical Director's Clinical Fellow Scheme, which provide successful applicants with a supported year in which to develop their knowledge and experience of medically related fields eg leadership, health management and policy or medical journalism. These are highly competitive, but will provide an excellent grounding in various 'portfolio career' activities.

LAT/LAS posts

Locum appointment for training (LAT) or locum appointment for service (LAS) posts are fixed-term contracts that enable NHS Trusts to cover vacancies. LAS posts may be up to 3 months in duration and cannot be counted towards specialist training, whilst a LAT can last from 3 to 12 months and may be given training recognition. However, the fixed-term nature of LATs means that if you run into training difficulties, your employer is not obliged to extend your contract as they are if you are employed in a regular specialist training post.

These posts allow for flexible clinical work, allowing you to gain an experience of different specialties, enjoy some medium-term job security and, in the case of a LAT, gain some accredited training experience should you decide to continue in that speciality. They can also be useful back-up options if you are unsuccessful in the national speciality recruitment rounds.

LAT/LAS posts are advertised in the second half of the medical year ie from March onwards, when trusts begin to work out their vacancies for the following year and applications take place via the national NHS online system Oriel. If you are interested in taking one of these posts in a particular speciality, it is a good idea to talk to local consultants and managers, who may also be able to give you an idea of whether a post is likely to exist and if so you can then express your interest at an early stage.

Case Study: Year out to study for a Master's degree

I chose to spend a year out of programme in advance of applying for core surgical training. As an F1 I approached a hand surgery department and asked if they would create a post for me to work as their research fellow helping them to set up a research department and in doing so a randomised clinical trial. I was most fortunate in that not only were they keen to have me but they also managed to get the post funded by the hospital.

I spent the year as a research fellow going through the stages of setting up an RCT; helping to develop the protocol, obtaining funding and ethics and setting up recruitment. My post was 80% research and 20% clinical (theatre and clinic). It was incredibly hard work, but in a very different way to clinical work, and I learnt an incredible amount and achieved a Master's in Trauma Science at the same time.

I would highly recommend taking time out after foundation training, but only if you can ensure that it will be an invaluable experience, and that you will have something to show for it at your ST3 and ideally CT interviews. I would strongly advise continuing with some clinical work during the year as it is a relatively early stage in your medical career to completely cease clinical practice for a whole year.

Travel and working abroad

The steady trickle of British junior doctors to Australia and New Zealand has recently become a heavy stream. Many doctors go for a limited period throughout their training in order to gain more clinical exposure, experience medicine in a different culture and enjoy the much-publicised favourable work-life balance. Although applications are becoming more competitive, it is still possible for organised UK doctors to successfully find vacancies to fill – often in general medicine, surgery or the emergency department. Other popular countries include South Africa, Canada, the US and other countries in the European Economic Area.

In addition to standard visa, health and qualification requirements, each country will have additional criteria that must be fulfilled in order to practice. For example, the US requires any doctor to have completed parts 1 and 2 of the USMLE and hold a satisfactory medical licence from the state or jurisdiction in which they wish to practise. Canada too has stringent conditions to be fulfilled. Given these requirements, early preparation for a year abroad is vital and there are several serious issues to consider before deciding on a year abroad after FY2.

Gaining a successful post abroad can be a costly process. Visa applications, compulsory health checks, official document verification and job application/ locum agency registration fees can all result in substantial initial costs – not to mention the flights, health insurance and other personal travel-related expenses. It is also crucial to think about student loan repayments, the NHS pension scheme, any mortgage repayments, tax implications and any differences in the cost of living that may influence your financial planning. It would be a good idea to discuss these issues with the relevant organisations.

The GMC needs to be notified of your intention to work abroad and you will need to re-register upon your return to the UK. In addition, it is essential to make sure you have valid medical indemnity cover whilst abroad, as some policies may not initially cover you. Whilst many countries have specific application schemes through which you must apply in order to gain a job, there are also many worldwide or country-specific locum agencies which will be able to help find appropriate posts. It is often a good idea to get some advice about good/bad agencies from any doctors who have previously used their services and online chat forums etc can be useful for this.

The decision about if and when to return to the UK is also an issue that requires careful consideration. If you wish to apply for a specialist training post for the following year, you will need to apply and return for any relevant selection interviews – this may be quite difficult from the other side of the world. Alternatively, some doctors choose to return to a LAT/LAS post and then apply in the following year. Obviously personal career and family circumstances may dictate at which point you leave and return to the UK, but the pull of the Antipodean sunshine has never been stronger.

Speciality training applications

Towards the end of the first Foundation Year 2 (FY2) rotation, applications for specialist training begin. Application processes differ between each speciality, although currently, national recruitment schemes exist for the majority at core or ST1 level, requiring completion of one online application. Part of this process requires you to preference rank the deaneries to which you wish to apply, and also, sometimes, the individual jobs. There will be a limited period during which these application forms must be completed and it is essential to be aware of these deadlines, which are well publicised online.

Each speciality has a person specification which outlines the features required for shortlisting. There is often also a guide to how applications and interviews are scored, and if available this can be found on the deanery websites. This is very helpful when structuring your answers to ensure you score highly.

Selection interviews may take place nationally (eg core surgical training) or locally (eg GP recruitment) and there may also be additional tests or selection procedures. Their exact structure is speciality specific. For example, core surgery consists of three 10-minute verbal stations: clinical scenarios, leadership and management and a portfolio station, whilst GP recruitment consists of a 30-minute written prioritisation task, followed by several 10- minute clinical roleplaying scenarios. You will be given further information at the time of shortlisting and the respective college websites are also very useful reference sources if you have further questions.

General advice

It is essential for any application or interview to include examples of personal experience and reflection as this is the only way you can make your answers stand out from other applicants. It is also crucial to be well structured and logical, to enable the recruiters to recognise your achievement and score you appropriately.

The first part of the application form will ask for personal details, your qualifications (both undergraduate and postgraduate), courses you have been on and details of at least two referees whom you wish to nominate; think carefully about whom you choose as your reference needs to support your application.

Why our speciality?

Every application is bound to ask why you are applying for that speciality and how you can demonstrate your commitment to it. It is important not to list generic reasons here; your answer will be much more effective if you outline three to four specific reasons and expand on these. For example, you may enjoy the challenge posed by the different levels of communication required in paediatrics or the mixture of surgical and medical skills required in obstetrics and gynaecology. Examples of commitment include audit work or research conducted within the speciality, undertaking postgraduate examinations, and attending courses in order to enhance your skills relevant to your chosen speciality.

Skills

Often within the application there will be at least one question asking for an example which illustrates a quality or skill you possess. Structuring this question is generally best with a concise description of the situation or example followed by an explanation of your actions – demonstrating the particular skill in question – and a reflection on what you gained from the experience. In particular, highlight how you developed as a result.

In addition, you may be asked what skills you possess that make you suitable for your chosen speciality. These will be generic eg time management, organisational skills, able to display initiative and decision-making, or speciality-specific. For the latter, it is important to use personal examples to highlight experiences or feedback that have allowed you to develop particular skillsets and why you are inspired to use these in the future. For example, you may have a logbook of procedures you have performed or you may have several DOPs in your e-portfolio, which could be used as evidence for development of specific skills or competencies.

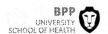

Audit or Quality Improvement (QI) projects

Assessing your involvement in audit and QI projects often forms part of the selection process. You need to demonstrate a sound understanding of the audit cycle and also demonstrate significant participation in the process – best if this involves completing the cycle ie implementing a change and demonstrating an improvement in clinical practice. Often, maximal points can potentially be scored where the audit has been presented regionally, published or resulted in changing a local/regional or national clinical guideline.

Research

Many applicants will have done a research project as part of a former undergraduate or Master's degree. Others will have made time to participate in 'extracurricular' research. Whatever your experience, make sure you describe: your specific role and contribution; particular skills you developed that are relevant to the application you are making; the eventual outcome of the project ie publication or presentation and plans you have for carrying out/ getting involved in future work.

Publications and presentations

Most applications will ask you to list any publications in a peer-reviewed journal of which you are an author and any presentations you have done. You score highly if you were first author on a publication or if you presented at a national or international level; however, you can also include regional or local/ departmental presentations.

Management/leadership

Pick a good example which illustrates your skills best, which may be medical or non-medical. You can use more than one example ensuring you describe the activity and how it enabled you to develop leadership/management skills as well as how these are relevant clinically. Roles include the running of medical committees and societies, involvement in rota co-ordination and sports team captain or local magazine editor.

It is also vital to demonstrate good teamworking skills. Good examples include scenarios where you have shown you are able to understand your role within a team and worked in co-ordination with others to achieve a common aim. Emphasise the importance of good communication skills, appreciation of the work performed by others and responsibility to perform your own role. In particular, demonstrate your involvement in multidisciplinary teams within clinical practice where optimal patient care is most important.

Teaching experience

Teaching is important. Try to structure your answer by dividing it into teaching experience of both a formal and an informal nature as well as any experience outside of medicine. Examples include teaching to undergraduates and being an OSCE examiner, being a course examiner (ALS/Advanced Trauma Life Support (ATLS)), and educating medical, social or charitable organisations (eg elective).

Discuss the different teaching methods you have used as well as the content of your teaching sessions. You will score highly if you have had formal training in teaching methods and hence it would be useful to attend a teaching course. Teaching at a regional level will also score higher than that at a local level.

Non-academic achievements

It is important to illustrate a good work-life balance with examples of achievements and commitment to activities outside the world of medicine; for example, sporting achievements and charity work as well as hobbies. Ensure you discuss the achievement itself, what makes you particularly proud of it and what skills you gained from it which will be relevant in your working life. The highest points will be scored where the achievement was within the context of a high level of competition as well as where you have shown your level of commitment. Always include some personal reflection of the achievement.

Conclusion

In order to score highly it is essential to make your answers structured and focused, illustrating personal examples and reflection where relevant. Ensure you are familiar with the scoring system and person specification for your speciality as well as the skills and qualities which are most relevant to it. Good luck!

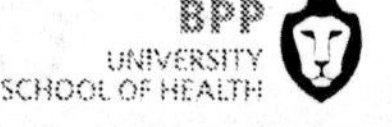

Further reading and references

1. McCartney, M. (2011) General Practice is the best job in the world. *BMJ* 2011; *350;h1721.*
2. Skills for Healthcare Workforce Portal. *Working Time Directive and Modernising Medical Careers 2009.* [Online] Available from: http://www.nhsemployers.org/~/media/Employers/Documents/SiteCollectionDocuments/WTD_FAQs_010609.pdf [Accessed 7 November 2016].
3. UK Foundation Programme Office. (2015) *F2 Career Destination Report 2015.* Birmingham: UK FPO.
4. NHS Higher Education England. (2016) *Medical Specialty Recruitment Handbook 2016.*
5. The Foundation Programme, www.foundationprogramme.nhs.uk.
6. NHS, www.specialtytraining.hee.nhs.uk.
7. Career advice, www.bma.org.uk/developing-your-career.
8. www.nihr.ac.uk/funding/academic-clinical-fellowships.html
9. Postgraduate study, www.prospects.ac.uk/postgraduate-study.
10. Oriel, www.oriel.nhs.uk.
11. Working abroad, www.bma.org.uk/advice/career/going-abroad/working-abroad.

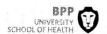

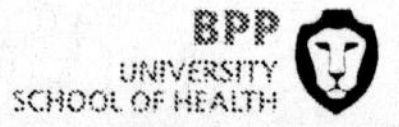
BPP
UNIVERSITY
SCHOOL OF HEALTH

Index

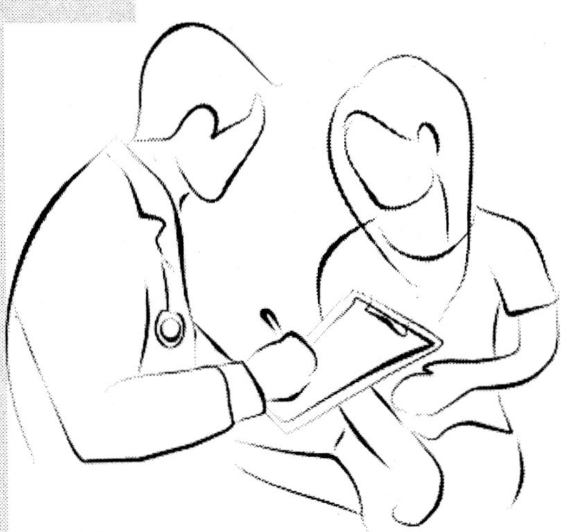

Index

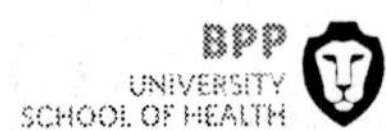
BPP
UNIVERSITY
SCHOOL OF HEALTH

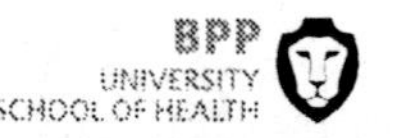
BPP
UNIVERSITY
SCHOOL OF HEALTH

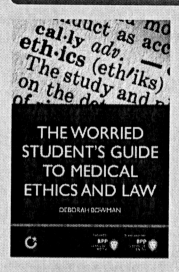

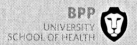